Behavioral Assessment in Schools

Second Edition

Behavioral Assessment in Schools

Second Edition

Theory, Research, and Clinical Foundations

Edited by

EDWARD S. SHAPIRO, Ph.D.
Lehigh University

THOMAS R. KRATOCHWILL, Ph.D.
University of Wisconsin–Madison

THE GUILFORD PRESS
New York *London*

Library of Congress Cataloging-in-Publication Data

Behavioral assessment in schools : theory, research, and clinical foundations / edited by
Edward S. Shapiro, Thomas R. Kratochwill.—2nd ed.
    p. cm.
  Includes bibliographical references and index.
  ISBN 1-57230-575-4 (cloth)
  1. Behavioral assessment of children—United States. 2. Handicapped
children—Education—United States. 3. Learning disabled children—Education—United
States. I. Shapiro, Edward S. (Edward Steven), 1951– II. Kratochwill, Thomas R.
LB1124 .B435 2000
370.15'3—dc21   99-044093

To Uncle Mike and Tom O.,
who probably don't know how much
they influenced me over the years. (E.S.S.)

To my best buddy, Tyler. (T.R.K.)

About the Editors

Edward S. Shapiro received his doctorate in school psychology from the University of Pittsburgh in 1978. He currently is Professor of School Psychology and Chairperson of the Department of Education and Human Services at Lehigh University, Bethlehem, Pennsylvania. In 1987, Dr. Shapiro received the Lightner Witmer Award from the Division of School Psychology of the American Psychological Association, in recognition for early career contributions to school psychology. From 1990 to 1995, he was editor of *School Psychology Review*, official journal of the National Association of School Psychologists. The author or coauthor of several books, including *Academic Skills Problems: Direct Assessment and Intervention* (second edition), *Academic Skills Problems Workbook*, and *Behavior Change in the Classroom: Self-Management Interventions*, all published by The Guilford Press, Dr. Shapiro has numerous publications in the areas of curriculum-based assessment, behavioral assessment, behavioral interventions, and self-management strategies for classroom behavior change. Currently, he is codirecting a project focused on training doctoral school psychologists as pediatric school psychologists. This model attempts to train students to integrate children's health care, psychological, and educational needs within school settings.

Thomas R. Kratochwill received his Ph.D. in educational psychology from the University of Wisconsin–Madison in 1973 with a specialization in school psychology. He joined the faculty at the University of Arizona in 1973 in the Department of Educational Psychology, School Psychology Program, serving as coordinator of the Office of Child Research. In 1983 he returned to the University of Wisconsin–Madison to direct the School Psychology Program and Psychoeducational Clinic.

Dr. Kratochwill has been associate editor of *Behavior Therapy*, *Journal of Applied Behavior Analysis*, and *School Psychology Review*. He was selected as the founding editor of the APA Division 16 journal *Professional School Psychology* (now *School Psychology Quarterly*) from 1984 to 1992. He is president of the Society for the Study of School Psychology and coauthor of the Task Force on Empirically Supported Interventions in School Psychology.

An active researcher and contributor to the scientific psychological literature, Dr. Kratochwill has written or edited 23 books and made more than 100 presentations at professional meetings. Among his books, several are classic contributions, including *Single Subject Research: Strategies for Evaluating Change* (1978); *Selective Mutism: Implications for Research and Treatment* (1981); a series devoted to advances in research, theory, and practice in school psychology (*Advances in School Psychology*, Volumes I through VIII, 1981–present); a book (with Richard J. Morris) on treatment of children's fears and phobias (*Treating Children's Fears and Phobias: A Behavioral Approach*, 1983); and (also with Richard J. Morris) a book on child therapy (*The Practice of Child Therapy*, 1983, and now in a third edition). He has also written (with John R. Bergan) a text on mental health consultation (*Behavioral Consultation and Therapy*, 1990) and is coeditor (with Karen Callan Stoiber) of the *Handbook of Group Interventions for Children and Families* (1998).

Contributors

Linda M. Bambara, Ph.D., Special Education Program, Department of Education and Human Services, Lehigh University, Bethlehem, Pennsylvania.

David W. Barnett, Ph.D., School Psychology Program, University of Cincinnati, Cincinnati, Ohio.

Barbara Rybski Beaver, Ph.D., Psychology Department, University of Wisconsin–Whitewater, Whitewater, Wisconsin.

Mary H. Bull, M.A., School Psychology Program, University of Massachusetts at Amherst, Amherst, Massachusetts.

R. T. Busse, Ph.D., School Psychology Program, Psychology Department, University of Wisconsin–Whitewater, Whitewater, Wisconsin.

Elisa M. Castillo, M.A., Department of Counseling Psychology, University of Wisconsin–Madison, Madison, Wisconsin.

Robin S. Codding, B.A., Department of Psychology, Syracuse University, Syracuse, New York.

Christine L. Cole, Ph.D., School Psychology Program, Department of Education and Human Services, Lehigh University, Bethlehem, Pennsylvania.

Edward J. Daly III, Ph.D., Department of Psychology, Western Michigan University, Kalamazoo, Michigan.

Karen I. Dittmer, M.S., School Psychology Program, Mississippi State University, Mississippi State, Mississippi.

Erin K. Dunn, M.S., Department of Psychology, Syracuse University, Syracuse, New York.

Tanya L. Eckert, Ph.D., School Psychology Program, Department of Psychology, Syracuse University, Syracuse, New York.

Ricardo B. Eiraldi, Ph.D., Center for Management of ADHD, Children's Hospital of Philadelphia, University of Pennsylvania School of Medicine, Philadelphia, Pennsylvania.

Douglas Fuchs, Ph.D., Peabody College, Vanderbilt University, Nashville, Tennessee.

Lynn S. Fuchs, Ph.D., Peabody College, Vanderbilt University, Nashville, Tennessee.

Maribeth Gettinger, Ph.D., Department of Educational Psychology, University of Wisconsin–Madison, Madison, Wisconsin.

Katie M. Guiney, B.A., Department of Psychology, Syracuse University, Syracuse, New York.

John M. Hintze, Ph.D., School Psychology Program, University of Massachusetts at Amherst, Amherst, Massachusetts.

Lorrie A. Howell, M.S., School Psychology Program, Mississippi State University, Mississippi State, Mississippi.

Thomas R. Kratochwill, Ph.D., Department of Educational Psychology, University of Wisconsin–Madison, Madison, Wisconsin.

Francis E. Lentz, Jr., Ph.D., School Psychology Program, University of Cincinnati, Cincinnati, Ohio.

F. Charles Mace, Ph.D., School of Psychology, University of Wales, Bangor, Wales.

Gregg Macmann, Ph.D., School Psychology Program, University of Kentucky, Lexington, Kentucky.

Ann M. Marquart, M.S., Department of Educational Psychology, University of Wisconsin–Madison, Madison, Wisconsin.

Jennifer J. McComas, Ph.D., Department of Education and Human Development, University of Minnesota, Minneapolis, Minnesota.

Stephanie H. McConaughy, Ph.D., Department of Psychiatry, University of Vermont, Burlington, Vermont.

Julia E. McGivern, Ph.D., Department of Educational Psychology, University of Wisconsin–Madison, Madison, Wisconsin.

Kenneth W. Merrell, Ph.D., School Psychology Program, Division of Psychological and Quantitative Foundations, The University of Iowa, Iowa City, Iowa.

Amy Murdoch, M.Ed., School Psychology Program, University of Cincinnati, Cincinnati, Ohio.

Stephen M. Quintana, Ph.D., Department of Counseling Psychology and Department of Educational Psychology, University of Wisconsin–Madison, Madison, Wisconsin.

Thomas J. Power, Ph.D., Center for Management of ADHD, Children's Hospital of Philadelphia, University of Pennsylvania School of Medicine, Philadelphia, Pennsylvania.

Jill K. Seibert, M.S., Department of Educational Psychology, University of Wisconsin–Madison, Madison, Wisconsin.

Edward S. Shapiro, Ph.D., School Psychology Program and Department of Education and Human Services, Lehigh University, Bethlehem, Pennsylvania.

Christopher H. Skinner, Ph.D, School Psychology Programs, Department of Educational Psychology, The University of Tennessee at Knoxville, Knoxville, Tennessee.

Gary Stoner, Ph.D., School Psychology Program, University of Massachusetts at Amherst, Amherst, Massachusetts.

Manuel X. Zamarripa, M.S., Department of Counseling Psychology, University of Wisconsin–Madison, Madison, Wisconsin.

Preface

When the first edition of this text was published in 1988, the field of behavioral assessment was burgeoning. Several texts that appeared at that time focused primarily on clinical assessment with children and adolescents. These books were targeted mainly toward the social/behavioral problems of children under different DSM diagnostic classifications. Very few volumes other than ours examined the use of behavioral assessment within school-based environments. Indeed, our text marked an important effort to bring much of the methodology of behavioral assessment that developed primarily for assessments in clinical settings to the schools.

The first edition was organized by method; each chapter examined both conceptual issues and practical implications of using a particular method. Authors provided detailed reviews of research and explained the implications of the research findings. The text incorporated discussions of issues specific to school settings, such as academic skills problems, as well as educational diagnosis.

In the revision of our first edition, we decided to embark on a somewhat different and bold direction. Given the amount of research since the publication of the first edition in 1988, and given the wide acceptance of behavioral assessment as common practice in school-based assessments, we believed that it would have been very difficult to provide a single current volume that could effectively address both the research and practice of behavioral assessment in school settings. At the same time, we wanted to provide continuity between research and practice.

The result is something a little different: two companion volumes with strong links between them. The current volume contains 16 chapters emphasizing the theory, research, and clinical foundations of behavioral assessment. In particular, the text offers descriptions and reviews of research that examines and evaluates each of the methods of behavioral assessment. Additional chapters look at complex issues in diagnosis, legal and ethical concerns, as well as the use of school-based behavioral assessment for individuals from culturally and linguistically diverse backgrounds. The companion volume is *Conducting School-Based Assessments of Child and Adolescent Behavior* (also published by The Guilford Press), and 10 authors of that text also authored chapters in the present volume. Written specifically with the practitioner in mind, that text provides case illustrations as well as discussions of the practical implications of behavioral assessment. Indeed, the combination of a text emphasizing theory, research, and foundations (this volume), alongside one emphasizing practice (*Conducting School-Based Assessments of Child and Adolescent Behavior*), offers a dual set of materials that are unique in our field.

Bringing together these two volumes simultaneously was quite a challenge. Many thanks to our current and past friends at Guilford who supported us in our venture. In addition, special appreciation goes to the authors of the chapters in this text who endured our editing recommendations and met due dates that were always too short. Finally, as in all of our efforts, special thanks go to our families (Sally, Dan, and Jay for Ed; Carol and Tyler for Tom), who again sacrificed some of our time with them so that we could produce this potentially important contribution to the literature.

We hope that you find the text stimulating.

Edward S. Shapiro
Thomas R. Kratochwill

Contents

III. ISSUES IN CHILD AND ADOLESCENT ASSESSMENT

CHAPTER 15

CHAPTER 16

Behavioral Assessment in Schools

Second Edition

PART I

Introduction

CHAPTER 1

Conceptual Foundations of Behavioral Assessment in Schools

THOMAS R. KRATOCHWILL
University of Wisconsin–Madison

EDWARD S. SHAPIRO
Lehigh University

The field of behavioral assessment has continued to grow rapidly in the areas of research, theory, and practice since the first edition of our assessment text. Recent developments in behavioral assessment of children in clinical and applied psychology have had important implications for the application of these procedures in schools and other applied settings. Behavioral assessment techniques and procedures have been offered as an alternative to traditional academic and social assessments conducted in psychology and education. As questions have been raised over the norms, reliability, validity, and utility of traditional assessment devices and procedures (e.g., projective tests, intellectual, and psychoeducational tests), assessors have looked for alternatives. Behavioral assessment frequently has been considered as an alternative to traditional testing in hope that the measures would provide a substitute for more traditional techniques where psychometric problems had not been solved.

Interest in behavioral assessment has also occurred as a result of the development of specific measures in outcome research on various adult and child disorders. Behavioral assessment has offered researchers a wide range of outcome measures that attest to the efficacy of treatment programs. For example, behavioral measures such as direct observation, psychophysiological recordings, and self-monitoring have advanced knowledge of what treatments are effective with what disorders, and what components of various treatments are active in certain therapeutic programs. In particular, behavioral outcome measures have provided alternatives to established outcome measures used in past research that were influenced by various sources of artifact and bias (e.g., self-report, global ratings). There have been many developments in behavioral assessment with advances in single-case or time-series research methodology used in clinical and educational research. In partnership with various designs, assessment schemes have helped document behavior change of great practical and social significance (Hayes, Barlow, & Nelson-Gray, 1999).

A prominent feature of behavioral assessment that has attracted a great deal of interest in applied fields is the conceptual and practical linking of assessment with treatment. Often psychologists practicing in educational settings have found that assessment techniques had little or no relation to establishing and monitoring an intervention program. Psychologists might have engaged in testing practices that were aimed at classification or diagnosis, but information related to designing a treatment procedure was frequently unavailable in such assessments. The role that assessment plays in designing an intervention program has been labeled "treatment validity" or utility (Nelson & Hayes, 1979). Nelson, Hayes, and Jarett (1986) provided an extensive discussion of methodologies to evaluate treatment validity, along with a review of the studies that examined some of these dimensions. Few applications of treatment validity, however, have appeared in child behavior assessment since our previous book on behavioral assessment (Shapiro & Kratochwill, 1987).

In behavioral assessment, assessment and treatment procedures can be linked in three ways: (1) designing the treatment program specific to the client's problem; (2) linking the assessment to environmental conditions of the individual's behavior; and (3) making assessment continuous throughout the treatment process so that decisions can be made to modify treatments if necessary. Although behavioral assessment may have been oversold on these dimensions of contribution early in the field, there is clear evidence that these techniques have led to the development and monitoring of treatment programs across many diverse childhood disorders and problems. The area of functional assessment provides one example of an assessment technology where assessment has led to treatment development and monitoring (Schill, Kratochwill, & Gardner, 1996).

These areas of growing interest in behavioral assessment of children convey something of the flavor of the continued enthusiasm in using these techniques in educational settings. Yet, many unresolved issues prevail in the field of behavioral assessment generally, and child behavior assessment in particular. In the next section we describe some of these issues. The text contains many excellent discussions that expand on issues in the field of assessment.

ISSUES IN CHILD BEHAVIORAL ASSESSMENT

Over the past two decades a number of books have been published that provide a discussion of issues relevant to the assessment of children (e.g., Breen & Fiedler, 1996; Ciminero, Calhoun, & Adams, 1977, 1986; Cone & Hawkins, 1977; Hersen & Bellack 1981; Shapiro, 1987, 1989; Shapiro & Kratochwill, 1987) and a growing number of chapters have appeared that focus exclusively on assessment of children in school psychology (e.g., Kratochwill, Sheridan, Carlson, & Lasecki, 1999; Stanger, 1996).

A major issue in the field of child behavioral assessment continues to be defining exactly is meant by "behavioral assessment" (Shapiro & Kratochwill, 2000). Anyone familiar with the recent literature on behavioral assessment can appreciate its remarkable variety, and that it is becoming even more diverse in a number of areas. In practice, behavioral assessors embrace a wide range of measures. A primary reason for the use of an increasing diversity of measures is that behavioral assessment is part of the larger domain of behavior therapy, or modification, known to be extraordinarily diverse in theoretical approaches, research methods, and therapy techniques (see Watson & Gresham, 1998; Witt, Elliott, & Gresham, 1988).

Behavioral assessment has always been linked closely with the development of behavior therapy (Kratochwill et al., 1999). Behavior therapy consists of certain subdomains, including applied behavior analysis, neo-mediational stimulus–response approaches, social learning theory, and cognitive behavior modification (Donahue & Krasner, 1995; Kazdin & Wilson, 1978; Nelson & Hayes, 1986; Wilson & Franks, 1982). It is beyond the scope of this brief introductory chapter to provide an overview of these areas and the reader should consult original writings for a review of some of the unique contributions of these areas to child behavioral assessment (see Chapters 5–8 in Wilson & Franks, 1982, for a review of conceptual foundations of the approaches).

Each of these major areas of behavior therapy has tended to include its own assessment techniques and procedures reflective of the theoretical position advanced. For example, individuals affiliated with applied behavior analysis have used the most specific conceptualization of behavior as compared, for example, with their cognitive behavior therapist counterparts. In applied behavior analysis, cognitive states or internal covert activities are generally not considered part of the assessment focus in research and applied work. Thus assessment involves, almost entirely, direct assessment measures of specific behaviors in analogue or naturalistic settings (see discussion below). In contrast, cognitive behavior therapists consider internal states or cognitions not only the proper focus for assessment and therapy, but also a major influence in directing behavior (e.g., Kendall & Braswell, 1985; Meichenbaum, 1977). Thus, assessors use measures that tap cognitions and so a heavy reliance on self-report measures is characteristic. It is therefore apparent that fundamental differences in assessment strategies have occurred across diverse theoretical approaches within the field of behavior therapy.

A related issue pertains to the actual techniques that are considered part of behavioral assessment. Keeping in mind these variations in theoretical approaches within behavior therapy, the number of different techniques and procedures subsumed under the rubric of behavioral assessment is extremely large. Defining what behavioral assessment is now and what it will be in the future will likely be determined by expanding theoretical perspectives rather than through some conceptual approach that maps specific techniques and procedures (Shapiro & Kratochwill, 2000). Behavioral assessment is generally regarded as a hypothesis-testing process about the nature of problems, causes of problems, and evaluation of treatment programs. This framework allows many techniques and methods of assessment. Although evolving theoretical conceptions of what is to be included within the domain of behavior therapy make the area of behavioral assessment difficult to define, some contrasts with so-called traditional techniques can be noted.

Generally, traditional assessment models that involve norm-referenced, psychosocial, psychoeducational, and cognitive assessments consider intraorganistic variables as essential in explaining the academic and behavioral performance of children. In traditional models, overt performance, either in the social or academic domain, is usually regarded as symptomatic of underlying dysfunction or psychic disturbance. In this context, the assessor assumes that something more fundamental than the overt behavioral performance of the client is an issue to be measured and assessed. One of the clearest examples of this feature is in the personality assessment domain where objective testing might be used to reveal unconscious factors or personality traits potentially related to client performance. In the assessment of academic performance processing dysfunctions, or minimal cerebral dysfunction, for example, might be a focus and assessment to measure these aspects of hypothesized functioning. More importantly, traditional assessors typically de-emphasize situational or environmental contextual variables during the assessment process and in interpretation of the data.

It is generally assumed among behavioral assessors that measurement must focus on a sample of overt behavior (and covert, depending on the theoretical orientation) in a variety of situations. In addition, assessors emphasize that the individual–environmental factors are assessed in multiple settings because environmental and ecological variables are said to influence performance in and across settings. Moreover, empirical data have often shown that an assessment of the functional relations between behavior and environment will identify factors that control deviant and challenging behaviors. The important issue is that the focus on individual and environmental factors in behavioral assessment is usually made without a primary reliance on underlying processes or hypothetical constructs.

Over the past decade, the distinctions between behavioral and nonbehavioral assessment have blurred considerably (Mash & Terdal, 1988; Shapiro & Kratochwill, 2000). Indeed, Mash and Terdal (1988) have argued that research in developmental psychopathology, combined with expansive interests in integrating family, cognitive, and environmental influences on behavior have moved the assessment process of children and youth toward a behavior systems assessment orientation. The interaction among factors impacting on child behavior must be understood to complete a fair and accurate evaluation. Such a conceptual approach to assessment requires that multiple methods, including those from behavioral and nonbehavioral frameworks, be considered in providing a best practice evaluation. Similarly, we (Shapiro & Kratochwill, 2000), have argued for behavioral assessment to be a multidimensional, problem-solving process.

A conceptual problem-solving approach to behavioral assessment may provide some consistency in defining the field, but expands considerably the range of possible techniques and procedures that can be included in child assessment. Behavioral assessment has usually been characterized as consisting of some general domains of assessment, including the interview, self-report, checklist and rating scales, self-monitoring, analogue assessment, and direct observational measures (see Cone, 1978). In this regard, behavioral assessment is conceptualized based on the contents assessed, the methods used to assess the contents, and the types of generalizability for scores on the measures that can be classified on the Behavioral Assessment Grid (Cone, 1978, 1979). The consideration of these three dimensions is presented in Figure 1.1. A tripartite response system (or content area) typically guides the behavioral assessment process, namely along the motor, cognitive, and physiological domains. Thus a learning or

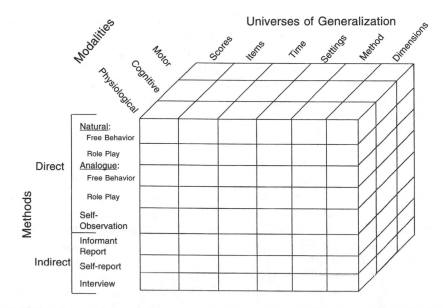

FIGURE 1.1 Behavioral Assessment Grid. From Cone (1978). Copyright 1978 by the Association for Advancement of Behavior Therapy. Reprinted by permission of the publisher and author.

academic problem would involve conceptualizing assessment along the lines of the three response systems insofar as they might contribute to the understanding and design of a treatment program for the child. For example, specific motor activities may be assessed, such as time spent working. In addition, cognitive components (e.g., positive or negative self-statements, cognitive rehearsal of specific skills) may be assessed as they relate to the solution of academic problems. Moreover, physiological arousal could be monitored, when possible, to understand further the child's reactions to the conditions of learning. When the three response systems are monitored, it is not assumed that they are highly correlated (Cone, 1979; Evans & Nelson, 1986).

Behavioral assessment methods mentioned above are usually presented along a continuum of directness/indirectness representing the extent to which they (1) measure the behavior of clinical relevance, and (2) measure it at the time and place of its natural occurrence (Cone, 1978). Thus, interviews, self-report, and ratings by others are considered *indirect* assessment strategies. For example, in the case of the interview and self-report measures, the behavior observed represents a verbal representation of activities taking place at some other time and place relative to the real time assessment occasions. When ratings are completed by other individuals (teachers, parents), the sample of behavior is considered a retrospective description that may or may not involve the clinical behavior of interest. The direct assessment category includes self-monitoring, analogue assessment, and naturalistic observation. These methods are direct in that the assessment takes place on some clinically significant target behavior at the time of its natural occurrence (see Shapiro & Kratochwill, 2000, for the discussion of these issues).

The expanding conceptualizations of child behavioral assessment within the context of the hypothesis testing approach and the conceptual framework for assessment allow many and diverse techniques to be considered as parts of the assessment scheme of the clinician. It is now conceded that behavioral assessors embrace a wide range of idiographic and nomothetic measures (Cone, 1986). For example, traditional tests could often be conceptualized as a format to provide standardized measures of skill performance, such as in the area of IQ or achievement tests (Kratochwill et al., 1999). Thus, assessments vary in their role in treatment selection, implementation, and monitoring.

A related issue in the field that remains to be resolved pertains to the psychometric features of behavioral assessment. In 1987 we noted that because of a rejection of the traditional assessment approaches and their associated measurement guidelines, and especially conceptual models embraced by traditional assessors, many of the psychometric features of child behavior assessment such as norming, reliability, validity, and generalizability had not been addressed adequately (Hartmann et al., 1979; Mash & Terdal, 1988). This issue still remains a prominent concern in the field. For example, there are still relatively few investigations examining the reliability of behavioral observation techniques. Behavioral assessors have been concerned primarily with establishing agreement measures, but have traditionally tended not to establish the reliability and validity of many assessment techniques with conventional psychometric criteria and especially the useful paradigm of treatment utility.

Generalizability theory has been proposed as an option to address psychometric properties of behavioral assessment. However, to date, little work has occurred in this area. To complicate matters even further, there has been a great deal of controversy regarding the appropriateness of traditional psychometric concepts (Cone, 1981, 1986; Strosahl & Linehan, 1986). Cone (1981) argued that psychometric research in the behavioral assessment field must focus on a paradigm radically different from the traditional nomothetic-trait psychometric model used for establishing the reliability, validity, and generalizability of tests. He argued that because behavioral assessment procedures are based on a different conceptual model of individual variability than traditional approaches (i.e., idiographic behavior), the traditional psychometric features vary widely in appropriateness depending on the type of reliability and validity being considered. As an alternative, Cone proposed that *accuracy* should be the primary method for establishing psychometric dimensions of behavioral assessment strategies. Nevertheless, it remains somewhat unclear as to what psychometric strategies might be used for behavioral assessment techniques and how the field will deal with various devices and procedures that have embraced traditional psychometric criteria.

The issues raised in the preceding paragraphs convey something of the concerns that are being addressed currently in child behavioral assessment, and behavioral assessment generally. The issues raised here reflect only some of the more general concerns that have emerged, but by no means do they represent a comprehensive overview. Each of the authors in this text addresses a broad spectrum of issues in the behavioral assessment field. The authors have provided a comprehensive overview of their own areas, taking into account diverse methods, techniques, and conceptual formats for practice.

OVERVIEW OF CHAPTERS

Direct observation has been the main stay of behavioral assessment technology since the beginning of the field. In Chapter 2, Skinner, Dittmer, and Howell review the application of direct observation in school settings within the context of a consultive problem-solving model (e.g., problem identification, problem analysis, and plan of evaluation). They review the advantages and limitations of direct observation within the theoretical context of behavioral psychology. Behavior observation focuses on both the target behaviors and variables related to the child's problematic behavior. The authors make an important point in emphasizing that comprehensive training in the conceptual foundations of behavioral assessment is critical in using these methods in applied settings.

Direct observational data assessment can be extended to academic skill problems. In Chapter 3, Daly and Murdoch provide an overview of standards and methods for measuring and evaluating academic performance outcomes. They are careful to point out that a variety of tactical and methodological issues remain unresolved in this domain of assessment. For example, an investigation of how fluency gains may contribute to generalized increases in performance needs to be addressed at the empirical level. The authors review a variety of issues surrounding fluency research and note that multiple concurrent measures of academic performance must be scheduled in assessments. An important part of the chapter focuses on descriptive and experimental functional analysis and its role in helping one to understand the contextual variables in academic skill problem assessment. Areas of research and, specifically, a focus on treatment utility research, are emphasized.

In recent years, functional assessment has become an important topic in psychology and education especially with the advent of the Individuals with Disabilities Education Act (IDEA) (1997). In Chapter 4, McComas and Mace discuss the theory and practice of conducting a functional analysis. Functional analysis is presented as a systematic analytic approach to understanding and treating severe behavioral problems, although it can be applied across a large dimension of challenging behaviors in children. The authors first emphasize that functional analysis can help in the understanding of underlying processes responsible for severe behavior problems. Second, they note that functional analysis can be used to help design specific intervention options and the probability that the intervention will be effective for severe difficulties. The authors review specific descriptive and experimental methods of functional assessment and emphasize heavily the use of functional analysis which involves experimental manipulation of antecedent and consequent events. The chapter provides a comprehensive overview of this technology as well as some needed areas of research in this important domain of behavioral assessment.

One important option to directly assessing behavior in the natural environment is to create an analogue assessment framework for assessment concerns. In Chapter 5, Hintze, Stoner, and Bull discuss the advantages of analogue assessment including the assessor's control over the environment for purposes of listening and observing low-frequency behaviors, eliminating the impact of extraneous stimuli that are of interest in assessment, and providing an option for assessment of behaviors otherwise difficult to observe. Although analogue assessment approaches are useful to the behavioral assessor, some significant issues have emerged in this area, especially with regard to the validity of these measures and their generalizability from the analogue to natural environments. Analogue procedures are said to often lack standardization such as in role-play enactments, behavioral avoidance tests, and so on. The authors also note that many analogue assessment strategies may not reflect social validity criteria for assessment of children's behavior. Analogue assessment tactics are also potentially reactive and many of the techniques are difficult to find because of unpublished sources. Despite these important limitations and issues, analogue assessment will likely continue to be a prominent aspect of behavioral assessment in the future.

Analogue assessment can also be extended to academic skill problems. In Chapter 6, Gettinger and Seibert discuss the application of analogue technology to a wide variety of academic skill problems. They note that in this application of analogue assessment, two procedural characteristics are prominent: (1) the role of examiners in analogue assessment is interactive in that there is typically some type of attempt to teach or prompt between the examiner and student, and (2) in analogue assessment a deliberate effort is made to change or improve performance of the skill to gain a better understanding of how the skill can be taught to the student or how the instructional environment can be improved. The authors discuss several implications of analogue assessment and review future research directions including the application of analogue assessment in screening young children who are at risk of academic problems, the application of analogue approaches in direct assessment of children's strategy use, analogue assessment's potential for identification of learners with special needs, application of analogue assessment in identification of gifted and talented learners, and the assessment of teacher perceptions in analogue assessment (e.g., teacher's perceptions of students and the instructional environment). The authors present a comprehensive overview of the applications of analogue assessment to diverse student problems in instructional environments.

Another form of analogue assessment of academic skills involves curriculum-based measurement and performance assessment. In Chapter 7, Fuchs and Fuchs present an overview of curriculum-based measurement (CBM) as a method for indexing academic competence and progress. CBM involves a sampling of curricula methods for administration and scoring and usually formats for summarizing and interpreting the database. The authors provide an overview of research and development underlying CBM and how CBM can merge with conventional and new formats of assessment. A case study is presented to illustrate how CBM can be used in decision making. The authors also provide an overview of CBM research and discuss limitations. The chapter offers some innovative procedures for integrating CBM with performance assessment methods. Performance assessment (PA) provides the assessor with a format for real-life problem solving and requires application and integration of multiple skills and strategies. Basically, PA informs the assessor of student strategy and processes and helps focus efforts on instructional techniques within a real-life context. The authors also discuss the limitations of PA for classroom assessment.

Among the many direct assessment options, self-monitoring has increasingly become a methodology for helping develop intervention programs in applied settings. In Chapter 8, Cole and Bambara review self-monitoring as applied in school settings. Self-monitoring involves two activities: self-observation, in which the individual becomes aware of his or her actions and whether a behavior of interest has occurred, and self-reporting, which refers to the actual recording process of some observed behavior (e.g., paper-and-pencil, mechanical device, etc.). Cole and Bambara note that although self-monitoring has been used both as an assessment and an intervention technique, its use in assessment has not been typical in schooling populations. Moreover, they review some of the major challenges that are likely to be encountered by the assessor using self-monitoring to gather data on academic and social behavioral problems. They carefully review the methodology of self-monitoring, provide numerous examples of how this recording occurs, and then discuss the methodological and conceptual issues surrounding its application in applied settings.

Several indirect methods of behavioral assessment can be used in applied settings. Child behavior rating scales fall into this domain. In Chapter 9, Merrell presents an overview of the use of these scales within child behavior assessment with a special emphasis on their applications in schools. He discusses three major areas including: (1) issues related to rater and instrument differences (e.g., cross-informant correlations, error of variance, situational factors); (2) issues regarding group differences in rating scales (e.g., gender, ethnicity, optimal sampling techniques, and practical considerations in generating norms); and (3) critical applications of behavior rating scales (e.g., screening, diagnosis, treatment selection, and progress monitoring). The use of behavior rating scales is increasing in behavioral assessment and individuals using these procedures in applied settings will find the chapter particularly useful in terms of the level of empirical knowledge available to guide practice.

Another indirect method of behavioral assessment involves the use of informant reports as specifically structured by interviews. In Chapter 10, Beaver and Busse present an historical and theoretical overview of interview methods for parents and teachers. They then discuss specific interview methods and formats while analyzing the current research on the use of behavioral interviews within applied settings. The authors note that significant advances have occurred in interviews including the areas of the psychometric properties of interviews, and conceptual advances have occurred in criterion-related and convergent validity. Despite many advances, considerable work needs to be done to elevate interviews to a level of high quality using standardized, reliable, and valid measures within the behavioral assessment field.

The use of self-report rating scales and checklists has increased in assessment activities in educational and other applied settings over the past decade. These measures have also increasingly played a prominent role in the techniques of individuals conducting behavioral assessment. In Chapter 11, Eckert, Dunn, Guiney, and Codding present an overview of self-report rating scale measures. They describe the use of these procedures within the context of a multi-method behavioral assessment framework. Specifically, they define self-report measures and provide an overview of some conceptual underpinnings in how these measures have been developed and used in applied settings. They then provide a review of the benefits of self-report measures and some of the practical and logical considerations in the application of these procedures in applied settings. Specific measures as used for two broad domains of behavior (externalizing and internalizing) are reviewed within the context of the psychometric properties of various scales. The chapter also includes a discussion of the advantages and limitations as well as future directions for the use of these scales in behavioral assessment.

In Chapter 12, McConaughy extends the discussion of the theory and practice of interviewing children. She begins the chapter by specifying some of the unique advantages of interviewing, including the opportunity to directly observe children's behavior, affect, and interaction style, the opportunity to assess children's perspectives on their own problems and competencies, clarifying the antecedent and consequences of specific problems, the feasibility of applying different interventions, and the opportunity to compare interview data with data obtained from other sources. The chapter focuses on a review of several structured and semi-structured diagnostic interviews for assessing child psychopathology. Thereafter, McConaughy describes a semi-structured clinical interview as part of a multimethod empirically based assessment system. In a final section of the chapter she reviews the application of behavioral interviewing with children. Readers will obtain a broad understanding of how interviews can be used in the diagnostic process and how empirically based assessment tactics can be integrated with other sources of data within behavioral assessment technology.

As behavioral assessors conduct assessment for diagnosis, treatment planning, and treatment monitoring, a variety of assessment issues are likely to emerge. In Chapter 13, Barnett, Lentz, and Macmann address a unique set of issues pertaining to the psychometric qualities of professional practice. The authors pose an important question: "What information about the quality of assessment data would be most useful to professionals as they make decisions during problem solving?" The authors review psychometric issues within the context of specific decisions during problem solving with a focus on the consequences of decisions emanating from the assessment process. The authors pose three ways in which professional decisions are affected by the psychometric quality of data gathered during the assessment process: (1) directly collecting data on the actual psychometric qualities of the measures that are used during problem solving; (2) reviewing published data on the psychometric qualities of assessment procedures to select the most appropriate procedure for some purpose; and (3) using information from previous research to project a range of possible errors associated with any assessment inference. Based on this conceptual framework, the authors provide an overview of psychometric concepts (e.g., reliability and validity of assessment). They then provide an overview of behavioral assessment as a psychometric model describing some unique features of this approach. Within the context of behavioral assessment the authors discuss consequences of assessment as a basis for problem solving. They then go on to advance a conceptual framework that incorporates a broadened view of assessment, taking into account the validity of decision making within behavioral assessment.

Among the important issues in the practice of assessment in educational and applied settings, legal and ethical concerns remain prominent for researchers and practitioners. In Chapter 14, McGivern and Marquart provide a comprehensive overview of the legal and ethical domain. Specifically, they provide a discussion of law and professional ethics including a definition of professional ethics, source of ethics, and major ethical principles. The sources of law are also reviewed in great detail. The authors also provide a discussion of legal issues for students with disabilities. An overview is also given of issues surrounding assessment of students from minority backgrounds including some guidelines for nonbiased assessment, bias in test use, and issues surrounding misclassification of students as well as assessing students with limited English proficiency. Some of the critical areas of legal and ethical concerns are discussed in the chapter, including child competence, informed consent as related to ethical codes, confidentiality of information, and privileged communication and its implications for practice. The authors conclude the chapter with a discussion of the technical adequacy of assessments, and the importance of addressing the reliability, validity, and treatment utility of assessment. A unique component of the chapter is the inclusion of a discussion of assessment accommodations for students with disabilities and the role that technology plays in assessing students with disabilities. Readers will find a comprehensive overview of legal and ethical considerations in the practice of behavioral assessment.

Among the most important issues to emerge in the behavioral assessment field is the assessment of ethnic and linguistic minority (ELM) children. Chapter 15 includes a comprehensive discussion of assessment of ethnic and linguistic minority children by Quintana, Castillo, and Zamarripa. The authors note that ethnic and racial minority children constitute the most rapidly growing segment of youth in the United States, now constituting about 35% of the public school population and 50% of the student population in many large urban school districts in various states. It is clear that anyone conducting assessment of children, whether behavioral or traditional, will need to attend to a variety of issues that emerge in applications of assessment techniques in this context. The authors provide an important overview of cultural and linguistic competencies that behavioral assessors should possess, including self-awareness of cultural background, awareness of the child's background, awareness of the cultural aspects of assessment procedures, and competencies for working with minority children. The authors also discuss in detail cultural and linguistic characteristics of children that are likely to have an important bearing on the assessment process. Next, the authors discuss the cultural nature of assessment procedures including such issues as normative data, innovative assessment procedures, and culturally centered assessment procedures. In the final part of the chapter the authors discuss the cultural nature of the assessment context including cultural aspects of school environments, the ELM community's reactions to school environments, and the relationship of these issues to the educational system. The chapter is comprehensive in providing an overview of this important domain and its relevance to the behavioral assessment field.

In the final chapter of the text, Power and Eiraldi discuss educational and psychiatric classification systems and their relevance to behavioral assessment. Specifically, the authors cover several issues including (1) the purposes of diagnostic classifications, (2) methods of assessment that can be used to make diagnostic decisions, (3) educational and psychiatric classification systems that may be useful to the behavioral assessor, (4) relationships among systems of classification, and (5) limitations of systems and a model for incorporating classification with functional approaches to problem solving. The latter area is particularly important and the authors provide an overview of how classification technology can be integrated into functional assessment methodology. They argue that the functional model is superior to a traditional classification model especially in the domain of intervention utility (i.e., intervention problem solving, plan selection, and monitoring). The authors extend our knowledge on how classification systems might be applied within a behavioral assessment framework.

The text incorporates a comprehensive overview of a variety of assessment technologies and issues that interface with the field of behavioral assessment. We are confident that readers of our text will find an extraordinarily large amount of useful information in their efforts to research and apply the technology of behavioral assessment. We now invite you to begin that journey and enjoy the information conveyed by a most talented group of scholars and writers in the field of behavioral assessment.

References

Breen, M. J., & Fiedler, C. R. (1996). *Behavioral approach to assessment of youth with emotional/behavioral disorders: A handbook for school-based practitioners*. Austin, TX: Pro-Ed.

Ciminero, D. R., Calhoun, K. W., & Adams, H. E. (Eds.). (1977). *Handbook of behavioral assessment*. New York: Wiley.

Ciminero, D. R., Calhoun, K. W., & Adams, H. E. (Eds.). (1986). *Handbook of behavioral assessment* (2d ed.). New York: Wiley.

Cone, J. D. (1978). The behavioral assessment grid (BAG): A conceptual framework and a taxonomy. *Behavior Therapy, 9*, 882–888.

Cone, J. D. (1979). Confounded comparisons in triple response mode assessment research. *Behavioral Assessment, 1*, 85–95.

Cone, J. D. (1981). Psychometric considerations. In M. Hersen & A. S. Bellack (Eds.), *Handbook of behavioral assessment* (2nd ed., pp. 38–68). Elmsford, NY: Pergamon Press.

Cone, J. D., (1986). Idiographic, nomothetic, and other perspectives in behavioral assessment. In R. O. Nelson & S. C. Hayes (Eds.), *Conceptual foundations of behavioral assessment* (pp. 111–128). New York: Guilford Press.

Cone, J. D., & Hawkins, R. (1977). *Behavioral assessment: New directions in clinical psychology*. New York: Brunner/Mazel.

Donahue, W. O., & Krasner, L. (1995). *Theories of behavior therapy*. Washington, DC: American Psychological Association.

Evans, I. M., & Nelson, R. O. (1986). Assessment of children. In A. R. Ciminero, K. S. Calhoun, & H. E. Adams (Eds.), *Handbook of behavioral assessment* (2nd ed., pp. 601–630). New York: Wiley.

Hartmann, D. P., Roper, B. L., & Bradford, D. C. (1979). Some relationships between behavioral and traditional assessment. *Journal of Behavioral Assessment, 1*, 3–21.

Hayes, S. C., Barlow, H. B., & Nelson-Gray, R. O. (1999). *The scientist practitioner: Research and accountability in the age of managed care*. Boston: Allyn & Bacon.

Hersen, M., & Bellack, A. S. (Eds.) (1981). *Behavioral assessment: A practical handbook* (2nd ed.). Elmsford, NY: Pergamon Press.

Individuals with Disabilities Education Act (1990, 1997), 20 U.S.C. Chapter 33, 1400 *et seq.*

Kazdin, A. E., & Wilson, G. T. (1978). *Evaluation of behavior therapy: Issues, evidence, and research strategies*. Cambridge, MA: Ballinger.

Kendall, P. C., & Braswell, L. (1985). *Cognitive-behavioral therapy for impulsive children*. New York: Guilford Press.

Kratochwill, T. R., Sheridan, S. M., Carlson, J., & Lasecki, K. L. (1999). Advances in behavioral assessment. In C. R. Reynolds & T. B. Gutkin (Eds.), *The handbook of school psychology* (3rd ed., pp. 350–382). New York: Wiley.

Mash, E. J., & Terdal, L. G. (1988). Behavioral assessment of child and family disturbance. In E. J. Mash & L. G. Terdal (Eds.), *Behavioral assessment of childhood disorders*, 2nd ed. (pp. 3–65). New York: Guilford Press.

Meichenbaum, D. (1977). *Cognitive behavior modification*. New York: Plenum Press.

Nelson, R. O., & Hayes, S. C. (1979). Some current dimensions of behavioral assessment. *Behavioral Assessment, 1*, 1–16.

Nelson, R. O., & Hayes, S. C. (Eds.). (1986). *Conceptual foundations of behavioral assessment*. New York: Guilford Press.

Nelson, R. O., Hayes, S. C., & Jarrett, R. B. (1986). Evaluating the quality of behavioral assessment. In R. O. Nelson & S. C. Hayes (Eds.), *Conceptual foundations of behavioral assessment* (pp. 463–503). New York: Guilford Press.

Schill, M. T., Kratochwill, T. R., & Cardner, W. I. (1996). Conducting a functional analysis of behavior. In M. J. Breen & C. R. Fielder (Eds.), *Behavioral approach to assessment of youth with emotional/behavioral disorders: A handbook for school-based practitioners* (pp. 83–179), Austin, TX: Pro-Ed.

Shapiro, E. S. (1987). *Behavioral assessment in school psychology*. Hillsdale, NJ: Erlbaum.

Shapiro, E. S. (1989). *Academic skills problems: Direct assessment and intervention*. New York: Guilford Press.

Shapiro, E. S., & Kratochwill, T. R. (1987). *Behavioral assessment in schools: Conceptual foundations and practical applications*. New York: Guilford Press.

Shapiro, E. S., & Kratochwill, T. R. (2000). Introduction: Conducting a multidimensional behavioral assessment. In E. S. Shapiro & T. R. Kratochwill (Eds.), *Conducting school-based assessments of child and adolescent behavior*. New York: Guilford Press.

Stanger, C. (1996). Behavioral assessment: An overview. In M. J. Breen & C. R. Fiedler (Eds.), *Behavioral approach to assessment of youth with emotional/behavioral disorders: A handbook for school-based practitioners* (pp. 3–21). Austin, TX: Pro-Ed.

Strosahl, K. D., & Linehan, M. M. (1986). Basic issues in behavioral assessment. In A. R. Ciminero, K. S. Calhoun, & H. E. Adams (Eds.), *Handbook of behavioral assessment* (2nd ed., pp. 12–46). New York: Wiley.

Watson, T. S., & Gresham, F. M. (1998). *Handbook of child behavior therapy*. New York: Plenum Press.

Wilson, G. T., & Franks, C. M. (Eds.). (1982). *Contemporary behavior therapy: Conceptual and empirical foundations*. New York: Guilford Press.

Witt, J. C., Elliott, S. N., & Gresham, F. M. (1988). *Handbook of behavioral therapy in education*. New York: Plenum Press.

PART II

Assessment Techniques

CHAPTER 2

Direct Observation
in School Settings

Theoretical Issues

CHRISTOPHER H. SKINNER
The University of Tennessee at Knoxville

KAREN I. DITTMER
LORRIE A. HOWELL
Mississippi State University

School psychology has long been associated with the administration and interpretation of standardized norm-referenced assessment instruments. These assessment instruments have been used to collect data that may assist education professionals in making a variety of decisions. Data collected may be used to screen students, to make decisions regarding referrals, to determine a students' eligibility for services, and to evaluate the effects of different interventions or placement procedures on a student's progress. Although research from the past three decades (i.e., mid-1970s through the mid-1990s) suggests that school psychologists spend about two-thirds of their professional time administering and interpreting standardized, norm-referenced assessment instruments (Reschly & Wilson, 1995), researchers and leaders in the field of school psychology have suggested and described how applying behavioral theory and behavioral assessment techniques within school settings can be used to assist with preventing and remedying student problems (Alessi, 1988; Gresham & Lambros, 1998; Shapiro, 1996).

Behavioral assessment procedures include a variety of data collection techniques (e.g., teacher and parent interviews, checklists, and rating scales). However, direct observation of behavior in the natural environment may be the most common behavioral assessment technique employed for addressing students' adaptive and maladaptive behaviors (Hops, Davis, & Longoria, 1995; Kratochwill, 1982, Shapiro, 1987). The theoretical assumptions and conceptual underpinnings of behavioral assessment procedures and, more specifically, direct observation procedures, differ from the assumptions and theory related to standardized assessment procedures (Hartmann, Roper, & Bradford, 1979). If school psychologists are to effectively employ direct observation in school environments, then they must understand the conceptual foundations associated with behavioral assessment procedures and the impact of these conceptual issues on assessment practices. Furthermore, both conceptual and applied differences between traditional assessment and direct observation procedures will reveal relative strengths associated with direct observation that may allow school psychologists to more effectively expand their assessment services and take a more active role in remedying school-based problems. Before discussing these conceptual issues, direct observation procedures will be defined and briefly described.

DIRECT OBSERVATION RECORDING PROCEDURES

Collecting direct observation data requires the observation and recording of behaviors. Behaviors have both physical and temporal characteristics. These characteristics include the topography or shape of a behavior, the intensity of a behavior, the frequency, duration, or rate of a behavior, and other temporal characteristics such as the latency between the beginning of a behavior and the end of a behavior (e.g., time required to finish an assignment). In addition to describing and measuring physical and temporal aspects of behaviors, behavioral assessment procedures can also be used to assess environmental conditions that may influence these behaviors.

In most instances, the intensity of a behavior cannot be precisely measured without the use of a technical instrument. Therefore, measures of behavioral intensity are rarely used during natural observation in school environments (see Greene, Bailey, & Barber, 1981, for an example of measuring and altering the intensity of student responses). However, other dimensions of behavior can be recorded in narrative and empirical forms by observers within educational environments (Shapiro & Skinner, 1990).

When narrative recording is being employed, observers write down, in narrative form, what they see occurring. There are several procedures for recording narrative data. Antecedent–behavior–consequence (ABC) narrative recording is a procedure where observers write descriptions of target behavior(s) (B), the antecedent (A) events and conditions that occurred prior to the observed behavior, and the consequent (C) events that occurred after the target behavior. When performing narrative recording procedures, observers should record what they directly observe, not inferences based on those behaviors. For example, rather than recording that the students appeared to be getting frustrated, the observer should record that the student moaned and slammed his pencil down while working on an independent seatwork assignment.

There are many procedures that can be used to record observations that result in quantitative or empirical data. Empirical data have many advantages relative to narrative recordings. Because written descriptions of behaviors and events are likely to differ across observers, it is difficult to verify these data unless quantitative recordings are collected in a systematic manner. Furthermore, quantitative data allow one to make comparisons within and across recording sessions and allow for the examination of trends, variability, and levels of observed behaviors (Barlow & Hersen, 1984; House, House, & Campbell, 1981; Shapiro & Skinner, 1990).

Quantitative data collection requires observers to operationally define behaviors and then record observed instances of those behaviors. Various procedures can be used to record observations. When event recording is used, each instance of a behavior is tallied. However, recording all events requires continuous observation rather than sampling behavior within observation intervals. Thus it is difficult to record each instance of discrete behaviors that occur at very high rates or behaviors that are more continuous rather than discrete (Lentz, 1988; Shapiro, 1987).

Event recording yields frequency count data that are often converted to rates or percentages. For example, a student may leave her/his seat five times during a 10-minute independent seatwork activity. Thus the student's rate of leaving her/his seat is once every two minutes. Similarly, during a group recitation session a teacher may ask the class 20 questions and a student may raise her/his hand 10 times. This student raised her/his hand 50% of the time following a question. By converting frequency counts to rate or percentage data observers report more precise data. These data are more useful than frequency counts alone because comparisons can be made across observation sessions that are unequal in length or across sessions in which the opportunities to engage in behaviors are unequal. These data often prove more useful than frequency counts for making psycho-educational decisions based on trends, variability, and behavior levels within-subjects and across phases in natural educational environments where opportunities to respond and session length tend to vary.

Direct observation data can also be collected using time-sampling procedures. Because it is difficult to collect duration data continuously, time sampling is often used to collect duration estimates (Lentz, 1988). The three basic time sample procedures are (1) whole interval time sampling, (2) partial interval time sampling, and (3) momentary time sampling. Each procedure requires observers to break observation sessions down into intervals. For example, a 20-minute observation system could be broken down to 120 ten-second intervals. Observers then record the presence or absence of target behaviors on an interval-by-interval basis. Whether intervals are scored depends upon the time-sampling technique employed. When whole interval time sampling is employed, intervals are only scored when the behavior is observed for the entire interval. Thus this procedure is most often used for behaviors that tend to occur continuously such as on-task behavior (e.g., head and eyes oriented toward material or in-seat behavior). With partial interval time sampling, if the behaviors occur any time during the interval, the interval is scored (Lentz, 1982). Finally, when momentary time sampling is employed, behaviors are recorded only if they are occurring at the moment when the interval begins (Powell, Martindale, Kulp, Martindale, & Bauman, 1977).

Time-sampling recordings yield data regarding the number of times a behavior occurred relative to the number of intervals observed (e.g., the student was on-task 60 of the 120 intervals observed). These data are then put into ratio format and used to estimate duration of occurrence (e.g., data suggest that the student was on-task 50% of the time). Researchers have shown that the quality of these estimates is affected by the time-sampling procedure employed (Lentz, 1982; Powell et al., 1977). Whole-interval time sampling tends to underestimate the duration of time a student spent engaged in a specific behavior, while partial-interval time sampling tends to overestimate the duration of time a student spent engaged in target behaviors. Momentary time sampling does not systematically alter duration estimates in one direction or the other.

The direct observation procedures briefly described can be used to collect data that are useful for making a variety of psychoeducational decisions and are often included as part of the assessment process. Both the conceptual basis for using direct observation and the issues surrounding the use of direct observation to make these decisions are complex. The next section will address these assumptions and then the following section will include implications that these assumptions have for problem-solving decisions.

CORE ASSUMPTIONS OF DIRECT OBSERVATION

There are two core assumptions associated with behavioral assessment procedures that differ from those associated with more traditional assessment procedures (Gresham, 1998; Hartmann et al., 1979; Kratochwill & Shapiro, 1988). One core assumption is concerned with how behavior is viewed. From a more traditional assessment perspective, behaviors are seen as symptoms of underlying problems that exist within the individual. Thus behaviors are used to infer underlying problems. However, behavioral psychologists tend to approach presenting behavior problems, both excesses and deficits, more directly. Changing or altering behaviors is often the goal associated with behavioral psychology.

Of all the behavioral assessment procedures, direct observation in the natural environment is often considered the most direct (Cone, 1978; Shapiro, 1987; Shapiro & Browder, 1989). The primary reason for this is that direct observation allows an outside observer to record data on the behavior of interest within the environment where the behavior is of concern and at the time the behavior actually occurs (Cone, 1978; Shapiro, 1987).

A second assumption that distinguishes behavioral from more traditional assessment is related to assumed causes of behavior. Traditional assessment paradigms often assume that behavior is caused by intrapsychic constructs or traits within the individual. These traits or intrapsychic causes or behaviors are often viewed as stable and relatively immutable (Hartmann et al., 1979). Under behavioral models, behaviors are assumed to be caused or maintained by current environmental conditions (Carr, 1993; Gresham, 1998; Hartmann et al., 1979). It is often possible to collect direct observation data on both the behaviors of interest and the environmental conditions that may be causing or maintaining these behaviors. Because stable behavior is dependent upon stable environmental conditions, the stability of behavior over time, settings, tasks, or environments is not assumed under a behavioral model (Shapiro, 1987). Because environmental causes of behavior are often alterable, the behaviors themselves are viewed as relatively more mutable or susceptible to change brought about by changing environmental conditions.

PROBLEM-SOLVING APPROACH

The assumptions regarding causes of behavior has had profound theoretical implications for school psychology practices. Reschly and Ysseldyke (1995) described the correlational and experimental disciplines associated with school psychology. The correlational discipline seeks to measure variations among people and use these variations to fit people into programs. For example, standardized assessment procedures (e.g., intelligence quotients) have often been used to differentially select students for different programs or placement. In contrast, the experimental discipline has sought to improve functioning by developing, implementing, evaluating, and disseminating effective interventions that improve a student's functioning. Reschly and Ysseldyke (1995) suggest that school psychologists need to shift away from the correlational discipline and begin to develop and apply theories, principles, and procedures more associated with the experimental discipline.

This shift toward a problem-solving approach is clearly in line with behavioral assumptions and procedures (Gresham, 1998). Because the behavioral model assumes that causes of behavior are relatively mutable, it suggests that education professionals can address problems by altering environmental conditions. Thus direct observation data can often be used to collect data on causes of behavior within the natural environment. These data can then be used to construct interventions based on alterations of causal conditions and lead to changes in behavior.

STAGES OF PROBLEM SOLVING

A variety of problem-solving models have been developed that are based on behavioral theory (Barrios & Hartmann, 1986; Bergan & Kratochwill, 1990; Kratochwill, 1982; Lentz & Shapiro, 1986). Although these models are similar, a modified version of the behavioral consultation model described by Bergan and Kratochwill (1990) will be used to provide a context in which to discuss conceptual issues related to direct observation in school settings. This model of behavioral consultation is divided into four sequential stages: (1) problem identification, (2) problem analysis, (3) plan implementation, and (4) treatment evaluation. It is important to note that direct observation of behaviors in natural environments is not required at each stage of this model and alternative behavioral and traditional assessment procedures both may be useful for making decisions across stages.

Problem Identification

The first step in most school psychology service delivery models is the referral. Following a referral, school psychologists must determine if a problem exists, describe the nature and extent of that problem, and help establish procedures for measuring this problem that can be used to evaluate the effects of interventions.

Traditional models of assessment and school psychology service delivery have been based on a nomothetic-trait approach. Using this approach, school psychologists have collected empirical data from standardized norm-referenced assessment instruments to help make these decisions. As previously mentioned, many of these measures were designed to assess intrapsychic traits (e.g., the child is passive–aggressive, impulsive, depressed, etc.). Thus the behavior for which the children were actually referred may have never been directly assessed (Shapiro, 1987). Determining whether the referred problem meets the criteria for services (e.g., treatment, programming, etc.) is often based on these standardized assessment scores. Criteria have been based typically on normative data and students falling outside expected ranges of scores (e.g., standard deviation units, abnormal scatter scores relative to the norm group).

The primary advantage to this system is that criteria could be precisely set and measured in a standardized manner. Identifying problems or students eligible for service is considered scientific and fair. However, in many instances this system was not meeting the needs of students (Reschly & Ysseldyke, 1995). The failure of a student to meet the criteria for having a problem that is severe enough to warrant services (e.g., meeting diagnostic criteria) does not mean that the student is not experiencing problems that should be addressed. As Lentz and Shapiro (1986) indicated, school-based problems should not be ignored merely because they do not fit into some criteria of a disorder.

Whereas traditional assessment procedures have largely been based on comparisons to normative sample data, behavioral psychologists have often employed an idiographic–behavioral approach to assessment. This approach differs from a nomothetic-trait approach in that behaviors and environmental conditions are assessed directly and repeatedly and comparisons are made within individuals, as opposed to across individuals (Cone, 1986, 1988; Johnston & Pennypacker, 1980).

While the focus on within-subject comparisons has many advantages, it makes it difficult to *empirically* determine if a problem behavior (excess or deficit) is severe enough to be considered a problem. Thus, in many instances, the determination of whether the behavior is considered severe enough to be a problem has been made based on qualitative data (e.g., teacher or parent interviews). However, direct observation procedures can still be useful at this stage of an assessment process.

Using Direct Observation to Specify the Target Behavior

In order to collect empirical data on a target behavior, the behavior must first be operationally defined. Operational definitions must be clear and precise enough so that observers can consistently or reliably record the presence or absence of the target behavior. Although teacher and parent interview data often help one establish operational definitions and construct recording procedures, observing behaviors empirically and in narrative format can help one refine and validate these reports and assist in determining the nature of the problem.

Problems include both behavior excesses and deficits and behaviors occurring at inappropriate times. Furthermore, these problems may be related to the topography, intensity, rate, or duration of the behavior of interest. However, referring agents (e.g., teachers or parents) do not always describe behaviors in these terms. Rather than saying the child does not follow directions, they will say the child is obstinate or disrespectful. Interview procedures can be used to elicit more precise definitions of problem behaviors (Bergan & Kratochwill, 1990). During this initial stage of problem identification, however, direct observation of the target behavior in the natural environment can help form operational definitions and validate reports of problems.

In the initial stage of forming operational definitions it is often difficult for people to describe the topography of behaviors of concern. This is especially true when behaviors are highly idiosyncratic or atypical. For example, someone may report that a child is engaging in inappropriate self-injurious behavior. However, the shape or topography of this behavior is likely to differ across students. Thus it is often useful for observers to enter the classroom and record narrative descriptions of the behavior. These narrative descriptions can then be used to form operational definitions of the behavior. Furthermore, by observing these behaviors, information regarding other characteristics of the behavior (e.g., rate, duration, continuous) can be gathered that allow for the development of empirical recording procedures.

Direct observation can also be used to validate referral problems. For example, a teacher may report that a child is constantly disrupting the class and never following directions. Entering the classroom and taking direct observation data on these behaviors may validate these concerns. Event data from a 20-minute observation may show that the teacher delivered ten directions and the student complied with these directions 50% of the time. Event recording could also show that the student initiated contact with classmates eight times in 20 minutes. Finally, momentary time sampling data may show that the student was engaged in social interactions with peers during 30 of the 60 intervals observed, or an estimated 50% of the time. After collecting the data, the observer could ask the teacher if the student's behavior was typical. If the teacher reported that the behavior was typical, then the direct observation data may both confirm teacher reports and suggest that the recording system being used is measuring valid behavior problems.

In other cases data may fail to confirm teacher reports. For example, a teacher may report that a student is constantly off-task during independent seatwork assignments. Direct observation data may show that the student is on-task during 85% of the intervals observed. The data may also show that the student did engage in disruptive behavior including leaving his seat, calling out, and throwing objects on eight occasions during the observation session. If the teacher confirms that the student's behavior was typical during this observation session, then these data suggest that duration of off-task behavior is not the primary problem. Rather, these data suggest that the teacher is primarily concerned with topographical aspects of behaviors that result in disruption in the classroom.

Normative and Comparison Child Data

Norm-referenced assessment instruments use standardized assessment procedures to collect data across students in order to form an empirical basis for comparison.

A variety of direct observation systems have been developed that could allow for standardized data-collection procedures within educational settings (Saudargas, 1992; Shapiro, 1996). Furthermore, numerous studies have shown that trained observers can record data in a reliable and consistent manner across school settings. However, normative data may not be useful for evaluating the extent of the behavioral excesses or deficits observed, because the situations in which behaviors are observed are likely to vary dramatically across educational environments. Because classroom environments are extremely fluid, normative data are likely to show a large degree of variance caused by situational variance across classroom environments.

Researchers who have developed behavioral assessment systems designed for use in the classroom have suggested that collecting data on a comparison child may provide useful information when identifying and validating problems and for setting intervention goals (Saudargas, 1992; Shapiro, 1996). These procedures include having the teacher identify one student whose behavior is acceptable, but not exceptional, and who is similar to the child in terms of sex, age, and perhaps cultural background (Alessi, 1988). The observer can then record direct observation data on the comparison student's behavior at predetermined intervals (e.g., every fourth interval). Observers could also record data sequentially on several comparison students at predetermined intervals. If the observation system is simple and behaviors are recorded at fairly low rates, it may also be possible for observers to record data on the target student's and comparison student's behavior simultaneously.

Because the comparison student's behavior is observed and measured in an environment that is similar to the target student's behavior, comparison student data may prove useful for identifying and validating problem behaviors. For example, direct observation data may show that a target student was off-task 40% of the intervals observed. If comparison student data show that this student was off-task on only 5% of the intervals observed, then these empirical data would support that off-task behaviors may be a problem. However, if comparison student behavior was off-task 35% of the intervals observed, then these data may suggest that the wrong target behavior has been identified or that the observation system may be inappropriate for measuring the target behavior (e.g., poor operational definitions, inappropriate recording procedures, observing behaviors at inappropriate times, observers positioning themselves in a manner that hinders direct observation).

Although comparison student data may prove useful for identifying problems, Alessi (1988) indicated several limitations with using this procedure. First, observations may be conducted during a time when the comparison child or children are engaged in unusually high levels of appropriate or inappropriate target behaviors. Second, the comparison child may not be accurately identified by the teacher in that the child may exhibit exceptional behavior or also be a child with similar behavior problems. Third, the wrong target behavior may have been identified or the target behavior may have been poorly defined. In addition to these problems, it may be impossible to collect comparison child data if the target behavior is idiosyncratic and no other student in the classroom engages in the target behavior.

Repeated Direct Observation Sessions

Testing effects refer to the impact that previous assessment procedures have had on subsequent assessment performance. Many standardized assessment instruments cannot be administered repeatedly over brief periods of time because testing effects cause changes in responding. One of the advantages of direct observation in natural settings is that observers can record behavior in natural environments repeatedly across conditions and the length of time between assessment sessions can be brief (Hartmann et al., 1979).

Repeated assessment has many advantages. With respect to problem identification, even when initial observations fail to identify or verify a problem, observers can return to the classroom almost immediately and collect data over several sessions, across activities, and settings, in order to help identify and verify referral problems. Repeated assessments also allow one to collect data on comparison student behavior over observation sessions. Thus, if during an observation session (1) the comparison child or children behave atypically, (2) the target child behaves atypically, (3) the target behavior is poorly defined or the observation system is inadequate, or (4) observations were made at a time or during activities when the target behaviors rarely occur, observers can return to collect data at another time with little delay between observation sessions.

Another advantage related to repeated assessment is that these procedures allow observers to collect baseline data on behavior levels, trends, and variability. These baseline data can then be used to evaluate the effects of intervention procedures. During the problem identification phase it is often advisable to collect a minimum of three data points, because this number is the minimum needed to establish a trend (Barlow & Hersen, 1984).

Multiple Target Behaviors

Using direct observation to identify target behaviors for interventions is a complicated process when a student is referred for just one primary problem. However, in many instances, students are referred for multiple problems. With these cases, merely verifying and measuring a problem may not be enough. It may also be necessary to select behaviors for intervention from a pool of possible behavior problems.

A variety of guidelines for selecting and prioritizing target behaviors for interventions have been identified (Ayllon & Azrin, 1968; Angle, Hay, Hay, & Ellinwood, 1977; Hawkins, 1986; Hintz & Shapiro, 1995; Kanfer & Grimm, 1977; Nelson & Hayes, 1986; O'Leary, 1972; Winett & Winkler, 1972). These guidelines included selecting target behaviors that

1. Pose a clear and immediate danger to the student, peers, parent, or staff;
2. Interfere with a broad array of functional daily activities;
3. Occur frequently or for long durations;

4. Disrupt daily routines and drain resources such as teacher and student time;
5. Are developmentally appropriate;
6. Are considered keystone behaviors in that these behaviors are necessary for the student acquiring, performing, or mastering a large array of other behaviors;
7. Will result in large, rapid, and sustained change when interventions are begun;
8. Occur early in a response chain;
9. Involve teaching appropriate behavior as opposed to inappropriate behavior;
10. Are more likely to be reinforced in the student's natural environment;
11. Are particularly annoying or troublesome to the referring agent.

When multiple problems are presented, direct observation may assist with identifying and prioritizing target behaviors. Direct observation may suggest that several behaviors are part of a behavior chain. For example, Greene, Bailey, and Barber (1981) found that students' inappropriate vocalizations may often occur before students engage in physical aggression. Reductions in physical aggression and inappropriate vocalization were achieved by implementing a procedure that directly targeted inappropriate vocalizations. Similarly, direct observation may suggest that a student is not engaging in a keystone behavior that is a necessary prerequisite for students to engage in a broad range of appropriate behaviors (e.g., following directions). Because altering this behavior may bring about changes in other identified target behaviors, this behavior may be selected as the primary target for intervention. Direct observation may also yield data that more clearly indicate the function of some behaviors more than other behaviors. In this case, it may be better to target a behavior that direct observation assessment data clearly indicate will be affected by an intervention procedure that is likely to be successful.

Even with these guidelines, the question of what constitutes a problem and decisions regarding how to choose and prioritize target behaviors is rarely based on precise empirical criteria. Thus for this initial stage and in all stages there is clearly the need to perform multi-method assessment procedures in order to make these decisions. During the problem identification stage of problem solving, interviews with teachers, parents, and even the children themselves could help identify and prioritize behavior problems (Bergan & Kratochwill, 1990; Kanfer & Grimm, 1977; Nelson & Hayes, 1986). Furthermore, having teams of interested individuals (e.g., teachers, parents, other school professionals, students) meet to share information and data may also help specify and prioritize problem behaviors (Fuchs, 1991).

Problem Analysis

The problem analysis stage follows target problem identification (Bergan & Kratochwill, 1990). The primary goal of this stage is to collect and analyze data that will allow for the construction of interventions designed to alter target behaviors. In this stage of problem solving, direct observation data are often used to collect data on natural environmental events that may be maintaining behaviors. A research base has developed that has clear implications for using direct observation in natural environments to identify the function of target behaviors, which then allows one to construct interventions based on the hypothesized function.

Functions of Behavior

One assumption associated with behavioral psychology is that behaviors are maintained by current environmental conditions and past learning history. It is the identification of current environmental conditions that function to maintain behaviors that allows one to link intervention procedures with assessment results under a behavioral model. Thus, from a problem-solving perspective, behavioral psychologists are as much concerned with the environmental variables that maintain target behaviors as the target behaviors themselves (Carr, 1993).

Operant behavioral psychology is based on the assumption that behaviors are maintained by contingencies of reinforcement. Contingencies describe and specify a relationship between antecedents, target behaviors, and consequences. When behaviors bring the student in contact with stimuli and that process increases the probability of the student engaging in that behavior again under similar situations, then the behavior has been positively reinforced (Sprague, Sugai, & Walker, 1998). Common positive reinforcing events in school settings include attention (e.g., smiles, praise, laughter) and obtaining access to activities (e.g., free time) or objects (e.g., gold stars, toys). When behaviors operate on the environment by removing stimuli and that process increases the probability of the student engaging in that behavior again under similar situations, then the behavior has been negatively reinforced. Common negatively reinforcing events in school settings include escaping or avoiding attention (e.g., being reprimanded or prompted by the teacher, being ridiculed by peers) and tasks or activities (e.g., mathematics seatwork).

Analysis of data collected via direct observation procedures can help one form hypotheses regarding the contingent relationship between target behaviors and consequent conditions that may be maintaining these behaviors under specific natural environmental conditions. For example, observers can use narrative ABC (antecedent, behavior, consequent) recording to help identify plausible positively and negatively reinforcing events. When this procedure is used, observers record the occurrence of the target behavior, events that immediately followed the target behaviors, and the conditions or antecedent events that preceded the target behaviors. This sequential analysis of events and conditions surrounding target behaviors may lead to the identification of the function of the behavior, or the event that may be serving to reinforce target behaviors under specific conditions.

Determining the function of a target behavior allows for the construction of interventions based on that function. For example, suppose a student is misbehaving to obtain attention (positive reinforcement). Then an intervention such as differential reinforcement (e.g., praise) for incompatible appropriate behavior (e.g., working on assigned tasks) is likely to be effective. However, if the same behavior is being

negatively reinforced by escaping or avoiding teacher attention, then the same intervention is likely to be ineffective and may actually strengthen the inappropriate target behavior.

Contiguity versus Contingency in Direct Observation

Contiguous events can be described as occurring in close proximity to the target
behavior (e.g., events or conditions that occur immediately before or immediately
after the target behavior). Events that occur contingent upon occurrence of the behavior do so as a result of the behavior. Direct observation of behavior in natural
environments and conditions surrounding that behavior only allows for the observation and determination of events contiguous to the target behavior. Events that follow a behavior may or may not be causally related to that behavior (e.g., they may
not reinforce the target behavior [Pierce & Epling, 1995; Rescorla & Wagner, 1972]).
Thus direct observation of behaviors in natural environments does not allow one to
unambiguously determine the function of a behavior. Rather, direct observation
allows one to form hypotheses with respect to the function of the behavior.

Precise determination of the function of a behavior would require experimental manipulation of hypothesized causal variables in order to rule out other causal
variables. Although direct observation is often used to assess the impact of these experimental manipulations (e.g., single-subject design research), the manipulations
themselves involve altering the natural environment. Therefore, procedures such as
experimental functional analysis and single-subject design procedures are beyond
the scope of this chapter.

Specifying Idiosyncratic Reinforcing Events

Some reinforcers are unconditioned whereas others are conditioned. Unconditioned
positive reinforcers are stimuli such as food and water, which typically act as reinforcers in the absence of any prior learning history (Sulzer-Azaroff & Mayer, 1986).
Unconditioned aversive stimuli that tend to occasion escape/avoidance behavior in
the absence of a prior learning history include events such as intense blows to the
head or sudden loud noises. If behaviors functioned solely to bring students into
contact with unconditioned reinforcers or to escape/avoid contact with unconditioned
aversive stimuli, then determining the function of behavior would be much simpler.
Observers could enter the classroom with a pre-established pool of reinforcers and
collect data designed to establish temporal relationships between students' behavior
and this *known* pool of reinforcing events.

In most instances reinforcers and aversive stimuli are conditioned or learned.
Because what is reinforcing or aversive is dependent upon a student's learning history, whether an event that occurs following a behavior is a reinforcer, a neutral
stimuli, or an aversive stimuli can vary across students, settings, and over time. One
historical example of idiosyncratic effects is related to attention. Barlow and Hersen

(1984) reviewed research related to the external validity of attention as a positively reinforcing event. Many researchers found that attention served as a positive reinforcer across people, settings, behavior, and time. However, some researchers investigating students who were considered conduct disordered or who engaged in self-injurious behavior found that attention was not an effective reinforcer (Wahler, Breland, & Coe, 1979). As researchers began to develop methods designed to test the function of specific behaviors, they found that specific events such as attention may serve as reinforcers in some cases, but in other cases a similar behavior may be reinforced by removal of attention (Iwata et al., 1994).

Researchers have shown that reinforcement tends to have a stronger impact on behavior when the consequences immediately follow that target behavior (e.g., Neef, Mace, & Shade, 1993; Neef, Shade, & Miller, 1994). This characteristic of reinforcement strengthens the assumption that events that occur contiguously (immediately following the target behavior) may be serving to positively or negatively reinforce target behaviors. Because specific stimuli may serve as reinforcers for some students in some situations and aversive or neutral stimuli for other students, or for the same student but in other situations, analysis of contiguous events may allow one to identify specific stimuli that are serving as positive and negative reinforcers. For example, if direct observation shows that target behaviors are followed by teacher reprimands, one may hypothesize that the target behavior is being positively reinforced by teacher reprimands. If a target behavior is followed by the removal of a demand, this procedure may help identify the specific stimuli the student is escaping or avoiding. For example, direct observation may show that a teacher changes a student's assignment to a briefer assignment (consequence) after he slams his textbook down and complains that he/she cannot do the assignment (target behavior). Because negative reinforcement involves the removal of a stimulus, it is especially important for observers to collect data on antecedent conditions or events that occur prior to the behavior.

Limitations for Determining Function via Direct Observation in Natural Environments

Observing and recording events that surround target behaviors can help identify the specific function of target behaviors, which, in turn, leads to interventions based on those direct observation data. However, researchers investigating operant models of behavior have conducted studies that indicate some limitations associated with using direct observation to identify the function of specific target behaviors within applied environments. Research on delayed reinforcers, intermittent reinforcement, extinction, competing schedules of reinforcement, and establishing operations all indicate limitations associated with using direct observation to determine the function of target behaviors.

Although immediate reinforcement tends to have a relatively stronger impact on behavior than delayed reinforcement (Neef et al., 1993, 1994), student behaviors may also be functionally related to reinforcing events that do not immediately follow the behavior that they are serving to reinforce (Baer, Osnes, & Stokes, 1983;

Fowler & Baer, 1981; Schwartz & Hawkins, 1970; Sluyter & Hawkins, 1972; Wilson, 1975). Delayed reinforcement is an important factor to consider when developing an intervention based on direct observation. If observers base their interventions on events that are contiguous or related by time to the target behavior, but not functionally related to the target behaviors, then these interventions may be ineffective. For example, suppose a student's misbehavior is being reinforced with peer attention that is delivered after school hours but never during school. Each time that Johnny acts out in class, observers may record events that immediately surround the behavior, but are not functionally related to the behavior. This may cause the observer to misidentify the function of the behavior (e.g., the misbehavior is being maintained by Johnny escaping the demand to do his school work).

Extinction occurs when a previously reinforced behavior is no longer being reinforced (Morgan, Morgan, & Toth, 1992). When a behavior that has been previously reinforced is undergoing extinction, the behavior may increase in rate, intensity, or duration. Another possibility is that extinction may lead to the performance of novel behaviors related to the previously taught behaviors (Lalli, Zanolli, & Wohn, 1994). The process of extinction also makes it difficult to use direct observation in natural environments to identify the function of a behavior. Suppose an observer is collecting data on an inappropriate behavior that has been previously reinforced by peer attention, but now peers are no longer attending to the behavior. Although the behavior may be occurring at fairly high rates, and perhaps even increasing in its occurrence, observers would not have the opportunity to assess (observe and record) the reinforcing condition that accounts for this behavior because the student's peers are no longer reinforcing the inappropriate behavior.

Intermittent reinforcement is the reinforcement of a particular behavior that is reinforced occasionally, as opposed to every time the behavior occurs (Pierce & Epling, 1995). Research on schedules of reinforcement has shown that in order to maintain a behavior, that behavior does not need to be reinforced following each occurrence of the behavior. Furthermore, this research suggests that behaviors that are maintained on thinner schedules of reinforcement may be more difficult to alter with procedures such as extinction (Baer, Blount, Detrich, & Stokes, 1987).

Intermittent reinforcement may also make it difficult to identify the function of target behaviors via direct observation in the natural environment. For example, suppose a target behavior is being maintained by occasional or intermittent peer attention. Even if that attention was delivered immediately, because it is delivered on an intermittent basis, observers may not be present during these intermittent instances of reinforcement. Thus they may be less likely to identify the actual function of the behavior and more likely to identify another event that may occur more frequently following the behavior (e.g., teacher reprimands) but have no contingent relationship to the target behavior.

Research on concurrent schedules of reinforcement also has implications for using direct observation data to determine the function of a behavior (Myerson & Hale, 1984). Classroom environments are extremely complex, with multiple schedules of reinforcement applied to multiple behaviors (McDowell, 1988). Research on what has become known as the Matching Law suggests that the presence or absence of an inappropriate target behavior is not merely dependent upon the rein-forcement procedures for that target behavior, but also dependent upon the re-inforcement procedures for competing incompatible behaviors (Herrnstein, 1961; Martens & Houk, 1989; Martens, Lochner, & Kelly, 1992). Variables that influence whether a child engages in incompatible behaviors include the *relative*, not abso-lute, quality, immediacy, and rate of reinforcement for the competing behaviors (Mace, McCurdy, & Quigley, 1990; Neef et al., 1993; Neef, Mace, Shea, & Shade, 1992; Neef et al., 1994). Furthermore, the relative amount of effort required to per-form each behavior can impact student choice of competing behaviors (Horner & Day, 1991; Mace, Neef, Shade, & Mauro, 1996; Skinner, 1998). Therefore, when attempting to identify variables that maintain target behaviors within school settings, it is often helpful to collect data on variables that influence competing behaviors. In many instances direct observation may allow one to identify these competing variables.

Temporally distant antecedent events also may be functionally related to be-haviors. Establishing operations are changes in the environment that have two ef-fects: they change the effectiveness of a reinforcing object or event as reinforcement and simultaneously alter the momentary frequency of the behavior that has been followed by that reinforcement (Michael, 1982). Using experimental functional analysis procedures, Ray (1997) investigated the effects of establishing operations on students' aggressive behavior and out-of-seat behavior under different consequent conditions. Results showed that when one child received less than 5 hours of sleep, tangibles were stronger reinforcers for out-of-seat behavior than when the child re-ceived more than 5 hours of sleep. When another student woke late, functional analy-sis indicated that his aggressive behavior was maintained by escape. However, when this student woke on time, the functional analysis indicated that access to tangible reinforcers maintained the aggressive behavior. Functional analysis data from a third student suggested that nocturnal enuresis was an establishing operation. When the establishing operation did not occur, the student's aggressive behavior was reinforced with access to tangible reinforcers. When the establishing operation did occur, the primary maintaining contingency for aggressive behavior was escape.

The Ray (1997) study demonstrated that temporally distal events may be func-tionally related to the specific target behavior. Because direct observation of contigu-ous behaviors in natural environments cannot be used to collect data on these tem-porally distant events, relying solely on direct observation data may not result in accurate hypotheses regarding the function of specific behaviors.

Within-Subject Variability

Because the traditional model of assessment attempts to measure constructs that are assumed to be stable, within-subject variability across repeated assessment is seen as measurement error. Under the behavioral model, this within-subject variability may prove critical for determining the functional relationship between behaviors and environmental events. As the Ray (1997) study indicates, through the use of repeated direct observation, it is possible to establish variability. Then direct observation procedures and other behavioral assessment procedures (e.g., parent interview) can be used to identify variables associated with that variability (e.g., temporally distant or proximally antecedent and consequent events). This type of analysis may allow one to determine under which conditions target behaviors occur and under what conditions they do not occur. Although this level of analysis is correlational, not experimental, it can still allow one to identify variables that are functionally related to the behavior.

Direct observation is a useful tool in the analysis of classroom behaviors. However, several issues regarding antecedent conditions and consequent events may lead to inaccurate results. These inaccurate results may, in turn, lead to implementation of an ineffective intervention. The use of additional assessments may ameliorate this problem. It may be helpful to conduct interviews with the teacher, parent, and/or the child in order to determine additional environmental variables that may be functionally related to target behaviors and account for the variability in direct observation data. Thus, even when environmental variables that maintain target behaviors cannot be observed, the variability that can be assessed via direct observation is critical to identifying the variables that may be better assessed using other procedures (e.g., Ray, 1997, used parent reports).

Plan Implementation and Evaluation

After a target behavior is identified and a treatment plan is developed, the next stage of a problem-solving process is to implement the planned treatment and evaluate the effects of this treatment. A treatment plan may be unsuccessful for a variety of reasons related to problem identification (e.g., wrong problem identified), problem analysis (e.g., wrong hypothesized function of target behavior), and a treatment being implemented inappropriately. Although direct observation data may not always allow for the determination of why a treatment failed or succeeded, repeated direct observation can at least allow one to evaluate the students' progress over time.

Treatment Evaluation: Possible Outcomes

The ability to collect data repeatedly over time is one of the primary procedural advantages of direct observation in the natural environment. Although this procedural advantage has implications for problem identification and analysis, from an applied perspective, repeated measurement may be most useful in the evaluation of treatment plans.

When single pre- and post-intervention measures of behavior are used to assess or evaluate intervention effects, only change in levels of the behavior can be detected. Using empirical data recording procedures, observers can collect pre-intervention and post-intervention data over repeated sessions. By comparing pre- and post-intervention data, it is possible to evaluate other aspects of within-subject behavior including variability and trend both within and across phases. These data also allow one to evaluate the immediacy of change brought about by an intervention. Evaluation of these data can help make data-based decisions with respect to the impact of an intervention procedure.

In order to help make decisions about the effects of an intervention, within-subject data are typically converted to time-series graphs that allow for visual analyses of the data (Johnston & Pennypacker, 1993). These graphs then serve as visual judgment aids that allow one to make decisions that guide the problem-solving process (Michael, 1974). Figure 2.1 provides hypothetical graphed data of three students' aberrant behaviors before (baseline or A phase) and after an intervention (treatment or B phase) was implemented.

Analysis of baseline data from Figure 2.1 shows that (1) Stew's baseline daily aberrant behavior rates are increasing, (2) Carlen's baseline daily aberrant behavior rates are neither increasing or decreasing, and (3) Sam's baseline daily aberrant behavior rates are decreasing. The amount of variability in the data influences trend analysis. Baseline data for Stew shows a clear increase in his daily aberrant behaviors, and baseline data for Sam shows a clear decreasing trend in Sam's aberrant behavior. Judging the trend in Carlen's aberrant behavior rates during baseline is more difficult because of the variability in that behavior.

As previously mentioned, analysis of baseline data can be used to make data-based decisions regarding interventions. With respect to the three students above, trend data suggest that Stew's aberrant behavior in baseline is a serious problem that may be in need of treatment. However, the decreasing trend in aberrant behavior associated with Sam's baseline data suggests that no intervention may be necessary. Thus the data from Stew and Sam may be useful for determining if an intervention should be implemented. However, with respect to determining the function of the behavior and developing intervention procedures, Carlen's data may prove even more useful. Under traditional models of assessment, within-subject variability over repeated assessment is seen as something negative (e.g., poor test–retest reliability). From a behavioral perspective, variability is assumed to be caused by variable environmental conditions. By attempting to identify events or conditions that correlate with the fluctuation in Carlen's data, it may be possible to identify the function of her behavior and develop an intervention based on that function. Thus, during behavioral assessment, within-subject variability may provide data that help one construct effective interventions.

Outcome data from an evaluation stage allow you to make decisions regarding the intervention's effectiveness. These data may show that following the intervention target behaviors (1) increased, (2) decreased, or (3) did not change. Furthermore, even when the data suggest that the intervention brought about change in the desired direction, analysis of trend data may suggest that the behavior is not changing rapidly enough and analysis of variability may suggest that intervention has not brought about a consistent change. This level of within-subject analysis allows practitioners to make decisions regarding whether (1) to continue with the intervention, (2) begin to fade the intervention and implement maintenance and/or generalization programming, or (3) to change intervention tactics by either implementing a new intervention or strengthening or modifying the current intervention.

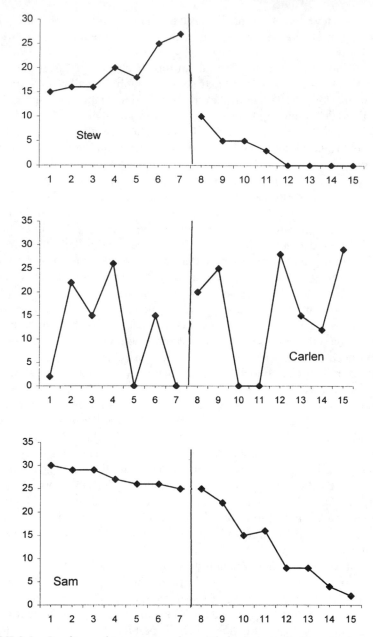

FIGURE 2.1   Baseline and intervention aberrant behavior rates for Stew, Carlen, and Sam.

Figure 2.1 also shows the impact of an intervention across phases. Stew's data show the most convincing change in the desired direction. When comparing Stew's data across phases, there is an immediate decrease in level (e.g., frequency of aberrant behaviors) following the implementation of the intervention. The data for Stew also show the trend reversed across phases, with a decreasing trend in aberrant behavior level in the treatment or B phase. Stew's data suggest that the behavior is no longer a problem. At this point, these data may suggest continuing the intervention or altering treatments in order to program for maintenance and generalization.

Following the intervention, Sam's data show little immediate change in level. However, the trend data show that the decreasing trend in inappropriate behavior rates has accelerated. Therefore, these data suggest that this intervention may also have been effective. However, Carlen's data suggest that the intervention was not effective in decreasing the level of her inappropriate behavior. Although Carlen's data series suggest earlier stages of the problem-solving process may need to be recycled, several conceptual issues prevent one from drawing firm conclusions related to intervention effectiveness.

Conceptual Issues Related to Cause-and-Effect Conclusions

There are several limitations associated with direct observation procedures that prevent one from drawing firm cause-and-effect conclusions with respect to the data series presented in Figure 2.1. First, with respect to Sam and Stew's data (Figure 2.1), no procedures have been implemented to control for threats to internal validity. This lack of experimental control makes it impossible to say that the intervention caused the change. Other procedures could be implemented that allow one to control for these threats to internal validity within natural environments (see Barlow & Hersen, 1984). However, there are other conceptual and applied issues that can make it difficult to use direct observation to evaluate the effects of interventions. To a large degree, additional direct observation procedures can be used to address these concerns.

Treatment Integrity

When visual analysis of direct observation data may suggest a treatment is ineffective and all goals associated with the first two stages of problem solving were met (e.g., the problem accurately identified, precise data-collection procedures developed, function of behavior identified and treatment based on that function is developed), the behavior may not change in the desired direction unless the plan is implemented as intended. Treatment integrity or treatment fidelity refers to the degree to which planned treatments are implemented as intended (Gresham, 1998). Although assessment of treatment integrity has often been a neglected component of the intervention stage of problem solving, direct observation may provide extremely useful for determining if the intervention is being implemented with integrity (Gresham, Gansle, & Noell, 1993; Peterson, Homer, & Wonderlich, 1982).

The professional literature suggests that there are many reasons why treatment plans may not be implemented with integrity. One reason why teachers may not implement interventions is that they find them unacceptable. Researchers have surveyed teachers and found that they prefer interventions that (1) require less time and resources, (2) are clear as opposed to complex, (3) are considered fair, and (4) increase appropriate behaviors as opposed to decrease inappropriate behavior (Clark & Elliott, 1988; Elliott, Witt, & Kratochwill, 1991; Martens, Peterson, Witt, & Cirone, 1986).

In some cases, interventions may not be implemented as intended because the person(s) responsible for implementing the intervention feels that the intervention is unacceptable. However, in other cases it may not be possible for the intervention to be implemented as intended. This may occur because the intervention is poorly described or the teacher does not have the resources or skills necessary to implement the intervention (Fuchs, 1991; Gresham, Gansle, Noell, Cohen, & Rosenblum, 1993; Sterling, Watson, Wildmon, Watkins, & Little, in press; Watson & Robinson, 1996).

Researchers have suggested a variety of variables that may impact treatment integrity. However, few studies have directly assessed the relationship between these variables and the degree of treatment integrity within natural environments (Witt, Gresham, & Noell, 1996). A research base does not exist that supports the assumption that any intervention will be implemented as planned. When evaluating the impact of a specific treatment, data should be collected to ensure that the treatment is being implemented as planned.

Several behavioral assessment techniques can be used to collect data on treatment integrity including teacher report (Wickstrom, Jones, LaFleur, & Witt, 1998), analysis of permanent product data (Witt, Noell, LaFleur, & Mortenson, 1997) and direct observation (Gresham, 1989). Although few studies have examined which behavior assessment procedures are superior for measuring treatment integrity, Wickstrom et al. (1998) found that teacher report data may overestimate the degree to which interventions are implemented with integrity. Direct observation of permanent products (see Witt et al., 1997) or direct observation in the natural environment may be more valid procedures for measuring treatment integrity.

Gresham (1989) outlines the procedures required for collecting treatment integrity data that are similar to the direct observation procedures used to record data on student behavior. First, the specific intervention components must be operationally defined. Next, a direct observation system should be constructed that allows one to record the occurrence or non-occurrence of each component. Observers then record occurrence or non-occurrence data and derive a treatment integrity index by computing the percentage of components implemented (e.g., converting data to a ratio).

CONCEPTUAL ISSUES RELATED TO THE QUALITY OF DIRECT OBSERVATION DATA

Behavioral theory does not assume that a student's behavior will be stable over repeated measurements. Just as the behavior of a student is not assumed to be stable, the recording behavior of observers may also fluctuate. This fluctuation in observers recording behavior introduces error that can adversely impact all decisions that are based on those data.

Inconsistent data collection can occur for a variety of reasons, including poorly trained observers, observer drift, poor operational definitions of target behaviors, and poorly constructed data-recording systems. Researchers investigating direct observation procedures have identified several procedures that may be used to measure and enhance the quality of direct observation data. The most common procedure involves having another trained observer collect data simultaneously with the primary observer. The data are then compared across observers and yield a measure of interobserver agreement.

Over the past 50 years, various methods of calculating interobserver agreement have been developed. Hops et al. (1995) reviewed the four most common methods of calculating interobserver agreement. The most easily calculated computes the percent of agreements out of the total number of agreements and disagreements. This method, however, does not control for chance agreement between observers. The second method, Cohen's kappa statistic, does correct for this chance agreement. However, it is difficult to calculate and no consensus has been reached on the Kappa level criteria necessary to conclude that the data are being collected consistently. The third method requires one to calculate a product–moment correlation coefficient, and is most commonly used with data that are collected on a single code category using an interval system. The primary weakness of this method is that it is insensitive to differences across observers in the average levels of coded behavior. Finally, a generalizability method has been suggested. Generalizability is based on a two-way analysis of variance procedure (Alessi, 1988; Hops et al., 1995). Regardless of the method used, interobserver agreement measures serve the same functions (Hawkins & Fabry, 1979). Low levels of interobserver agreement may be caused by (1) inadequate operational definitions, (2) poorly constructed data recording procedures, or (3) inadequate training of observers. Early detection of these problems can prevent observers from collecting imprecise data that might lead to faulty judgments based on these data throughout the problem-solving process.

Obtaining initially high levels of interobserver agreement data early in the direct observation process does not ensure that the person collecting the data will remain consistent in their recording procedure over time. Observer drift occurs when observers alter their recording behavior across sessions (Kratochwill & Wetzel, 1977). Kazdin (1977) offered suggestions to help control for observer drift including (1) continuous training of observers, (2) monitoring recording behaviors using direct observation of identical videotapes early and later during the data-collection process and comparing the recordings (e.g., calculate within-observer intraobserver agreement on the same tape over time to provide feedback with respect to drift), and (3) training a third observer early on but having them collect data infrequently along with the other observers so that interobserver agreement can be calculated across experienced observers versus observers who may not be as susceptible to drift.

Standard psychometric concepts such as criterion-related and construct validity may not be applicable to direct observation data because these data are not used to make inference regarding traits or constructs (Cone, 1988). However, interpreting direct observation does require observers to infer that what occurred would have occurred in a non-assessment situation (Gresham, 1998). Because of a phenomenon known as reactivity, validity is still an important consideration when collecting and interpreting direct observation data. Reactivity occurs when the process of collecting data alters the general ecology of the classroom and the behaviors of those being observed.

Reactivity is related to several variables including personal attributes of the observer, conspicuousness of the observer, and the rationale provided for the observation. Several recommendations have been made for reducing students' reactivity during classroom observation including (1) providing students with a vague rationale regarding the presence of the observer, (2) having the observer avoid staring at target students, (3) having the observer make no direct contact with students, (4) utilizing equipment such as one-way mirrors and video camera, (5) having the observer sit in an inconspicuous area of the room, and (6) having the observer enter the classroom before the students enter (Johnson & Bolstad, 1973; Saudargas, 1992; Shapiro, 1996).

While attempts can be made to minimize student reactivity, it may be more difficult to minimize teacher reactivity. Because teachers often play a role in the referral, problem identification, problem analysis, and plan implementation stages it is often difficult to reduce reactivity. Reactivity of teacher behavior may be a problem when direct observation is used to collect data on treatment integrity, as teachers may be more likely to carry out each aspect of an intervention when observers are present. Insofar as teacher behavior influences student behavior, reactivity from teachers can, in turn, cause students to behave in a manner that differs from how they would have behaved in a non-assessment situation. Although observing behaviors through one-way mirrors and video cameras at unspecified intervals can reduce teacher reactivity, in many educational environments these options are not available.

Reactivity can threaten the validity of data collected via direct observation. Furthermore, because it is difficult to predict whether reactivity will occur or to measure changes in behavior brought about by reactivity, steps should be taken that are designed to reduce reactivity. Clearly more research is needed on this phenomenon in order to better understand the causes of reactivity and to identify procedures designed to reduce reactivity. Within school settings, it may be particularly important for researchers to begin investigating teacher reactivity because changes in teacher behavior owing to direct observation can also alter target student behavior.

SUMMARY

Within the field of school psychology, there has been a shift away from traditional assessment models that focus on classification of students and toward models of assessment that lead to interventions (Hintze & Shapiro, 1995). In this chapter, we indicated how direct observation data can prove useful for each stage of problem solving (e.g., problem identification, problem analysis, and plan evaluation). To some degree, both the advantages and limitations of using direct observation data within a problem solving model are impacted by the core assumptions of behavioral psychology. The assumption that behaviors are legitimate problems allows for the direct assessment of problems and for the direct evaluation of treatment effects. The assumption that behaviors are caused by environmental conditions means that observers can record data on both the target behaviors and variables that cause those behaviors. Thus direct observation data can be used to indicate effective intervention procedures.

Although observing and recording behaviors appears to be a simple method of collecting data, the underlying theory associated with direct observation is complex. School psychologists who do not understand the conceptual foundations of behavioral psychology and who are not exposed to the research base on direct observation procedures may be less likely to employ direct observation procedures and/or more likely to make fundamental errors in their application of these procedures. Therefore, school psychologists should receive training in both behavioral assessment procedures and the underlying theory and assumptions associated with these procedures (Hintze & Shapiro, 1995). Furthermore, given the potential benefit of direct observation data for preventing and remedying problems, school psychology researchers should participate in the development of the research base needed to better understand and apply direct observation procedures within a problem-solving framework.

References

Alessi, G. (1988). Direct observation methods for emotional/behavior problems. In E. S. Shapiro & T. R. Kratochwill (Eds.), *Behavioral assessment in schools* (pp. 14–75). New York: Guilford Press.

Angle, H. V., Hay, L. R., Hay, W. M., & Ellinwood, E. H. (1977). Computer assisted behavioral assessment. In J. D. Cone & R. P. Hawkins (Eds.), *Behavioral assessment: New directions in clinical psychology* (pp. 369–380). New York: Brunner/Mazel.

Ayllon, T. & Azrin, N. (1968). *The token economy.* New York: Appleton–Century–Crofts.

Baer, R. A., Blount, R. L., Detrich, R., & Stokes, T. F. (1987). Using intermittent reinforcement to program maintenance of verbal/nonverbal correspondence. *Journal of Applied Behavior Analysis, 20,* 179–184.

Baer, R. A., Osnes, P. G., & Stokes, T. F. (1983). Training generalized correspondence between verbal behavior at school and nonverbal behavior at home. *Education and Treatment of Children, 6,* 379–388.

Barlow, D. H., & Hersen, M. (1984). *Single case experimental designs: Strategies for studying human behavior.* New York: Pergamon Press.

Barrios, B., & Hartmann, D. (1986). The contributions of traditional assessment: Concepts, issues and methodologies. In R. Nelson & S. Hayes (Eds.), *Conceptual foundations of behavioral assessment* (pp. 81–110). New York: Guilford Press.

Bergan, J. R., & Kratochwill, T. R. (1990). *Behavioral consultation in applied settings.* New York: Plenum Press.

Carr, E. G. (1993). Behavior analysis is not ultimately about behavior. *Behavior Analyst, 16,* 47–49.

Clark, L., & Elliott, S. N. (1988). The influence of treatment strength information on knowledgeable teachers' pretreatment evaluations of social skills training methods. *Professional School Psychology, 3,* 241–251.

Cone, J. D. (1978). The Behavioral Assessment Grid (BAG): A conceptual framework and a taxonomy. *Behavior Therapy, 9,* 882–888.

Cone, J. D. (1986). Idiographic, nomothetic, and related perspectives in behavioral assessment. In R. O. Nelson & S. C. Hayes (Eds.), *Conceptual foundations of behavioral assessment* (pp. 111–128). New York: Guilford Press.

Cone, J. D. (1988). Psychometric considerations and the multiple models of behavioral assessment. In A. Bellack & M. Hersen (Eds.), *Behavioral assessment: A practical handbook* (pp. 42–66). New York: Pergamon Press.

Elliott, S. N., Witt, J. C., & Kratochwill, T. R. (1991). Selecting, implementing, and evaluating classroom interventions. In G. Stoner, M. R. Shinn, & H. M. Walker (Eds.), *Interventions for achievement and behavior problems* (pp. 99–135). Silver Spring, MD: National Association of School Psychologists.

Fowler, S. A., & Baer, D. M. (1981). "Do I have to be good all day?" The timing of delayed reinforcement as a factor in generalization. *Journal of Applied Behavior Analysis, 14,* 13–24.

Fuchs, D. (1991). Mainstream assistance teams: A prereferral intervention system for difficult-to-teach students. In G. Stoner, M. R. Shinn, & H. M. Walker (Eds.), *Interventions for achievement and behavior problems* (pp. 241–268). Silver Spring, MD: National Association of School Psychologists.

Greene, B. F., Bailey, J. S., & Barber, F. (1981). An analysis and reduction of disruptive behavior on school buses. *Journal of Applied Behavior Analysis, 14,* 177–192.

Gresham, F. M. (1989). Assessment of treatment integrity in consultation and prereferral intervention. *School Psychology Review, 18,* 37–50.

Gresham, F. M. (1998). Designs for evaluating behavior change: Conceptual principles of single-case methodology. In T. S. Watson & F. M. Gresham (Eds.), *Handbook of child behavior therapy* (pp. 23–40). New York: Plenum Press.

Gresham, F. M., Gansle, K. A., & Noell, G. H. (1993). Treatment integrity in applied behavior analysis with children. *Journal of Applied Behavior Analysis, 26,* 257–263.

Gresham, F. M., Gansle, K. A., & Noell, G. H., Cohen, S., & Rosenblum, S. (1993). Treatment integrity in school-based behavioral intervention studies: 1980–1990. *School Psychology Review, 22,* 254–272.

Gresham, F. M., & Lambros, K. M. (1998). Behavioral and functional assessment. In T. S. Watson & F. M. Gresham (Eds.), *Handbook of child behavior therapy* (pp. 3–22). New York: Plenum Press.

Hartmann, D. P., Roper, B. L., & Bradford, C. C. (1979). Some relationships between behavioral and traditional assessment. *Journal of Behavioral Assessment, 1,* 3–21.

Hawkins, R. P. (1986). Selection of target behaviors. In R. O. Nelson & S. C. Hayes (Eds.), *Conceptual foundations of behavioral assessment* (pp. 331–385). New York: Guilford Press.

Hawkins, R. P. & Fabry, B. D. (1979). Applied behavioral analysis and interobserver reliability: A commentary on two articles by Birkimer and Brown. *Journal of Applied Behavior Analysis, 12,* 545–552.

Herrnstein, R. J. (1961). Relative and absolute strength of response as a function of frequency of reinforcement. *Journal of the Experimental Analysis of Behavior, 4,* 267–272.

Hintz, J. M., & Shapiro, E. S. (1995). Systematic observation of classroom behavior. In A. Thomas & J. Grimes (Eds.), *Best practices in school psychology—III* (pp. 651–660). Washington, DC: National Association of School Psychologists.

Hops, H., Davis, B., & Longoria, N. (1995). Methodological issues in direct observation: Illustrations with the Living in Familial Environments (LIFE) coding system. *Journal of Clinical Child Psychology, 24,* 193–203.

Horner, R. H., & Day, H. M. (1991). The effects of response efficiency on functionally equivalent competing behaviors. *Journal of Applied Behavior Analysis, 24,* 719–732.

House, A. E., House, B. J., & Campbell, M. B. (1981). Measures of interobserver agreement: Calculation formulas and distribution effects. *Journal of Behavioral Assessment, 3,* 37–58.

Iwata, B. A., Pace, G. M., Dorsey, M. F., Zarcone, J. R., Vollmer, T. R., Smith, R. G., Rodgers, T. A., Lerman, D. C., Shore, B. A., Mazaleski, J. L., Goh, H. L., Cowdery, G. L., Kalsher, M. J., McCosh, K. C., & Willis, K. D. (1994). The functional analysis of self-injurious behavior: An experimental-epidemiological analysis. *Journal of Applied Behavior Analysis, 27,* 215–240.

Johnson, S. M., & Bolstad, O. D. (1973). Methodological issues in naturalistic observation: Some problems and solutions. In L. A. Hamerlynck, L. E. Handy, & E. J. Mash (Eds.), *Behavior change: Methodology, concepts, and practices* (pp. 7–68). Champaign, IL: Research Press.

Johnston, H., & Pennypacker, H. (1980). *Strategies for human behavior research.* Hillsdale, NJ: Erlbaum.

Johnston, H., & Pennypacker, H. (1993). *Strategies and tactics of behavioral research.* Hillsdale, NJ: Erlbaum.

Kanfer, F. H., & Grimm, L. G. (1977). Behavioral analysis: Selecting target behaviors in the interview. *Behavior Modification, 1,* 7–28.

Kazdin, A. E. (1977). Artifact, bias, and complexity of assessment: The ABC's of reliability. *Journal of Applied Behavior Analysis, 10,* 141–150.

Kratochwill, T. R. (1982). Advances in behavioral assessment. In C. R. Reynolds & T. B. Gutkin (Eds.), *The handbook of school psychology* (pp. 314–350). New York: Wiley.

Kratochwill, T. R. & Shapiro, E. S. (1988). Introduction: Conceptual foundations of behavioral assessment in schools. In E. S. Shapiro & T. R. Kratochwill (Eds.), *Behavioral assessment in schools: Conceptual foundations and practical applications* (pp. 1–13). New York: Guilford Press.

Kratochwill, T. R., & Wetzel, R. J. (1977). Observer agreement, credibility, and judgement: Some considerations in presenting observer agreement data. *Journal of Applied Behavior Analysis, 10,* 133–139.

Lalli, J. S., Zanolli, K., & Wohn, T. (1994). Using extinction to promote response variability in toy play. *Journal of Applied Behavior Analysis, 27,* 735–736.

Lentz, F. E. (1982). *An empirical examination of the utility of partial interval and momentary time sampling as measurements of behavior.* Unpublished doctoral dissertation, University of Tennessee, Knoxville.

Lentz, F. E. (1988). On-task behavior, academic performance, and classroom disruptions: Untangling the target selection problem in classroom interventions. *School Psychology Review, 17,* 243–257.

Lentz, F. E. & Shapiro, E. S. (1986). Functional assessment of the academic environment. *School Psychology Review, 15,* 346–357.

Mace, F. C., McCurdy, B., & Quigley, E. A. (1990). A collateral effect of reward predicted by matching theory. *Journal of Applied Behavior Analysis, 23,* 197–205.

Mace, F. C., Neef, N. A., Shade, D., & Mauro, B. C. (1996). Effects of problem difficulty and reinforcer quality on time allocated to concurrent arithmetic problems. *Journal of Applied Behavior Analysis, 29,* 11–24.

Martens, B. K., & Houk, J. L. (1989). The application of Herrnstein's law of effect to disruptive and on-task behavior of a retarded adolescent girl. *Journal of the Experimental Analysis of Behavior, 51,* 17–27.

Martens, B. K., Lochner, D. G., & Kelly, S. Q. (1992). The effects of variable-interval reinforcement on academic engagement: A demonstration of matching theory. *Journal of Applied Behavior Analysis, 25,* 143–151.

Martens, B. K., Peterson, R. L., Witt, J. C., & Cirone, S. (1986). Teacher perceptions of school-based interventions. *Exceptional Children, 53,* 213–223.

McDowell, J. J. (1988). Matching theory in natural human environments. *Behavior Analyst, 11,* 95–109.

Michael, J. L. (1974). Statistical inference for individual organism research: Mixed blessing or curse? *Journal of Applied Behavior Analysis, 7,* 647–653.

Michael, J. L. (1982). Distinguishing between discriminative and motivational functions of stimuli. *Journal of the Experimental Analysis of Behavior, 37,* 149–155.

Morgan, D. L., Morgan, R. K., & Toth, J. M. (1992). Variation and selection: The evolutionary analogy and the convergence of cognitive and behavioral psychology. *Behavior Analyst, 15,* 129–138.

Myerson, J., & Hale, S. (1984). Practical implications of the matching law. *Journal of Applied Behavior Analysis, 17,* 367–380.

Neef, N. A., Mace, F. C., & Shade, D. (1993). Impulsivity in students with serious emotional disturbance: The interactive effects of reinforcer rate, delay, and quality. *Journal of Applied Behavior Analysis, 26,* 37–52.

Neef, N. A., Mace, F. C., Shea, M. C., & Shade, D. (1992). Effects of reinforcer rate and reinforcer quality on time allocation: Extensions of matching theory to educational settings. *Journal of Applied Behavior Analysis, 25,* 691–699.

Neef, N. A., Shade, D., & Miller, M. S. (1994). Assessing the influential dimensions of reinforcers on choice in students with serious emotional disturbance. *Journal of Applied Behavior Analysis, 24,* 575–583.

Nelson, R. O., & Hayes, S. C. (1986). The nature of behavioral assessment. In R. O. Nelson & S. C. Hayes (Eds.), *Conceptual foundations of behavioral assessment* (pp. 1–35). New York: Guilford Press.

O'Leary, K. D. (1972). The assessment of psychopathology in children. In H. C. Quay & J. S. Werry (Eds.), *Psychopathological disorders of childhood* (pp. 234–272). New York: Wiley.

Peterson, L., Homer, A., & Wonderlich, S. (1982). The integrity of independent variables in behavior analysis. *Journal of Applied Behavior Analysis, 15,* 477–492.

Pierce, W. D., & Epling, W. F. (1995). *Behavior Analysis and Learning.* Englewood Cliffs, NJ: Prentice-Hall.

Powell, J., Martindale, B., Kulp, S., Martindale, A., & Bauman, R. (1977). Taking a closer look: Time sampling and measurement error. *Journal of Applied Behavior Analysis, 10,* 325–332.

Ray, K. P. (1997). *Experimental analysis of the effects of temporally distant events on school behavior.* Unpublished doctoral dissertation, Mississippi State University, Starkville.

Reschly, D. J., & Wilson, M. S. (1995). School psychology practitioners and faculty: 1986 to 1991–92 trends in demographics, roles, satisfaction, and system reform. *School Psychology Review, 24,* 62–80.

Reschly, D. J., & Ysseldyke, J. E. (1995). School psychology paradigm shifts. In A. Thomas & J. Grimes (Eds.), *Best Practices in School Psychology–III* (pp. 17–31). Washington, DC: National Association of School Psychologists.

Rescorla, R. A., & Wagner, A. R. (1972). A theory of Pavlovian conditioning: Variations in the effectiveness of reinforcement and nonreinforcement. In A. H. Black & W. F. Prokasy (Eds.), *Classical conditioning II: Current research and theory* (pp. 64–69). New York: Appleton–Century–Crofts.

Saudargas, R. A. (1992). *State-Event Classroom Observation System* (SECOS). Knoxville: University of Tennessee, Department of Psychology.

Schwartz, M. L., & Hawkins, R. P. (1970). Application of delayed reinforcement procedures to the behavior of an elementary school child. *Journal of Applied Behavior Analysis, 3,* 85–96.

Shapiro, E. S. (1987). *Behavioral assessment in school psychology.* Hillsdale, NJ: Erlbaum.

Shapiro, E. S. (1996). *Academic skills problems: Direct assessment and intervention,* (2nd. ed.). New York: Guilford Press.

Shapiro, E. S., & Browder, D. M. (1989). Behavioral assessment: Applications for persons with mental retardation. In J. Matson (Ed.), *Handbook of mental retardation* (2nd ed.) New York: Plenum Press.

Shapiro, E. S., & Skinner, C. H. (1990). Best practices in observational/ecological assessment. In A. Thomas & J. Grimes (Eds.), *Best Practices in School Psychology–II* (pp. 507–518). Washington, DC: National Association of School Psychologists.

Skinner, C. H. (1998). Preventing academic skills deficits. In T. S. Watson & F. M. Gresham (Eds.), *Handbook of child behavior therapy* (pp. 59–82). New York: Plenum Press.

Sluyter, M. A., & Hawkins, R. P. (1972). Delayed reinforcement of classroom behavior by parents. *Journal of Learning Disabilities, 5,* 20–28.

Sprague, S., Sugai, G., & Walker, H. (1998). Antisocial behavior in schools. In T. S. Watson & F. M. Gresham (Eds.), *Handbook of child behavior therapy* (pp. 451–474). New York: Plenum Press.

Sterling, H. E., Watson, T. S., Wildmon, M., Watkins, C. & Little, S. (in press). Treatment acceptability, direct training, and treatment integrity: Applications to consultation. *School Psychology Quarterly.*

Sulzer-Azaroff, B., & Mayer, G. R. (1986). *Achieving educational excellence using behavioral strategies.* New York: Holt, Rinehart & Winston.

Wahler, R. G., Breland, R. M., & Coe, T. D. (1979). Generalization processes in child behavior change. In B. B. Lahey & A. E. Kazdin (Eds.), *Advances in clinical child psychology* (pp. 36–72). New York: Plenum Press.

Watson, T. S., & Robinson, S. L. (1996). Direct behavioral consultation: An alternative to traditional behavioral consultation. *School Psychology Quarterly, 11*, 76–92.

Wickstrom, K. F., Jones, K. M., LaFleur, L. H., & Witt, J. C. (1998). An analysis of treatment integrity in school-based behavioral consultation. *School Psychology Quarterly, 13*, 141–154.

Wilson, L. R. (1975). Learning disability as related to infrequent punishment and limited participation in delay of reinforcement tasks. *Journal of School Psychology, 13*, 255–263.

Winett, R. A., & Winkler, R. C. (1972). Current behavior modification in the classroom: Be still, be quiet, be docile. *Journal of Applied Behavior Analysis, 5*, 499–504.

Witt, J. C., Gresham, F. M., & Noell, G. H. (1996). What's behavioral about behavioral consultation? *Journal of Educational and Psychological Consultation, 7*, 327–344.

Witt, J. C., Noell, G. N., LaFleur, L. H., & Mortenson, B. P. (1997). Teacher use of interventions in general education settings: Measurement and analysis of the independent variable. *Journal of Applied Behavior Analysis, 30*, 693–696.

CHAPTER 3

Direct Observation in the Assessment of Academic Skills Problems

EDWARD J. DALY III
Western Michigan University

AMY MURDOCH
University of Cincinnati

The winds of educational reform that have been blowing over the past 30 years have not subsided. They have merely taken a different direction. School reform debates continue with the same intensity, but in broader arenas and with a revised agenda. Whereas the educational reform mandate in the 1970s focused efforts on improving schools' ability to provide equal educational opportunities for poor and minority children (those most at risk for academic failure), since the 1980s the educational reform mandate has been for an overhaul of the entire system (Bickel, 1999). This mandate, born of growing concern about the educational level of the entire nation, has been the impetus for what is referred to as the "restructuring" period. According to Bickel (1999), popular reform initiatives include "national and state standards, state curriculum frameworks and alignments, and assessment innovations" (p. 968). For example, the National Assessment of Educational Progress (National Center for Educational Statistics, 1998) routinely conducts and publishes the results of national-level assessments, self-described as "an important source for obtaining information on what students know and can do" (p. 1). In the state of Ohio, schools now receive report cards from the Department of Education. State-level proficiency test results weigh heavily in the Department of Education's evaluations of school districts (Ohio Department of Education, 1998). These standards and assessments are increasing expectations for schools. Increasing expectations for schools are also visible in the 1997 reauthorization of the Individuals with Disabilities Education Act (IDEA), which now requires functional assessments to address students' needs. To meet these demands, educators must have greater sophistication with assessment and intervention for remediating academic performance problems.

The purpose of this chapter is to describe assessment methods for improving instructional decision making for students with academic skills problems. To this end, we begin with a discussion of the conceptual foundations for the direct observation of academic skills problems, which lays the groundwork for sections on choosing and measuring academic performance targets and conducting functional assessments of academic performance problems. We approach this topic from a behavior-analytic framework because of its demonstrated utility for individual decision making through the use of repeated measurements and efforts to identify controlling variables on an individual basis.

CONCEPTUAL FOUNDATIONS FOR THE DIRECT OBSERVATION OF ACADEMIC SKILLS PROBLEMS

Behavioral assessment distinguishes itself from other forms of assessment in its standards for measurement (and consequently the types of data that are generated for decision making) and how variability in the data is treated. Nelson and Hayes (1979) point out that, "The novelty of the field of behavioral assessment lies then, not in its goals or strategies, but rather in its deliberate attempt to improve the identification and measurement of dependent variables, to increase the probability of selecting successful treatment techniques, and to refine the evaluation of those intervention procedures" (p. 2). The foundation for this approach is rooted in over 40 years of basic and applied experimental research using methods that are gaining prominence in the behavioral assessment of students (Martens, Witt, Daly, & Vollmer, 1999; Reschly & Ysseldyke, 1995). A review of the field's standards for measurement and its approach to evaluating variability serves to clarify the defining features of behavioral assessment. These standards are then used as a basis for discussing and evaluating contemporary trends in the direct observation and assessment of academic skills problems.

A fundamental task of any science is the quantification of the phenomena that make up its subject matter. Skinner (1938) sought to give shape to how psychology, then a young discipline struggling to define itself as a science, should quantify its subject matter by arguing that *rate of responding* should serve as the basic datum. Because rate of responding is directly observable and sensitive to environmental changes, it has the advantage of allowing for accounts of interrelationships between variables (i.e., dependent and independent variables) through experimental manipulation. When a discipline can provide systematic accounts of the effects of independent variables on dependent variables (i.e., the dependent variables vary in predictable ways according to the strength, the frequency, or the types of independent variables), empirically derived principles emerge. These principles then serve as tools for further refining our understanding of how and under what circumstances they can be invoked to produce changes in behavior. As a basic datum, rate of responding reflects a combination of accurate and fluent responding which, when measured continuously, can also provide an account of the durability and generality of responding (Binder, 1996). These qualities make it particularly appealing for quantifying observations of behavior for individualized assessment and intervention.

A consequence of defining rate of responding as the primary datum of the subject matter of psychology is that potential sources of data are limited to direct observations of behavior. Whereas many efforts are expended in psychology and education in indirect measurement strategies (e.g., surveys, checklists, global estimates of functioning on norm-referenced measures), from a behavioral assessment viewpoint good decision making relies on *direct measurement* of the learner's responses. The learner either emitted the correct response under the appropriate circumstances (e.g., wrote the digit "7" when presented with the problem "15 – 8 = ____" on a piece of paper) or not. Patterns of responding can be examined across time. Conclusions drawn are relative to the environmental conditions (i.e., setting, instructions, task demands, and response formats) under which they were observed.

This approach is vastly different from making decisions about student functioning based on their ranking in a distribution. Johnston and Pennypacker (1980, 1993) describe the former approach as *idemnotic* measurement and the latter approach as *vaganotic* measurement. In the case of idemnotic measurement, the units of measurement are standard and absolute (insofar as the response class is adequately defined). As in the natural sciences, the accuracy of these measurements can be scrutinized because the phenomenon itself is independent of how it's being measured. In the case of vaganotic measurement, the units of measurement are variable depending on the sample making up the distribution and how the items interact with the individuals on whom the test was standardized. Assumptions have to be made regarding how representative the sample is of the larger population. However, the validity of these assumptions is not generally investigated (Sidman, 1960). Furthermore, the accuracy of these measures cannot be assessed because the units of measurement are not reflective of the occurrence or nonoccurrence of actual responses; rather, they are anchored in the distribution itself, which could change, depending on which participants make up the sample and which tasks are administered. For example, if a student scores at the 12th percentile on a standardized norm-referenced test of academic achievement, the score reflects an inferred construct (i.e., "academic achievement"), which means that it is not a phenomenon that exists separately from the units of measurement themselves. As such, it has no temporal or physical referent. Inferences about the role of an inferred construct in an individual's learning profile rely on a more basic substrate of a set of observations of behavior. For this reason, a psychometric tradition of evaluating the consistency of scores within and across measures of the same type has emerged. These criteria are not, however, sufficient for assuring the accuracy of the data for describing student functioning and how it is affected by environmental events like how the classroom is arranged or how instructions are presented (Cone, 1995). Indeed, there are measurement problems intrinsic to the analysis of correlated variables that make the database unreliable for individual decision making (Macmann & Barnett, 1997, 1999).

Rate of responding implies features of behavior that can be further analyzed into quantifiable dimensions for which units of measurement must be assigned (Johnston & Pennypacker, 1980, 1993). The properties of a response class must be measurable. The units of measurement must assign the same quantity to each occurrence of the response class and the unit of measurement must be sensitive to changes in behavior (Wolery, Bailey, & Sugai, 1988). For example, if the response class of interest is correctly written letters when randomly chosen letter sounds are dictated orally at 5-second intervals to a first-grade student for a 2-minute period, a score of "1" might be assigned to each correctly written letter. The unit of measurement, therefore, is a correctly written letter.

The fundamental properties of behavior that permit quantification include (1) when they occur in time ("temporal locus"), (2) for how long they occur ("temporal extent"), and (3) how frequently they occur in time ("repeatability") (Johnston & Pennypacker, 1980, 1993). If, for example, a student takes too long to respond to calculation questions during the math lesson, the *latency* of responding to teacher-generated calculation questions may be the most desirable dimension to measure (assessing the "temporal locus" of the response class). Alternately, if a student spends too little time looking in the direction of the teacher who is reading a story during story time, the *duration* of responding during story reading time may be the most desirable dimension to measure (assessing the "temporal extent" of the response class). Finally, if a student writes too few words during journal writing time, the *countability* of responding (e.g., the number of words or letters written) may be the most desirable dimension to measure (assessing the "repeatability" of the response class).

By measuring the combination of when a behavior occurs ("temporal locus") and how frequently it occurs ("repeatability"), rate of responding can be obtained. In the journal writing example, if there is a standard amount of time devoted to journal writing on a daily basis (e.g., 20 minutes), the frequency of the behavior per time unit—rate—can be described (e.g., 10 words written per 20 minutes prior to classroom modifications). When rate is examined across time, the celeration (i.e., changes in behavior across time) can be examined by displaying the data graphically (Lindsley, 1990). If classroom modifications were made that successfully improved the rate of responding to 145 words written per 20 minutes, a graphic display should reveal an increasing trend in the behavior across time (acceleration). If, however, the goal of classroom modifications is to decrease behaviors (e.g., inappropriate verbalizations during teacher lectures), a visual display of the data would permit analysis of whether there is a decreasing trend (deceleration). The graphic analysis of data is the standard for decision making within a behavioral assessment framework because it permits analysis of behavior across time and under different conditions. It also happens to be a more conservative approach to data interpretation than the statistical analysis of data, which forces investigators to pursue more robust behavior–environment relationships (Parsonson & Baer, 1978, 1986, 1992).

It is precisely the variability of behavior that is of most interest to experimental analysts and behavioral assessors alike. The assumption is made that variability in behavior is caused by environmental conditions that can be controlled and whose effects on behavior can be observed. In other words, variability is suggestive of behavior–environment relationships. Rather than treating variability in the data statistically, an effort is made to identify potential sources of variability and attempts are made to directly manipulate them (Sidman, 1960). Because behavior is measured across time, both short-term and long-term effects of changes in environmental conditions can be observed and the need for modifications to the intervention protocol can be inferred from the patterns in the data. For instance, if a student's reading improves across time to an acceptable level following an instructional program, plans for modifying the intervention may be warranted. Within this approach, behaviors are only expected to vary together to the degree that they share the same *controlling variables* (Hayes, Nelson, & Jarrett, 1986). These assumptions represent a *functional approach* to the evaluation of behavior (Nelson & Hayes, 1986). They lead the investigator to ask why a behavior occurs or fails to occur in a particular context. The answer to this question relies on a direct manipulation of variables (i.e., an experimental analysis) to identify their effects for the purpose of *prediction* and *control*. A functional approach sets a rigorous standard for how conclusions are drawn about the interaction of variables. Nelson and Hayes (1986) comment, "For behaviorists in touch with functional-analytic roots, it seems more appropriate to evaluate the quality of behavioral assessment devices and procedures in terms of their accuracy and the *functions that are served*" (p. 6).

These measurement issues have important implications for the choice of which behaviors to measure, an area referred to as target selection (Hawkins, 1986). Quantifying rate of academic responding in the manner described above is a *low inference* approach to target selection that should help the investigator avoid the problems associated with assuring the accuracy of measurement for high-inference constructs. Choosing academic behaviors (and their successful resolution) over the elimination of disruptive behaviors should increase the learner's capacity to function adaptively in the classroom environment and beyond. When academic targets are individualized, the evaluation meets the learner's needs better by improving the evaluator's understanding of controlling variables. Targeting academic behaviors that are precursors for the acquisition of more complex academic behaviors increases the likelihood of the student acquiring more difficult skills. Essentially, targeting and improving academic behaviors amounts to a differential reinforcement strategy which has potential benefits across environments and with tasks of increasing complexity. Finally, targeting academic behaviors has *socially meaningful consequences* for the learner because of the outcomes produced and how they are valued by parents, educators, and the community.

THE NATURE OF ACADEMIC RESPONDING AND ITS RELATIONSHIP TO THE INSTRUCTIONAL ENVIRONMENT

Frequently, variables such as socioeconomic status (SES), education of parents, measured IQ, and category of disability are used to explain poor achievement. Unfortunately, reliance on unalterable variables over which educators do not have control does not provide guidance about what can be done to improve student achievement. An alternate approach is to focus on variables over which educators do have control and that have been shown to affect student achievement. In order to assess academic performance in a way that is ultimately helpful to improving student learning it is necessary to understand the nature of academic performance, those observable and reliable patterns of behavior that are clear indices of learning (i.e., how behavior changes across time), and the processes governing their occurrence (i.e., how they change in response to environmental manipulations). In this section, key variables that are useful for describing learning and principles governing academic learning are discussed.

Academic Engagement and Active Responding

Academic engagement, the proportion of time that a student is actively responding to relevant academic tasks (writing, reading aloud, answering academic questions, etc.), is a variable under the control of educators that is directly related to student achievement (Greenwood, Terry, Marquis, & Walker, 1994). Descriptive studies of how students spend time in the classroom suggest that large differences exist in the amount of time students spend actively engaged in relevant curricular tasks across classrooms (Rosenshine, 1980). Longitudinal studies examining the amount of time students spend actively engaged in classrooms have found large differences across socioeconomic levels, differences favoring students of higher socioeconomic status over students of lower socioeconomic status (Greenwood, Hart, Walker, & Risley, 1994). These cumulative differences (amounting to more than one-and-a-half years of schooling by the end of middle school) help to explain the gap in achievement that widens as students of differing socioeconomic status progress through school. Increasing academic engaged time of lower SES students through classwide peer tutoring has been shown to reduce the achievement gap for these students (Greenwood, 1991).

Clearly, academic engagement is a construct of primary importance in the assessment of students. A large database has emerged in the literature, demonstrating that increasing the quantity of academic engagement can be expected to increase measured achievement (Greenwood, 1996). The effects of academic engagement are not, however, independent of instruction; rather, academic engagement mediates the effects of instruction on student achievement (Greenwood, Terry, et al., 1994). Academic engagement and other similar constructs like academic learning time are directly affected by classroom variables such as teacher behavior and instructional materials (Greenwood, 1991; Ysseldyke & Christenson, 1993).

Academic engagement is also an important indicator of whether student responding is occurring in classrooms; as such it may be used as an outcome measure. There is a direct correspondence between behaviors constituting academic engagement (i.e., those sampled under observation conditions) and those measured to infer achievement. Active engagement as a performance target has been shown to lead to greater generalized improvements in overall achievement than when the target behavior is "on-task" (Hoge & Andrews, 1987; Lentz, 1988a). A student who is passively looking in the direction of the teacher or instructional materials could be "on-task" but not actively engaged in the instructional activity. The Ecobehavioral Assessment Systems Software (EBASS; Greenwood, Carta, Kamps, & Delquadri, 1995) and the Behavioral Observation of Students in Schools (BOSS; Shapiro, 1996a, 1996b) are recent innovations in the assessment of academic engagement. They represent an improvement over other discontinuous observation systems because they do not confound "on-task" behavior with academic engagement. However, because they are time-based, they are not entirely satisfactory for measuring outcomes. They merely provide an estimate of the duration of responding but do not permit the accurate quantification of the rate or celeration of responding. Furthermore, the behaviors sampled indicate whether responses are occurring or not but do not indicate whether they are the types of responses desired for meeting the instructional objectives.

A more direct measure of engagement that is amenable to calculating rate is active student responding. Heward (1994) defines active student responding as occurring "when a student emits a detectable response to ongoing instruction" (p. 286). The observer, therefore, must define the specific responses relevant to the task (e.g., verbal responses during the lesson closure portion of a science lesson, written words during journal writing time, etc.). There are several advantages to quantifying active student responding for assessment purposes. First, measures are easy to construct and can be used to describe rate of responding. It is necessary to specify a priori the types of responses expected during the observational period, to note the beginning and ending time of the observational period and, finally, to record each occurrence of the relevant responses. Measuring active student responding in the classroom provides an index of the behaviors of interest in the natural environment under the effects of typical classroom factors, allowing teachers to assure that appropriate responses are occurring so that they can provide corrective feedback during the lesson as needed. Also, it is sensitive to changes in the classroom. It has been useful for comparing the effects of different instructional techniques in research (e.g., see Heward, 1994, Narayan, Heward, Gardner, Courson, & Omness, 1990, and Sterling, Barbetta, Heron & Heward, 1997) and can be readily incorporated into functional assessments of students' academic performance problems. Using rate of responding under natural classroom conditions or within the curriculum as an outcome metric is likely to increase student achievement by providing important feedback to teachers, which may prompt them to adjust instruction according to the student's needs (Heward, 1994). For all of these reasons, we view the quantification of active student responding as *the* central construct that should drive the direct observation and measurement of academic skills.

Environmental Determinants of Academic Responding

A key assumption of a functional approach to assessment is that student responses occur as a result of environmental events. Therefore, an understanding of the mechanisms that control the occurrence of student responding is critical for assessment and decision making. From a behavior-analytic perspective, academic responses are discriminated operant behaviors that have been brought under the control of relevant stimuli. Stimulus control is a basic behavioral process whereby a change in environmental stimuli occasions a response (Rilling, 1977). Stimulus control develops as a result of differential reinforcement applied to properties of the stimuli (Catania, 1998). In the classroom, the teacher works to bring student behavior under the control of curricular materials (Vargas, 1984). For instance, the teacher may expect a flashcard with the letter "a" to produce the verbal response "*ah*." Some features of curricular stimuli should become critical to making the correct response. For example, the sequence and configuration of letters in the word "bat" are critical features for occasioning a response (student reads "bat") that differs from other responses (e.g., reading "cat") occasioned by yet other stimuli. On the other hand, some features of stimuli should become irrelevant to the development of a discrimination (e.g., the font type of the text).

Schools have curricula that define the "skills" necessary to graduate. Curricular objectives are descriptions of the types of tasks students should master. As such, they outline the stimuli that should occasion responding and the types of responses that should be obtained (as well as the conditions under which they should be obtained). Teachers must sequence tasks and stimulus materials carefully and provide repeated opportunities to respond while reinforcing correct responses to help students master curricular objectives, bringing student behavior under the control of critical stimuli. When students are initially learning a particular skill, teaching items should be narrowly configured to help students make correct discriminations (e.g., teaching a phonics rule and having students read words like "map," "tap," and "tad"; Gersten, Carnine, & White, 1984; Grossen & Carnine, 1991). As students become proficient, teaching items should more closely approximate real world tasks (e.g., filling out a job application). Learning occurs across a gradient of responding and teachers should plan instruction to facilitate the generalization of academic responding across stimulus gradients.

Precision teaching has produced superior educational results by making measurement along a gradient of responding the core of instructional decision making. Curricular tasks are broken down into component behaviors (e.g., number writing, multiplication, division, addition, etc.) which are assessed and then targeted for instruction if necessary. Johnson and Layng (1994) report that when component behaviors reach high fluency levels, more complex skills (e.g., problem solving, calculus, etc.) are easier to teach and that they are actually able to spend less time teaching harder skills. Indeed, students' prerequisite skill level prior to instruction has been shown to account for at least as much variance in student outcomes as teachers' actions themselves (Howell, Fox, & Morehead, 1993). Assessment is used to diagnose proficiency with both prerequisite skills and global curricular objectives to draw conclusions about fluency rates of behaviors along a gradient of response repertoires from more isolated responses (like writing numbers) to sequences of responses (like writing answers to calculus problems). Having examined how measurement can be used to improve instructional decision making, let's now turn to how instruction can be delivered to improve learning.

Effective teaching increases the probability of the development of stimulus control by orienting the learner to features of the environment (and sources of reinforcement) that may not be readily apparent, and increasing the speed with which stimulus control is developed. The learning trial is the basic unit of instruction for accomplishing this task (Albers & Greer, 1991; Heward, 1994; Skinner, Fletcher, & Henington, 1996). The teacher presents instructional antecedents, reinforcement for responding (when the natural environment is not likely to do so as readily), and error correction. Although there are slight variations in how different behavior-analytic instructional models elaborate the learning trial, these approaches are compatible with one another and have revealed consistent predictable effects of instructional procedures on student responding. For example, one model is based entirely on discrete learning trials—the Comprehensive Application of Behavior Analysis to Schools (CABAS; Greer, 1994, 1997). The success of Direct Instruction is partly attributable to its close adherence to some basic principles of curricular design that amount to a general teaching protocol for promoting stimulus control (Gersten et al., 1984; Kinder & Carnine, 1991). The Instructional Hierarchy (IH; Haring, Lovitt, Eaton, & Hansen, 1978) has been shown to be useful for choosing instructional components based on student's level of proficiency (Daly, Lentz, & Boyer, 1996; Daly & Martens, 1994). Other useful sources include reviews of effective instruction that can be found in Heward, Heron, Hill, and Trap-Porter (1984), Howell et al. (1993), Wolery et al. (1998), Martens and Kelly (1993), McKee and Witt (1990), and Ysseldyke and Christenson (1993), as well as Lentz and Shapiro's (1986) functional model for examining the instructional environment. It is beyond the scope of this chapter to review all of these sources in detail. However, a general framework that integrates empirically validated instructional practices is presented in Table 3.1. Table 3.1 identifies five domains of instruction as well as teaching actions that should be associated with each domain.

Lindsley (1996) has suggested that complex behaviors may be response chains where an environmental stimulus (e.g., teacher directions to complete the long-division problems on p. 56 of the workbook) leads to a series of interrelated responses in which each response (e.g., dividing one number into another) occasions the next response (dividing the next number). If Lindsley's (1996) conjectures are correct, academic responses are only likely to emerge as discriminative stimuli if they are of sufficient strength as response classes to be high-probability behaviors, which means that they must have been adequately reinforced themselves. In the classroom, students and teachers alike engage in complex sequences of behaviors that should be interlocking links in a continuous chain, ultimately leading to elaborate student responses following teacher-presented problems (or even student-generated problems). Student behaviors should be largely determined by teacher behaviors. Likewise, teacher behaviors should also be determined by student behaviors. When there is a rupture in the interlocking sequence of behaviors (i.e., teacher behaviors are not functionally related to student behaviors) problems arise. Academic intervention involves realigning instructional practices so that they lead to more rapid accelerations in student academic behavior, creating or strengthening functional relationships between teacher behavior and student behavior.

FUNCTIONAL ASSESSMENT OF ACADEMIC SKILLS

Good quality assessment methods will allow the evaluator to make decisions about various sources of variability in student performance and link those decisions to treatment strategies to remediate academic skill problems. Functional relations are inferred from patterns of variability in the data. For example, one source of variability might be differences between a referred student and peers in curricular materials, information that might have utility for operationalizing a problem. This source of variability, however, is not likely to explain why a problem is occurring. Another source of variability might be variability in daily performance in the classroom or with different materials. This information could yield useful information about instructional or classroom factors that appear to be affecting student performance. Yet

TABLE 3.1 Effective Teacher Actions for Promoting Student Learning

Instructional domain	Teacher actions
Instructional planning	The curricular objective is identified. Prerequisite skills are identified and there is an appropriate match between instructional activities and students' skill level. Instructional materials and activities that teach the general case and promote good stimulus control are chosen. There is a performance monitoring system for knowing how well students are progressing. Sufficient time for teaching and student responding is allocated.
Classroom environment and behavior management	Rules are posted. There are obvious classroom routines that make it easier for students to know where to be and what to do. The teacher actively supervises students by scanning, walking around the room, stopping inappropriate behavior as it is just beginning, and consequating disruptive behavior. The teacher delivers a higher proportion of attention for student responding than for competing behaviors.
Instruction for promoting accuracy	There is a description of (a) a rationale for instructional activities and (b) contingencies for performance. There are clear directions for how to complete tasks and modeling of instructional items that includes • Explicit demonstration of how to use previously learned skills, • Step-by-step problem solving with verbal descriptions, and • Non-examples (so students learn when to use and when *not* to use the skill). There is guided practice with • A wide variety of item types, • Items sequenced so that examples and non-examples are minimally different at the beginning, • Questions to elicit descriptions of steps used to get the answer as well as answers, and • A feedback ratio of 1:1 for responses (including error correction) and correct use of steps. Contingencies for accurate performance are delivered.
Instruction for promoting fluency	There is a description of (1) how to complete fluency activities and (2) contingencies for performance. There are frequent response opportunities to practice the skill(s). There is fluency feedback. Students self-monitor performance. Contingencies for fluent performance are delivered.
Instruction for promoting generalization	Instructional activities allow students to respond to a wide variety of instructional items and in natural contexts. Instructional activities that introduce newly learned skills to natural incentives are used. Application activities that allow skills to be combined in novel ways and that incorporate newly learned skills in more complex skills are used. Students self-monitor performance.

another source of variability is variability in student performance across time. Each of the following topics outlines a general approach to assessing, describing, and interpreting variability in the data for academic skills problems. A descriptive analysis attempts to elucidate natural patterns of variability in the classroom. Functional analysis attempts to directly control variability in a prescribed manner as a basis for verifying hypothesized relationships. Formative evaluation, or ongoing progress monitoring, usually has a longer time frame. Formative evaluation examines patterns of variability across time following instructional modifications.

Descriptive Analysis

Descriptive analysis is the process of gathering information about the natural setting to generate hypotheses about how some variables affect other variables. Various sources of information (e.g., interviews, assessments, and observations) are used to make statements about what typically happens in the classroom when a particular problem is most likely to occur. For example, interview information, direct assessment data, and classroom observation data might suggest that the reading passages used during reading instruction are too difficult. These statements describe sequences of behavior (e.g., "During the independent seatwork portion of language arts, Alex only completes 35% of the items on his phonics worksheets correctly on average and frequently stares around the room, plays with objects, and talks with peers.") from which hypothesized causes are inferred (e.g., "The instructional material may be too difficult and Alex receives insufficient feedback on his performance. As a result, he doesn't complete his work and engages in high rates of competing behaviors during independent seatwork."). The purpose of a descriptive analysis is to identify *presumed controlling variables* that affect student performance. Descriptive analysis does not, however, involve a direct manipulation of classroom events. Therefore, one must be cautious about drawing firm conclusions.

   Methods for conducting descriptive analyses for academic performance problems should include interviews, direct assessments of student performance, and direct observations of the student in the classroom. Shapiro (1996a) provides interviews that are useful for describing instructional routines, how decisions are made, and teacher perceptions of student performance. The Instructional Environment System II (Ysseldyke & Christenson, 1993) contains both teacher interview and student interview questions related to empirically validated instructional practices.

   Direct assessments of student performance can be conducted with curriculum-based measures. Writing, spelling, and math can be assessed in a whole group format in the classroom. Reading is assessed individually. When peer data from the same classroom are also collected, comparisons of fluency rates can be made between a referred child and the average or median performance in the peer group. This information can be used for identifying deficits in basic skills that may be contributing to academic performance problems. For example, if a target student who is having difficulty in math with double-digit by double-digit multiplication problems writes answers to single-digit multiplication problems at one-fourth the rate of the average peer, fluency with the more basic skill can be targeted for intervention. If a target student does not display low fluency rates relative to peers in basic academic skills, the evaluator might then turn to the classroom to examine whether another skill should be targeted for intervention or whether there may be other factors adversely affecting a student's academic performance (e.g., a lot of teacher attention for disruptive behavior but little to no feedback on academic performance).

Direct observation of the target behavior(s) in the natural setting is perhaps the most important part of descriptive analysis. The classic and seminal example of descriptive analyses is Bijou, Peterson, and Ault's (1968) report of methods for integrating descriptive and experimental analyses. Bijou et al. (1968) outline four steps for observing and describing events and their occurrence. First, it is necessary to specify the situation in which the study is being conducted. Second, behavioral and environmental events must be defined in observable terms. Third, there must be measurements of observer reliability to assure the accuracy of the data. Finally, there must be procedures for collecting, analyzing, and interpreting the data. They describe procedures for conducting observations based on the three-term contingency (antecedent–behavior–consequence).

Mace, Lalli, and Pinter-Lalli (1991) point out that descriptive analysis information provides an empirical basis for formulating and testing hypotheses via functional analyses, which increases the likelihood that analogue conditions will reflect actual environmental circumstances and decreases the likelihood that a problem behavior will come under the control of new contingencies. Recent descriptive analysis methods reported in the literature have typically targeted aberrant or disruptive behaviors. For example, Lalli, Browder, Mace, and Brown (1993) identified and confirmed the operant function of students' problem behaviors in a pretreatment assessment that included descriptive analyses followed by experimental analyses. Dunlap, Kern-Dunlap, Clarke, and Robbins (1991) used descriptive analysis and experimental analysis methods to identify antecedent curricular revisions that were incorporated in a treatment package that led to increases in on-task behavior and decreases in disruptive behaviors.

The studies conducted to date have targeted behaviors that are at a free operant level (e.g., disruptive behaviors, on-task), meaning that the behaviors occur in response to already established functional relations. Unfortunately, students are generally referred for academic performance problems because academic behaviors are *not* at a free operant level. Therefore, observation results cannot be expected to suggest already existing functional relationships that are maintaining behavior. They can, however, be tailored to identifying whether there are enough instructional antecedents and consequences of the right type for the student's skill proficiency to promote active student responding. What is needed is a conceptual framework for sorting through possible instructional or classroom variables that might be affecting student performance. Daly, Witt, Martens, and Dool (1997) recommended that simple explanations for academic performance problems be sought first and identified five reasons why students have academic performance problems. These five reasons include the following: (1) They do not want to do it; (2) They have not spent enough time doing it; (3) They have not had enough help to do it; (4) They have not had to do it that way before; and (5) It is too hard. Behavioral assessors could organize descriptive analyses to identify one or more of these reasons before developing interventions to address them (e.g., see Daly et al., 1997).

The evaluator should request permission to observe in the classroom during the time when the student is having the most difficulties. Next, the observer must define student and environmental events in measurable terms. Table 3.2 contains a list of suggested antecedents, academic behaviors, and consequences that classroom observers should look for when conducting classroom observations. To gather data, teacher and student behaviors can be recorded continuously. We suggest making four columns, one for time, one for antecedents, one for student behaviors, and one for consequences (see Bijou et al., 1968). If the time column is broken down into small time intervals (e.g., 1 minute), it will be easier to identify and summarize which antecedents preceded which behaviors and which behaviors preceded which consequences. For example, if each row is 1 minute of observation time, the behaviors in Table 3.2 could be recorded as they occur during the observation. The observer should note beginning time and ending time so that rates of behavior can be calculated. When teacher and student behaviors are summarized as rate data, they can be used in conjunction with interview and direct assessment data to answer the questions in Table 3.3. The questions in Table 3.3 are based on the five reasons described by Daly et al. (1997). Although certainly not exhaustive, it can be used as a basis for identifying robust instructional strategies that have been shown to improve student achievement as potential treatment components and may be appropriate for the referred student.

TABLE 3.2 Descriptive Analysis Categories for Student Behaviors and Instructional Antecedents and Consequences

Instructional antecedents	Student behaviors	Consequences
1. Teacher provides directions for how to do the instructional activity.	1. Student writes a response.	1. Teacher praises individual student.
2. Teacher describes contingencies for completing the instructional activity.	2. Student gives a verbal response.	2. Teacher praises the group.
	3. Student matches one item to another.	3. Teacher reprimands the student.
3. Teacher asks a question.	4. Student selects a correct response.	4. Teacher redirects the student.
4. Teacher presents an item.	5. Student manipulates objects to give a response.	5. Teacher corrects a student error.
5. Teacher demonstrates or models.	6. Student raises hand.	6. Peers respond to student's behavior.
6. Teacher prompts a student to respond.	7. Student engages in competing behaviors.	7. Teacher delivers a contingency.

TABLE 3.3   Descriptive Analysis of Academic Performance:
Questions to Investigate and Data Sources

Questions to investigate	Data sources
1. What are the incentives for doing it?	1. Teacher report, student report, direct observation.
2. Are there incentives for the student to do other things?	2. Teacher report, student report, direct observation.
3. Is it aversive to do it?	3. Teacher report, student report, direct observation.
4. Is there a clear rationale for why it's important to do it?	4. Direct observation of directions delivered at the beginning of activities.
5. Does the student have frequent *opportunities* to do it?	5. Teacher report of allocated time, direct observation of student responding.
6. Does the student do it enough?	6. Direct observation of student responding.
7. Are there too few instructional antecedents?	7. Direct observation of sequences of teacher and student behavior.
8. Are they the wrong types of antecedents?	8. Direct observation of sequences of teacher and student behavior.
9. Does the student receive sufficient feedback?	9. Direct observation of sequences of student and teacher behavior.
10. Is the student being asked to do the wrong thing?	10. Examination of permanent products.
11. Does the student have the prerequisite skills to do it?	11. Direct assessments of student performance in prerequisite skills.
12. Is it too hard for the student to do?	12. Examination of permanent products, direct assessments of student performance in instructional tasks, direct observation of student behavior.

Functional Analysis

The purpose of a functional analysis is to identify controlling variables through the systematic evaluation of the effects of an independent variable on a dependent variable (Martens, Eckert, Bradley, & Ardoin, 1999). Since Iwata, Dorsey, Slifer, Bauman, and Richman's (1982/1994) pioneering study in the development of functional analysis methods for self-injurious behavior, extensive work has been done on the application of this technology to other types of behaviors and other settings. Although functional analysis procedures have been successfully applied in classrooms to develop treatments for disruptive behavior (e.g., Broussard & Northup, 1995; Kern, Childs, Dunlap, Clarke, & Falk, 1994), the procedures for conducting functional analyses of academic behaviors are just being developed (Daly et al., 1997; Hendrickson, Gable, Novak, & Peck, 1996). One reason why the technology of functional analysis has not previously been used in schools to analyze academic performance problems is probably related to the amount of time and resources necessary for collecting the data. Recently, however, a number of studies have demonstrated that brief functional analysis procedures can be successfully used to develop treatments for children's disruptive behaviors (Cooper et al., 1992; Derby et al., 1992; Harding, Wacker,

Cooper, Millard, & Jensen-Kovalan, 1994). The use of brief experimental conditions for developing treatments is likely to make functional analysis more efficient and more applicable in schools.

We suspect that another reason why functional analysis has not been previously developed for academic performance problems is that the existing model of functional analysis is not readily applicable to academic behaviors. In the case of aberrant social behaviors, evaluators are faced with behavioral excesses for which previous learning has already occurred. The stimulus conditions are designed to elicit, occasion, or reinforce already existing response classes. When clearly discriminable differences in behavior are obtained across stimulus conditions, results are interpretable because functional relations have been *directly* tested. Discriminable differences can be detected when there are existing functional relations between at least one set of stimulus conditions and the target behavior and non-existent functional relations with the other set(s) of stimulus conditions. Intervention components such as differential reinforcement, extinction, and shaping procedures are *indirectly* inferred, based on identified functional relations between response classes and environmental events. In the case of academic behaviors, evaluators are often faced with behavioral deficits that exist because previous learning has failed to occur. Students' academic performance is not under the stimulus control of the instructional activities and materials (or, as in the case of a performance deficit, is under the stimulus control of instructional activities under very restricted conditions; see Lentz, 1988b). As such, academic behaviors will not appear in a functional analysis unless stimulus conditions create functional relations that can be measured. Therefore, another approach is necessary if a functional analysis technology is to be developed for academic performance problems. It would be more useful to know how much work it will take to create functional relations between student behavior and academic stimuli.

To date, few studies have been conducted that apply brief functional analysis procedures to academic behaviors. In these studies, treatments were applied directly to academic targets. A preliminary study by McComas et al. (1996) used a brief multielement design to analyze students' academic responding in the areas of spelling and reading comprehension. The results of this study suggested that brief experimental analyses of instructional strategies might be helpful for identifying effective instructional components if they include design and procedures that allow the evaluator to produce clear, discriminable, and reliable response rates across "test" conditions. More recently, Daly, Martens, Dool, and Hintze (1998) applied test conditions that consisted of baseline (i.e., no assistance) and treatment conditions (i.e., assistance was provided) to students having difficulty learning how to read. Using a brief multielement design, test conditions were administered until a visible increase in oral reading fluency was observed. Next, a mini-reversal was conducted by repeating the last ineffective treatment or baseline condition and the first effective treatment condition to confirm the initial results. The object of these brief test conditions was to identify interventions that produce the largest outcomes in the most efficient manner possible; the easiest test conditions were applied first. Although the results do not guarantee that an effective treatment will be identified, they are at least useful for eliminating interventions that will probably be ineffective because they did not even produce immediate effects.

Daly et al. (1998) attempted to evaluate instructional components separately. Test conditions in the study were presented under the assumption that instructional components functioned independently to improve performance. Actually, the development of academic skills requires a sequence of instructional activities that build upon one another. The strategies that teachers use to facilitate the mastery of specific skills are often interrelated (e.g., modeling and error correction for acquisition also increase a student's opportunities to respond to the instructional materials), and teachers generally do a variety of things at once. Therefore, test conditions that sequentially add or "stack" instructional components to prior conditions should be expected to produce greater performance gains more quickly while informing subsequent instructional programming in a manner that is more like what teachers actually do.

More recently, Daly, Martens, Hamler, Dool, and Eckert (1999) conducted brief experimental analyses of oral reading fluency where instructional components were sequentially "stacked" (i.e., added on) across test conditions. For example, if increasing opportunities to respond through repeated practice did not lead to a visible improvement in student performance, modeling was *added* to the next test condition. Different response patterns were observed across participants, suggesting that effective combinations of instructional components were identified. Additionally, this approach required fewer test conditions than the one reported by Daly et al. (1998), making the process more efficient. These investigations indicated that brief functional analyses can be conducted successfully with interventions targeting students' oral reading fluency.

A number of conditions related to the instructional materials must be met when using this format. First, to ensure that outcome differences are indeed due to the treatment conditions, assessment materials of equal difficulty level should be used across test conditions unless a test condition is designed to examine difficulty level specifically. Second, assessment materials should be independent of one another across test conditions to minimize overlapping content across materials. Overlapping content between conditions increases the chances of multiple-treatment interference affecting the results. Third, the assessment materials should reflect the content of what was instructed during each test condition so that the assessment will be sensitive to any effects produced by instruction. Curriculum-based measures of oral reading, math computation, written expression, and spelling are particularly well suited to academic performance problems when students are having difficulty with basic academic skills.

This approach is more appropriate for certain types of treatment than others. Martens et al. (1999) suggest that treatments that are likely to produce more immediate changes in behavior and/or that provide sufficient opportunities for the behavior to occur are more appropriate for this type of analysis. Additional research is necessary to determine whether the results of brief analyses produce reliable results in more extended analyses and whether they lead to long-term outcomes that justify the resources and time necessary to conduct the analyses. We turn now to two case examples where brief experimental analyses were conducted and an attempt was made to confirm the results of the brief analyses with more extended analyses.

Case Examples

Both students—Latasha and Andrew—were in the second grade and were being instructed at a first-grade reading level. They had both been referred for reading problems and were in the same classroom. They were 7 years old at the time of referral. To obtain screening information, they read a first-grade passage from the Burns and Roe Informal Reading Inventory (Burns & Roe, 1989) aloud. Next, the examiner asked comprehension questions related to the passage. The number of correctly read words (CRW) per minute, errors, and percent correctly answered comprehension questions were calculated. Latasha read 22 CRW per minute with 5 errors and answered 25% of the questions correctly. Andrew read 9 CRW per minute with 7 errors and answered 12.5% of the comprehension questions correctly.

Analyses were conducted in an attempt to identify effective instructional components. A series of test conditions consisting of baseline and treatment conditions was administered to each student until a visible change in performance was observed. The treatment conditions were administered in order from easiest to implement (i.e., required the least amount of adult supervision and feedback) to most difficult to implement (i.e., required extensive adult supervision, assistance, and feedback). When an effective treatment condition was identified, the last two conditions (i.e., baseline or the last unsuccessful treatment condition and the successful treatment condition) were alternated repeatedly. In each test condition, two separate passages were administered for assessment purposes: an instructional passage (i.e., the passage in which instruction was provided) and a high-content overlap passage (HCO; a passage containing approximately 80% of the words in the instructional passage written as a different story). Instructional passages were taken from the first-grade level of the Silver-Burdett, and Ginn reading series (Pearson et al., 1989). The HCO passages were written to contain many of the same words as a corresponding instructional passage but constitute a different story. They were administered immediately following treatment to probe for generalization of responding across passages.

For the brief analysis, two conditions were administered to Latasha: baseline (in which she received no assistance from the examiner) and repeated readings (RR; in which she read the instructional passage aloud four times and was told how quickly she read the passage after each reading). The results for Latasha are displayed in Figure 3.1. The results of the brief analysis are on the left side of the figure. In the baseline condition, Latasha read at a rate of 40 correctly read words per minute (CRW/min) in the instructional passage and 42 CRW/min in the HCO passage. In the RR condition, Latasha read 68 CRW/min in the instructional passage and 58 CRW/min in the HCO passage, suggesting that she benefited from the additional practice afforded by RR and that her improved reading fluency generalized to the HCO passage. Therefore, a decision was made to alternate baseline and RR conditions to deter-

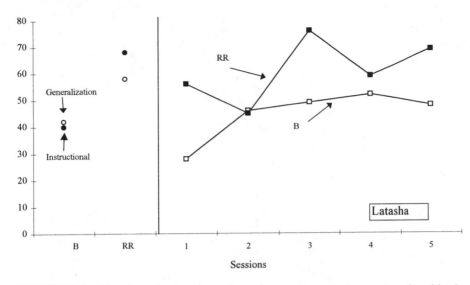

FIGURE 3.1 Number of correctly read words per minute in instructional and high-content overlap (HCO) passages for Latasha.

mine whether the results were reliable. The results for the HCO passages only are displayed on the right side of the graph. Baseline and RR were alternated and the order of administration was counterbalanced across five sessions. In all but one case (session 2), Latasha's reading fluency was superior in the RR condition to the baseline condition even though treatment was provided only in the instructional passages and not in the HCO passages. Interestingly, there is an increasing trend in the baseline data. This increasing trend occurred in spite of the fact that independent passages were used for each administration. It is possible that Latasha was so responsive to the treatment that generalized increases in performance began to occur in untreated instructional materials. The results suggest that Latasha would probably benefit from repeated practice in instructional materials with feedback about rate of responding.

More elaborate procedures were necessary to identify instructional components for Andrew. For the brief analysis, four test conditions were administered to Andrew: (1) baseline, (2) RR (as described above), (3) listening passage preview plus repeated readings (LPP/RR; in which the examiner read the passage aloud to Andrew before Andrew read it aloud three times while receiving feedback on how quickly he read the passage), and (4) LPP/RR plus sequential modification (LPP/RR/SM). SM is a generalization strategy in which a treatment is applied sequentially across settings (Stokes & Bear, 1977). In this case, the LPP/RR treatment was applied to both the instructional passage and the HCO passages. Each of the treatment conditions added an instructional component to the prior condition. Treatments were applied until there was a visible increase in Andrew's performance. The results of the brief analysis are displayed on the left panel of Figure 3.2. In the baseline condition, Andrew read at a rate of 19 CRW/min in the instructional passage and 27 CRW/min in the

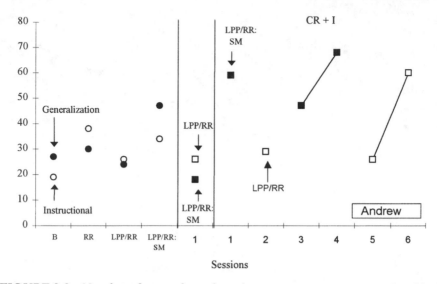

FIGURE 3.2 Number of correctly read words per minute in instructional and high-content overlap (HCO) passages for Andrew.

HCO passage. Andrew's reading fluency improved in the instructional passage in the RR condition (to 38 CRW/min) but not in the HCO passage (30 CRW/min). It was decided to proceed with additional treatment conditions to determine whether additional instructional components could further improve Andrew's rate of responding. His reading fluency did not, however, improve in the following condition—LPP/RR. In this condition, he read 26 CRW/min in the instructional passage and 24 CRW/min in the HCO passage. A decision was made to proceed further by applying the treatment (LPP/RR) to both the instructional and generalization passages (SM). In this condition, Andrew read 34 CRW/min in the instructional passage and 47 CRW/min in the HCO passage. His reading performance in the generalization almost doubled in this condition relative to baseline. It appeared that Andrew benefited from the sequential application of LPP/RR to both the instructional and HCO passages.

An attempt was made to confirm the results of the brief analysis by administering the effective treatment and the last ineffective treatment in counterbalanced order in independent passages (middle panel of Figure 3.2). The purpose of this phase was to determine whether the results of the brief analysis could be replicated in independent instructional materials. Andrew's performance dropped precipitously during this phase, failing to confirm the previous hypothesis regarding the effects of LPP/RR/SM. Andrew's performance in the LPP/RR/SM condition was below all prior conditions. We reasoned that applying the treatment in both passages may have made the condition too long, requiring a greater response effort on Andrew's part. It was hypothesized that adding reinforcement to the instructional conditions might improve his performance. This hypothesis was examined in the third part of the analysis. For this phase, a reward was offered for meeting a criterion fluency rate of 60 CRW/min (defined as Mastery level by Shapiro, 1996a). The two treatment condi-

new instructional content. Teachers rely on skill hierarchies that are logically but not necessarily empirically derived and must make frequent measurement shifts to continuously assess student learning. By way of contrast, the other approach, general outcome measurement, involves the use of materials that are representative of the entire school year's curriculum and global outcome indicators like passage reading fluency that produce reliable and valid samples of student proficiency. In this measurement approach, long-term goals can be developed and measurement is not necessarily tied to an instructional sequence (e.g., teaching long vowel words before teaching r-controlled words). Advantages of this approach include (1) the ability to obtain estimates of students' generalized performance across curricular materials and time, (2) independence of measurement and instruction (which allows for a more rigorous test of instructional methods), and (3) stronger content and criterion validity (because the focus of decision making is on proficiency in critical behaviors in annual curricular domains rather than on the analysis of sequential mastery of specific subskills; Fuchs & Deno, 1991).

As a form of general outcome measurement, formative evaluation is the analysis of student performance using repeated measures of student performance that are sensitive to instructional modifications (Deno, 1986; Fuchs & Fuchs, 1986). Formative evaluation data can be used to modify instruction through goal setting, graphic displays of data, and systematic data-evaluation rules. Program modification is treated empirically. In other words, the data are used for deciding whether instruction was effective after instruction was provided rather than for predicting what or how to teach. Large treatment gains have been found for the use of formative evaluation by teachers (Fuchs & Fuchs, 1986), including an average effect size of .70 for progress monitoring and an average effect size of .91 when systematic data-evaluation rules were used in conjunction with routine progress monitoring. In an investigation of teacher behaviors, Fuchs, Fuchs, and Stecker (1989) found that the use of formative evaluation led teachers to develop more specific acceptable goals for student performance, less optimism about goal attainment, more objective data sources, and more frequent instructional modifications. By allowing the evaluator to examine celeration and make decisions regarding students' generalized performance in the curriculum, formative evaluation is useful for prompting data-based decision making about the effectiveness of instruction and student performance over time.

Within this framework, practitioners are faced with decisions regarding the format for assessment, which materials to use for monitoring, how to set goals, and expected growth rates. All of these factors are likely to affect measured outcomes and, hence, decision making about instruction. The purpose of this section is to address methodological issues in direct assessment practices that have bearing on these questions. There is a growing database on formative evaluation assessment formats and how stimulus materials are likely to affect estimates of students' responsiveness to instruction. This research should help to guide these decisions. To accomplish the first task, deciding how to assess student performance, it is necessary to calibrate behaviors, an issue described earlier as defining properties of a response class. The reader is reminded of the earlier calibration example of correctly written letters in response to orally dictated letter sounds. Calibrating behaviors has been done most extensively by precision teachers (Binder, 1996; Johnson & Layng, 1992, 1994; Lindsley, 1990; West, Young, & Spooner, 1990; White & Haring, 1980).

As an extension of the methods developed by precision teaching, curriculum-based measurement has been investigated for purposes of formative evaluation (Shinn, 1989; Shinn & Hubbard, 1992). Curriculum-based measures have been developed to assess fluency in basic skills in the areas of oral reading, math computation, spelling, and written expression. In reading, the student reads three passages chosen randomly from curricular materials for 1 minute and the number of correctly read words and errors per minute are calculated. In math, the student writes answers to computation questions for 2 minutes and the number of correctly written *digits* per 2 minutes is calculated. In spelling, words are dictated for 2 minutes to the student who writes responses. The number of correctly written *letter sequences* per 2 minutes is calculated. In written expression, students are given a story starter, 1 minute to think about a story to write, and 3 minutes to write. Student performance can be evaluated in several ways. Calculating the total number of words, the total number of correctly spelled words, and/or the total number of correct word sequences per 3 minutes are the most common scoring methods.

A unique characteristic of curriculum-based measurement relative to other forms of academic assessment is that samples of student responding can be obtained in the curriculum in which the child is being instructed. The same cannot be said for commercial norm-referenced tests. Indeed, depending on the test one chooses and the amount of content overlap that exists between test items and curricular materials ("test-teach" overlap), different scores are likely to result from different tests administered to the same child (Bell, Lentz, & Graden, 1992; Good & Salvia, 1988; Shapiro & Derr, 1987). Commercial tests yield a thin sample of student responding for any given area in an attempt to assess skills broadly, all for the purpose of describing student performance within a distribution of scores. If, however, student performance differs depending on the amount of test–teach overlap, decisions about student proficiency or the effectiveness of instruction may be unreliable. Alternately, because curriculum-based measures can be used to obtain estimates of student proficiency in curricular materials repeatedly over time, they should be more useful for instructional decision making.

The necessity of sampling from the curriculum, however, has been questioned. Fuchs and Deno (1992) found strikingly similar correlation coefficients between students' oral reading samples in two different basal reading series and their performance on a norm-referenced test of comprehension. Hintze, Shapiro, Conte, and Basile (1997) had a similar finding using the same methodology; albeit lower correlations were obtained. Fuchs and Deno (1992) also found similar growth rates across series, and concluded, "users of CBM need not worry extensively about the possibility of curriculum bias" (p. 240). Fuchs and Deno (1994) argued that the key pattern in the data for assessing instructional effects is the trend across time *within* the series and that differences across series are less relevant for deciding whether instruction was effective. For these reasons, they recommend that it is not necessary to use curricular materials for progress monitoring as long as repeated measures of valid indicators of the critical outcomes of instruction are used.

A closer examination of the implications of this recommendation, however, should cause practitioners to regard it with some skepticism. First, if there are differences in trend within reading series across different reading series, the results may prompt the evaluator to make different decisions depending on the series chosen for assessment. Fuchs and Deno (1994) do acknowledge that factors like variability of item difficulty within a reading series and the generalizability of results are likely to affect instructional decisions. It is therefore necessary to understand how *accurately* measurement in different reading series affects trends *over time* and whether the differences actually affect decision making and subsequent student achievement (i.e., generalized growth to independent stimulus materials). In the data reported by Fuchs and Deno (1992) there are large absolute differences for some grade levels in average fluency rates across basal reading series. For instance, at the second-grade level the average performance in one series was approximately 31 CRW/min and the average performance in the other series was approximately 49 CRW/min for the same students, representing a difference of 18 CRW/min in *average* performance across reading series (which amounts to a difference of between one-third to one-half of the observed rates of responding, depending on the series used). A similar pattern was found for one of the books at the third-grade level. The difference in average reading fluency rates for third-grade students in the second-grade materials was 31 CRW/min, which might lead an evaluator conducting a survey-level assessment to very different conclusions regarding student performance, depending on the series used. Although Hintze et al. (1997) also obtained similar correlation coefficients with a comprehension measure across series, they found differences in oral reading rates across grade levels as a function of series used for assessment. The question of whether these differences affect teacher behaviors and student achievement is a methodological issue requiring experimental analyses. Correlational data are inadequate to draw firm conclusions about whether it is necessary to use materials from the curriculum.

The recommendation by Fuchs and Deno (1992, 1994) is an empirical hypothesis that can only be adequately tested by looking at differences in performance over time across series. One way to do this is to compare students' slopes of improvement across series. For instance, Hintze, Shapiro, and Lutz (1994) compared slopes of improvement in a literature-based basal and a traditional basal reading series at the students' instructional level. One group was receiving literature-based reading instruction and another group was receiving traditional reading instruction. In all, repeated measures were gathered on 48 students in the third grade over a nine-week period. Hintze et al. (1994) found *negative* slopes of improvement in the literature-based basal across *both* instructional methods (i.e., for both groups of students) and *positive* slopes of improvement in the traditional basal reader. In a similar investigation, Hintze and Shapiro (1997) compared slopes of improvement in a literature-based basal and a traditional basal at *one grade level above* the level at which students were being instructed for 160 students at the second-, third-, fourth-, and fifth-grade levels and found significantly greater growth in the literature-based passage probes on average across grade levels and negative slopes of improvement for second-grade students. The results of these investigations clearly indicate that measured outcomes themselves may be influenced by the materials in which student performance is measured, which may, in turn, influence instructional decisions like placement in the curriculum or the adequacy of student progress over time.

The grade level of the material within the curriculum is another issue that has been recently investigated. The difficulty level of the materials may be expected to influence measured outcomes. Shinn, Gleason, and Tindal (1989) examined student trends over time in two different measurement conditions: (1) one grade level below and one level above students' current placements, and (2) two and four grade levels above instructional placements. Thirty students in grades 3 through 8 participated and their progress was monitored over four weeks. Shinn et al. (1989) found no significant differences in slope of improvement as a function of difficulty level of the materials used for monitoring. As a result, Shinn et al. (1989) recommended using goal level material for progress monitoring. Goal level material refers to passages from one grade level above the student's instructional placement. An advantage of this approach is that the monitoring materials allow the evaluator to assess generalized growth to passages that are different from those being used for instruction. In addition, by monitoring in goal level material it is possible to assure that students reach an acceptable proficiency level before placing them in those materials for instruction.

The validity of this recommendation, however, has come into question in light of more recent investigations of student progress across instructional and goal level (or "challenging" level) material. Hintze et al. (1998) pointed out that Shinn et al.'s (1989) sample was composed only of students having difficulty learning to read. Also, Shinn et al. (1989) did not measure student growth in instructional-level materials. Hintze, Shapiro, and Daly (1998) monitored student performance in instructional-level and challenging-level materials for a group of 80 first-, second-, third-, and fourth-grade students over an 11-week period. They found that students in grades 1 and 2 performed significantly better on average in instructional-level rather than challenging-level material but that students in grades 3 and 4 did not display such significant differences across monitoring levels. The difficulty level of the materials used for progress monitoring does appear to be an important factor that is likely to influence outcomes for some students. The average growth rates across instructional and challenging materials for three studies (Fuchs, Fuchs, Hamlett, Walz, & Germann, 1993; Hintze & Shapiro, 1997; Hintze et al., 1998) are displayed in Table 3.4. The most striking result of a comparison of the three studies is the differences within monitoring levels as well as across monitoring levels. For example, Hintze et al. (1998) obtained growth estimates for first-grade students at the instructional level that were more than one-and-a-third the size of the estimates obtained by Fuchs et al. (1993); whereas the estimates for second-grade students at the instructional level were one-half the estimates obtained by Fuchs et al. (1993). At the third-grade level, Hintze et al.'s growth estimates were less than one-fifth the rates obtained by Fuchs et al. (1993). Curriculum-based measures of reading fluency appear to be extremely sensitive measures of student proficiency. In fact, environmental factors like who administers passages and where they are administered (factors that should be extraneous to instructional decision making) have been shown to influence the results (Derr & Shapiro, 1989; Derr-Minneci & Shapiro, 1992). In order for these measures to be

TABLE 3.4   Research-Based Estimates of Typical Rates of Improvement across Monitoring Levels

Grade	Instructional level material[a]	Challenging level material[b]	Instructional level material[c]	Challenging level material[c]
1	2.10		3.29	1.95
2	1.46	0.14	0.72	0.30
3	1.08	1.13	0.16	0.06
4	0.84	2.26	1.57	1.85
5	0.49	1.98		
6	0.32			

[a]Fuchs et al. (1993).
[b]Hintze and Shapiro (1997).
[c]Hintze, Shapiro, and Daly (1998).

useful for validly describing trends in performance, the variables affecting student performance must be accounted for and considered when decisions are being made about which materials to use for progress-monitoring purposes. Adequate answers to these methodological questions require experimental analyses that permit accurate conclusions about sources of behavioral variability.

In an attempt to experimentally investigate the role of content overlap and difficulty level on instructional outcomes, Daly, Martens, Killmer, and Massie (1996) directly manipulated the amount of content overlap and the difficulty level of instructional materials. High- versus low-content overlap depended on the proportion of words appearing in assessment passages that also appeared in passages in which students were instructed. High-content overlap passages had a larger percentage of words that appeared in instructional passages than low-content overlap passages. Student performance in both high- and low-content overlap passages was assessed following instruction. Difficulty level was manipulated by using two sets of instructional and assessment materials. In the materials that were more appropriately matched to the students' skill levels, students displayed higher accuracy and fluency rates prior to exposure to the experimental conditions than in more difficult materials. This comparison yielded four conditions: (1) high-content overlap/appropriate instructional match, (2) low-content overlap/appropriate instructional match, (3) high-content overlap/instructional mismatch, and (4) low-content overlap/instructional mismatch. The instructional procedures were the same across all conditions. Daly, Martens, et al. (1996) found that students displayed higher performance levels in the high-content overlap/appropriate instructional match condition than in the other conditions. There was a clear interaction of difficulty level and content overlap for all participants in the study. Although this study did not measure rates of progress across time, these results in combination with the other investigations described above are important because the students who are referred for reading problems will probably have more difficulty generalizing from instruction in the first place. Therefore, if the materials used for progress monitoring are different or more difficult than those in which the students are being instructed, smaller growth rates (i.e., lower trends in performance) can be expected. If, however, content overlap is maximized (which means also that the student is being monitored at the instructional level), larger growth rates (i.e., higher trends in performance) can be expected.

The earlier discussion of stimulus control has bearing on these issues. Assessment materials should accurately reflect appropriate generalization gradients. When the materials are not configured to reflect what was taught, changes in performance can only be observed if there are broad generalization effects. If, however, the student is having difficulty generalizing in the first place, the instruction may be increasing response rates but only more narrowly. On the other hand, the disadvantage to measuring only in the materials in which students are being instructed is that it may be difficult to determine whether more generalized improvements are occurring in materials different from those in which instruction is being carried out (Fuchs & Deno, 1994). It is possible that these issues are less relevant for students who are beyond just acquiring initial reading skills. You will recall that Hintze et al. (1998) found no significant differences between difficulty level for third- and fourth-grade regular education students.

Further research is necessary on the effects of the proximity of assessment materials to instructional materials (i.e., the amount of content overlap) on decision making and students' actual generalized performance as a result of the use of different data sources. Also, additional research is necessary on the priority that should be given to variables like the level of controlled vocabulary in reading passages. This research should be conducted to help practitioners understand how these factors are likely to interact. In addition, more direct experimental analyses of the interaction between instruction and content overlap with students of differing proficiency levels at baseline are necessary. Finally, investigations of the generalizability of these findings to other assessment areas should be conducted. This research should provide more direction to practitioners on methodological issues like which materials to use, how to set goals, and how much growth should be expected.

A cautionary note is in order, however. Although it is useful to know what typical rates of improvement are for different types of students, research based parameters for setting goals and expected rates of improvement should be developed through empirical investigations of how different goals actually affect student achievement and not based merely on typical rates of improvement for regular education students (Binder, 1996). Precision teachers are critical of the latter approach to goal setting because the development of goals based on average levels of performance for regular education students may actually underestimate the proficiency levels necessary to improve generalized performance. If norm-based criteria are used for developing goals (e.g., the average peer reads aloud at a rate of 92 CRW/min in the curriculum), goals may not be high enough to promote the levels of fluency necessary to achieve generalized responding. Binder (1996) argues that competency-based aims, empirically derived levels of performance necessary to permit generalized responding, are what educators should use. If precision teachers are correct, the use of norm-based criteria may actually perpetuate cumulative skill deficiencies, making it harder for students to learn more complex skills later. This issue promises to be an especially challenging one for educators and researchers to resolve because of the way schools are currently organized and the prevailing paradigms that are guiding instructional design.

CONCLUSION

Positive educational outcomes are more likely to occur when the evaluator's behavior is under the control of the data (Bushell & Baer, 1994). For a professional to bring his or her behavior under the control of the data, he or she must maintain rigorous standards for measurement, attend carefully to patterns of variability in the data, and continuously seek to evaluate decisions with further data. This chapter provided an overview of standards and some methods for measuring and evaluating academic performance outcomes. Much more research needs to be done, however, to bring more clarity to the tactical and methodological issues discussed in this chapter. Binder (1996) outlines an extensive agenda for fluency research, not the least of which is a recommendation for investigating how fluency gains may contribute to generalized increases in performance. Also, precision teaching's claims of improved endurance are intriguing and, yet, should be amenable to careful experimental analyses.

With respect to the issues raised in this chapter, one salient area where additional fluency research should be conducted is in the development of more formats for measuring fluency in classroom behaviors and content areas like social studies and history (examples of subject areas where middle and high school students often display academic problems). More research in fluency gains in basic academic skills will provide important baserate information regarding typical rates of improvement and also help to illuminate how different variables should be accounted for in instructional decision making. Instructional decision making itself should also be the target for experimental analyses. Multiple, concurrent measures of academic performance could be gathered. By identifying students' baseline levels of proficiency with target skills and controlling the types of data reported to teachers, it may be possible to determine which data sources produce the best learning outcomes or whether there are key variables that should be taken into consideration when developing monitoring methods for intervention design.

More work needs to be done in the areas of linking descriptive analyses of academic performance to functional analyses. Also, different approaches to conducting functional analyses of academic performance in more academic subjects should be pursued. If researchers can balance demands placed on practitioners with the exigencies of experimental control, further developments may help to make this area a technological innovation that can be widely used by school psychologists. Relatedly, the treatment utility of functional analyses should be a guiding theme in this research. The purpose of this research would be to determine whether the achievement results obtained following their use justify the costs associated with gathering the information.

References

Albers, A. E., & Greer, R. D. (1991). Is the three-term contingency trial a predictor of effective instruction? *Journal of Behavioral Education, 1,* 337–354.

Bell, P. F., Lentz, F. E., & Graden, J. L. (1992). Effects of curriculum-test overlap on standardized achievement test scores: Identifying systematic confounds in educational decision making. *School Psychology Review, 21,* 644–655.

Bickel, W. E. (1999). The implications of the effective schools literature for school restructuring. In C. R. Reynolds & T. B. Gutkin (Eds.), *The handbook of school psychology* (3rd ed., pp. 959–983). New York: Wiley .

Bijou, S. W., Peterson, R. F., & Ault, M. H. (1968). A method to integrate descriptive and experimental field studies at the level of data and empirical concepts. *Journal of Applied Behavior Analysis, 1,* 175–191.

Binder, C. (1996). Behavioral fluency: Evolution of a new paradigm. *The Behavior Analyst, 19,* 163–197.

Broussard, C. D., & Northup, J. (1995). An approach to functional assessment and analysis of disruptive behavior in regular education classrooms. *School Psychology Quarterly, 10,* 151–164.

Burns, P. C., & Roe, B. D. (1989). *Burns/Roe informal reading inventory: Preprimer to twelfth grade.* Boston: Houghton Mifflin.

Bushell, D., & Baer, D. M. (1994). Measurably superior instruction means close, continual contact with the relevant outcome data. Revolutionary! In R. Gardner III, D. M. Sainato, J. O. Cooper, T. E. Heron, W. L. Heward, J. W. Eshleman, & T. A. Grossi (Eds.), *Behavior analysis in education: Focus on measurably superior instruction* (pp. 3–10). Pacific Grove, CA: Brooks/Cole.

Catania, A. C. (1998). *Learning* (4th ed.). Upper Saddle River, NJ: Prentice-Hall.

Cone, J. D. (1995). Assessment practice standards. In S. C. Hayes, V. M. Follette, R. M. Dawes, & K. E. Grady (Eds.), *Scientific standards of psychological practice: Issues and recommendations* (pp. 201–224). Reno, NV: Context Press.

Cooper, L. J., Wacker, D. P., Thursby, D., Plagmann, L. A., Harding, J., Millard, T., & Derby, M. (1992). Analysis of the effects of task preferences, task demands, and adult attention on child behavior in outpatient and classroom settings. *Journal of Applied Behavior Analysis, 25,* 823–840.

Daly, E. J., III, Lentz, F. E., & Boyer, J. (1996). The instructional hierarchy: A conceptual model for understanding the effective components of reading interventions. *School Psychology Quarterly, 11,* 369–386.

Daly, E. J., III, & Martens, B. K. (1994). A comparison of three interventions for increasing oral reading performance: Application of the instructional hierarchy. *Journal of Applied Behavior Analysis, 27,* 459–469.

Daly, E. J., III, Martens, B. K., Dool, E. J., & Hintze, J. M. (1998). Using brief functional analysis to select interventions for oral reading. *Journal of Behavioral Education, 8,* 203–218.

Daly, E. J., III, Martens, B. K., Hamler, K. R., Dool, E. J., & Eckert, T. L. (1999). A brief experimental analysis for identifying instructional components needed to improve oral reading fluency. *Journal of Applied Behavior Analysis, 32,* 83–94.

Daly, E. J., III, Martens, B. K., Kilmer, A., & Massie, D. (1996). The effects of instructional match and content overlap on generalized reading performance. *Journal of Applied Behavior Analysis, 29,* 507–518.

Daly, E. J., III, Witt, J. C., Martens, B. K., & Dool, E. J. (1997). A model for conducting a functional analysis of academic performance problems. *School Psychology Review, 26,* 554–574.

Deno, S. L. (1986). Formative evaluation of individual student programs: A new role for school psychologists. *School Psychology Review, 15,* 358–374.

Derby, K. M., Wacker, D. P., Sasso, G., Steege, M., Northup, J., Cigrand, K., & Asmus, J. (1992). Brief functional assessment techniques to evaluate aberrant behavior in an outpatient setting: A summary of 79 cases. *Journal of Applied Behavior Analysis, 25,* 713–721.

Derr, T. F., & Shapiro, E. S. (1989). A behavioral evaluation of curriculum-based assessment of reading. *Journal of Psychoeducational Assessment, 7,* 148–160.

Derr-Minneci, T. F., & Shapiro, E. S. (1992). Validating curriculum-based measurement in reading from a behavioral perspective. *School Psychology Quarterly, 7,* 2–16.

Dunlap, G., Kern-Dunlap, L., Clarke, S., & Robbins, F. R. (1991). Functional assessment, curricular revision, and severe behavior problems. *Journal of Applied Behavior Analysis, 24,* 387–397.

Fuchs, L. S., & Deno, S. L. (1991). Paradigmatic distinctions between instructionally relevant measurement models. *Exceptional Children, 57,* 488–500.

Fuchs, L. S., & Deno, S. L. (1992). Effects of curriculum within curriculum-based measurement. *Exceptional Children, 58,* 232–242.

Fuchs, L. S., & Deno, S. L. (1994). Must instructionally useful performance assessment be based in the curriculum? *Exceptional Children, 57*, 488–500.

Fuchs, L. S., & Fuchs, D. (1986). Effects of systematic formative evaluation: A meta-analysis. *Exceptional Children, 53*, 199–208.

Fuchs, L. S., Fuchs, D., Hamlett, C. L., Walz, L., & Germann, G. (1993). Formative evaluation of academic progress: How much growth can we expect? *School Psychology Review, 22*, 27–48.

Fuchs, L. S., Fuchs, D., & Stecker, P. M. (1989). Effects of curriculum-based measurement on teachers' instructional planning. *Journal of Learning Disabilities, 22*, 51–59.

Gersten, R., Carnine, D., & White, W. A. T. (1984). The pursuit of clarity: Direct instruction and applied behavior analysis. In W. L. Heward, T. E. Heron, D. S. Hill, & J. Trapp-Porter (Eds.), *Focus on behavior analysis in education* (pp. 38–57). Columbus, OH: Charles E. Merrill.

Good III, R. H., & Salvia J. (1988). Curriculum bias in published norm-referenced reading tests: Demonstrable effects. *School Psychology Review, 17*, 51–60.

Greenwood, C. R. (1991). A longitudinal analysis of time, engagement, and achievement in at-risk versus non-risk students. *Exceptional Children, 57*, 521–535.

Greenwood, C. R. (1996). The case for performance-based instructional models. *School Psychology Quarterly, 11*, 283–296.

Greenwood, C. R., Carta, J. J., Kamps, D. M., & Delquadri, J. (1995). *Ecobehavioral assessment systems software: Technical manual and software*. Kansas City, KS: Juniper Gardens Children's Project, University of Kansas.

Greenwood, C. R., Hart, B., Walker, D., & Risley, T. (1994). The opportunity to respond and academic performance revisited: A behavioral theory of developmental retardation and its prevention. In R. Gardner III, D. M. Sainato, J. O. Cooper, T. E. Heron, W. L. Heward, J. W. Eshleman, & T. A. Grossi (Eds.), *Behavior analysis in education: Focus on measurably superior instruction* (pp. 213–224). Pacific Grove, CA: Brooks/Cole.

Greenwood, C. R., Terry, B., Marquis, J., & Walker, D. (1994). Confirming a performance-based instructional model. *School Psychology Review, 23*, 652–668.

Greer, R. D. (1994). The measure of a teacher. In R. Gardner III, D. M. Sainato, J. O. Cooper, T. E. Heron, W. L. Heward, J. W. Eshleman, & T. A. Grossi (Eds.), *Behavior analysis in education: Focus on measurably superior instruction* (pp. 161–172). Pacific Grove, CA: Brooks/Cole.

Greer, R. D. (1997). The education crisis. In M. A. Mattaini & B. A. Thyer (Eds.), *Finding solutions to social problems: behavioral strategies for change* (pp. 113–146). Washington, DC: American Psychological Association.

Grossen, B., & Carnine, D. (1991). Strategies for maximizing reading success in the regular classroom. In G. Stoner, M. R. Shinn, & H. M. Walker (Eds.), *Interventions for achievement and behavior problems* (pp. 333–356). Silver Spring, MD: National Association of School Psychologists.

Harding, J., Wacker, D. P., Cooper, L. J., Millard, T., & Jensen-Kovalan, P. (1994). Brief hierarchical assessment of potential treatment components with children in an outpatient clinic. *Journal of Applied Behavior Analysis, 27*, 291–300.

Haring, N. G., Lovitt, T. C., Eaton, M. D., & Hansen, C. L. (1978). *The fourth R: Research in the classroom*. Columbus, OH: Merrill.

Hawkins, R. P. (1986). Selection of target behaviors. In R. O. Nelson & S. C. Hayes (Eds.), *Conceptual foundations of behavioral assessment* (pp. 331–385). New York: Guilford Press.

Hayes, S. C., Nelson, R. O., & Jarrett, R. B. (1986). Evaluating the quality of behavioral assessment. In R. O. Nelson & S. C. Hayes (Eds.), *Conceptual foundations of behavioral assessment* (pp. 463–503). New York: Guilford Press.

Hendrickson, J. M., Gable, R. A., Novak, C., & Peck, S. (1996). Functional assessment as strategy assessment for teaching academics. *Education and Treatment of Children, 19*, 257–271.

Heward, W. L. (1994). Three "low-tech" strategies for increasing the frequency of active student response during group instruction. In R. Gardner III, D. M. Sainato, J. O. Cooper, T. E. Heron, W. L. Heward, J. W. Eshleman, & T. A. Grossi (Eds.), *Behavior analysis in education: Focus on measurably superior instruction* (pp. 283–320). Pacific Grove, CA: Brooks/Cole.

Heward, W. L., Heron, T. E., Hill, D. S., & Trapp-Porter, J. (Eds.). (1984). *Focus on behavior analysis in education*. Columbus, OH: Charles E. Merrill.

Hintze, J. M., & Shapiro, E. S. (1997). Curriculum-based measurement and literature-based reading: Is curriculum-based measurement meeting the needs of changing reading curricula? *Journal of School Psychology, 35,* 351–375.

Hintze, J. M., Shapiro, E. S., Conte, K. L., & Basile, I. M. (1997). Oral reading fluency and authentic reading material: Criterion validity of the technical feature of CBM survey-level assessment. *School Psychology Review, 26,* 535–553.

Hintze, J. M., Shapiro, E. S., & Daly, E. J., III. (1998). An investigation of the effects of passage difficulty level on outcomes of oral reading fluency progress monitoring. *School Psychology Review, 27,* 433–445.

Hintze, J. M., Shapiro, E. S., & Lutz, J. G. (1994). The effects of curriculum on the sensitivity of curriculum-based measurement in reading. *Journal of Special Education, 28,* 188–202.

Hoge, R. D., & Andrews, D. A. (1987). Enhancing academic performance: Issues in target selection. *School Psychology Review, 16,* 228–238.

Howell, K. W., Fox, S. L., & Morehead, M. K. (1993). *Curriculum-based evaluation: Teaching and decision making* (2nd ed.). Belmont, CA: Brooks/Cole.

Iwata, B. A., Dorsey, M. F., Slifer, K. J., Bauman, K. E., & Richman, G. S. (1994). Toward a functional analysis of self-injury. *Journal of Applied Behavior Analysis, 27,* 215–240. (Reprinted from *Analysis and Intervention in Developmental Disabilities, 2,* 1–20, 1982.)

Johnson, K. R., & Layng, T. V. J. (1992). Breaking the structuralist barrier: Literacy and numeracy with fluency. *American Psychologist, 47,* 1475–1490.

Johnson, K. R., & Layng, T. V. J. (1994). The Morningside model of generative instruction. In R. Gardner III, D. M. Sainato, J. O. Cooper, T. E. Heron, W. L. Heward, J. W. Eshleman, & T. A. Grossi (Eds.), *Behavior analysis in education: Focus on measurably superior instruction* (pp. 173–198). Pacific Grove, CA: Brooks/Cole.

Johnston, J. M., & Pennypacker, H. S. (1980). *Strategies and tactics of human behavioral research.* Hillsdale, NJ: Erlbaum.

Johnston, J. M., & Pennypacker, H. S. (1993). *Strategies and tactics of behavioral research* (2nd ed.). Hillsdale, NJ: Erlbaum.

Kern, L., Childs, K. E., Dunlap, G., Clarke, S., & Falk, G. D. (1994). Using assessment-based curricular intervention to improve the classroom behavior of a student with emotional and behavioral challenges. *Journal of Applied Behavior Analysis, 27,* 7–19.

Kinder, D., & Carnine, D. (1991). Direct instruction: What it is and what it is becoming. *Journal of Behavioral Education, 1,* 193–213.

Lalli, J. S., Browder, D. M., Mace, F. C., & Brown, D. K. (1993). Teacher use of descriptive analysis data to implement interventions to decrease students' problem behaviors. *Journal of Applied Behavior Analysis, 26,* 227–238.

Lentz, F. E. (1988a). On-task behavior, academic performance, and classroom disruptions: Untangling the target selection problem in classroom interventions. *School Psychology Review, 17,* 243–257.

Lentz, F. E. (1988b) Effective reading interventions in the regular classroom. In J. L. Graden, J. Zins, & M. J. Curtis (Eds.), *Alternative educational delivery systems: Enhancing instructional options for all students* (pp. 351–370). Washington, DC: National Association of School Psychologists.

Lentz, F. E., & Shapiro, E. S. (1986). Functional assessment of the academic environment. *School Psychology Review, 15,* 346–357.

Lindsley, O. R. (1990). Precision teaching: By teachers for children. *Teaching Exceptional Children, 22,* 10–15.

Lindsley, O. R. (1996). Is fluency free-operant response-response chaining? *Behavior Analyst, 19,* 211–224.

Mace, F. C., Lalli, J. S., & Pinter-Lalli, E. (1991). Functional analysis and treatment of aberrant behavior. *Research in Developmental Disabilities, 12,* 155–180.

Macmann, G. M., & Barnett, D. W. (1997). Myth of the master detective: Reliability of interpretations for Kaufman's "intelligent testing" approach to the WISC-III. *School Psychology Quarterly 12,* 197–234.

Macmann, G. M., & Barnett, D. W. (1999). Diagnostic decision making in school psychology:

Understanding and coping with uncertainty. In C. R. Reynolds & T. Gutkin (Eds.), *The hand-book of school psychology* (3rd ed., pp. 519–548). New York: Wiley.

Martens, B. K., Eckert, T. L., Bradley, T. A., & Ardoin, S. P. (1999). Identifying effective treatments from a brief experimental analysis: Using single-case design elements to aid decision making. *School Psychology Quarterly, 14*, 163–181.

Martens, B. K., & Kelly, S. Q. (1993). A behavioral analysis of effective teaching. *School Psychology Quarterly, 8*, 10–26.

Martens, B. K., Witt, J. C., Daly, E. J., III, & Vollmer, T. R. (1999). Behavior analysis: Theory and practice in educational settings. In C. R. Reynolds & T. B. Gutkin (Eds.), *The handbook of school psychology* (3rd ed., pp. 638–663). New York: Wiley.

McComas, J. J., Wacker, D. P., Cooper, L. J., Asmus, J. M., Richman, D., & Stoner, B. (1996). Brief experimental analysis of stimulus prompts for accurate responding on academic tasks in an out-patient clinic. *Journal of Applied Behavior Analysis, 29*, 397–401.

McKee, W. T., & Witt, J. C. (1990). Effective teaching: A review of instructional, and environmental variables. In T. B. Gutkin & C. R. Reynolds (Eds.), *The handbook of school psychology* (2nd ed., pp. 821–846). New York: Wiley.

Narayan, J. S., Heward, W. L., Gardner, R., Courson, F. H., Omness, C. K. (1990). Using response cards to increase student participation in an elementary classroom. *Journal of Applied Behavior Analysis, 23*, 483–490.

National Center for Educational Statistics. (1998). *National assessment of educational progress* [online]. Available Internet: http://www.nces.ed.gov/naep

Nelson, R. O., & Hayes, S. C. (1979). Some current dimensions of behavioral assessment. *Behavioral Assessment, 1*, 1–16.

Nelson, R. O., & Hayes, S. C. (Eds.). (1986). *Conceptual foundations of behavioral assessment*. New York: Guilford Press.

Ohio Department of Education. (1998). *School district report card* [online]. Available Internet: http://www.ode.ohio.gov/reptcard/report_card.html

Parsonson, B. S., & Baer, D. M. (1978). The analysis and presentation of graphic data. In T. R. Kratochwill (Ed.), *Single-subject research: Strategies for evaluating change* (pp. 101–165). New York: Academic Press.

Parsonson, B. S., & Baer, D. M. (1986). The graphic analysis of data. In A. Poling and R. W. Fuqua (Eds.), *Research methods in applied behavior analysis: Issues and advances* (pp. 157–186). New York: Plenum Press.

Parsonson, B. S., & Baer, D. M. (1992).The visual analysis of data, and current research into the stimuli controlling it. In T. R. Kratochwill & J. R. Levin (Eds.), *Single-case research design and analy-sis* (pp. 15–40). Hillsdale, NJ: Erlbaum.

Pearson, P. D., Johnson, D. D., Clymer, T., Indirsano, R., Venezky, R. L., Baumann, J. F., Hiebert, E., & Toth, M. (1989). *Silver, Burdett, and Ginn*. Needham, MA: Silver, Burdett, and Ginn.

Reschly, D. J., & Ysseldyke, J. E. (1995). School psychology paradigm shift. In A. Thomas & J. Grimes (Eds.), *Best practices in school psychology III* (pp. 17–32). Washington, DC: National Associa-tion of School Psychologists.

Rilling, M. (1977). Stimulus control and inhibitory processes. In W. K. Honig & J. E. R. Staddon (Eds.), *Handbook of operant behavior* (pp. 432–480). Englewood Cliffs, NJ: Prentice-Hall.

Rosenshine, B. V. (1980). How time is spent in elementary classrooms. In C. Denham, & A. Lieberman (Eds.), *Time to learn* (pp. 107–126). Washington, DC: U.S. Department of Education.

Shapiro, E. S. (1996a). *Academic skills problems: Direct assessment and intervention* (2nd ed.). New York: Guilford Press.

Shapiro, E. S. (1996b). *Academic skills problems workbook*. New York: Guilford Press.

Shapiro, E., & Derr, T. (1987). An examination of overlap between a reading curricula and standard-ized achievement tests. *Journal of Special Education, 21*, 59–76.

Shinn, M. R. (1989). *Curriculum-based measurement: Assessing special children*. New York: Guilford Press.

Shinn, M. R., Gleason, M. M., & Tindal, G. (1989). Varying the difficulty of testing materials: Impli-cations for curriculum-based measurement. *Journal of Special Education, 23*, 223–233.

Shinn, M. R., & Hubbard, D. (1992). Curriculum-based measurement and problem-solving assessment: Basic procedures and outcomes. *Focus on Exceptional Children, 24,* 1–20.

Sidman, M. (1960). *Tactics of scientific research: Evaluating experimental data in psychology.* New York: Basic Books.

Skinner, B. F. (1938). *The behavior of organisms.* Acton, MA: Copley.

Skinner, C. H., Fletcher, P. A., & Henington, C. (1996). Increasing learning rates by increasing student response rates: A summary of research. *School Psychology Quarterly, 11,* 313–325.

Sterling, R., Barbetta, P. M., Heron, T. E., & Heward, W. L. (1997). A comparison of active student response and on-task instruction on the acquisition and maintenance of health facts by students with learning disabilities. *Journal of Behavioral Education, 7,* 151–166.

Stokes, T. F., & Baer, D. M. (1977). An implicit technology of generalization. *Journal of Applied Behavior Analysis, 10,* 349–367.

Vargas, J. S. (1984). What are your exercises teaching? An analysis of stimulus control in instructional materials. In W. L. Heward, T. E. Heron, D. S. Hill, & J. Trapp-Porter (Eds.), *Focus on behavior analysis in education* (pp. 126–141). Columbus, OH: Merrill.

West, R. P., Young, K. R., & Spooner, F. (1990). Precision teaching: An introduction. *Teaching Exceptional Children, 22,* 4–9.

White, O. R., & Haring, N. G., (1980). *Exceptional teaching* (2nd ed.). Columbus, OH: Charles E. Merrill.

Wolcry, M., Bailey, D. B., Jr., & Sugai, G. M. (1988). *Effective teaching: Principles and procedures of applied behavior analysis with exceptional children.* Boston: Allyn & Bacon.

Ysseldyke, J., & Christenson, S. (1993). *The instructional environment system II.* Longmont, CO: Sopris West.

CHAPTER 4

Theory and Practice in Conducting Functional Analysis

JENNIFER J. McCOMAS
University of Minnesota

F. CHARLES MACE
University of Wales

A behavior-analytic approach to addressing severe and persistent behavior problems relies on a systematic inquiry into behavior–environment relationships. This approach requires that the behavior analyst occasionally review the methods that have proven to be successful, revise those that have not, and pursue new directions that may result in more efficacious approaches to assessment and intervention.

Before applied behavior analysts had a systematic methodology to identify the environmental variables or conditions maintaining severe problem behavior, the underlying behavioral processes that are responsible for maintenance of the problem behavior were largely ignored when seeking treatment. Without an understanding of the underlying processes, in other words, *why* the behavior was occurring, clinicians relied on potent putative reinforcers, punishers, or both to change problem behavior. This approach, known as behavior modification, relied on "best guesses" regarding reinforcers and punishers. Although effective in many cases of previously intractable and unmanageable behavior (Neuringer, 1970), this strategy led to concerns about an overreliance on the default technologies of contingent aversive stimulation and artificial positive reinforcement (Iwata, 1988).

Behavior modification research has generally limited itself to procedural questions such as: "What procedures produce behavior change?" and "What is the relative efficacy of various procedures in treating the same problem behavior?" Although these questions are clearly relevant for individual cases, the focus of this type of question is limited to technical application rather than the identification and specification of the variables that control an individual's behavior under natural conditions. The behavior modification approach has resulted in a large number of interventions that can be effective in many situations. Unfortunately, behavior problems in schools and homes continue to exist, and are frequently unresponsive to attempted treatments. Moreover, this approach has often failed to affect durable change. In general, under this approach to treatment, interventions are judged to be effective or ineffective, although the effects are rarely this distinct; more often the treatment may be somewhat, but not entirely effective. Unfortunately, the treatments are not typically "fine-tuned" to improve their efficacy. Instead, if a particular intervention fails to produce behavior change, it is abandoned and increasingly intrusive treatments are implemented, often including default procedures such as punishment (e.g., time-out, over-correction, mediation essays). Further, treatment failures are seldom analyzed to identify the conditions necessary and sufficient to result in behavior change.

This failure to identify effective and durable treatments may be attributed to the absence of a systematic, individualized rationale for selecting a particular treatment for a given individual. In fact, a number of studies have shown that the inefficacy of some treatments may be caused by the mismatch between treatment and the underlying behavioral process responsible for maintenance of the problem behavior (Durand & Carr, 1987; Iwata, Pace, Condery, & Miltenberger 1994; Repp, Felce, & Barton, 1988). Thus there are two interrelated problems with the behavior-modification approach to treating behavior problems: (1) they do not offer information about the nature of behavior–environment relationships maintaining problem behaviors, and (2) interventions tend toward reliance on default technologies that are often intrusive and sometimes unacceptable to consumers.

Applied behavior analysis holds two general assumptions: (1) behavior occurs in a context of environmental events, and (2) it occurs for a reason (i.e., it has a function). The vast majority of these "reasons" are believed to follow operant paradigms of positive and negative reinforcement. Thus a methodology of functional analysis that specifies the context of environmental events and the behavior–environment relationships responsible for the occurrence of problem behavior is needed.

Although the first comprehensive and standardized functional analysis methodology was formulated by Iwata, Dorsey, Slifer, Bauman, and Richman (1982/1994), the roots of functional analysis can be traced to the earliest years of applied behavior analysis and systematic evaluation of behavior–environment relations (e.g., Ayllon & Michael, 1959; Bijou, Petersen, & Ault, 1968; Thomas, Becker, & Armstrong, 1968). Carr (1977) introduced the conceptual framework for considering that rather than psychodynamic constructs, operant processes, specifically reinforcement, serve to maintain problem behaviors such as self-injury. Building on that concept, Iwata et al. (1982/1994) provided a methodology for systematically testing hypotheses regarding the effects of specific classes of reinforcement. This methodology, initially applied to the analysis of self-injurious behavior, was soon adapted to analyze behavior–environment interactions that maintained a wide range and variety of behavior problems, including aggression, disruption, property destruction, reluctant speech, and obsessive–compulsive behaviors.

The primary goal of functional analysis is to identify environmental conditions that are correlated with the occurrence and nonoccurrence of specified problem behavior. Functional analysis provides a systematic, analytic method for identifying the variables or conditions that support or maintain problem behavior. It is based on a well-conceptualized model of the possible operant influences on problem behavior (Carr, 1977) and involves controlled conditions that represent those influences within single-case experimental designs. This method of assessment involves analogue conditions and permits an experimentally rigorous analysis of the conditions that maintain problem behavior. Thus the methodology provides a more precise analysis of the conditions or variables affecting problem behavior than previous approaches to the treatment of problem behavior. The resultant information is used to design or select interventions that interrupt or alter the conditions that support or maintain problem behaviors. Thus a successful functional analysis yields two benefits: (1) information about the nature of the environmental variables affecting the problem behavior, and (2) a clear direction for treatment based on a systematic analysis of the problem.

Wacker (1996) suggested that the widespread acceptance of this methodology by practitioners, as well as by applied researchers, is noteworthy because it illustrates the power of basing practice on direct links to basic underlying behavioral processes or mechanisms. The results provide information that practitioners can use to develop highly effective treatments, and have led to changes in the way that clinical services are provided (Wacker et al., 1994). Although identification of the operant function of an individual's problem behavior does not *guarantee* successful treatment, over a decade of research has demonstrated the general effectiveness of this treatment model and encouraged its widespread endorsement (Axelrod, 1987). For example, at the 1989 National Institutes of Health Consensus Conference, a panel convening on the treatment of destructive behaviors associated with developmental disabilities recommended that treatment of severe behavior disorders be based on the results of a pretreatment functional analysis (National Institutes of Health, 1989). Additionally, the Amendments of 1997 (PL 105–17) to the Individuals with Disabilities Education Act (IDEA) require by law that functional behavioral assessment be conducted and a behavioral intervention plan be implemented prior to disciplinary action for children with disabilities. Taken together, these legislative acts support the investment of resources necessary for a systematic analysis of problem behavior.

The purpose of this chapter is to feature the conceptual and research literature pertaining to the current status of a functional analysis approach to treating problem behavior. The behavioral processes maintaining behavior problems, technical approaches to functional analysis, and function-based interventions will be highlighted. Additionally, some discussion of experimental designs and issues related to validity will be presented. Finally, some directions for the future development and application of this technology will be indicated.

BEHAVIORAL PROCESSES MAINTAINING
BEHAVIOR PROBLEMS

Behavior has been characterized as that part of an individual's interaction with the environment that results in a measurable change in at least one aspect of the environment (Johnston & Pennypacker, 1994). Environmental changes that produce benefits for the individual result in a strengthening, or reinforcement of the behavior that produced those consequences. Reinforcers are either positive (i.e., their presentation increases the likelihood of responses that produce it) or negative (i.e., their removal or postponement increases the likelihood of responses that have that effect). Any behavior may be maintained by positive or negative reinforcement. In addition to the consequences of behavior, other stimuli might also be functionally related to problem behavior.

Antecedent events or stimuli may serve as establishing operations (i.e., they momentarily alter the reinforcing effectiveness of a consequent stimulus), or as discriminative stimuli (i.e., they signal the availability of a reinforcing consequence). These four events, (1) the establishing operation (EO), (2) the discriminative stimulus (SD), (3) the behavioral response (R), and (4) the reinforcing consequence (SR) comprise the four-term contingency. An analysis of conditions under which problem behavior occurs should take into consideration these terms (Smith & Iwata, 1997). It has been argued that the clearest assessment results are expected to occur under conditions in which each element is carefully considered (Iwata, Pace, Kalsher, Cowdery, & Cataldo, 1990). Specifically, the following are arranged: (1) relative deprivation of the reinforcer, (2) a pairing of each contingency with a distinct stimulus, (3) continuous reinforcement of the target behavior, and (4) no reinforcement for competing responses.

Establishing Operations

Establishing operations are those events that momentarily alter the reinforcing effectiveness of specific consequences and, therefore, the momentary probability of responses that have previously produced those consequences (Keller & Schoenfeld, 1950; Michael, 1982). Thus, in the presence of the three-term contingency, the probability of the occurrence of a response may be increased or decreased by the presence or absence of EOs that increase or decrease the reinforcing effectiveness of that consequence. For example, the presence of aversive stimulation (e.g., loud noises, tedious tasks, a toothache) can increase the likelihood of a response that has been previously negatively reinforced by escape from that stimulation. The effects of establishing operations such as appetite-surpressing medications, otitis media, duration of tasks, and rate of task presentation have been experimentally evaluated and documented by researchers (Northup, Fusilier, Swanson, Roane, & Borrero, 1997; O'Reilly, 1997; Smith, Iwata, Goh, & Shore, 1995).

Discriminative Stimuli

Discriminative stimuli are those events that are differentially correlated with a specific contingency of reinforcement (Skinner, 1953). In the presence of these stimuli, the probability of reinforcement is either increased or decreased. Thus the presence of a discriminative stimulus increases the likelihood that a response will occur. For example, a neon "Open" sign in the window of a store signals the availability of reinforcement contingent on a chain of responses composed of entering the store, selecting, and paying for the merchandise. The effects of discriminative stimuli on problem behavior have been experimentally isolated, controlled, and demonstrated (e.g., Carr, Yarborough, & Langdon, 1997; Lalli, Mace, Livezey, & Kates, 1998).

Behavior

Public behavior (i.e., actions) or private behavior (i.e., thoughts or feelings) that cause concern or distress to an individual or those around him or her are the focus of functional analysis. Questions such as "Why is the behavior currently occurring?" or "What environmental variables are responsible for maintaining this behavior" pave the way for an analysis of the behavior–environmental, or functional, relationships that are responsible for the ongoing occurrence of problem behavior. Of importance is the focus on function rather than form (topography) of the behavior. The topography of the behavior does not suggest the behavioral process responsible for the occurrence of the response and leads to a behavior-modification approach rather than a behavior-analytic approach to treatment. It has been well documented that a single topography of behavior often is maintained by multiple or different reinforcing contingencies across different individuals (e.g., Iwata, et al., 1994), and frequently within individuals (Richman, Wacker, Asmus, & Casey, 1998; Smith, Iwata, Vollmer, & Zarcone, 1993).

Reinforcing Stimuli

Reinforcers are consequent events produced by the response (i.e., "reaction" to response) that results in an increase in the frequency or likelihood of the response that produced them.

Positive Social Reinforcement (Attention)

Positive reinforcement in the form of attention occurs when problem behavior produces attention (from adults, peers, or siblings). Attention can take many forms including praise, reprimands, sympathy, redirection, consolation, restraint, smiles, frowns, or eye contact. Regardless of the form, any of these stimuli are referred to as positive reinforcement if they serve to increase the likelihood of the response that produces it. Attention is a common reinforcer for problem behavior (Frea & Hughes, 1997; Northup et al., 1995; Piazza et al., 1998; Thompson, Fisher, Piazza, & Kuhn, 1998). During any given period of time, attention can vary in its capacity to function as a reinforcer. The circumstances that establish attention as a positive reinforcer are known as establishing operations (EOs). In general, the EOs for attention-maintained behavior are periods of low levels of attention, such as when an adult is preoccupied with another activity. These conditions constitute the environmental context in which behavioral intervention for attention maintained behavior is targeted.

Positive Social Reinforcement (Materials)

Positive reinforcement (materials) occurs when problem behavior results in items or preferred activities. Food, toys, music, television, and specific articles of clothing are among the materials that can maintain maladaptive behavior. Several researchers have found that a variety of problem behaviors are positively reinforced when they provide access to objects or activities that are otherwise restricted (Day, Rae, Schussler, Larsen, & Johnson, 1988; Durand & Kishi, 1987; Goh et al., 1995; Lalli, Casey, & Kates, 1997). Relative states of deprivation or restricted access to these types of stimuli can establish the items as reinforcers for problem behavior. For example, EOs that are related to problem behavior maintained by this type of positive reinforcement are situations in which a preferred item or activity is unavailable (e.g., a favorite toy is being washed or broken) or access is restricted (e.g., video games during homework time or snacks just before dinner). These conditions comprise the environmental context within which intervention is targeted.

Negative Social Reinforcement

Escape or avoidance of aversive events is a powerful reinforcer and occurs when a response is strengthened because it results in the removal or avoidance of an aversive stimulus. The performance of basic self-care, academic, or vocational tasks appears to be aversive for many individuals. Presentation of these tasks often sets the occasion for problem behavior that may terminate or postpone a caregiver's expectations for performance. When problem behavior serves to escape or avoid performance demands, the behavior is said to be negatively reinforced. Numerous experimental analyses have identified negative reinforcement as the maintaining contingency for problem behavior (Northup et al., 1991; O'Reilly, 1997; Piazza et al., 1997; Steege et al., 1990; Vollmer, Marcus, & Ringdahl, 1995). Iwata and his colleagues (1994) conducted an epidemiological study of 152 single-subject functional analyses of self-injurious behavior. Results indicated that negative reinforcement accounted for the largest proportion of the sample population. In general, duration of tasks, novel tasks, or other sources of aversive stimuli can function to establish escape or avoidance as a reinforcer for an individual's problem behavior (Smith et al., 1995). Thus those specific situations are targeted for treatment.

Nonsocial Automatic Reinforcement

Behavior is said to be automatically reinforced when it occurs at elevated levels in alone or control conditions. For a small proportion of persons who engage in problem behavior, generally self-injurious or stereotypic behavior, the results of a functional analysis of social reinforcers may be inconclusive. Specifically, an individual might engage in high rates of problem behavior in a low-stimulation condition. Similarly, the occurrence of the behavior may be undifferentiated by condition (Iwata et al., 1982/94). That is, the controlling variables for the maladaptive behavior have not been isolated. Although the controlling variables are unclear in these cases, a number of researchers have proposed that some of the topographies of self-injurious and stereotypic behavior suggest that the responses may be maintained by sensory or perceptual consequences that are automatically produced by the behavior itself (Cataldo & Harris, 1982; Kennedy & Souza, 1995; Lovaas, Newsom, & Hickman, 1987). When these consequences are stimulating, the behavior producing these effects may be positively reinforced. Similarly, if the consequences attenuate an aversive physiologic condition (e.g., pain), the response may be negatively reinforced. An alternative account of undifferentiated results is that a biological mechanism may be responsible for the occurrence of the behavior. Although this assessment outcome is inherently ambiguous, effective interventions are still available and are selected based on a hypothesis-testing approach to direct assessment (Kennedy & Souza, 1995; Piazza et al., 1998; Thompson et al., 1998). It should be noted that until methodologies are developed that facilitate distinguishing operant from biologic processes, considerable caution is needed in interpreting the results of undifferentiated functional analyses (see Wacker et al., 1996).

APPROACHES TO FUNCTIONAL ANALYSIS

There are a number of approaches to the functional assessment of behavior problems. These approaches for specifying the behavioral process maintaining problem behavior can be divided into three general categories: (1) indirect, (2) direct, and (3) experimental.

Indirect

This type of assessment involves gathering information reported by the individual or his or her care providers, including parents, teachers, or employers. These reports provide information about the form, frequency, intensity, and conditions under which the behavior is likely to occur. When gathering indirect information, the assessor seeks specific information pertinent to the potential events maintaining the problem behavior (e.g., specific antecedents and consequences, physical and social environments, activities, physiological conditions). Sources of indirect information can include historical records, interviews, rating scales, and checklists (Aberrant Behavior Checklist [Aman & Singh, 1986, 1994] the Child Behavior Checklist [Achenbach & Edelbrock, 1981], and the Conners Parent Rating Scales—Revised (S) [Conners, 1997]). While indirect assessment can provide valuable information that can be used in generating hypotheses about the behavior–environment relations, it generally is not sufficient for the prescription of interventions.

Direct

Direct observation provides data on the occurrence of the behavior within the context of the natural environmental events within which it occurs. The assessor simultions—LPP/RR/SM and LPP/RR—were administered in independent passages under reinforcement conditions. The LPP/RR/SM treatment was administered in one set of instructional and HCO passages (repeatedly if necessary) until Andrew met the criterion rate to earn a reward. The LPP/RR condition was yoked to the prior LPP/RR/SM condition: this treatment was administered in an independent passage the same number of times that it took Andrew to reach criterion in the previous LPP/RR/SM condition. Each administration of treatment conditions was done on a different day.

The results for the HCO passages only are displayed in the right panel of Figure 3.2. Andrew met the criterion in one trial in the first administration of the LPP/RR/SM condition. He read 59 CRW/min in the HCO passage. (Andrew received the reward in spite of the fact that he read 1 fewer than 60 CRW/min because the criterion was based on how quickly he read the entire passage. Overall, he read the passage faster than the criterion rate.) The LPP/RR condition was administered once with the offer of a reward for meeting the criterion. In this condition, Andrew did not earn the reward. He read only 29 CRW/min. The LPP/RR/SM condition was repeated in another passage. This time he met the criterion in two trials. On the first trial he read at a rate of 47 CRW/min. On the second trial he read at a rate of 68 CRW/min, his best performance to date. In the LPP/RR condition, Andrew also met the criterion in two trials. On the first trial he read 26 CRW/min, and on the second trial he read 60 CRW/min. These results indicate that rewards interacted with the instructional components to improve his performance. Andrew's performance was highest in the reward plus LPP/RR/SM condition: both initial and final levels of responding were higher for this condition than for the reward plus LPP/RR condition. The combination of rewards for fluency rate and instructional components comprised of LPP/RR applied to both instructional and generalization passages led to the highest fluency gains for Andrew.

Both analyses identified intervention components that improved students' reading fluency in the HCO passages. In the case of Latasha, generalized improvements were observed with the RR condition only. In the case of Andrew, a more explicit generalization component and rewards in conjunction to LPP and RR were necessary to improve his performance. Promising instructional components were identified relatively quickly. Yet, very different interventions were indicated for each student.

Formative Evaluation and Data-Based Decision Making

Fuchs and Deno (1991) describe two general approaches to assessment for instructional decision making: *specific subskill mastery measurement* and *general outcome measurement*. In the former approach, curriculum objectives are broken down into subskills and ordered hierarchically by the teacher or a curricular scope and sequence chart. Student performance on short-term instructional objectives is monitored through the use of criterion-referenced tests. When outcome data suggest that a student has mastered a set of subskills, a new subskill is introduced for instruction and student progress is again monitored using a different set of materials that reflect the taneously observes and records the behavioral and environmental events as they occur. This approach to assessment produces information that can help to specify the environmental events that may be correlated with the occurrence of problem behavior. Thus direct observation can aid in the generation of hypotheses regarding environmental events that may be responsible for the occurrence of an individual's problem behavior. Three ways to conduct direct observations include: (1) ABC, (2) scatterplot, and (3) descriptive assessments. In antecedent–behavior–consequence (ABC) assessments (Bijou et al., 1968; O'Neill, Horner, Albin, Storey, & Sprague, 1990), the behavior and the events before and after are directly observed and a description of those events is recorded. The assessor reviews the record of a number of instances of the behavior and seeks similarities in the kinds of stimuli or events that typically precede and follow the target behavior. An example of a form for recording ABC information is shown below in Figure 4.1. Similarly, patterns of responding throughout the day can be documented using a scatterplot assessment (Touchette, MacDonald, & Langer, 1985), shown below in Figure 4.2. Scatterplots involve recording the time of day the problem behavior occurs across successive days. This method of recording the occurrence of the problem behavior allows for a visual analysis of possible

Student: _____   Observer: _____

Date	Time	Antecedent	Behavior	Consequence	Comments

FIGURE 4.1   Sample form for recording antecedent–behavior–consequence (ABC) data.

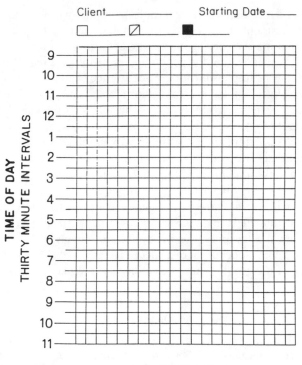

FIGURE 4.2   Sample form for recording scatterplot data. From Touchette, MacDonald, and Langer (1985). Copyright 1985 by the Society for the Experimental Analysis of Behavior, Inc. Reprinted by permission.

correlations between the occurrence of problem behavior and time of day or specific activities. A final method of collecting direct observation data is via real-time recording of establishing operations, behavior, and subsequent events. This is referred to as a descriptive assessment (Bijou et al., 1968; Lalli & Goh, 1993; Lalli, Browder, Mace, & Brown, 1993; Mace & Lalli, 1991) and is also conducted by directly observing the behavior as it occurs in the natural environment. The occurrences of behavior are recorded as they occur in relation to ongoing antecedent and consequent events. Conditional probabilities of the occurrence of each behavioral response recorded are then calculated under the specific environmental conditions that were observed and recorded. These probabilities, like the information derived from the other methods of direct observation, are used to generate a hypothesis about the environmental conditions in which the problem behavior is most likely to occur.

This approach to naturalistic observation without manipulating the variables that are associated with problem behavior is used to identify variables that appear to influence behavior (i.e., are correlated with behavior). However, information gathered without systematically isolating and manipulating environmental variables is only suggestive of functional relations. To make definitive statements about functional relations, it is necessary to conduct a more precise experimental (functional) analysis in which environmental events are systematically manipulated and examined within a single-subject experimental design.

Experimental

Based on the information gathered from both indirect and direct sources, one or more hypotheses about the maintaining contingencies for problem behavior are generated. Those hypotheses are then tested within a single-subject experimental design in which the individual serves as his or her own control, and experimental conditions are introduced and withdrawn repeatedly to demonstrate their effects on behavior. The purpose of this approach is to isolate and determine the influence of particular variables on the individual's target behavior. To do this, short (5-, 10-, or 15- minute) conditions are arranged that are simulations of the naturally occurring conditions, but which control for extraneous variables. Specifically, analogue conditions are conducted in which the variable being tested is directly manipulated while all other variables are held constant. The occurrence of problem behavior is examined across conditions to determine the effects of specific environmental variables. Both antecedents and consequences can be manipulated and evaluated within an experimental analysis.

Antecedent Manipulation

As we have indicated, consequent-based functional analysis procedures (Iwata et al., 1982/94) involve the systematic isolation and evaluation of the effects consequences have on problem behavior. It allows the professional to both (1) identify the reason (i.e., reinforcers) that problem behavior is occurring, and (2) match an intervention to the results of the analysis. However, antecedent variables also influence behavior and knowledge of these influences can be useful in the design of effective interventions (Wacker et al., 1998).

   In an antecedent analysis, specified antecedent variables are presented systematically to the individual in a series of analogue conditions within a single-case experimental design. Consequences for problem behavior are either not arranged or are held constant for each condition. These analyses, sometimes referred to as "structural analyses" (Axelrod, 1987), can produce idiosyncratic but predictable changes in problem behavior (Carr & Durand, 1985; Dunlap, Kern-Dunlap, Clarke, & Robbins, 1991; Mace, Yankanich, & West, 1989). While this type of analysis might suggest control by a specific antecedent event, consideration of the consequences for behavior is still warranted. The assumption that certain antecedent events are uniformly correlated with certain consequences may prove to be erroneous for an individual (Iwata, 1994). That is, problem behavior that occurs in the presence of task demands is not necessarily maintained by negative reinforcement (i.e., escape from task demands); it may be maintained by positive reinforcement (i.e., attention in the form of assistance in completing the task). Further, if no consequence is delivered during sessions of the antecedent analysis, the behavior may be exposed to extinction, thus compromising an evaluation of the effects of the antecedents. Thus, when conducting an antecedent analysis, it is preferable to provide a consistent consequence across all conditions of an antecedent analysis (see Smith et al., 1995).

Consequent Manipulation

Although knowledge of antecedent influences can be useful for designing effective interventions, an evaluation of the response–reinforcer relationship maintaining the target behavior provides the most direct assessment of behavioral function (Wacker, Berg, Asmus et al., 1998). In a consequent analysis, a different consequence is arranged for problem behavior in different EO conditions. For example, restricted access to tangible items serves as the establishing operation for positive reinforcement in the form of tangible items. The conditions are presented in a single-case experimental design by alternating the conditions in a randomized or counterbalanced order (multielement design), or by presenting a series of a given test condition (e.g., attention or escape) followed by a series of control sessions (reversal design). The occurrence of problem behavior is then compared across conditions to determine the effects of each consequence on problem behavior. Elevation in an experimental condition suggests a behavior–environment relationship.

SINGLE-CASE EXPERIMENTAL DESIGNS
FOR EVALUATING FUNCTIONAL RELATIONSHIPS

The effects of antecedents and consequences can be evaluated within brief analyses, extended multi-element analyses, or extended reversal analyses. Experimental control is demonstrated in all three approaches via repeated measures within a single-case design. If high rates of problem behavior are consistently correlated with a particular test condition, then the antecedent or consequent stimuli of that test condition are considered to be functionally related to the problem behavior.

    Brief functional analyses involve a very small number of analogue sessions. Brief analyses were initially developed to meet the time restrictions imposed in outpatient clinics and were used for children with behavior disorders (Cooper et al., 1990; Northup et al., 1991). These designs have been further refined to allow for inferences to be made about the maintaining contingencies for problem behavior and evaluation of the effects of preliminary treatment recommendations (Harding, Wacker, Cooper, Millard, & Jensen-Kovalan, 1994; Millard et al., 1993). Brief analyses are typically conducted in two phases: (1) initial analogue assessment of two or more conditions (e.g., attention and escape), and (2) replication, in which the "best" and "worst" conditions are repeated. Control over behavior is established when marked differences in the rate of target behavior are apparent across analogue conditions, and are replicated within a "mini-reversal" design (Cooper et al., 1992). Although brief experimental analyses allow for replication of effects and produce differentiated outcomes over half of the time, they do not permit an evaluation of stability within conditions (Derby, Wacker, Sasso, Steege, Northup, Cigrand, & Asmus, 1992; Kahng & Iwata, 1999). A case example involving a 10-year-old boy with developmental disabilities who displayed severe aggression at home and at school is shown in Figure 4.3. The occurrence of aggressive behavior was recorded in four conditions: (1) control (free play), (2) escape from task demands contingent on aggression, (3) divided attention with attention provided contingent on aggression, and (4) restricted access to preferred tangible items (the computer) with access provided contingent on aggression. Within seven sessions, the results of the experimental analysis (with replication of "best" and "worst" conditions in "mini-reversals") indicated that his aggressive behavior was a function of two reinforcers: escape from task demands and access to preferred items. Treatment focused on differential reinforcement of appropriate requests for work breaks and for access to the computer.

An *extended functional analysis* is necessary to obtain an indication of behavioral stability within and between conditions. The first comprehensive and standardized functional analysis methodology was presented by Iwata et al. (1982/94). Extended analyses most frequently involve multi-element experimental designs in which the occurrence of problem behavior is compared across a number of sessions in each condition to examine the effects of specific environmental variables on the problem behavior. A number of sessions of each condition are rapidly alternated (Sidman, 1960) in a counterbalanced or randomized order. A visual analysis is conducted to examine patterns of responding within conditions to determine which, if any, of the variables

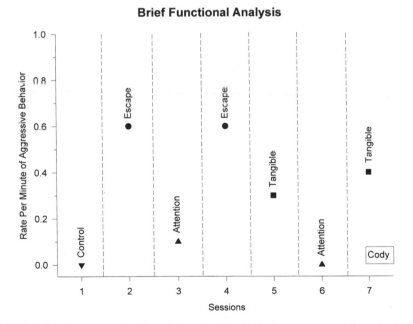

FIGURE 4.3   Case example of brief functional analysis. Results suggested aggression was maintained by negative and positive reinforcement: escape and tangible items.

are responsible for the occurrence of the problem behavior. However, a subject's failure to discriminate between experimental conditions (Vollmer, Iwata, Duncan, & Lerman, 1993) or the presence of interaction effects across conditions (Higgins-Hains & Baer, 1989) can render functional analysis data difficult to interpret. In these cases, the multi-element design can be extended to a reversal design to facilitate interpretation of the behavior–environment relationships (Vollmer et al., 1993; Vollmer, Marcus, Ringdahl, & Roane, 1995; Vollmer and Van Camp, 1998). A case example of a 4-year-old boy with pervasive developmental disabilities and severe destructive behavior at his preschool is shown in Figure 4.4. The occurrence of destructive behavior was recorded in four conditions: (1) control (free play), (2) escape from task demands, (3) divided attention with attention provided contingent on aggression, and (4) restricted access to preferred tangible items (floor puzzles and blocks) with access provided contingent on aggression. The results of the multi-element experimental design indicate that his destructive behavior was positively reinforced by attention. Treatment focused on differential reinforcement of socially appropriate behavior.

An *extended reversal design* involves several consecutive sessions of a single test condition to allow the individual's behavior to adjust to the contingencies and occur in a predictable pattern. Following an extended number of sessions of one variable, typically the control (A), a test variable (B) is introduced in isolation for an extended number of sessions. Following this sequence, these two conditions are repeated to form an ABAB, or reversal design.

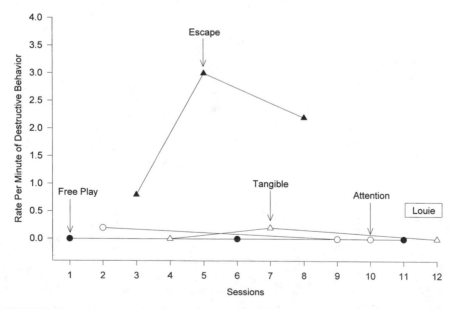

Extended Functional Analysis

FIGURE 4.4 Case example of extended functional analysis. Results suggested destructive behavior was maintained by negative reinforcement in the form of escape from academic tasks.

Finally, Vollmer, Marcus, Ringdahl, and Roane (1995) have suggested a systematic progression from brief to multi-element to extended reversal designs for conducting functional analyses. This progression could quickly yield response differentiation, and thus specification of functional relationships within an experimentally controlled analysis.

All methods of behavioral assessment that involve sampling behavior out of the natural context will depend on inferences drawn from those samples. As with any assessment technique, issues of internal and external validity should be considered when conducting and interpreting functional analyses. Of all the assessment techniques described above, the analogue experimental manipulations that are involved in functional analyses produce the most internally valid assessment results. Specifically, by arranging the full four-term contingency (EO, SD, response, and reinforcer) over repeated observations, it has the capacity to rule out alternative explanations for results. To evaluate the external validity of the analysis (i.e., how representative the analogue conditions are of naturally occurring events), the correlation between the occurrence of behavior in individualized analogue conditions experimental analysis with the occurrence of behavior in a descriptive assessment can be examined (e.g., Sasso et al., 1992). Finally, three things should be emphasized here: (1) functional analysis is not capable of and was not designed to tell us anything about the etiology of behavior; rather it specifies the environmental variables responsible for the maintenance of an individual's behavior, (2) the results of a functional analysis only apply to the individual with whom the analysis was conducted; only the methodology of functional analysis will generalize to other individuals and populations, the results will not, and (3) the utility of an analysis should be evaluated by examining the effects of the intervention implemented for an individual based on the results of the analysis (Nelson & Hayes, 1979).

SELECTING AND IMPLEMENTING APPROPRIATE INTERVENTIONS BASED ON FUNCTION

The product of a successful functional analysis is the identification of one or more behavior–environment relations (e.g., reinforcement contingencies) that serve to maintain an individual's problem behavior. When intervention is based on the identified reinforcer of problem behavior, the general approach to treatment involves both weakening the maintaining contingency for problem behavior and strengthening a concurrently available alternative response. Problem behavior, arguably like most behavior, can be conceptualized as a choice (Myerson & Hale, 1984). Specifically, in the case of behavior problems, the important choice is whether the individual engages in problem behavior or one or more concurrently available adaptive responses.

Treating Problem Behavior as Choice

Because problem behavior and adaptive behavior can be viewed as choices among concurrently available options, matching theory provides a general conceptual framework for intervention selection that is applicable across operant functions (Mace & Roberts, 1993; McDowell, 1988; Myerson & Hale, 1984; Pierce & Epling, 1983). Matching theory refers to the predictable and robust effects of concurrent schedules of reinforcement on allocation of behavior (deVilliers, 1977; Herrnstein, 1961, 1970). In research on matching theory, the individual has two or more response options, or choices, simultaneously available. Each alternative is uniquely paired with a discriminative stimulus and an independent schedule of reinforcement. The effects of those schedules of reinforcement on an individual's allocation of behavior among the response alternatives are examined. Results of basic research on response allocation with human and non-human animals (Davison & McCarthy, 1988; Lowe & Horne, 1985; Pierce & Epling, 1983), as well as applied research (Conger & Killeen, 1974; Mace, McCurdy, & Quigley, 1990; Mace, Neef, Shade, & Mauro, 1996; Martens, Lochner, & Kelly, 1992; Neef, Shade, & Miller, 1994; Peck et al., 1996), have demonstrated that response allocation is lawful and affected by at least four major factors: (1) rate of reinforcement, (2) quality of reinforcement, (3) immediacy of reinforcement, and (4) response effort.

First, there is a direct relationship between the rate of obtained reinforcement and the rate of responding to each response alternative (Herrnstein, 1961, 1970). Specifically, the rate of responding on each alternative tends to "match" (or be proportional to) the rate of reinforcement delivered for each response alternative. These effects have been demonstrated for different sets of math problems (Neef, Mace, Shea, & Shade, 1992), on- and off-task behavior (Martens & Houk, 1989; Martens et al., 1992), and conversation between a subject and two experimenters (Conger & Killeen, 1974).

Similarly, quality of reinforcement affects choice. Consequent events can vary greatly in their capacity to reinforce behavior. When one consequent event or stimulus is preferred over another, that preferred event is said to possess a higher quality of reinforcement than the other. The availability of different quality reinforcers for different response options can affect the allocation of behavior across response alternatives (Hollard & Davison, 1971; Miller, 1976). This influence can occur either independent of the effects of rate of reinforcement, or reinforcer quality may interact with the rate of reinforcement (Neef et al., 1992) or amount (magnitude) of reinforcement (Peck et al., 1996) to jointly determine response allocation. It should be noted that the quality of reinforcement is not necessarily constant and stable; in fact, in most cases, the quality or value of a reinforcer is relative to other available options and can change from one minute to the next, depending on levels of deprivation and satiation, among other things.

The third variable that affects choice is delay to reinforcement. Delay to reinforcement refers to the time between completion of a response and access to the reinforcer. Individuals reliably allocate their behavior toward that alternative that provides the shorter delay to reinforcement. Delay to reinforcement is such a strong influence that studies have demonstrated that individuals will choose immediately available reinforcement that is of lower value or quality than higher quality reinforcement that is delayed (Neef, Mace, & Shade, 1993). In applied situations, a child with developmental disabilities might engage in property destruction or other problem behavior rather than saying, "Come here," because the problem behavior results in a markedly more immediate response from adults (even if it involves a reprimand) than the appropriate verbal request for attention.

Finally, the effort required by each response alternative to earn reinforcement affects choice. In basic research, the effect of response effort on choice behavior has been studied by varying the pressure required to depress a response key (e.g., Bauman, Shull, & Brownstein, 1975). The results of these studies on response effort generally show a preference for the alternative with the lower response effort. In applied situations, wrist weights have been used to increase the response effort required to engage in problem behavior, thereby decreasing the occurrence of problem behavior and increasing the occurrence of adaptive behavior (Hanley, Piazza, Keeney, Blakeley-Smith, & Worsdell, 1998). Similarly, task difficulty might be conceptualized as response effort. Level of task difficulty has been shown to affect how individuals allocate behavior between appropriate (e.g., task engagement) and problem behavior (e.g., Center, Deitz, & Kaufman, 1982; Cooper et al., 1992; Durand & Carr, 1987; Gaylor-Ross, Weeks, & Lipner, 1980; Horner, Day, Sprague, O'Brien, & Heathfield, 1991). Results have suggested that in some cases, difficult tasks resulted in less task engagement and more problem behavior compared with easy tasks.

In sum, patterns of response allocation across concurrent alternatives are predictable (Herrnstein, 1961; 1970) and a function of relative reinforcer rates and amounts, reinforcer quality, reinforcer delay, and response force or effort (Davison & McCarthy, 1988). When the effects of deprivation and satiation of reinforcement are also considered, it becomes apparent that problem behavior is influenced by several variables that should be considered when selecting an intervention. For example, a functional analysis may reveal that a child's destructive behavior is maintained by intermittent teacher attention in the form of reprimands. To decrease disruption and increase adaptive behavior, a treatment could be designed that arranged more frequent attention (e.g., high-rate) and high-quality teacher attention (enthusiastic praise) for appropriate behavior, while discontinuing the contingency between destruction and attention (i.e., extinction). The treatment could be further strengthened by teaching the student to recruit attention during periods of low adult attention (e.g., Connell, Carta, & Baer, 1993; Peck et al., 1996). The general approach to intervention suggested here is to steer response-allocation patterns away from problem behavior and toward adaptive replacement responses through systematic manipulation of relevant antecedent and consequent stimuli identified via a systematic, comprehensive functional analysis.

Treatment Options

Interventions should relate directly to the response–reinforcer relation specified in the functional analysis (Iwata et al., 1994; Iwata et al., 1990); thus it is important to precede intervention with a hypothesis-testing approach to assessment (e.g., a functional analysis). There are two fundamental aspects of treatment matched to the operant function of problem behavior: (1) weakening the maintaining response–reinforcer relationship, and (2) building or strengthening a response–reinforcer relationship for an adaptive response class that replaces the function of the problem one. In addition, antecedent-based approaches focus on altering the establishing operations (EOs) and changing the discriminative stimuli (SDs) that set the occasion for problem behavior. Thus three distinct approaches to intervention are commonly considered: (1) extinction, (2) alternative reinforcement, and (3) antecedent manipulations. Some of these approaches will not be appropriate or feasible for all individuals, therefore careful consideration should be given to selection and implementation of interventions for each individual. These three approaches can be combined and individualized and tailored to an individual and his or her environment in any number of ways to increase their effectiveness. Some examples are provided within each approach; however, it is beyond the scope of this chapter to describe in detail all specific interventions.

Consequent-Based Approaches: Extinction

One means of effectively weakening the response–reinforcer contingency is via extinction. With extinction, the reinforcement contingency maintaining the problem behavior is discontinued (see Iwata et al., 1994). Specifically, the response no longer results in the reinforcer (i.e., attention is no longer provided in response to attention-maintained problem behavior; access to materials is no longer available as a result of problem behavior maintained by access to materials; task demands are not interrupted when escape-maintained problem behavior occurs). For instance, extinction of attention-maintained behavior might consist of planned ignoring (Repp et al., 1988), whereas extinction of escape-maintained behavior might involve continuation of instruction (Mace, Browder, & Lin, 1987). Because extinction involves the termination of the response–reinforcer contingency, it is critical to have identified the maintaining reinforcer via a functional analysis. For example, withholding attention following a negatively reinforced problem behavior would not be expected to have a therapeutic effect (Iwata et al., 1994).

Sensory extinction has been attempted in the treatment of various automatically reinforced responses, such as hand-flapping and toy-spinning. Frequently the response cannot be completely discontinued because the response itself provides sensory reinforcement. Treatments have focused on altering the sensations produced by the behavior. For example, Rincover, Cook, Peoples, and Packer (1979) carpeted table-tops to reduce auditory stimulation from plate-spinning and placed gloves on a child's hands to reduce the stimulation of hand-rubbing. Both procedures reduced problem behavior, perhaps because the sensory consequences were attenuated.

It should be noted that extinction alone can produce undesirable side effects (Lovaas & Simmons, 1969; Sajwaj, Twardosz, & Burke, 1972). These side effects include initial increases in the occurrence of the target problem behavior; the emergence, or induction, of new topographies of problem behavior; and emotional reactions such as crying, screaming, and aggression. However, combining extinction with alternative reinforcement can prevent or attenuate most adverse reactions to extinction (Lerman, Iwata, & Wallace, 1999).

Consequent-Based Approaches: Alternative Reinforcement

There are numerous operations, both within and across maintaining functions, that can provide an alternative source of reinforcement. Alternative reinforcement involves the presentation of the maintaining reinforcer on some schedule that is not contingent on problem behavior. Differential reinforcement can be provided contingent on an appropriate or communicative response (e.g., DRA, DRC), contingent on the omission of the target problem behavior (DRO), or independent of problem behavior on a fixed or variable time schedule (FT, VT).

In many cases it is desirable to provide reinforcement contingent on an appropriate alternative response. When the operant function of problem behavior is known, differential reinforcement of alternative responses is possible. This strategy is based on the assumption that the problem behavior serves a function (Carr & Durand, 1985; Wacker et al., 1990). Therefore, perhaps one of the most common interventions involves differential reinforcement of a replacement response that produces the same functional reinforcer. This intervention is designed to preserve the operant function for the individual but importantly, to replace the problem behavior with other more adaptive responses. This type of alternative reinforcement can be arranged in numerous ways, including contingent on a specific alternative behavior such as in DRA schedules, on a communicative gesture such as in DRC schedules (e.g., Steege et al., 1990; Wacker et al., 1990), or on the omission of the problem behavior for a specified period of time, such as in DRO schedules (e.g., Mazeleski, Iwata, Vollmer, Zarcone, & Smith, 1993).

One particularly effective arrangement of alternative reinforcement is DRC, or teaching a communicative response. A distinct advantage of teaching individuals a communicative response is that, to some extent, the individual can control the timing and rate of reinforcement, thereby avoiding periods of deprivation that may occasion problem behavior. For example, if a functional analysis indicates that a specific problem behavior is maintained by attention, the individual could be taught to appropriately solicit attention in any number of ways. She could be taught to say, "Come here, please," or to hand someone a 2" × 2" card that says, "Hugs please," or to press a microswitch that is connected to a tape-recorded message that says, "Come here, please." Identical methods can be used for escape-maintained problem behavior, with the message being "Give me a break, please."

Alternately, the reinforcer maintaining the problem behavior can be arranged on a non-contingent basis. Specifically, reinforcers are delivered based on the passage of a fixed (FT) or variable (VT) amount of time, regardless of the individual's behavior. This may operate to decrease the individual's motivation to engage in problem behavior because the problem behavior no longer has to be produced to obtain the reinforcer (i.e., the reinforcer is "free"). FT or VT schedules may also operate to decrease behavior because the reinforcer is available in the absence of the behavior, thus the response–reinforcer relationship is weakened and ultimately eliminated. Thus if attention-maintained problem behavior occurs when the teacher has been working on another activity for long periods of time, brief but frequent non-contingent positive comments to the student might decrease the occurrence of attention-maintained problem behavior.

Antecedent-Based Approaches

Interventions for problem behavior are not limited to consequences; treatment can be directed at the antecedent events. Like consequent-based interventions, antecedent interventions are also most effective if they are related to the maintaining variables for problem behavior (Wacker et al., 1998). When operant function and treatment are matched, there are numerous specific treatment options available from two broad classes of antecedent variables: establishing operations (EOs) and discriminative stimuli (SDs).

The events or stimuli that establish consequences as reinforcing (EOs) can be proactively manipulated to decrease the likelihood of problem behavior. For example, if a student displays attention-maintained problem behavior when the teacher is occupied working with other students, the teacher might engage in a few minutes of social interaction with the student prior to turning her attention to the other students (e.g., Berg, Peck, Wacker, Derby, Asmus, & Richman, 1994). General enrichment of the environment with a variety of stimulating objects may decrease the motivation to engage in problem behavior maintained by access to materials. Some evidence for this proposition comes from studies by Horner (1980) and Finney, Russo, and Cataldo (1982), showing that the availability of toys, attractive materials, and alternative activities can considerably reduce the occurrence of maladaptive behavior. This finding is also consistent with basic studies with non-human animals reporting decreased response rates following noncontingent delivery of reinforcement (Nevin, 1974). For escape-maintained problem behavior that occurs when difficult tasks are presented, instructional strategies could be provided to the student to provide assistance in successful task completion, thereby decreasing the unpleasantness of the task and the motivation to avoid or escape it (McComas, Hoch, Goddard, & Vintere, 1998). Finally, an approach to diminishing the establishing operations for automatically reinforced problem behavior has been to provide a high rate of noncontingent alternative sensory stimulation. A number of studies have shown that simply increasing the level of stimulation in the environment, via social interaction (e.g., Mace & Knight, 1986), visual displays (Forehand & Baumeister, 1970; Kennedy & Souza, 1995), or music (Mace et al., 1989), is correlated with lower levels of automatically reinforced problem behavior. The presumption is that noncontingent stimulation diminishes the establishing conditions for behavior maintained by automatic positive reinforcement.

The environmental events that occur prior to problem behavior and signal the availability of reinforcement for problem behavior (SDs) can be altered to decrease the likelihood of future occurrences of problem behavior. The availability for reinforcement in the form of attention for problem behavior may be signaled by a teacher turning her attention to the problem behavior of another student. In this case, the teacher's turning her attention to the other student constitutes the discriminative stimulus (SD) for reinforcement. To change this, the teacher might say, "I am going to work with Brian. When I am finished with that, if you work quietly while I am away, I will play a round of your favorite game with you." This proactive antecedent-based approach arranges SDs for appropriate behavior rather than problem behavior. Similar manipulations could be arranged for problem behavior maintained by access to materials. For example, a student may display problem behavior when told it is someone else's turn to play a computer game. In this case, the teacher might say, "It is Jill's turn to play on the computer now, but if you quietly read your book, you can have another turn when the timer rings." Again, this approach is geared toward arranging signals for the availability of reinforcement for appropriate rather than inappropriate behavior. Finally, if escape-maintained problem behavior occurs when a student is told that it is time to complete a task, the teacher could say, "Its time for math. If you finish your math without any problem behavior, you can take a break before the next assignment."

Because specific treatment components are selected based on their likelihood to disrupt maintaining contingencies or reinforce adaptive replacement behavior for an individual, it is important to individualize parameters of the reinforcement schedules and idiosyncratic discriminative stimuli pertinent to that individual and his environment (e.g., Carr et al., 1997).

FUNCTIONAL ANALYSIS AS A RESEARCH TOOL TO STUDY BASIC BEHAVIORAL PROCESSES MAINTAINING SOCIALLY SIGNIFICANT HUMAN BEHAVIOR

Finally, functional analysis methods may contribute to the integration of basic and applied research by permitting applied behavior analysts to incorporate advances in basic research into the analysis and treatment of behavior problems (Kerwin, Ahern, Eicher, & Burd, 1995; Mace, Mauro, Boyajian, & Eckert, 1997; Neef et al., 1994; Wacker, 1996). Knowing the operant function of problem behavior allows applied researchers to conceptualize severe problem behavior as a function of environment–behavior interactions (i.e., specific basic operant processes). Research that isolates the variables influencing these processes may then prove to be highly relevant to applied work (Hineline & Wacker, 1993; Iwata & Michael, 1994; Mace, 1994; Pierce & Epling, 1983; Smith & Iwata, 1997).

SUMMARY

Functional analysis is a systematic, analytic, and effective approach to understanding and treating severe behavior problems. With ongoing development, this approach continues to provide fertile ground for the analysis and treatment of a wide variety of behavior problems with a wide range of populations. It serves two important and related purposes in the treatment of severe and persistent problem behavior. First, it aids in better understanding the underlying processes responsible for the ongoing occurrence of problem behavior. Second, that understanding of the responsible processes is used to narrow the range of appropriate treatment options and increase the likelihood that a selected intervention will be effective at decreasing the occurrence of problem behavior. Although experts at behavior modification continue to develop highly refined and effective interventions, behavior analysts using functional analysis technologies will continue to learn about the variables that maintain problem behavior and the conditions under which specific interventions are appropriate for a given individual.

Acknowledgment

We would like to express our gratitude to Hannah Hoch for her assistance with the graphs in Figures 4.3 and 4.4.

References

Achenbach, T. M., & Edelbrock, C. S. (1981). *Behavioral problems and competences reported by parents of normal and disturbed children aged four through sixteen.* Monograph on Social Research in Child Development, 46 (1, Serial No. 188).

Aman, M. G., & Singh, N. N. (1986). *The Aberrant Behavior Checklist and Manual.* East Aurora, NY: Slosson.

Aman, M. G., & Singh, N. N. (1994). *The Aberrant Behavior Checklist: Community.* East Aurora, NY: Slosson.

Axelrod, S. (1987). Functional and structural analyses of behavior: Approaches leading to reduced use of punishment procedures? *Research in Developmental Disabilities, 8,* 165–178.

Ayllon, T., & Michael, J. (1959). The psychiatric nurse as a behavioral engineer. *Journal of the Experimental Analysis of Behavior, 2,* 323–334.

Bauman, R. A., Shull, R. L., & Brownstein, A. J. (1975). Time allocation on concurrent schedules with asymmetrical response requirements. *Journal of the Experimental Analysis of Behavior, 24,* 53–57.

Berg, W. K., Peck, S. M., Wacker, D. P., Derby, K. M., Asmus, J., & Richman, D. M. (May 1994). The effects of setting events on responding during assessment and intervention for attention maintained behavior problems. In K. M. Derby (Chair), *Applications of behavioral assessments and treatments with toddlers and preschoolers.* Symposium presented at the annual conference of the Association for Behavior Analysis, Atlanta.

Bijou, S. W., Petersen, R. F., & Ault, M. F. (1968). A method to integrate descriptive and experimental field studies at the level of data and empirical concepts. *Journal of Applied Behavior Analysis, 1,* 175–191.

Carr, E. G. (1977). The motivation of self-injurious behavior: A review of some hypotheses. *Psychological Bulletin, 84,* 800–816.

Carr, E. G., & Durand, M. V. (1985). Reducing behavior problems through functional communication training. *Journal of Applied Behavior Analysis, 18,* 111–126.

Carr, E. G., Yarbrough, S. C., & Langdon, N. A. (1997). Effects of idiosyncratic stimulus variables on functional analysis outcomes. *Journal of Applied Behavior Analysis, 30,* 673–685.

Cataldo, M. F., & Harris, J. (1982). The biological basis for self-injury in the mentally retarded. *Analysis and Intervention in Developmental Disabilities, 2,* 21–39.

Center, D. B., Deitz, S. M., & Kaufman, M. (1982). Student ability, task difficulty, and inappropriate classroom behavior. *Behavior Modification, 6,* 355–374.

Conger, R., & Killeen, P. (1974). Use of concurrent operants in small group research. *Pacific Sociological Review 17,* 339–416.

Connell, M. C., Carta, J. J., & Baer, D. M. (1993). Programming generalization of in-class transition skills: Teaching preschoolers with developmental delays to self-assess and recruit contingent teacher praise. *Journal of Applied Behavior Analysis, 26,* 345–352.

Conners, K. C. (1997). *Conners Parent Rating Scale — Revised* (S). North Tonawanda, NY: Multi-health Systems.

Cooper, L. J., Wacker, D. P., Sasso, G. M., Reimers, T., & Donn, L. (1990). Using parents as therapists to evaluate appropriate behavior of their children: Application to a tertiary clinic. *Journal of Applied Behavior Analysis, 23*, 285–296.

Cooper, L. J., Wacker, D. P., Thursby, D., Plagmann, L. A., Harding, J., Millard, T., & Derby, M. (1992). Analysis of the effects of task preferences, task demands, and adult attention on child behavior in outpatient and classroom. *Journal of Applied Behavior Analysis, 25*, 823–840.

Davison, M., & McCarthy, D. (1988). *The matching law: A research review.* Hillsdale, NY: Erlbaum.

Day, R. M., Rae, J. A., Schussler, N. G., Larsen, S. E., & Johnson, W. L. (1988). A functionally based approach to the treatment of self-injurious behavior. *Behavior Modification, 12*, 565–589.

Derby, K. M., Wacker, D. P., Sasso, G., Steege, M., Northup, J., Cigrand, K., & Asmus, J. (1992). Brief functional assessment techniques to evaluate aberrant behavior in an outpatient setting: A summary of 79 cases. *Journal of Applied Behavior Analysis, 25*, 713–721.

deVilliers, P. A. (1977). Choice in concurrent schedules and a quantitative formulation of the law of effect. In W. K. Honig & J. E. R. Staddon (Eds.). *Handbook of operant behavior* (pp. 233–287). Englewood Cliffs, NJ: Prentice-Hall.

Dunlap, G., Kern-Dunlap, L., Clarke, S., & Robbins, F. R. (1991). Functional assessment, curricular revision, and severe behavior problems. *Journal of Applied Behavior Analysis, 24*, 387–397.

Durand, V. M., & Carr, E. G. (1987). Social influences on "self-stimulatory" behavior: Analysis and treatment application. *Journal of Applied Behavior Analysis, 20*, 119–132.

Durand, V. M., & Kishi, G. (1987). Reducing severe behavior problems among persons with dual sensory impairments: An evaluation of a technical assistance model. *Journal of the Association for Persons with Severe Handicaps, 12*, 2–10.

Finney, J., Russo, D., & Cataldo, M. (1982). Reduction of pica in young children with lead poisoning. *Journal of Pediatric Psychology, 7*, 197–207.

Forehand, R., & Baumeister, A. A. (1970). The effect of auditory and visual stimulation on stereotyped rocking behavior and general activity of severe retardates. *Journal of Clinical Psychology, 26*, 426–429.

Fisca, W. D., & Hughes, C. (1997). Functional analysis and treatment of social communicative behavior of adolescents with developmental disabilities. *Journal of Applied Behavior Analysis, 30*, 701–704.

Gaylord-Ross, R., Weeks, M., & Lipner, C. (1980). An analysis of antecedent, response, and consequence events in the treatment of self-injurious behavior. *Education and Training of the Mentally Retarded, 15*, 35–42.

Goh, H-L., Iwata, B. A., Shore, B. A., DeLeon, I. G., Lerman, D. C., Ulrich, S. M., & Smith, R. G. (1995). An analysis of the reinforcing properties of hand mouthing. *Journal of Applied Behavior Analysis, 28*, 268–284.

Hanley, G. P., Piazza, C. C., Keeney, K. M., Blakeley-Smith, A. B., & Worsdell, A. S. (1998). Effects of wrist weights on self-injurious and adaptive behaviors. *Journal of Applied Behavior Analysis, 31*, 307–310.

Harding, J., Wacker, D. P., Cooper, L. J., Millard, T., & Jensen-Kovalan, P. (1994). Brief hierarchical assessment of potential treatment components with children in an outpatient clinic. *Journal of Applied Behavior Analysis, 27*, 291–300.

Herrnstein, R. J. (1961). Relative and absolute strength of response as a function of frequency of reinforcement. *Journal of the Experimental Analysis of Behavior, 4*, 267–272.

Herrnstein, R. J. (1970). On the law of effect. *Journal of the Experimental Analysis of Behavior, 13*, 243–266.

Higgins-Hains, A., & Baer, D. M. (1989). Interaction effects in multi-element designs: Inevitable, desirable, and ignorable. *Journal of Applied Behavior Analysis, 22*, 57–69.

Hineline, P. N., & Wacker, D. P. (1993). JEAB, November '92: What's in it for the JABA reader? *Journal of Applied Behavior Analysis, 26*, 269–274.

Hollard, V., & Davison, M. C. (1971). Preference for qualitatively different reinforcers. *Journal of the Experimental Analysis of Behavior, 16*, 375–380.

Horner, R. D. (1980). The effects of an environmental "enrichment" program on the behavior of insti-
tutionalized profoundly retarded children. *Journal of Applied Behavior Analysis, 13*, 473–491.

Horner, R. H., Day, H. M., Sprague, J. R., O'Brien, M., Heathfield, L. T. (1991). Interspersed requests:
A nonaversive procedure for decreasing aggression and self-injury during instruction. *Journal
of Applied Behavior Analysis, 24*, 265–278.

Iwata, B. A. (1988). The development and adoption of controversial default technologies. *Behavior
Analyst, 11*, 149–157.

Iwata, B. A. (1994). Functional analysis methodology: Some closing comments. *Journal of Applied
Behavior Analysis, 27*, 413–418.

Iwata, B. A., Dorsey, M. F., Slifer, K. J., Bauman, K. E., & Richman, G. S. (1994). Toward a functional analysis of self-injury. *Journal of Applied Behavior Analysis, 27*, 197–209. (Reprinted from
Analysis and Intervention in Developmental Disabilities, 2, 3–20, 1982.)

Iwata, B. A., & Michael, J. L. (1994). Applied implications of theory and research on the nature of
reinforcement. *Journal of Applied Behavior Analysis, 27*, 183–193.

Iwata, B. A., Pace, G. M., Cowdery, G. E., & Miltenberger, R. G. (1994). What makes extinction work:
An analysis of procedural form and function. *Journal of Applied Behavior Analysis, 27*, 131–
144.

Iwata, B. A., Pace, G. M., Dorsey, M. F., Zarcone, J. R., Vollmer, T. R., Smith, R. G., Rodgers, T. A.,
Lerman, D. C., Shore, B. A., Mazaleski, J. L., Goh, H-L., Cowdery, G. E., Kalsher, M. J.,
McCosh, K. C., & Willis, K. D. (1994). The functions of self-injurious behavior: An experi-
mental-epidemiological analysis. *Journal of Applied Behavior Analysis, 27*, 215–240.

Iwata, B. A., Pace, G. M., Kalsher, M. J., Cowdery, G. E., & Cataldo, M. F. (1990). Experimental
analysis and extinction of self-injurious escape behavior. *Journal of Applied Behavior Analysis,
23*, 11–27.

Johnston, J. M., & Pennypacker, H. S. (1993). *Strategies and Tactics of Behavioral Research*. Hillsdale,
NJ: Erlbaum.

Kahng, S., & Iwata, B. A. (1999). Correspondence between outcomes of brief and extended functional
analyses. *Journal of Applied Behavior Analysis, 32*, 149–159.

Keller, F. S., & Schoenfeld, W. N. (1950). *Principles of psychology*. New York: Appleton–Century–
Crofts.

Kennedy, C. H., & Souza, G. (1995). Functional analysis and treatment of eye poking. *Journal of Applied
Behavior Analysis, 28*, 27–38.

Kerwin, M., Ahern, W., Eicher, P., & Burd, D. (1995). The costs of eating: A behavioral economic
analysis of food refusal. *Journal of Applied Behavior Analysis, 28*, 245–260.

Lalli, J. S., Browder, D. M., Mace, F. C., & Brown, D. K. (1993). Teacher use of descriptive analysis
data to implement interventions to decrease students' problem behaviors. *Journal of Applied
Behavior Analysis, 26*, 227–238.

Lalli, J. S., Casey, S. D., & Kates, K. (1997). Noncontingent reinforcement as treatment for severe
behavior: Some procedural variations. *Journal of Applied Behavior Analysis, 30*, 127–137.

Lalli, J. S., & Goh, H-L. (1993). Naturalistic observations in community settings. In J. Reichle & D. P.
Wacker (Eds.), *Communicative alternatives to challenging behavior: Integrating functional
assessment and intervention strategies* (pp. 11–39). Baltimore: Paul H. Brookes.

Lalli, J. S., Mace, F. C., Livezey, K., & Kates, K. (1998). Assessment of stimulus generalization gradients
in the treatment of self-injurious behavior. *Journal of Applied Behavior Analysis, 31*, 479–483.

Lerman, D. C., Iwata, B. A., & Wallace, M. D. (1999). Side effects of extinction: Prevalence of burst-
ing and aggression during the treatment of self-injurious behavior. *Journal of Applied Behavior
Analysis, 32*, 1–8.

Lovaas, O. I., Newsom, C., & Hickman, C. (1987). Self-stimulatory behavior and perceptual reinforcement. *Journal of Applied Behavior Analysis, 20*, 45–68.

Lovaas, O. I., & Simmons, J. Q. (1969). Manipulation of self-destruction in three retarded children.
Journal of Applied Behavior Analysis, 2, 143–157.

Lowe, C. F., & Horne, P. J. (1985). On the generality of behavioral principles: Human choice and the
matching law. In C. F. Lowe (Ed.), *Behavior analysis and contemporary psychology* (pp. 97–
115). London: Erlbaum.

Mace, F. C. (1994). The significance and future of functional analysis methodologies. *Journal of Applied Behavior Analysis, 27*, 385–392.

Mace, F. C., Browder, D. M., & Lin, Y. (1987). Analysis of demand conditions associated with stereotypy. *Journal of Behavior Therapy and Experimental Psychiatry, 18*, 25–31.

Mace, F. C., & Knight, D. (1986). Functional analysis and treatment of severe pica. *Journal of Applied Behavior Analysis, 19*, 411–416.

Mace, F. C., & Lalli, J. S. (1991). Linking descriptive and experimental analyses in the treatment of bizarre speech. *Journal of Applied Behavior Analysis, 24*, 553–562.

Mace, F. C., Mauro, B. C., Boyajian, A. E., & Eckert, T. L. (1997). Effects of reinforcer quality on behavioral momentum: Coordinated applied and basic research. *Journal of Applied Behavior Analysis, 30*, 1–20.

Mace, F. C., McCurdy, B., & Quigley, E. A. (1990). A negative side-effect of reward predicted by the matching law. *Journal of Applied Behavior Analysis, 23*, 197–206.

Mace, F. C., Neef, N. A., Shade, D., & Mauro, B. C. (1996). Effects of problem difficulty and reinforcer quality on time allocated to concurrent arithmetic problems, *Journal of Applied Behavior Analysis, 29*, 11–24.

Mace, F. C., & Roberts, M. L. (1993). Factors affecting selection of behavioral interventions. In D. P. Wacker & J. Reichle (Eds.), *Communicative alternatives to challenging behavior: Integrating functional assessment and intervention strategies.* Baltimore: Paul H. Brookes.

Mace, F. C., Yankanich, M. A., & West, B. (1989). Toward a methodology of experimental analysis and treatment of aberrant classroom behaviors. *Special Services in the School, 4*, 71–88.

Martens, B. K., & Houk, J. L. (1989). The application of Herrnstein's law of effect to disruptive and on-task behavior of a retarded adolescent girl. *Journal of the Experimental Analysis of Behavior, 51*, 17–28.

Martens, B. K., Lochner, D. G., & Kelly, S Q. (1992). The effects of variable-interval reinforcement on academic engagement: A demonstration of matching theory. *Journal of Applied Behavior Analysis, 25*, 143–152.

Mazeleski, J. L., Iwata, B. A., Vollmer, T. R., Zarcone, J. R., & Smith, R. G. (1993). Analysis of the reinforcement and extinction components in DRO contingencies with self-injury. *Journal of Applied Behavior Analysis, 26*, 143 156.

McComas, J. J., Hoch, H., Goddard, C., Vintere, P. (1998). *Escape behavior during academic tasks: A preliminary analysis of establishing operations.* Paper presented at the annual conference of the Association for Behavior Analysis, Orlando, May.

McDowell, J. J. (1988). Matching theory in natural human environments. *Behavior Analyst, 11*, 95–109.

McDowell, J. J. (1989). Two modern developments in matching theory. *Behavior Analyst, 12*, 153–166.

Michael, J. (1982). Distinguishing between discriminative and motivative functions of stimuli. *Journal of the Experimental Analysis of Behavior, 37*, 149–155.

Millard, T., Wacker, D. P., Cooper, L. J., Harding, J., Drew, J., Plagmann, L. A., Asmus, J., McComas, J., & Jensen-Kovalan, P. (1993). A brief component analysis of potential treatment packages in on outpatient clinic setting with young children. *Journal of Applied Behavior Analysis, 26*, 475–476.

Miller, J. T. (1976). Matching-based hedonic scaling in the pigeon. *Journal of the Experimental Analysis of Behavior, 26*, 335–347.

Myerson, J., & Hale, S. (1984). Practical implications of the matching law. *Journal of Applied Behavior Analysis, 17*, 367–380.

National Institutes of Health. (1989). *Consensus development conference statement on treatment of destructive behaviors in persons with developmental disabilities.* Bethesda, MD: Author.

Neef, N. A., Mace, F. C., & Shade, D. (1993). Impulsivity in students with serious emotional disturbance: The interactive effects of reinforcer rate, delay, and quality. *Journal of Applied Behavior Analysis, 26*, 37–52.

Neef, N. A., Mace, F. C., Shea, M. C., & Shade, D. B. (1992). Effects of reinforcer rates and reinforcer quality on time allocation: Extension of matching theory to educational settings. *Journal of Applied Behavior Analysis, 25*, 691–700.

Neef, N. A., Shade, D. B., & Miller, M. S. (1994). Assessing influential dimensions of reinforcers on choice in students with emotional disturbance. *Journal of Applied Behavior Analysis, 27*, 575–584.

Nelson, R. O., & Hayes, S. C. (1979). Some current dimensions of behavioral assessment. *Behavioral Assessment, 1*, 1–16.

Neuringer, C. (1970). Behavior modification as the clinical psychologist views it. (pp. 1–9). In C. Neuringer & J. L. Michael (Eds.), *Behavior Modification in Clinical Psychology.* New York: Appleton–Century–Crofts.

Nevin, J. A. (1974). Response strength in multiple schedules. *Journal of the Experimental Analysis of Behavior, 21*, 389–408.

Northup, J., Broussard, C., Jones, K., George, T., Vollmer, T. R., & Herring, M. (1995). The differential effects of teacher and peer attention on the disruptive classroom behavior of three children with a diagnosis of attention deficit hyperactivity disorder. *Journal of Applied Behavior Analysis, 28*, 227–228.

Northup, J., Fusilier, I., Swanson, V., Roane, H., & Borrero, J. (1997). An evaluation of methylphenidate as a potential establishing operation for some common classroom reinforcers. *Journal of Applied Behavior Analysis, 30*, 615–625.

Northup, J., Wacker, D. P., Sasso, G., Steege, M., Cigrand, K., Cook, J., DeRaad, D. (1991). A brief functional analysis of aggressive and alternative behavior in an outclinic setting. *Journal of Applied Behavior Analysis, 24*, 509–522.

O'Neill, R. E., Horner, R. H., Albin, R. W., Storey, K., & Sprague, J. (1990). *Functional analysis of problem behavior: A practical assessment guide.* Sycamore, IL: Sycamore Press.

O'Reilly, M. F. (1997). Functional analysis of episodic self-injury correlated with recurrent otitis media. *Journal of Applied Behavior Analysis, 30*, 165–167.

Peck, S. M., Wacker, D. P., Berg, W. K., Cooper, L. J., Brown, K. A., Richman, D., McComas, J. J., Frischmeyer, P., & Millard, T. (1996). Choice-making treatment of young children's severe behavior problem. *Journal of Applied Behavior Analysis, 29*, 263–289.

Piazza, C. C., Fisher, W. W., Hanley, G. P., Remick, M. L., Contrucci, S. A., & Aitken, T. L. (1997). The use of positive and negative reinforcement in the treatment of escape-maintained destructive behavior. *Journal of Applied Behavior Analysis, 30*, 279–298.

Piazza, C. C., Fisher, W. W., Hanley, G. P., LeBlanc, L. A., Worsdell, A. S., Lindauer, S. E., & Keeney, K. M. (1998). Treatment of pica through multiple analyses of its reinforcing functions. *Journal of Applied Behavior Analysis, 31*, 165–189.

Piazza, C. C., Hanley, G. P., Bowman, L. G., Ruyter, J. M., Lindauer, S. E., & Saiontz, D. M. (1997). Functional analysis and treatment of elopement. *Journal of Applied Behavior Analysis, 30*, 653–672.

Pierce, W. D., & Epling, W. F. (1983). Choice, matching and human behavior: A review of the literature. *Behavior Analyst*, 57–76.

Repp, A. C., Felce, D., & Barton, L. E. (1988). Basing the treatment of stereotypic and self-injurious behaviors on hypotheses of their causes. *Journal of Applied Behavior Analysis, 21*, 281–290.

Richman, D. M., Wacker, D. P., Asmus, J. A., & Casey, S. D. (1998). Functional analysis and extinction of different behavior problems exhibited by the same individual. *Journal of Applied Behavior Analysis, 31*, 475–478.

Rincover, A., Cook, R., Peoples, A., & Packer, D. (1979). Sensory extinction and sensory reinforcement principles for programming multiple adaptive behavior change. *Journal of Applied Behavior Analysis, 12*, 221–233.

Sajwaj, T., Twardosz, S., & Burke, M. (1972). Side effects of extinction procedures in a remedial preschool. *Journal of Applied Behavior Analysis, 5*, 163–175.

Sasso, G. M., Reimers, T. M., Cooper, L. J., Wacker, D. P., Berg, W., Steege, M., Kelly, L., & Allaire, A. (1992). Use of descriptive and experimental analyses to identify the functional properties of aberrant behavior in school settings. *Journal of Applied Behavior Analysis, 25*, 809–822.

Sidman, M. (1960). *Tactics of scientific research.* New York: Basic Books.

Skinner, B. F. (1953). *Science and human behavior.* New York: Macmillan.

Smith, R. G., & Iwata, B. A. (1997). Antecedent influences on behavior disorders. *Journal of Applied Behavior Analysis, 30,* 343–375.

Smith, R. G., Iwata, B. A., Goh, H.-L., & Shore, B. A. (1995). An analysis of establishing operations for self-injury maintained by escape. *Journal of Applied Behavior Analysis, 28,* 433–445.

Smith, R. G., Iwata, B. A., Vollmer, T. R., & Zarcone, J. R. (1993). Experimental analysis and treatment of multiply controlled self-injury. *Journal of Applied Behavior Analysis, 26,* 183–196.

Steege, M. W., Wacker, D. P., Cigrand, K. C., Berg, W. K., Novak, C. G., Reimers, T. M., Sasso, G. M., & DeRaad, A. (1990). Use of negative reinforcement in the treatment of self-injurious behavior. *Journal of Applied Behavior Analysis, 23,* 459–467.

Thomas, D. R., Becker, W. C., & Armstrong, M. (1968). Production and elimination of disruptive classroom behavior by systematically varying teacher's behavior. *Journal of Applied Behavior Analysis, 1,* 35–45.

Thompson, R. H., Fisher, W. W., Piazza, C. C., & Kuhn, D. (1998). The evaluation and treatment of aggression maintained by attention and automatic reinforcement. *Journal of Applied Behavior Analysis, 31,* 103–116.

Touchette, P. E., MacDonald, R. F., & Langer, S. N. (1985). A scatter plot for identifying stimulus control of problem behavior. *Journal of Applied Behavior Analysis, 18,* 343–351.

Vollmer, T. R., Iwata, B. A., Duncan, B. A., Lerman, D. L. (1993). Extensions of multielement treatment analyses using reversal-type designs. *Journal of Developmental and Physical Disabilities, 5,* 311–325.

Vollmer, T. R., Marcus, B. A., & Ringdahl, J. E. (1995). Noncontingent escape as treatment for self-injurious behavior maintained by negative reinforcement. *Journal of Applied Behavior Analysis, 28,* 15–26.

Vollmer, T. R., Marcus, B. A., Ringdahl, J. E., & Roane, H. S. (1995). Progressing from brief assessments to extended experimental analyses in the evaluation of aberrant behavior. *Journal of Applied Behavior Analysis, 28,* 561–576.

Vollmer, T. R., & Van Camp, C. M. (1997). Experimental designs to evaluate antecedent control. (pp. 87–111) In J. K. Luiselli & M. J. Cameron (Eds.), *Antecedent control procedures for the behavioral support of persons with developmental disabilities.* Baltimore: Paul H. Brookes.

Wacker, D. P. (1996). Behavior analysis research in JABA: A need for studies that bridge basic and applied research. *Experimental Analysis of Human Behavior Bulletin, 14 (1),* 11–14.

Wacker, D. P., Berg, W. K., Asmus, J. A., Harding, J. W., & Cooper, L. J. (1998). Experimental analysis of antecedent influences on challenging behavior. In J. K. Luiselli & M. J. Cameron (Eds.), *Antecedent control: Innovative approaches to behavioral support* (pp. 67–86). Baltimore: Paul H. Brookes.

Wacker, D. P., Berg, W. K., Cooper, L. J., Derby, K. M., Steege, M. W., Northup, J., & Sasso, G. (1994). The impact of functional analysis methodology on outpatient clinic services. *Journal of Applied Behavior Analysis, 27,* 405–407.

Wacker, D. P., Berg, W. K., Harding, J. W., Derby, K. M., Asmus, J. M., & Healy, A. (1998). Evaluation and long-term treatment of aberrant behavior displayed by young children with disabilities. *Developmental and Behavioral Pediatrics, 19 (4),* 260–266.

Wacker, D. P., Harding, J., Cooper, L. J., Derby, K. M., Peck, S., Asmus, J., Berg, W. K., & Brown, K. A. (1996). The effects of meal schedule and quantity on problematic behavior. *Journal of Applied Behavior Analysis, 29,* 79–92.

Wacker, D. P., Steege, M. W., Northup, J., Sasso, G., Berg, W., Reimers, T., Cooper, L., Cigrand, K., & Donn, L. (1990). A component analysis of functional communication training across three topographies of severe behavior problems. *Journal of Applied Behavior Analysis, 23,* 417–429.

CHAPTER 5

Analogue Assessment
Research and Practice in Evaluating Emotional and Behavioral Problems

JOHN M. HINTZE
GARY STONER
MARY H. BULL
University of Massachusetts at Amherst

As an alternative to direct observation measures, analogue assessment has been used increasingly for gathering observational information. Although direct observation within the natural setting probably provides the most ecologically valid data for behavioral assessment (Cone, 1978), certain behaviors or classes of behaviors do not always lend themselves to be observed directly. In these situations, analogue methods offer many benefits not found in direct measures of assessment. For example, some behaviors may be highly situation specific, by which the observer may not be at the right time or place to observe the target behavior (e.g., during recess or lunch). Similarly, some behaviors pose accessibility problems such that directly observing the behavior of interest would be extremely difficult for the observer (e.g., a school bus). Third, some behaviors occur at such a low frequency that continuous direct observation would not prove time or cost efficient. Finally, analogue assessment may help simplify and reduce complex constructs, thereby allowing assessors to observe isolated features of what is considered more global behavioral repertoires (e.g., anxiety) (Kratochwill, Sheridan, Carlson, & Lasecki, 1999; Shapiro & Kratochwill, 1988).

Analogue assessment measures refer to a set of indirect measurement procedures that reflect how an individual might behave in a real-life situation. In its most typical form, analogue measures assess behavior in a simulated or hypothetical situation that is set up to mimic the real-life situation in which the behavior of interest occurs. The assessor, using analogue measures, assumes some overlap in the similarity between the behavior and the setting in the analogue arrangement, and how the individual behaves and responds in the actual real-life environment (Prout & Ferber, 1988). The observation of the behavior in the analogue setting then is used to predict the individual's behavior in the real-life environment. Because of this, analogue assessment procedures are less direct than observation within the natural setting, with the level of inference varying as a function of the extent to which the analogue procedure deviates from the real-life setting.

Analogue assessment procedures may be conceptualized according to the method of presentation of the analogue situations and the manner in which participants are asked to respond (Gettinger, 1988). McFall (1977) proposed that analogue procedures be considered with respect to the particular dimension of the natural environments that were being simulated—subjects, treatment procedures, specific settings, or specific responses. Subject analogues refer to those in which the target subjects are considered equivalent to subjects outside the analogue setting to whom the results of the analogue assessment are generalized. For example, results of a reinforcement preference menu from a randomly selected group of third-grade students may be used to decide the types of reinforcers other third-grade students would like. Treatment analogues refer to procedures by which the response to brief simplified interventions is used to generalize to analogous but more complex and extensive treatment procedures. For example, responses to an analogue experimental manipulation of reinforcement contingencies—as typically conducted in functional analysis—could give the assessor vital information about how a client may respond to a more elaborate treatment package based on the principles tested within the functional analysis. This may be the case when it is found that a student's problematic behavior is maintained by social attention. A generalized treatment package could be arranged so that social attention is made contingent on desired behavior, while at the same time withheld for unwanted behavior.

Third, situational analogues refer to structured or controlled assessment situations considered equivalent to the natural environments they simulate. Again, because of the control needed to formulate functional hypotheses most functional analytic procedures involve the use of contrived settings, thereby eliminating or reducing the variables in the natural environment that can contaminate assessment results. Similarly, many social skill assessments involve an element of situational control necessary because of the difficulty in directly observing specific social interactions without significantly altering them. Finally, response analogues refer to those assessments where one response is considered equivalent to similar responses to which the results are generalized. For example, high levels of aggression in highly structured small group play activities could suggest similar response patterns when the student is in unstructured play situations such as recess or at home.

In a different manner, Nay (1977) categorized analogue procedures according to the method of presentation of the analogue procedure—or the way in which the subjects were asked to respond. In doing so, four general categories of analogue assessment methods are identified: (1) paper-and-pencil, (2) audiotape, (3) videotape, and (4) enactment or role-play analogues. Paper-and-pencil, audiotape, and videotape all refer to the manner in which the analogue procedure is presented. For example, paper-and-pencil analogues require the subject to respond to a stimulus situation presented in a written format. Once read, the subject is asked to respond with either a written, verbal, or physical response, or any combination of the three. Similarly, audiotaped and videotaped analogues require that the subject listen to an auditory stimulus and/or watch a visual stimulus. In each case, subjects are typically required to respond with either a verbal or physical response, or both.

The final and perhaps most common type of analogue requires the subject to respond to contrived situations in an ongoing manner. With enactments, typical situations are recreated to mirror the stimuli that are present in the natural environment. For example, a family therapist may recreate a mealtime scenario in a clinical setting and simply observe the interaction patterns that result. Little attempt is made to control the responses of the subjects. Conversely, role plays make an attempt to contrive the responses of the subject by requiring or requesting a specific response. For example, in an assessment of social skills a subject may be asked to respond as he or she would upon meeting a person for the first time. Unlike enactments where response patterns are free to vary, role plays require the subject to respond in a delineated fashion.

Although analogue assessment procedures offer many distinct advantages in comparison to direct observation in the natural environment, the methods are not without their shortcomings. Perhaps most important, because many analogue procedures are not standardized, questions are raised with respect to the reliability and validity of the information gathered. In comparison to other forms of assessment used to evaluate emotional and behavioral problems, the psychometric properties of most analogue procedures are far less established. In fact, some experts argue that by relying on analogue measures of behavior, clinicians sacrifice the well-established technical properties of standardized measures (Gettinger, 1988). One very salient validity issue relates to the generalizability and accuracy of decisions based on data generated in a highly structured and controlled environment, to situations where the control of the environmental contingencies are less pronounced. Although the establishment of stimulus control is a desired feature of any behavior-change strategy, duplicating the equivalent degree of structure obtained in analogues, in the natural classroom environment, is often very difficult. As such, a major limitation of analogue measures is that they never perfectly replicate the natural setting, calling into question the accuracy and validity of such procedures. Reliability is also a major concern of analogue procedures (Barrios, Hartmann, & Shigetomi, 1981; Johnson & Melamed, 1979; Morris & Kratochwill, 1983). Besides a lack of traditional forms of reliability (e.g., test–retest, alternate form), the treatment integrity of the procedures also remains wanting. For example, clinicians are likely to vary considerably in their use and interpretation of many analogue measures. Finally, as with any type of assessment procedures, clinicians may fail to acknowledge or fully appreciate the difference between assessing and intervening in a contrived setting versus programming for behavior change in the natural environment. Although targeted behavior change in the analogue setting can serve as a critical first step in many intervention plans, a "train-and-hope" generalization strategy is likely to be unsuccessful (Stokes & Baer, 1977). Indeed, clinicians need to be mindful of the lack of generalization of such approaches and actively program for the transfer of skills (DuPaul & Eckert, 1994).

The purpose of this chapter is to present an overview of the use of analogue measures in the assessment of emotional, social-behavioral, social-cognitive, and peer status domains. As previously discussed, the spectrum of analogue assessment measures is extensive and could easily fill an entire volume. Consequently, the chapter will attempt to highlight a sampling of enactment, role-play, and paper-and-pencil strategies used in the assessment of social, emotional, and behavioral domains. Although by definition, behavior rating scales and informant reports could fit easily within this discussion, their use will be covered only briefly. For a more extensive discussion of these topics the reader is referred to Eckert, Dunn, Guiney, and Codding (Chapter 11, this volume) and Merrell (Chapter 9, this volume).

EMOTIONAL CONCERNS

Anxieties, Fears, and Phobias

Anxiety disorders have been widely recognized as the most common class of emotional disorders affecting children and youth (Albano, Chorpita, & Barlow, 1996; Bell-Dolan & Brazeal, 1993; Kashani & Orvaschel, 1988). Although passing fears and anxieties are considered part of normal development, for a significant number of children anxieties and fears become a debilitating aspect of their daily lives (Albano et al., 1996; Kendall & Ronan, 1990; March, 1995; Morris & Kratochwill, 1985). Common forms of impairment include an avoidance of activities such as schooling, peer involvement, and autonomous activities (Bell-Dolan & Brazeal, 1993; Kendall & Ronan, 1990).

For purposes of clarity, it is first important to define what is meant by fears, phobias, and anxieties. Too often, these terms are used interchangeably, leading to confusion. As defined, fear is a natural response to some real or imagined threatening stimuli (King & Ollendick, 1989). Developmentally normal fear has an adaptive and protective function. However, occasionally a child's fear is beyond what would be expected for his or her given age and persists, or even worsens, over time. These excessive, abnormal fears are often referred to as phobias, and can impede social and academic functioning (King & Ollendick, 1989). Anxiety, on the other hand, refers to the overriding, unpleasant sensation involving subjective apprehension and is associated with severe impairment in functioning (Albano et al., 1996; King & Ollendick, 1989).

Assessment studies of children in this area, therefore, have primarily focused on anxieties and phobias, that is, fears and reactions to feared stimuli that are not age appropriate and/or impair normal functioning (cf. Beidel, 1988; Glennon & Weisz, 1978; Van Hasselt, Hersen, Bellack, Rosenblum, & Lamparski, 1979; Zatz & Chassin, 1983).

The direct assessment of anxieties, fears, phobias, and avoidant behaviors overall has been proven to be problematic for several reasons. First, because these problems are often related to private events that are accessible only through verbal self-report, responses to feared or anxiety-producing stimuli may be subject to a social desirability bias. Second, and perhaps more important, reactions to feared and anxiety-producing stimuli are highly susceptible to negative reinforcement by which the avoidance of those situations and thoughts that occasion unpleasant feelings is reinforcing to the child. As such, any attempt to make a direct observation of the child's reaction to a feared or anxiety-producing stimulus in the natural setting becomes extremely difficult (Shapiro & Kratochwill, 1988).

With children, the difficulty of assessing avoidant behaviors is compounded. Often children's self-reports may not accurately reflect their internal states. Anxious children, in particular, often present in an outwardly apparent nondistressed manner. That is, a part of the fearful and anxious child's interpreting of social and evaluative situations includes perceiving threat and responding in a nonfearful or nonanxious manner to reduce the threat (Kendall & Ronan, 1990). Given the assessment problems inherent in such situations, the continued use of self-report rating and interviews is most likely attributable to the economy and convenience involved in their administration and scoring and utility as a screening device. However, without corroborating information from other response channels (e.g., motoric), the assessment and treatment of avoidant disorders are hindered.

Overall, three types of analogue measures have typically been used in the assessment of anxiety, fears, and phobias. First, enactment and role-playing tasks place children in a simulated condition in which they come into contact with the feared or anxiety-producing stimulus. Outcome measures usually involve the recording of responses of some predetermined target behaviors. A second type of analogue assessment—self-report measures—asks the child to respond in a paper-and-pencil format to descriptions of specific stimuli that usually describe fearful or anxiety-arousing situations. Typically respondents are asked to rate their level of fear or anxiety rather than produce a written response in a narrative manner. Finally, informant reports, another type of paper-and-pencil measure, ask caretakers (usually parents and teachers) to report the degree of fear or anxiety of a specific child. Like self-reports, informant reports typically require ratings rather than detailed written accounts of a child's behavior.

Enactment and Role Plays

Enactment and role-playing analogues have typically involved simulating an anxiety-provoking situation for the subjects and then rating their behavioral responses using a measure or scale, on which specific behaviors that reflect fear are operationally defined and recorded (King & Ollendick, 1989).

One quite common enactment method that measures motoric components of fears and anxiety is the Behavioral Avoidance Test (BAT; Hamilton & King, 1991; Lang & Lazovik, 1963; Van Hasselt et al., 1979). Most typically, the BAT involves some variation of bringing a subject in proximity or contact with the feared or anxiety-arousing stimuli and observing the resultant behavior. Measures of time spent with the object, proximity to the object, and handling of the object are just a few of the behaviors that can be observed or rated. In a different variation, the clinician instructs the subject to perform each step of a graded hierarchy that brings the subject closer and closer to the feared or anxiety-producing stimulus. In this instance, the subject's compliance with the graded hierarchy or self-ratings may serve as the primary outcome datum.

As one example, Lang and Lazovik (1963) used a variation of a BAT to study the effects of desensitization on snake phobia. Using a fear thermometer, 13 college student volunteers were asked to rate their anxiety on a ten-point scale before and after systematic desensitization training. In addition, a direct estimate of the subjects' avoidance behavior was obtained by confronting each subject with the phobic object. In each instance, the subject was informed that a nonpoisonous snake was confined in a glass case in a nearby laboratory. Upon entering the laboratory, the experimenter removed a grill that covered the top of the glass case and encouraged the subject to come forward. Through a series of steps, the subject was brought closer to the snake and, if possible, told to touch the snake. Immediately following the experiment the subject was asked to rate his anxiety again. Effectiveness of the intervention was assessed by comparing the two BAT ratings.

In another use of the BAT, Hamilton and King (1991) examined the temporal stability of the measure with 14 participants (ranging in age from 2 to 11 years) who exhibited a phobia to dogs. In this instance, the BAT consisted of a series of 14 performance tasks requiring increasingly closer interactions with a dog. Two test administrations were conducted seven days apart before treatment. This was done to partial out or examine any gains that might be attributable to the BAT itself (i.e., gains in approach scores should be attributable to the treatment process, rather than to repeated assessments). Overall, high test–retest reliability was obtained ($r = .97$). Ten children obtained identical total approach scores on each test, and within subtask test–retest agreement over all subjects was 97%. Four children showed slight increases in approach behavior at retesting. The authors report that these children had relatively high initial scores, showing that they were more amenable to close contact with the dog at the outset. Findings suggest that the BAT was a clinically useful assessment tool that did not appear to be overly susceptible to reactivity.

In an example of a role-play analogue, Esveldt-Dawson, Wisner, Unis, Matson, and Kazdin (1982) treated a 12-year-old girl for phobias of school and unfamiliar males. A combined treatment package that consisted of instructions, performance feedback, participant modeling, and social reinforcement was introduced in a multiple baseline format across several phobic and prosocial behaviors. Treatment outcomes were assessed based on responses to ten role-play situations. Five of the role plays pertained to unfamiliar males—including asking a man for a donation to a children's hospital, asking a salesperson about trying on a new pair of shoes, meeting a new male therapist, welcoming a peer's father to the treatment session, and sitting next to an usher at a wedding reception dinner. Anxiety-provoking school situations consisted of picking up a graded semester report with a poor mark, being excluded by peers during an art project, speaking in front of a class, being accused of cheating by the teacher, and being sent to the principal because of tardiness. Each role-play analogue lasted approximately 15 minutes.

In each session direct observations were made of several target behaviors that included both avoidance and prosocial behaviors. Avoidance behaviors included stiffness of movements, nervous mannerisms, and a self-rating of anxiety. Prosocial behaviors consisted of eye contact, appropriate affect, appropriate body movement, and a rating of overall social skills. Results showed a rapid reduction in the frequency and rate of avoidance behaviors during all role plays. Furthermore, the frequency of prosocial behavior also increased. Follow-up role-play and anecdotal reports suggested that treatment effects were maintained and transferred to everyday situations.

Finally, Evans and Garfield (1981) observed the approach behavior of children to spiders. Seventeen children were brought to an analogue room and invited to sit close to a jar containing a harmless garden spider. Instructions were open-ended, in that the children were permitted and even mildly encouraged to try to touch the spider and included the clear alternative of merely talking about the situation. Data were collected on approach behaviors, including the time taken to initiate the first contact (latency) and the cumulative total time in contact with the spider (contact). Results of the quasi-experimental study showed that boys evidenced higher approach behaviors than girls as a group; however, all children showed increases in approach behavior with repeated experience.

Paper-and-Pencil Measures

Besides enactment and role-play techniques, paper-and-pencil informant and self-report measures also are frequently used in the assessment of anxieties, fears, and phobias. (For a more detailed discussion of informant and self-report measures, see Breen, 1996; Eckert, Dunn, Guiney, & Codding, Chapter 11, this volume; Eckert & DuPaul, 1996; and Merrell, Chapter 9, this volume.) Although less direct than enactment and role plays, paper-and-pencil techniques present a number of advantages in comparison to more direct approaches. First, paper-and-pencil informant and self-report measures are less expensive in terms of the professional time and training needed to administer and score responses. Although specific training is still needed to accurately interpret the assessment results, the ease with which information is gathered makes them extremely time and cost efficient. Second, unlike other forms of direct assessment, paper-and-pencil informant and self-report measures can provide useful data on behaviors occurring relatively infrequently. As such, respondents can make use of observations conducted over a longer period of time as compared with enactment and role-play measures. With enactment and role-play measures, the clinician can only hope that structuring the environment will occasion the behavior or response of interest. Although less precise, informant- and self-reports allow for the summary of observations in settings like those of the analogue situations. The overlap between the two methodologies lies in the operational and behavioral description of how the questions are presented. Thus questions that are low in specificity will most likely share little variability with results from an enactment or role play. Third, paper-and-pencil informant and self-reports make use of judgements by persons who are highly familiar with the child. Parents, teachers, and even children themselves are asked to provide the type of information needed. Finally, because of the way in which they are developed, informant- and self-reports are generally more reliable, from a psychometric perspective, than most enactment and role-play methodologies.

On the downside, informant- and self-reports afford only a global description of behavior and do not provide any actual direct observational data. Because they are completed by informants, paper-and-pencil measures are subject to response and source bias (e.g., halo effects, leniency or severity in reporting, or central tendency effects) that may obfuscate or contradict findings derived from direct measures. Finally, from a treatment perspective, informant- and self-reports may be less sensitive to the situational specificity and temporal variability of behavior. As such, clinicians may have difficulty in differentiating between change that is caused by the actual treatment and that caused by the actual measurement system itself (i.e., error).

Still, paper-and-pencil informant and self-report measures are widely accepted in clinical use in the assessment of anxieties and fears. Although an exhaustive review is beyond the scope of this chapter, some more popular measures include the Child Behavior Checklist/4-18 (CBCL/4-18; Achenbach, 1991a), the Teacher's Report Form (TRF; Achenbach, 1991b), the Youth Self-Report (YSR; Achenbach, 1991c), and the Behavior Assessment System for Children (BASC; Reynolds & Kamphaus, 1992). Characterized as "broadband" behavior rating scales, these measures facilitate information gathering from multiple informants across a variety of problem areas including anxieties, fears, and phobias. One of their limitations, however, is that a relatively small sample of behavior (i.e., only about six to eight questions) is used to describe behavioral functioning across time and situations. This, as noted above, can be problematic in interpretation and does not speak directly to a child's functioning in any one setting or time.

Besides broad measures of behavioral functioning, a number of paper-and-pencil informant reports exist that allow clinicians to more closely assess, specifically, anxiety symptomatology in children. Included are the Fear Survey Schedule for Children—Revised (FSSC-R; Ollendick, 1983), the Revised Children's Manifest Anxiety Scale (RCMAS; Reynolds & Richmond, 1985), the State–Trait Anxiety Inventory for Children (STAIC; Spielberger, 1973), the Social Anxiety Scale for Children—Revised (LaGreca & Stone, 1993), the Social Phobia and Anxiety Inventory for Children (Beidel et al., 1995), and the Children's Anxiety Survey (CAS; Passarello, Hintze, Owen, & Gable, 1999; Passarello & Hintze, 1999). Finally, a somewhat unique self-report, The Fear Thermometer (Kelly, 1976) asks children to identify their level of anxiety or fear by selecting a specific color that corresponds to a facial representation of how he or she feels during a specific situation. Overall, the Fear Thermometer appears to have significant clinical utility in helping children describe, in quantifiable terms, their internal physiological states (Shapiro & Kratochwill, 1988).

Videotape Measures

Although less popular in use, videotape measures have also been used in the assessment of anxieties and fears (Dowrick, 1991, 1999). More typically used as part of an overall treatment package, the videotaping of individuals also has been used in assessing initial or baseline levels of behavioral functioning, the generalization and transfer of setting-specific skills to natural settings, assessing the amount of hidden support required to prompt a desired behavior, and the engagement or disuse of low-frequency behaviors (Dowrick, 1999).

For example, Dowrick and Dove (1980) used videotape to assess and treat the anxiety-related swimming fear of a child with spina bifida. Because spina bifida leaves a child paralyzed from the waist down, swimming and many physical activities can occasion fearful and anxiety-like signs and symptoms. In this specific case, an enactment was created using a swimming therapist as a hidden support (i.e., she was hidden from the camera angle and not part of the video). This analogue then served as the desired outcome for treatment. Progress toward goal-level performance (i.e., independent swimming) was assessed throughout the program by videotaping the child. The creation of the initial enactment analogue serves as a form of positive self-review by which clients can see and assess for themselves the ultimate or goal behavior.

Similar to real-time enactments and role plays, the use of videotape allows clinicians to assess behavioral performance in a direct manner. Its use, however, may be somewhat limited in situations where the clinician wishes to remain unobtrusive in his or her observations. Without specific assessment arrangements such as the use of a one-way mirror, the videotaping itself may be reactive and create an expectancy for behavior change that might not otherwise occur in more natural observation conditions. Nonetheless, videotaping could help in addressing some of the psychometric concerns noted earlier with enactment and role plays from an interrater perspective. That is, a subject's behavior could be videotaped and then two independent raters could score the assessment protocol based on the videotaped performance to assess interrater reliability. Clearly, further research is warranted; however, preliminary evidence suggests that videotape can be useful as an adjunct analogue assessment measure for fears and anxieties.

Depression

As with anxiety and fear, the direct assessment of depression and other mood disorders has been generally proven to be problematic. This is perhaps even more difficult with constructs such as depression—which tends to be less clearly situation specific and environmentally controlled, as many fears and anxieties tend to be— and more pervasive across a variety of situations and contexts. While some symptoms of depression are best observed directly (e.g., psychomotor agitation/retardation, weepiness, negative self-statements, social withdrawal/isolation, etc.), others, by the very nature of the definition of depression, require more indirect measures (e.g., feelings of hopelessness, dysphoric mood, irritability, etc.) (Semrud-Clikeman, 1990; Stark, 1990). Given this range of symptoms, the assessment of depression has relied most heavily on the use of direct observation in natural settings, paper-and-pencil informant reports, and interview methods. As with the assessment of anxiety, private events account for much of that which is considered to contribute to the makeup of depression.

Enactment and Role Plays

A review of the literature suggests limited use of enactments and role plays in the assessment of depression. Again, this corroborates the general notion that the signs and symptoms that contribute to the diagnosis of depression may be best accounted for in direct observations and the use of self- or informant reports. Interestingly, however, role plays and enactments have been used in the cognitive–behavioral treatment of depression. For example, Butler, Miezitis, Friedman, and Cole (1980) used role-play techniques in a treatment comparison study also involving cognitive restructuring, attention–placebo, and control conditions. Role-play sessions focused on acceptance and rejection by peers, success and failure, guilt and self-blame, and loneliness. Each session focused on sensitizing the child to personal thoughts and feelings, and to those of others; teaching skills to facilitate social interaction; and teaching a problem-solving approach to threatening or stressful situations by learning to generate multiple potential solutions to the problem. Results suggested a significant reduction in depressive symptoms for those children who received either role-play or cognitive restructuring treatments when compared with attention–placebo or control conditions, with those children who received role-play that displayed the greatest reduction in symptom relief.

In another behaviorally oriented case study, Frame, Matson, Sonis, Fialkov, and Kazdin (1982) used role plays in the treatment of a 10-year-old boy who had been hospitalized for major depression and suicidal ideation. As part of an overall treatment package, poor eye contact, inaudible speech, one-word answers, bland facial expressions, and body posturing were targeted for intervention. Treatment consisted of direct instruction, modeling, rehearsal, and feedback. Training was conducted daily for 20-minute intervals in enactment and role-play situations. Targeted behaviors were treated sequentially in a multiple baseline design across behaviors. Results suggested substantial improvement in targeted behaviors that were maintained over a 12-week period.

Finally, Bellak, Kay, and Murrill (1989) reported on the use of an apparatus similar to the Fear Thermometer, called the Dysphorimeter. Based on the premise that it is sometimes difficult for an individual to communicate verbally the exact severity of a subjective state such as depression, anhedonia, pain, or anxiety, the Dysphorimeter in its simplest form contains a tube that sits on a base plate. A slot in the tube permits a selector-slide to be moved up and down. This lateral slot is marked off into ten equidistant marker stops with the number 1 at the top of the meter and the number 10 at the bottom of the meter. Furthermore, each marker stop is paired with an audible tone. For example, a neutral tone is presented at the number 1 and an increasingly unpleasant, screeching tone for each successive movement of the selector-slide toward the number 10. The basic instructions to the individual are to move the selector-slide down until it matches the experienced degree of depression (anxiety, pain, etc.). At each assessment occasion, the subject indicates the level of discomfort three times in succession with the mean of the three ratings serving as the outcome datum for that session. Measures are taken repeatedly during treatment as an evaluation of treatment outcomes. Test–retest reliability of the Dysphorimeter is reportedly strong (ranging from .82 to .98). However, criterion-related validity estimates were found to be highly variable with self-report measures ranging from .37 to .70 for depression, and .27 to .35 for anxiety-related disorders (Bellak et al., 1989).

Paper-and-Pencil Measures

As with the assessment of anxiety and fears, there are currently available a number of paper-and-pencil informant report measures in the area of depression. Besides the broadband informant rating scales noted previously (Achenbach Scales and the BASC), a number of narrowband instruments aimed specifically at assessing depression have been developed. To date, most measures are self-report in format and include the Children's Depression Inventory (CDI; Kovacs, 1992), the Reynolds Child Depression Scale (RCDS; Reynolds, 1989), the Reynolds Adolescent Depression Scale (RADS; Reynolds, 1987), and the Child Behavior Checklist Depression Scale (CBCL-D; Clarke, Lewinsohn, Hops & Seeley, 1992).

Besides informant and self-report, several sociometric methods are available for the assessment of depression. The foremost instrument for peer identification is the Peer Nomination Inventory for Depression (PNID; Lefkowitz & Tesiny, 1980). This measure consists of 14 items for depressive behaviors, two items for popularity, and two items for happiness. For each PNID item, the child's score is his or her number of peer nominations divided by the total number of students in the classroom. Factor analytic research on the PNID suggests the presence of four separate factors. Three of the factors are related to depression (i.e., inadequacy, loneliness, and dejection) and the other factor to happiness. Using a similar methodology, the Teacher Nomination Inventory for Depression (TNID; Lefkowitz & Tesiny, 1980) provides teacher ratings of all children in the classroom and can be used in screening much like the PNID.

Videotape Measures

As with anxiety and fears, recent use of videotape is also found in the area of depression. However, as with role plays and enactments, the use of videotape has typically been used as both an assessment device and an intervention aid. For example, as part of a larger treatment comparison study, Kahn, Kehle, Jenson, and Clark (1990) used both enactments and videotape in the assessment and treatment of depression of adolescent boys and girls. Through coaching and enactments, subjects were videotaped looking nondepressed (e.g., were well dressed with hair combed and told to smile, talk in an optimistic manner, etc.), which served as a template for intervention and continued assessment. Results suggested that the use of enactments and videotape was equally effective as compared with cognitive–behavioral therapy and relaxation training in the reduction of depressive symptomatolgy.

Similarly, Dowrick and Jesdale (1990; as cited in Dowrick, 1999) videotaped five- to 10-minute conversations of 32 mildly depressed women. Subjects were encouraged to choose topics of conversation that were pleasant to them while an interviewer socially reinforced smiles, animated speech, and other indications of pleasure. As in the Kahn et al. study, the videotaped enactment served as both an initial self-assessment device and a template for use in ongoing assessment and intervention. Once videotaped, half the women were instructed to view their videotape while the other half were given a videotape of a pleasant countryside and soothing music. Results suggested significant improvements in mood for those women who viewed videotapes of themselves versus those who watched nonspecific videotapes.

Summary and Conclusions

The use of a variety of analogue measures is quite common in the assessment of emotional problems such as anxiety, depression, fears, and phobias. Interestingly, a review of the literature suggests a possible decrease in the use of enactment and role-play measures with a concomitant rise in the use of paper-and-pencil measures and videotape methodologies. One plausible explanation for this observation may be a leveling-off of originality and innovation in the areas of enactments and role plays. That is, once described in sufficient detail, replications of their use may not find their way into the research literature. Furthermore, the last decade has witnessed a veritable explosion of self- and informant-report measures in the areas of emotional concern. Besides the time and cost involved with analogue measures, psychometric advances in test development have now enabled a new generation of paper-and-pencil measures previously unavailable. Whereas previous paper-and-pencil measures of child functioning were of dubious psychometric quality (and often modified versions of adult measures), contemporary behavioral assessment allows for a wide range of psychometrically sound instruments designed specifically for use in child assessment.

Nevertheless, the use of enactments and role plays continues to provide a vital source of direct assessment information not available by other means. Generally less intrusive and more time efficient than systematic direct observation, enactment and role-play assessment methodologies lend themselves quite well to use by a variety of school-based professionals. Standardization of the procedures, however, continues to be a main weakness and calls into question the reliability of the measures (Barrios et al., 1981; Johnson & Melamed, 1979; Morris & Kratochwill, 1983). The fact that most investigations create their own enactments and role plays procedures makes comparisons across studies quite difficult (Kendall & Ronan, 1990). Other problems include the lack of specific instructions provided to assessors, format for arranging the environment, and scoring procedures (Barrios & Shigetomi, 1985). Furthermore, some have questioned the validity of the procedures themselves. That is, to what extent can a child's response under a highly controlled assessment situation be generalized to the natural environment? This weakness in external validity—common across all analogue measures—clearly suggests the need for other types of assessment procedures (cf. Shapiro & Kratochwill, 1988).

Limitations aside, enactments and role plays offer several advantages not found in other assessment strategies. Because the assessment situation is highly structured and controlled, the internal validity of observed outcomes is enhanced. Since possible confounding variables and artifacts of bias are held to a minimum, functional relationships are more likely to be captured between observed behavior and the operating environmental contingencies. As such, enactments and role plays are more likely to be sensitive to behavioral changes over time. Since such procedures are often linked to intervention—behavioral changes are a direct result of treatment effects and little inference needs be made between what has been done and observed. Clearly, when combined with other measures functioning (e.g., systematic direct observation informant and self-report) enactments and role plays provide a strong source of multimethod information that can be used across a variety of emotional concerns.

SOCIAL–BEHAVIORAL CONCERNS

Noncompliance

Broadly conceptualized, noncompliance refers to the basic refusal to initiate or complete a request made by another person or the refusal to follow direct or implied rules or accepted standards of behavior (Forehand & McMahon, 1981). Although a quite common behavior pattern of most children from time to time, severe manifestation of noncompliance (and other similar forms of conflict between caregivers and children) has been found to have a strong relationship with the development of adolescent and adult psychological problems (Patterson, Reid, & Dishion, 1992).

As with emotional difficulties, the direct assessment of compliance in the natural setting may be problematic. Like anxiety disorders—which often share a strong functional relationship with specific environmental conditions—the frequency with which episodes of noncompliance are observed may be infrequent. In addition, like anxiety, noncompliance is often maintained by negative reinforcement. That is, a child is likely to engage in any one of a number of behaviors in order to escape or avoid something that they perceive as aversive—often a demand or request. Consequently, enactments and role plays are often well suited to the assessment of noncompliance because the clinician can structure scenarios that have a high probability of occasioning the noncompliant response.

Enactments and Role Plays

Several procedures have been developed for recording parent–child interactions in analogue settings. Of the earliest, the Child's Game and the Parent's Game (Forehand & McMahon, 1981) involve a parent and a child being observed in a playroom that contains various age-appropriate toys, such as building blocks, toy trucks and cars, dolls, puzzles, crayons, and paper. In the Child's Game, the parent is instructed to engage in any activity that the child chooses and to allow the child to decide the nature and rules of play. Thus the Child's Game serves as a free-play situation. In the Parent's Game, the parent is instructed to engage the child in activities whose rules and nature are determined by the parent. In this instance, the Parent's Game serves as a command situation. Each situation is observed for five minutes and inter-actions are systematically recorded. Parent behaviors of interest include: approval statement and physical attention; social attention; questioning; commands; warnings; and time-outs. Child behaviors of note include compliance, noncompliance, and inappropriate behaviors, including whining, yelling, tantrums, aggression, and devi-ant talk. Overall, the assessment system demonstrates adequate reliability and has been shown to discriminate between clinic-referred and nonclinic-referred children, besides being highly related to and predictive of behavior at home.

In a modified version of Forehand and McMahon's analogue assessment, Barkley (1987) has developed a similar parent–child enactment, titled the Response Class Matrix, which requires the parent to issue a series of ten commands. Both parent and child are taken to a playroom that contains a sofa, coffee table, armchair, several small worktables, an adult's desk chair, and a child's desk chair. Toys are set out on a table for play purposes. In addition, magazines are provided on a coffee table. After an initial five-minute habituation period, the parent is instructed to issue a series of commands (e.g., "Give me one of those toys," "Put the toys and their boxes on the shelves," etc.). Data are recorded in one-minute samples. Within each minute the observer notes that a command was issued, whether and how often a command needed to be reissued, whether or not the child complied with the directive, and if the child displayed opposition, refusal, whining, complaining, or behavior resistant to the command, and whether the parent reinforced compliance or yelled, reprimanded, or behaved negatively toward the child. Once collected, data are summarized by (1) number of parents' commands per minute, (2) number of repeat commands per original command, (3) child compliance percent, (4) percent of child negative be-haviors per command, (5) number of parent approvals per minute, and (6) number of parent negative behaviors per minute. Although sensitive to parent–child inter-actions in clinic settings, the Response Class Matrix requires a high level of training. In addition, reliability information is missing, although the instrument has been found to be sensitive to treatment gains (Barkley, 1990).

Another enactment analogue, The Compliance Test (CT; Roberts & Powers, 1988) also involves the use of standardized instructions and commands. Like other compliance analogues, parent and child are placed in a playroom stocked with distractor toys, instruction-designated toys (e.g., animals, cars, blocks, dolls), and instruction-designated containers (e.g., cardboard box, doll house, toy truck). Fol-lowing a habituation period, the child is told by the parent that they are going to be asked to do things and that doing them right away is important for them. Following this, 30 standardized instructions are presented to the child (e.g., "[Johnny,] put the [toy] in the [container]"). This is facilitated by having the parent wear an earpiece in order to hear the directions provided by a clinician stationed behind a one-way mir-ror. After presentation of the instruction, the behavior of the child is observed for five seconds and initiation of compliance is noted. Compliance is defined as a con-tinuous motor behavior initiated within the five-second postinstruction interval that terminated in grasping the instruction-designated toy. A child's compliance ratio is defined as the number of compliant responses divided by 30, (the number of instructions issued). In comparison to other role-play or enactment procedures, the CT is well researched and presents strong psychometric characteristics. In a study of 231 children, Roberts and Powers reported interobserver agreement ratios greater than 97% and an internal consistency reliability of .99 (KR – 20 = .99). Criterion-related validity is reportedly high with other measures of within session behavior (e.g., –.553 with negative child verbalizations) and with other clinic-based analogues $r = .537$).

For adolescents, the Parent–Adolescent Interaction Coding System (PAICS; Robin & Foster, 1989) allows for the observation of parent–teen interactions in a role-play arrangement. As conducted, the parent and the adolescent are asked to engage in a problem-centered discussion of three topic areas: (1) a neutral discussion (e.g., where to go on vacation), (2) a discussion of an area of disagreement (e.g., curfew time), and (3) a positive discussion (e.g., the most positive characteristic of the other discussant). Discussions may be audiotaped or videotaped. Following discussions, data are summarized using simple global behavioral codes (i.e., positive, negative, neutral) for each participant, or in more detail using six mutually exclusive categories (i.e., "puts down/commands," "defends/complains," "facilitates," "problem solves," "defines/evaluates," and "talks"). The PAICS shows adequate interobserver agreement and has been shown to discriminate between distressed and nondistressed families (Robin & Foster, 1989). Like the Response Class Matrix, however, the PAICS requires considerable observer training for everyday use. Nonetheless, observation of communication patterns provides useful information for both initial assessment and ongoing monitoring of treatment progress.

Paper-and-Pencil Measures

Besides enactments and role plays a number of paper-and-pencil measures are currently available for the assessment of compliance. In addition to the broadband informant rating scales noted previously (Achenbach Scales and the BASC), a number of narrowband instruments aimed specifically at assessing compliance have been developed. Included are the Disruptive Behavior Disorders Rating Scale—Parent Form, the Disruptive Behavior Disorders Rating Scale—Teacher Form, the Home Situations Questionnaire, and the School Situations Questionnaire, all available in Barkley (1997). Finally, both the Eyberg Child Behavior Inventory (ECBI; Eyberg, 1980) and the Conflict Behavior Questionnaire (CBQ; Robin & Foster, 1989) have subscales designed to measure the degree of conflict and, with the CBQ, the quality of communication in parent–child relationships.

Aggressive Behavior

Aggressive behavior toward peers is a common complaint of parents and teachers of young children (Campbell, 1998). Although overlapping considerably with compliance issues noted previously, aggression typically refers to verbal and physical hostility directed toward others. With noncompliance, aggression is often considered an early critical indicator for adolescent maladjustment (Patterson et al., 1992). Existing research suggests that the mechanism for the development and maintenance of aggression in children may occur as a result of the combination of early negative temperament (e.g., irritability, quickness to anger, low frustration tolerance) with disordered parental and family functioning (Barkley, 1990). For instance, the work of Patterson and colleagues (Patterson, 1982; Patterson et al., 1992) suggests that the use of coercion (unpredictable, often noncontingent aversive verbal and physical exchanges) in parent–child interactions lead to the child's adopting an aggressive behavioral repertoire as a means of successfully escaping or avoiding unwanted, tedious, or aversive intrusions of others. Like compliance, the strong relationship between aggression and the environment make it well suited to analogue assessment methodologies.

Enactments and Role Plays

In behaviorally oriented assessment, the most common approach to assessing aggression involves the use of a standardized functional analysis enactment methodology (Gable, Hendrickson, & Sasso, 1995). The goal of such assessment is to determine the operant variables in the environment that control aggressive and other aberrant behavior. Based on the work of Iwata and colleagues (1982, 1990) and Carr and Durand (1985), the analogue conditions consist of a number of different arrangements, each designed to test a specific hypothesized relationship between the environment and resultant aggressive behavior.

For example, Gable et al. (1995) describe the use of five different arrangements or analogue conditions. In the *attention (gain)* condition, the examiner and the child together enter a therapy room that contains a wide variety of preferred toys. The child is instructed to play alone while the examiner, seated several feet away, pretends to do some work (i.e., read or write). Contingent on each instance of an aggressive target behavior (e.g., throwing a toy, yelling at the examiner), the examiner provides social attention in the manner of a reprimand or disapproving statement (e.g., "Don't throw your toys, you'll break them."). All other behaviors are ignored by the examiner. This condition is designed to assess social attention as a variable that maintains aggression. In the second condition, *tangible (gain)*, the child is directed to engage in a specific task (e.g., write the alphabet) with preferred toys, edibles, or desired activities with view. Each occurrence of the aggressive target behavior (e.g., throwing, hitting) results in the preferred items being made available to the child. In this condition, if the aggressive behavior occurs at a high rate it is likely controlled by tangible reinforcers. The third condition, *demand (escape)*, the child and the examiner are seated at a table. Tasks are selected that the child is capable of completing but finds difficult to do. A three-step, least-to-most-guided compliance procedure is employed with the presentation of each task. If the child engages in the aggressive target behaviors at any time during task presentation, the task is removed and the examiner walks away. Following termination of the aggressive behavior, the examiner reintroduces the task. The condition assesses the role of negative reinforcement or escape in the maintenance of aggressive responses.

The fourth condition in the evaluation process attempts to assess whether aggression varies as a function of being ignored. Termed the *ignore* condition, the child and the examiner are placed into the therapy room with no sources of potential reinforcement (e.g., toys, etc.). The examiner does not respond to the child under any circumstances. The rationale for this condition is that some behaviors may be maintained by a lack of sensory stimulation. If the frequency of aggressive target behaviors is high, lack of sensory stimulation is inferred. Finally, the fifth condition, *toy play (control)*, once again places the examiner and child together with access to a number of preferred toys. The child is allowed to play alone or cooperatively and is occasionally prompted to engage in play activities. Rather than provide social disapproval contingent on aggressive behaviors, the examiner ignores the child each time an aggressive behavior is exhibited. In addition, the examiner provides frequent (approximately every 30 seconds) social praise and attention for behaving appropriately. This condition is designed to act as a control condition to the other phases of assessment.

Each assessment condition is conducted for 10 minutes. The examiner can determine the order of presentation of the conditions. Data are summarized for each condition using either frequency/event or interval recording. Visual representation of the data for each condition provides the basis for assessment and treatment recommendations. To account for order effects or more closely inspect variability in data, replication of specific conditions enable the examiner to place greater confidence in the assessment results.

An example of a functional analytic enactment assessment is provided by Northup et al. (1991). Three individuals who exhibited aggressive and self-injurious behaviors were assessed in an analogue arrangement that focused on identifying maintaining contingencies for aggressive behavior. Results of each analogue assessment showed that each individual displayed substantially greater frequency of aggressive behavior during one condition than during any other. Analogue conditions were similar to those proposed by Gable et al. (1995). For example, one individual displayed aggressive behavior during escape conditions only, the second individual during tangible and escape conditions, and the third during escape and attention conditions. Once maintaining contingencies were identified, a contingency reversal phase was instituted such that the contingency that produced the highest percentage of aggressive behavior was presented for the occurrence of specific alternative prosocial behaviors. Results of continuous analogue assessments showed that when contingencies were reversed, each individual displayed substantial reductions in aggressive behaviors and increases in alternative prosocial behaviors.

In an interesting arrangement using teachers as the examiners, Sasso et al. (1992) evaluated the aggressive behavior of two children with autism. Once trained, teachers conducted analogue assessments using conditions again similar to Gable et al. (1995). Results of the analogue functional assessments showed that for both students, aggression was maintained primarily by escape from task demands to engage in more preferred activities. Importantly, reliability data indicated that for the dependent measures (i.e., measures of aggression) the average agreement was 84% (range, 71.3%–91.1%). Furthermore, the procedural reliability (the extent to which teachers were able to effectively implement the analogue procedures) averaged 90% (range, 85.2%–100%). Once maintaining contingencies were identified for each student, an intervention was designed such that aggressive behavior was no longer reinforced using a combination of positive reinforcement, response cost, and guided compliance. Results showed reductions in aggressive behaviors with concomitant increases in on-task behavior. Acceptability ratings completed by the teachers suggested high acceptability for the analogue assessment methodologies. Reportedly, teachers' acceptability ratings were influenced most by the effectiveness of the analogue procedures in identifying the maintaining contingencies for aggression and the resultant decreases in the rated level of classroom disruption.

Paper-and-Pencil Measures

As with emotional concerns and compliance issues, a variety of paper-and-pencil measures are available for the assessment of aggression. Again, perhaps the most common are the broadband behavior rating scales, which include factors related to the construct of aggression (e.g., Achenbach and BASC scales). In addition, the Conner's teacher, parent, and adolescent long report forms all contain constructs that represent oppositional, aggressive, and anger-control problems (CTRS-R:L, CPRS-R:L, CASS:L; Conners, 1997).

Finally, the use of peer nominations has also been suggested using a typical format by which children are asked to nominate the child in the class who "starts fights the most." Peer nominations of aggression have been shown to be correlated with psychiatric diagnoses of conduct disorder and are highly stable over time. For example, Huesmann, Eron, Lefkowitz, and Walder (1984), in a study spanning 22 years, found that early aggressiveness was predictive of later serious antisocial behavior, including criminal behavior, spousal abuse, traffic violations, and socialized acts of aggression. Using a peer nomination index of aggression, more than six-hundred subjects beginning in the third grade were asked to report on peer aggression by nominating other children, "Who push or shove other children?" and similar questions. Each child's aggression score was calculated by a percentage of how many questions they were nominated for. Internal consistency estimates for the procedures were reported to be extremely high (coefficient alpha = .96) with concomitant test–retest reliability of .91. In a similar study, Coie, Dodge, and Coppotelli (1982) found social preference to be inversely related to aggression. Furthermore, those children identified by their peer as aggressive were more likely to be of controversial status, that is, they were perceived as being disruptive and aggressive, as well as viewed in some manner as leaders.

Summary and Conclusions

As with emotional concerns, the use of analogue measures may be quite useful for social–behavioral concerns such as noncompliance and aggression. However, unlike some emotional disorders (e.g., anxiety and depression), the use of enactments and role plays continues to be quite common in the assessment of clinical treatment outcomes. At least one reason for this may be that, comparatively speaking, the behavioral treatment of externalizing disorders such as noncompliance and aggression is relatively more recent than that of internalizing disorders overall. Indeed, the work of Barkley (1987, 1997) and Forehand and McMahon (1981) represent some of the earliest and most often cited work in the field. This, combined with the burgeoning work in the experimental analysis of behavior (e.g., Carr & Newsome, 1985; Northup et al., 1991) has led to a reconceptualization of the nature of social and behavioral concerns that fully appreciates the interactional nature of the problem. Given this perspective, more direct forms of assessment that include various forms of enactments and role plays provide a type of data that cannot be gathered from paper-and-pencil measures alone.

SOCIAL RELATIONSHIP CONCERNS

Social Skills and Competence

Over the past several decades children and adolescents with emotional and behavior problems have been shown to experience social relationship difficulties at higher rates than their typically developing peers. This relationship has been particularly well documented with children presenting with aggressive and antisocial behavior patterns (Patterson et al., 1992) and children presenting with attention-deficit/hyperactivity disorder (ADHD) (Barkley, 1990). These social difficulties can lead to impairments in developing and maintaining relationships with parents, teachers, peers, and others.

The term *social skills* has been defined in a variety of ways. More recently, a differentiation has been made between what are referred to as "social skills" versus "social competence." Simply, social skills are defined as discrete, learned behaviors exhibited by an individual for the purpose of performing a task (Sheridan & Walker, 1999). Children with social skill deficits do not have the necessary social skills in their repertoires or have not learned the critical steps in the performance of a behavioral sequence (Gresham, 1988). For example, a child may not know how to take turns in playing a game, join into a group, or greet someone. Social competence, however, is primarily concerned with the evaluative judgements of others (Gresham, 1986). In practice, social competence has generally referred to the global judgements and descriptions used by others to describe the behavior of a child.

Although it remains unclear whether the nature of the relationship between emotional/behavior problems and social difficulties is primarily causal, correlational, or simply concomitant (see Gresham, 1992, for a discussion of these types of relations), the importance of social problems among these children is quite clear. Impaired social relationships are highly correlated with suboptimal academic, social, emotional, and occupational outcomes (Elliott, Sheridan, & Gresham, 1989). In addition, poor peer relationships have been shown to be relatively stable over time (Coie et al., 1982) and predictive of later adult psychopathology. Moreover, social skill and competence difficulties have been linked to poor academic adjustment for children both with (McKinney & Speece, 1983) and without disabilities (Hoge & Luce, 1979).

Enactment and Role Plays

As with the assessment of other emotional and behavioral concerns, situational role plays and enactments have demonstrated practical utility in the assessment of social skills. As with other types of role-play measures, in its most typical form, a child is presented with a specific interpersonal situation and is asked to respond as if the situation were actually occurring. The response of the target child is then observed and recorded with respect to some predetermined set of response alternatives. Role plays are created which represent the types of situations with which the target child has difficulty (Shapiro & Kratochwill, 1988). In one excellent example, Bornstein, Bellack, and Hersen (1977) developed the Behavioral Assertiveness Test for Children (BAT-C). The BAT-C consists of nine scenes—five of which involve a same-sex role model and four of which involve an opposite-sex role model. As conducted, the child is first presented with an initial practice scene and description of what the role play will entail. Following this, the nine assessment scenes are presented as follows: (1) the narrator presents the scene, (2) the role model presents a prompt (a standard lead-in line), (3) the child then responds to the role model. For example, in one scene designed for a male target child the narrator describes a scene in which "You're in school and you brought your chair to another classroom to watch a movie. You go out to get a drink of water. When you come back, Mike is sitting in your seat." Once set, the role play continues with the role model (typically a confederate to the situation) exclaiming, "I'm sitting here." The response of the target child is observed and scored along four dimensions: (1) the ratio of eye contact to speech duration, (2) loudness of speech, (3) requests for new behavior, and (4) an overall assertiveness rating.

   More recent examples of situational role plays are offered by Elliott and Gresham (1991). As one part of a multimethod approach to the assessment of social skills, the authors have identified five specific domains of generalized social behavior that should be assessed in children suspected of exhibiting social skill problems. The first domain, *Cooperation*, is subdivided into a working and playing domain and a classroom interaction domain. Role plays here include ignoring distractions from classmates when doing classwork and paying attention to and following the teacher's instructions. The second domain, *Assertion*, includes both conversation and joining and volunteering subdomains. Examples of role plays here include giving a compliment to a peer, introducing oneself to a new person, and inviting others to join an activity. The *Responsibility* domains asks the target child to respond to situations such as questioning rules that may be unfair and refusing unreasonable requests from others. The *Empathy* domain is once again subdivided and assesses various prosocial skills such as nonverbally greeting and acknowledging others and listening to others when they are talking. The final, and fifth domain examines various *Self-Control* skills and is subdivided into conflict-resolution and anger-control skills. For each role play the target child is asked to (1) define the skill being prompted, (2) tell why the skill is important, (3) state the skill steps and repeat them with the examiner, and (4) demonstrate the skill within the context of the situational analogue. Although no specific scoring rules are employed, data are recorded using naturalistic observation skills on each of the four child-prompted requests.

In addition to role plays, enactments can also be used in the assessment of social skills. However, unlike role plays where targeted responses are prompted and highly contrived, enactments allow response patterns to vary freely in a more naturalistic environment. Typically enactment assessments of social skills would involve systematic observations of social behavior within the natural environment. Using the methods of systematic direct observation and behavioral assessment, specific target behaviors are operationally defined and measured within an ongoing, natural context. Walker and Severson (1992) illustrated the use of such enactments in a multiple-gating procedure for identifying children with social and behavioral concerns. As part of the assessment, target children are systematically observed on the playground and the frequency of positive and negative social behaviors recorded. For example, *social-engagement* is defined as the exchange of social signals between the target child and another that involves either verbal or nonverbal interaction. *Participation* is coded when the target child is observed participating in a game or activity, with two or more peers, that has a clearly specified and agreed-upon set of rules. *Parallel play* is noted each time the target child is observed engaged in some activity within five feet of another child, but is not interacting either verbally or nonverbally with him/her.

Of the two, enactment has been found to be a more valid and sensitive measure of overall social behavior (Gresham, 1998). Because it reflects the behavior as it occurs in the naturally occurring environment, direct observation of social behavior correlates better than role plays with other behavioral assessment strategies such as interviews, informant reports, and peer nominations and ratings. In general, social skill role plays have been found to have low external validity in comparison to naturalistic observation and lower reliability (DuPaul & Eckert, 1994; Van Hasselt, Hersen, & Bellack, 1981).

Paper-and-Pencil Measures

In addition to role plays and enactments, various paper-and-pencil measures have been frequently used to assess the peer status and social acceptance of children (Asher, 1990). Perhaps the most common of the paper-and-pencil techniques are the sociometric assessment strategies. In its most typical use, sociometric techniques involve the use of either peer nominations or ratings.

The basic procedure in using peer nominations is to have children nominate peers according to certain nonbehavioral criteria (Gresham & Elliott, 1984). For example, children are asked to nominate other children along dimensions such as best friends, preferred play partners, work partners, or physical attributes. As such, nomination procedures assess children's attitudes or preferences for engaging in certain activities with specified peers rather than specific behaviors or target children (Gresham & Elliott, 1984). Peer nomination can also be used to evaluate negative criteria such as least-liked peers, or least-preferred play or work partners.

One of the most frequently used sociometric models was developed by Coie et al. (1982). Based on the use of standard scores derived from peer nominations using both positive and negative evaluative statements, children are classified along one of five sociometric status groups: (1a) popular, (2) neglected, (3) rejected, (4) controversial, and (5) average. Simply, each child in a class is asked to select from all other children in the class, three peers they like most and three peers that they like least. For each student, all peer nominations are summed to yield a like most (LM) and liked least (LL) scores. These scores are then used to calculate social preference (SP) and social impact (SI) scores. Social preference is found by subtracting the liked least score from the liked most score (SP = LM – LL). Social impact is derived by adding the liked most score to the liked least score (SI = LM + LL).

Responses are interpreted by standardizing the scores for the entire class on each variable (standardized scores should have a mean [M] of 0 and a standard deviation [SD] of 1). Once standardized, an individual child's score can be determined relative to other students in the class. Sociometric status groups are classified according to the following criteria: (1) *popular* includes children receiving a social preference (SP) score greater than 1.00, a liked most (LM) score of greater than 0, and a liked least (LL) score of less than 0; (2) *controversial* consists of children who receive social impact (SI) scores greater than 1.00, and liked least (LL) and liked most (LM) scores greater than 0; (3) *neglected* consists of children who receive a social impact (SI) score of less than –1.00 and an absolute liked most (LM) score of 0; (4) *rejected* includes children receiving a social preference (SP) score less than –1.00, a liked least (LL) score greater than 0, and a liked most (LM) score less than 0; and (5) *average* refers to children who fall at or around the mean of the social preference (SP) and social impact (SI) dimensions.

In another example, Bower (1969) described the use of The Class Play. In this assessment technique, children are asked to assign other class members to various roles, both positive and negative, in an imaginary play. For example, children might be asked to cast peers in the part of a character who is "too bossy," "a born leader," and so forth. In the original scoring, the total number of negative roles assigned to a child is divided by the total number of assigned roles overall. High percentages indicate elevated levels of peer rejection and lower percentages suggest higher social status.

The "guess who" technique is another sociometric measure whereby brief descriptive personality characteristic statements are provided to children. Each child is then asked to write down the names of other children in their class who fit the description (Merrell, 1999). For example, a child may be asked to list who "is the teacher's pet," "fights with other children," or "does best in their schoolwork." The content of the descriptive statements can be developed by the teacher or practitioner, based on the specific characteristics that they are interested in identifying. Scoring is completed by a simple frequency count for each child on each descriptive statement.

In comparison to peer nomination procedures, peer rating procedures require each child within the class to respond to a sociometric question for each and all other children in the class. In its most typical form, each child in the class is provided with a class roster and a list of sociometric statements. Each child in the class is then asked to rate all other children in the class on each sociometric statement on a five-point scale (Connolly, 1983). For example, a child may be asked to evaluate the extent to which they would like to "play with" or "work with" each other child in the class, on a scale from (1) "not at all" to (5) "very much" (Merrell, 1999).

In an extension of peer ratings, teachers are asked to rank-order each child in the class according to some sociometric criteria (Merrell, 1999). For example, all the children in the class might be rank-ordered from highest to lowest on attributes such as "popularity" or "disruptiveness." As an alternative, a teacher might be first asked to identify all those children who fit a particular social or behavioral description (e.g., disruptiveness), and then to rank-order those children from highest to lowest with respect to the particular attribute. In this case, not all children are ranked.

In addition to sociometrics, a number of informant- and self-report rating scales are available for the assessment of social behavior and skills. As with other emotional and behavioral areas of development, informant and self-ratings represent a useful and efficient method for summarizing social behavior. One in particular, The Social Skills Ratings System (SSRS; Gresham & Elliott, 1990) requires raters to rate both the frequency and importance of particular social skills. Importance ratings are made based on how important the informant feels the behavior is for success in the classroom (teacher version), toward the child's development (parent version), or to relationships with other children (student version).

Besides the SSRS, other ratings scales are also available. However, unlike the SSRS, these scales employ only teachers as informants, which limits the scope of what is reported. Included here are the Walker–McConnell Scale of Social Competence and School Adjustment (WMS; Walker & McConnell, 1988), the School Social Behavior Scales (SSBS; Merrell, 1993), the Social Behavior Assessment Inventory (SBAI; Stephens & Arnold, 1992), the School Social Skills Rating Scale (S³; Brown, Black, & Downs, 1984); and the Waksman Social Skills Rating Scale (WSSRS; Waksman, 1985). An excellent comprehensive review of social skills rating scales can be found in Demaray et al. (1995).

Videotape Measures

In an example of the use of videotape in the analogue assessment of social skills, Hughes et al. (1989) created a pool of 28 social vignettes whereby a child model was videotaped delivering a social prompt. Half of the vignettes represent scenes calling for positive assertion (e.g., giving and receiving positive compliments), with the other half calling for negative assertion (e.g., standing up for one's own rights and denying an unreasonable request) on the part of the target child. The response to each scene is rated on the basis of how effective the response is relative to children of similar age as the target child. A rating of 3 indicates an effective response, a 2 indicates a response that is neither effective nor ineffective, and a 1 indicates an ineffective response. The authors report that the test has been validated on 157 fourth- and fifth-grade boys and girls who had been classified as popular, average, neglected, or rejected on the basis of sociometric testing. Overall, the videotape vignettes evidenced good interrater ($r = .99$), test–retest ($r = .84$ over a 3- to 4-week period), and internal consistency reliabilities ($r = .79$). In addition, children's role-play responses correlated significantly with teacher ratings of social competence ($r = .–.29$), and with peer sociometric ratings ($r = .22$ for popularity and $r = .21$ for sustaining friendships). Interestingly, however, like standard situational role plays, teacher ratings of children's social behavior continues to differentiate among social status groups better than the videotaped role plays.

In a similar manner, Irvin et al. (1992) developed a videodisc assessment device that assesses domains of social behavior such as peer group entry, teasing and provocation, and compliance with teacher directives. Each domain is then further subdivided into different configurations. For example, the peer group entry domain is subdivided into peer free activity: group competitive—drop-the-flag game; dyadic competitive—darts game; and dyadic cooperative—puzzle completion. Each vignette is shown to the target child. The first response assessed is labeled *cue recognition*, which represents the target child's assessment of when is the "best time" to join into the ongoing video. For example, any natural break in the activity would be a correct time to try to join in, where, for example, during an argument over the rules would not be a good time to join in. Once done, the assessment focuses on response alternatives. For instance, target children are asked to choose from five different possible joining-in strategies—two externalizing (e.g., aggress, brag), two internalizing (e.g., hover, wait until too late), and one appropriate (ask at first natural break). Each alternative is presented on the video in an interactive manner. For each strategy, target children are asked, "Would you do this?" and are asked to respond on the video screen to "yes," "no," or "maybe." Following this, the video tests knowledge of likely consequences. For example, target children are asked, "Would other kids let you join in if you did this?" for each selected strategy. Finally, for each option to which the target child responded "yes" or "maybe", the assessment asks the examinee to make judgements as to how other children would react if the particular joining-in strategy were used and about the relative friendliness or hostility of the potential reaction. Reliability for the videodisc test are reported as .70 to .90 for total and subscale scores for 2-week to 6-month time intervals. Moreover, an internal consistency (alpha) of .90 is reported. Validity work on the test, however, is still being conducted.

Social–Cognitive and Interpersonal Problem Solving

Social–cognitive functioning in children involves their beliefs and perceptions surrounding daily interactions with others, including how successful or unsuccessful they are being in given situations, how others perceive their social acumen, and how others experience and react to given situations. The accuracy (or inaccuracy) of these perceptions, and the degree to which they correspond with those of peers, parents, and teachers appears to play an important role in shaping the social behavior and functioning of children with emotional and behavior problems (Dodge, Pettit, McClaskey, & Brown, 1986; Lochman, Dunn, & Klimes-Dougan, 1993). For example, aggressive children have been shown to misinterpret a peer's intent as hostile during social interactions (Patterson et al., 1992), and children with ADHD appear to consistently overrate their social acumen and social status (Diener & Milich, 1997; Milich & Okazaki, 1991). Such inaccurate judgments in the context of social relationship development can produce disastrous effects on decisions, choices, and outcomes for these children (see Rachlin, 1989 for a cognitive–behavioral discussion of the relationship between judgment, decision, choice, and outcomes).

Enactments and Role Plays

In comparison to most of the work compiled in the area of social skills, the use of situational analogues in the area of social-cognition and interpersonal problem solving has been focused more in the area of intervention than assessment. However, given the lack of bifurcation with respect to these two areas in behavioral assessment, a review of some of the intervention literature in this area may be helpful. Perhaps the best example of the use of situational analogues in the area of social–cognitive interpersonal problem solving comes from the extensive work of Goldstein (1999). Over the course of 20 years, Goldstein has developed a number of enactments and role plays aimed at the assessment and treatment of social misperception, anger control, moral reasoning, stress management, problem solving, and empathy training. The most recent rendition of this work is represented in The Prepare Curriculum (Goldstein, 1999), which contains a compilation of situational role plays for use in social cognition and interpersonal problem solving. In one example of situational perception training titled "The Right Time and Place," two students and the teacher act out a scene where one child observes the other stealing money from the teacher's purse while she is out of the room. When the teacher returns to the room the child who observes the stealing publicly announces what he saw. The boy accused of stealing is sent to the principal's office. While leaving the classroom he makes a fist at the accuser and says, "You are dead today after school. I'm going to kill you. Just wait!" Once the role play is conducted, the whole class answers questions such as: (1) Do you think it was right for the boy to tell the teacher about the other boy's stealing of the money? (2) Do you think the accuser chose the right time and place to tell his teacher?, and (3) How could the accuser have been more discreet when he told his teacher?

    In another example, students are presented with a scenario and asked to answer a series of questions, first silently to themselves, and then collectively as a group. In one example, a situation is described where a teacher leaves the class while a math test is being administered. When leaving she exclaims to the students that they are on their honor not to cheat. Once out of the room, one boy whispers to another, "Let me see your answers." Questions regarding the situation are first answered individually (e.g., "Should Antonio let Ed copy his answers?" "What if Ed whispers that cheating is no big deal and that he knows plenty of guys who cheat all the time. Then should Antonio let Ed cheat?"), and are then discussed as a group.

In another example, Elias and Tobias (1996) describe the "Classroom Constitution." The goal of this situational analogue is to teach students the importance of rules and to give them an experience in group decision making. First, the group leader discusses the United States Constitution in a general manner and how a class constitution would be helpful to the class. Next, the class generates a list of "articles" for appropriate classroom behavior. This list may include both "do's" and "don'ts." Once an initial list is completed, a discussion of each "article" ensues, with some rules kept, some amended, and others discarded. The final product is a set of "laws" for the class.

Other examples of interpersonal problem-solving curricula which contain numerous examples of situational enactments and role plays include the ACCEPTS program (Walker et al., 1983), the Social Skills in the Classroom program (Stephens, 1992), and the Think Aloud program (Camp & Bash, 1981), to name just a few. Each of these provides numerous examples of role plays that can be used in the treatment of interpersonal problem solving.

Paper-and-Pencil Measures

Besides the use of situational enactments and role plays, analogue assessments of children's social cognition and relations have included paper-and-pencil techniques. These include standardized assessment instruments such as the Assessment of Interpersonal Relations, interview strategies such as the Children's Inventory of Social Support, as well as peer sociometric nominations and ratings.

The Assessment of Interpersonal Relations (AIR; Bracken & Kelley, 1993) questionnaire is designed for use in evaluating children's perceptions of their social interactions. Consisting of 35 items, the AIR requires respondents to rate the degree to which they agree or disagree with statements describing interactions with five different categories of people: peers (both male and female), parents (mother and father), and teachers. Statements include, for example, "I am treated fairly," and "When I am in trouble, I talk to my parents." Administration involves children/adolescents in considering the list of statements relative to each of the five relationships noted.

According to the manual, the AIR was normed on a sample of 2,500 children and is suitable for use with children between the ages of 9 and 19. The AIR possesses technically adequate test–retest and internal consistency reliability, as well as construct and discriminant validity characteristics. For example, a study by Kelley (1990) showed that a sample of clinically referred inpatient adolescents scored less well across each of the five relationship areas on the AIR when compared with a nonclinical comparison group. Overall, the AIR is a well-supported, easily administered instrument for measuring the self-perceptions of children and adolescents regarding their interpersonal relations.

The Children's Inventory of Social Support (CISS; Wolchik, Beals, & Sandler, 1989) is another, more detailed approach to examining children's social relations using a paper-and-pencil approach. The CISS involves a structured interview designed to assess children's social networks and friendships, and the benefits children perceive to derive from them. Suitable for use with children between the ages of 8 and 15 years, the CISS involves asking children to consider situations within several domains, and to report their social support and contacts within them. Domains covered include: recreation/play (e.g., people you go to the movies with), advice and information (e.g., people who tell you what you could do to solve a problem), goods and services (e.g., people who give us things we need or do things for us that we have trouble doing ourselves), emotional (e.g., people who we share our feelings with), positive feedback (people who tell us that they like the things that we have done), negative interactions (e.g., people who make us feel very bad, unhappy, upset, or angry), and friendships (e.g., things you may or may not do with friends, and about feeling you may or may not have toward them).

Children being administered the CISS first are asked to list all the people, both family and non-family, who have provided each type of support within a given time (e.g., the past three months). Then children rate their satisfaction with the support provided by each listed person, and their feelings about spending time with each. Children's scores are derived by tallying the number of persons providing each function within the relationship categories.

The content and format of the CISS were derived from the Arizona Social Support Interview Schedule (Barrera, 1980). Both theoretically and practically, the CISS was developed to yield information about the structure and function of children's social networks. The authors report initially interviewing 285 children and adolescents between the ages of 8 and 16, in approximately equal groups of three. One group was made up of children who had experienced the death of a parent in the previous two years; another consisted of children whose parents had divorced in the previous two years; and the third group contained children diagnosed with chronic asthma. The technical properties of the CISS are in need of development, however, the authors do present data that suggest high satisfaction with support is correlated with higher numbers of functions provided by family members, and that higher levels of satisfaction with family support are negatively correlated with depression and conduct problems.

Videotape Measures

Social cognition and peer status have also been assessed through a variety of role-play and enactment approaches, some of which have used videotape of children interacting for use in making cognitive judgments. For example, in one of the seminal works of Kenneth Dodge and colleagues that examined social competence in children (Dodge et al., 1986), videotaped vignettes were shown to children in order to assess social cognitions in two related studies.

The first involved a two-phase study of children's cognition regarding peer group entry. Forty-three children in kindergarten through second grade participated. As measured by sociometric nominations, 18 of the children were low-peer-status children, and 25 were classified as having high peer status. Initially, children were individually shown videotaped scenes, depicting paid child actors engaged in playing a board game. Further, the children shown were seated at a table and took turns several times during the scene. Then the video's narrator asked the viewer to imagine himself or herself wanting to join the children on the tape in playing the game. Child participants then were asked a series of questions tapping into interpretation of social cues (e.g., How much would the children on the tape want you to play with him or her?). Then children were asked the rationale for their answers, again to determine whether children depended on internally generated, video-generated, or irrelevant cues to guide their decisions. Third, the children were asked to think of as many ways as possible to join the group.

The third and fourth steps of this initial study began with the researchers showing the participants five more videotaped scenarios, each involving a third child attempting to join the original group. In each of these scenarios the entering child used one of five joining strategies: (1) competent, (2) aggressive, (3) self-centered, (4) passive, and (5) authority intervention. Participating children then were asked a series of questions involving the likely success of the depicted children, the likely success of the strategies, and the child's preferred strategy from the ones depicted. Finally, children were asked to demonstrate how they would attempt to join an ongoing play group.

In the second phase of this study, children participating in the first phase of the study were engaged in a peer group entry situation, by which they were instructed to join an ongoing play group of two children. The children's interactions were videotaped for 7 minutes, and later the target children were interviewed about their entry strategies.

Briefly, results of the studies provided empirical support for three important hypothesized relationships between social information processing and social behavior. First, children's social information-processing patterns predicted their competence and success in the peer group entry task. Second, children's peer group entry behavior predicted peers' judgments and perceptions about them. Finally, host children's perceptions about the entry children were related to their actions toward them.

A follow-up study replicated the procedures just described and then extended them by engaging child participants with videotaped vignettes involving what they referred to as a provocative situation. Here, a child actor was depicted seated on the floor, building a tower out of wooden blocks. Then, a second child is depicted entering the room and knocking over the blocks "in as ambiguous a manner as possible." Child participants then were asked a series of questions regarding their perceptions of the depicted situation. Initially, children were asked whether the blocks were knocked over accidentally, on purpose, or in an ambiguous manner. Then they were asked how they could tell, regarding their first answer. Children then were asked to identify as many ways as possible to respond to the provocation.

In the next phase of this study, children were shown scenarios of two children playing with blocks, until one ambiguously knocks them over. The child whose blocks were knocked over then is shown responding using aggressive, competent, or passive strategies. Following the scenes, each child was interviewed about the likely outcomes and success of the various strategies, and about how they would respond in a similar situation.

The results of the second study replicated those of the first and extended them in several ways. First, it was shown that social behaviors regarding both group entry and response to provocation could be predicted from social cognition information. Second, using direct observations of classroom and playground behavior, the authors were able to predict actual social behavior in these settings from the children's social-information patterns of responding to interview questions.

In summary, Dodge and colleagues have used videotaped vignettes and role playing in conjunction with the other methods in the study of children's social–cognitive functioning. Their work provides an excellent example of the use of these types of analogue assessment, and could be used as a model for investigating social cognition in children presenting with emotional and behavioral problems.

Summary

The various analogue measures presented here for assessing the social skills, social cognition, and interpersonal problem solving of children include well-developed, psychometrically sound measures with a long and rich history of use in research on the development of social competence and antisocial behavior. However, it appears that some less well-documented measures may warrant continued investigation on several accounts.

For example, some measures are extremely naturalistic (e.g., playground observation) and may tap into critical features of social development not addressed by the others (e.g., CISS). Ultimately, however, each measure is lacking in one critical feature necessary to support its use in a behavioral assessment paradigm—treatment utility. That is, to what degree does the information gathered contribute to improvements in treatment efficacy? An answer to this question, and further pursuit of questions of accuracy and generalizability of results regarding these analogue techniques (Hayes, Nelson, & Jarrett, 1989) is a much needed future direction for work in this area.

CONCLUSIONS

The purpose of this chapter has been to provide an overview of the variety of analogue procedures available for use in the behavioral assessment of school-aged children and youth. Although analogue measures have provided an alternative to direct forms of assessment, clearly such procedures present a number of problems that limit their frequent use. Notably, most analogue assessment procedures carry a great deal of inference in drawing conclusions regarding actual behavior. In practice, many questions are likely to arise with respect to the validity of the obtained data. Despite many of the measures having adequate internal validity, almost all measures suffer from problems with limited external validity. Indeed, studies that have compared results obtained from analogue and direct-assessment measures show only a moderate to slight association between the two (Shapiro & Kratochwill, 1988). Given the fact that analogue assessment measures were developed to serve as a simulation of the natural environment, the lack of correspondence between analogue and direct-assessment outcome data proves to be problematic. Because of this it is recommended that analogue measures be used to supplement rather than supplant more direct forms of assessment.

In addition to problems with validity, many of the analogue measures lack procedural standardization. This is most apparent with situational analogues such as role plays and enactments. In comparison to other forms of assessment (e.g., paper-and-pencil), which pay close attention to technical adequacy issues, analogue assessment procedures frequently lack any type of reliability or integrity information. Because of this, information gained from analogues must be interpreted with a certain degree of caution (Gettinger, 1988). In a related manner, issues of social validity must also be considered when adopting analogue measures (Wolf, 1978). That is, to what extent do the behaviors required of the analogue reflect socially valued and important skills for subject? Although it might appear important to some to assess the degree of fear associated with strangers, for a given child such fear may actually be adaptive and protective in function. Third, as with just about any form of assessment, careful consideration must be paid to the role of reactivity in observed outcomes (Sulzer-Azaroff & Mayer, 1991). Because the subject is often aware of being assessed, their behavior and performance may reflect what they think they should do rather than what they would otherwise do naturally. Finally, a problem facing the clinician when using analogue assessment procedures is the accessibility to these instruments (Shapiro & Kratochwill, 1988). Many of the measures are unpublished or have been developed to assess very specific clinical outcomes, lacking applicability to a wide range of problems.

Despite these limitations and concerns, analogue assessment strategies do possess some advantages. As noted in the beginning of the chapter, one of the main advantages of analogue measures it that the clinician has much greater control over the environment than with naturalistic observation. In doing so the clinician increases the opportunities for eliciting and observing important, but low-frequency behaviors. Similarly, by controlling the environment, clinicians can reduce or eliminate the impact of extraneous stimuli and its resultant affect on the behavior of interest. Doing so increases the internal validity of the observed findings; however, the issue of generalizability continues to be a concern. Finally, analogue procedures provide an alternative assessment strategy for behaviors that are difficult to observe naturally.

References

Achenbach, T. M. (1991a). *Manual for the child behavior checklist/4–18 and 1991 profile*. Burlington: University of Vermont, Department of Psychiatry.

Achenbach, T. M. (1991b). *Manual for the teacher's report form and 1991 profile*. Burlington: University of Vermont, Department of Psychiatry.

Achenbach, T. M. (1991c). *Manual for the youth self-report and 1991 profile*. Burlington: University of Vermont, Department of Psychiatry.

Albano, A. M., Chorpita, B. F., & Barlow, D. H. (1996). Childhood anxiety disorders. In E. J. Mash & R. A. Barkley (Eds.), *Childhood psychopathology* (pp. 196–241). New York: Guilford Press.

Asher, S. R. (1990). Recent advances in the study of peer rejection. In S. R. Asher & J. D. Coie (Eds.), *Peer rejection in childhood* (pp. 3–14). New York: Cambridge University Press.

Barkley, R. A. (1987). *Defiant children: A clinician's manual for parent training.* New York: Guilford Press.

Barkley, R. A. (1998). *Attention-deficit hyperactivity disorder: A handbook for diagnosis and treatment.* (2nd ed.). New York: Guilford Press.

Barkley, R. A. (1997). *Defiant children. A clinician's manual for assessment and parent training.* New York: Guilford Press.

Barrera, M., Jr. (1980). A method for the assessment of social support networks in community survey research. *Connections, 3,* 8–13.

Barrios, B. A., Hartmann, D. P., & Shigetomi, C. C. (1981). Fears and anxieties in children. In E. J. Mash & L. G. Terdal (Eds.), *Behavioral assessment of childhood disorders* (pp. 259–304). New York: Guilford Press.

Barrios, B. A., & Shigetomi, C. C. (1985). Assessment of children's fears: A critical review. In T. R. Kratochwill (Ed.), *Advances in school psychology* (Vol. IV, pp. 80–132). Hillsdale, NJ: Erlbaum.

Beidel, D. C. (1988). Psychophysiological assessment of anxious emotional states in children. *Journal of Abnormal Psychology, 97,* 80–82.

Beidel, D. C., Turner, S. M., & Morris, T. L. (1995). A new inventory to assess childhood social anxiety and phobia: The Social Phobia and Anxiety Inventory for Children. *Psychological Assessment, 7,* 73–79.

Bell-Dolan, D., & Brazeal, T. J. (1993). Separation anxiety disorder, overanxious disorder, and school refusal. *Child and Adolescent Psychiatric Clinics of North America, 2,* 563–580.

Bellak, L., Kay, S. R., & Murrill, L. M. (1989). The Dysphorimeter: An objective analogue for the assessment of depression, anxiety, pain, and other dysphoric states. *American Journal of Psychotherapy, 43,* 260–268.

Bornstein, M. R., Bellack, A. S., & Hersen, M. (1977). Social-skills training for unassertive children: A multiple-baseline analysis. *Journal of Applied Behavior Analysis, 10,* 183–195.

Bower, E. M. (1969). *Early identification of emotionally handicapped children in school* (2nd. Ed.). Springfield, IL: Charles C Thomas.

Bracken, B. A., & Kelley, P. (1993). *Assessment of Interpersonal Relations.* Austin, TX: Pro-Ed.

Breen, M. J. (1996). Parent-, teacher-, and youth-completed child-behavior questionnaires. In M. J. Breen & C. R. Fiedler (Eds.), *Behavioral approach to assessment of youth with emotional/behavioral disorders: A handbook for school-based practitioners* (pp. 243–288). Austin, TX: Pro-Ed.

Brown, L. J., Black, D. D., & Downs, J. C. (1984). *School Social Skills Rating Scale.* New York: Slosson Educational Publications.

Butler, L., Miezitis, S., Friedman, R., & Cole, E. (1980). The effect of two school-based intervention programs on depressive symptoms in preadolescents. *American Educational Research Journal, 17,* 111–119.

Camp, B. W., & Bash, M. A. (1981). *Think aloud.* Champaign, IL: Research Press.

Campbell, S. B. (1998). Developmental perspectives. In T. H. Ollendick & M. Hersen (Eds.), *Handbook of child psychopathology* (3rd ed, pp. 3–35). New York: Guilford Press.

Carr, E. G., & Durand, V. M. (1985). Reducing behavioral problems through functional communication training. *Journal of Applied Behavior Analysis, 18,* 111–126.

Carr, E. G., & Newsom, C. D. (1985). Demand-related tantrums: Conceptualization and treatment. *Behavior Modification, 9,* 403–426.

Clarke, G. N., Lewinsohn, P. M., Hops, H., & Seeley, J. R. (1992). A self- and parent-report measure of adolescent depression: The Child Behavior Checklist Depression Scale. *Behavioral Assessment, 14,* 443–463.

Coie, J. D., Dodge, K. A., & Coppotelli, H. (1982). Dimensions and types of social status: A cross-age perspective. *Developmental Psychology, 18,* 557–570.

Cone, J. D. (1978). The behavioral assessment grid (BAG): A conceptual framework and taxonomy. *Behavior Therapy, 8,* 411–426.

Conners, C. K. (1997). *Conners' rating scales—revised: Technical manual.* North Tonawanda, NY: Multi-Health Systems.

Connolly, J. A. (1983). A review of sociometric procedures in the assessment of social competencies in children. *Applied Research in Mental Retardation, 4*, 315–327.

Demary, M. K., Ruffalo, S. L., Carlson, J., Busse, R. T., Olson, A. E., McManus, S., & Leventhal, A. (1995). Social skills assessment: A comparative evaluation of six published rating scales. *School Psychology Review, 24*, 648–671.

Diener, M. B., & Milich, R. (1997). Effects of positive feedback on the social interactions of boys with attention deficit hyperactivity disorder: A test of the self-protective hypothesis. *Journal of Clinical Child Psychology, 26*, 256–265.

Dodge, K. A., Pettit, G. S., McClaskey, C. L., & Brown, M. M. (1986). Social competence in children. *Monographs of the Society for Research in Child Development, 51* (2, Serial No. 213).

Dowrick, P. W. (Ed.). (1991). *Practical guide to using video in the behavioral sciences.* New York: Wiley.

Dowrick, P. W. (1999). A review of self modeling and related interventions. *Applied & Preventative Psychology, 8*, 23–39.

Dowrick, P. W., & Dove, C. (1980). The use of self-modeling to improve the swimming performance of spina bifida children. *Journal of Applied Behavior Analysis, 13*, 51–56.

DuPaul, G. J., & Eckert, T. L. (1994). The effects of social skills curricula: Now you see them, now you don't. *School Psychology Quarterly, 9*, 113–132.

Eckert, T. L., & DuPaul, G. J. (1996). Youth-completed and narrow-band child-behavior questionnaires. In M. J. Breen & C. R. Fiedler (Eds.), *Behavioral approach to assessment of youth with emotional/behavioral disorders: A handbook for school-based practitioners* (pp. 289–354). Austin, TX: Pro-Ed.

Elias, M. J., & Tobias, S. E. (1996). *Social problem solving: Interventions in the schools.* New York: Guilford Press.

Elliott, S. N., & Gresham, F. M. (1991). *Social skills intervention guide: Practical strategies for social skills training.* Circle Pines, MN: American Guidance Services.

Elliott, S. N., Sheridan, S. M., & Gresham, F. M. (1989). Assessing and treating social skills deficits: A case study for the scientist-practitioner. *Journal of School Psychology, 27*, 197–222.

Esveldt-Dawson, K., Wisner, K. L., Unis, A. S., Matson, J. L., & Kazdin, A. E. (1982). Treatment of phobias in a hospitalized child. *Journal of Behavior Therapy and Experimental Psychiatry, 13*, 77–83.

Evans, P. D., & Garfield, H. (1981). Children's self-initiated approach to spiders. *Behavior Research & Therapy, 19*, 543–546.

Eyberg, S. M. (1980). Eyberg Child Behavior Inventory. *Journal of Clinical Child Psychology, 9*, 22–28.

Forehand, R. L., & McMahon, R. J. (1981). *Helping the noncompliant child: A clinician's guide to parent training.* New York: Guilford Press.

Frame, C., Matson, J. L., Sonis, W. A., Fialkov, M. J., & Kazdin, A. E. (1982). Behavioral treatment of depression in a prepubertal child. *Journal of Behavior Therapy and Experimental Psychiatry, 3*, 239–243.

Gable, R. A., Hendrickson, J. M., & Sasso, G. M. (1995). Toward a more functional analysis of aggression. *Education and Treatment of Children, 18*, 226–242.

Gettinger, M. (1988). Analogue assessment: Evaluating academic abilities. In E. S. Shapiro & T. R. Kratochwill (Eds.), *Behavioral assessment in schools: Conceptual foundations and practical applications* (pp. 247–289). New York: Guilford Press.

Glennon, B., & Weisz, J. R. (1978). An observational approach to the assessment of anxiety in young children. *Journal of Consulting & Clinical Psychology, 46*, 1246–1257.

Goldstein, A. P. (1999). *The Prepare Curriculum* (rev. ed.) Champaign, IL: Research Press.

Gresham, F. M. (1986). Conceptual issues in the assessment of social competence in children. In P. S. Strain, M. J. Guralnick, & H. M. Walker (Eds.), *Children's social behavior: Development, assessment, and modification* (pp. 143–179). New York: Academic Press.

Gresham, F. M. (1988). Social skills: Conceptual and applied aspects of assessment, training, and social validation. In J. C. Witt, S. N. Elliott, & F. M. Gresham (Eds.), *Handbook of behavior therapy in education* (pp. 523–546). New York: Plenum Press.

Gresham, F. M. (1992). Social skills and learning disabilities: Causal, concomitant, or correlational? *School Psychology Review, 21*, 348–360.

Gresham, F. M. (1998). Social skills training with children. In T. S. Watson & F. M. Gresham (Eds.), *Handbook of child behavior therapy* (pp. 475–497). New York: Plenum Press.

Gresham, F. M., & Elliott, S. N. (1984). Assessment and classification of children's social skills: A review of methods and issues. *School Psychology Review, 13,* 292–301.

Gresham, F. M., & Elliott, S. N. (1990). *The Social Skills Rating System.* Circle Pines, MN: American Guidance Services.

Hamilton, D. I. & King, N. J. (1991). Reliability of a behavioral avoidance test for the assessment of dog phobic children. *Psychological Reports, 69,* 18.

Hayes, S. C., Nelson, R. O., & Jarrett, R. B. (1989). The applicability of treatment utility. *American Psychologist, 44,* 1242–1243.

Hoge, R. D., & Luce, S. (1979). Predicting academic achievement from classroom behavior. *Review of Educational Research, 49,* 479–496.

Huesmann, L. R., Eron, L. D., Lefkowitz, M. M., & Walder, L. O. (1984). Stability of aggression over time and generations. *Developmental Psychology, 20,* 1120–1134.

Hughes, J. N., Boodoo, G., Alcala, J., Maggio, M., Moore, L., & Villapando, R. (1989). Validation of a role-play measure of children's social skills. *Journal of Abnormal Child Psychology, 17,* 633–646.

Irvin, L. K., Walker, H. M., Noell, J., Singer, G. H. S., Irvine, A. B., Marques, K., & Britz, B. (1992). Measuring children's social skills using microcomputer-based videodisc assessment. *Behavior Modification, 16,* 475–503.

Iwata, B., Dorsey, M., Slifer, K., Bauman, K., & Richman, G. (1982). Toward a functional analysis of self-injury. *Analysis and Intervention in Developmental Disabilities, 2,* 3–20.

Iwata, B., Pace, G., Kalsher, M., Cowdery, G., & Cataldo, M. (1990). Experimental analysis and extinction of self-injurious escape behavior. *Journal of Applied Behavior Analysis, 23,* 11–27.

Johnson, S. B., & Melamed, B. G. (1979). The assessment and treatment of children's fears. In B. B. Lahey & A. E. Kazdin (Eds.), *Advances in clinical child psychology* (Vol. 2, pp. 107–139). New York: Plenum Press.

Kahn, J. S., Kehle, T. J., Jenson, W. R., & Clark, E. (1990). Comparison of cognitive–behavioral, relaxation, and self-modeling interventions for depression among middle-school students. *School Psychology Review, 19,* 196–211.

Kashani, J. H., & Orvaschel, H. (1988). Anxiety disorders in midadolescence: A community sample. *American Journal of Psychiatry, 145,* 960–964.

Kelley, P. A. (1990). *Relationship between self-esteem, family environment, and interpersonal relations in a clinical and nonclinical sample of male and female adolescents.* Unpublished doctoral dissertation, Memphis State University, Memphis, TN.

Kelly, C. K. (1976). Play desensitization of fear of darkness in preschool children. *Behaviour Research and Therapy, 14,* 79–81.

Kendall, P. C., & Ronan, K. R. (1990). Assessment of children's anxieties, fears, and phobias: Cognitive–behavioral models and methods. In C. R. Reynolds & R. W. Kamphaus (Eds.), *Handbook of psychological and educational assessment of children: Personality, behavior, and context* (pp. 223–244). New York: Guilford Press.

King, N. J., & Ollendick, T. H. (1989). Children's anxiety and phobic disorders in school settings: Classification, assessment, and intervention issues. *Review of Educational Research, 59,* 431–470.

Kovacs, M. (1992). *Children's Depression Inventory.* Los Angeles: Multi-Health Systems.

Kratochwill, T. R., Sheridan, S. M., Carlson, J., & Lasecki, K. L. (1999). Advances in behavioral assessment. In C. R. Reynolds & T. B. Gutkin (Eds.), *The handbook of school psychology* (pp. 350–382). New York: Wiley.

La Greca, A. M., & Stone, W. L. (1993). The Social Anxiety Scale for Children—Revised: Factor structure and concurrent validity. *Journal of Clinical Child Psychology, 22,* 17–27.

Lang, P. J., & Lazovik, A. D. (1963). Experimental desensitization of a phobia. *Journal of Abnormal and Social Psychology, 66,* 519–525.

Lefkowitz, M. M., & Tesiny, E. P. (1980). Assessment of childhood depression. *Journal of Consulting and Clinical Psychology, 48,* 43–50.

Lochman, J. E., Dunn, S. E., & Klimes-Dougan, B. (1993). An intervention and consultation model from a social cognitive perspective: A description of the Anger Coping Program. *School Psychology Review, 22,* 458–471.

March, J. S. (Ed.). (1995). *Anxiety disorders in children and adolescents.* New York: Guilford Press.

McFall, R. M. (1977). Analogue methods in behavioral assessment: Issues and prospects. In J. D. Cone & R. P. Hawkins (Eds.), *Behavioral assessment: New directions* (pp. 152–177). New York: Brunner/ Mazel.

McKinney, J. D., & Speece, D. C. (1983). Classroom behavior and the academic progress of learning disabled students. *Journal of Applied Developmental Psychology, 4,* 149–161.

Merrell, K. W. (1993). *School social behavior scales.* Bradon, VT: Clinical Psychology.

Merrell, K. W. (1999). *Behavioral, social, and emotional assessment of children and adolescents.* Mahwah, NJ: Erlbaum.

Milich, R., & Okazaki, M. (1991). An examination of learned helplessness among attention deficit hyperactivity disordered boys. *Journal of Abnormal Child Psychology, 19,* 607–623.

Morris, R. J., & Kratochwill, T. R. (1983). *Treating children's fears and phobias: A behavioral approach.* New York: Pergamon Press.

Morris, R. J., & Kratochwill, T. R. (1985). Behavioral treatment of children's fears and phobias: A review. *School Psychology Review, 14,* 84–93.

Nay, W. R. (1977). Analogue measures. In A. R. Ciminero, K. S. Calhoun, & H. E. Adams (Eds.). *Handbook of behavioral assessment* (pp. 233–277). New York: Wiley.

Northup, J., Wacker, D., Sasso, G., Steege, M., Cigrand, K., Cook, J., & DeRaad, A. (1991). A brief functional analysis of aggressive and alternative behavior in an outclinic setting. *Journal of Applied Behavior Analysis, 24,* 509–522.

Ollendick, T. H. (1983). Reliability and validity of the revised Fear Survey Schedule for Children (FSSC-R). *Behaviour Research and Therapy, 21,* 395–399.

Passarello, D. J., & Hintze, J. M. (1999). *Further development of the Child Anxiety Survey (CAS): An examination of construct validity via a multitrait–multimethod matrix.* Unpublished manuscript.

Passarello, D. J., Hintze, J. M, Owen, S. V., & Gable, R. K. (1999). Exploratory factor analysis of parent ratings of child and adolescent anxiety: A preliminary investigation. *Psychology in the Schools, 36,* 89–102.

Patterson, G. R. (1982). *Coercive family process.* Eugene, OR: Castalia.

Patterson, G. R., Reid, J. B., & Dishion, T. J. (1992). *Antisocial boys: A social interactional approach.* Eugene, OR: Castalia.

Prout, H. T., & Ferber, S. M. (1988). Analogue assessment: Traditional personality assessment measures in behavioral assessment. In E. S. Shapiro & T. R. Kratochwill (Eds.), *Behavioral assessment in schools: Conceptual foundations and practical applications* (pp. 322–350). New York: Guilford Press.

Rachlin, H. (1989). *Judgment, decision, and choice: A cognitive/behavioral synthesis.* New York: W. H. Freeman.

Reynolds, C. R., & Kamphaus, R. W. (1992). *Behavior assessment system for children.* Circle Pines, MN: American Guidance Service.

Reynolds, C. R., & Richmond, B. O. (1985). *Revised children manifest anxiety scale (RCMAS).* Los Angeles: Western Psychological Services.

Reynolds, W. M. (1987). *Professional manual for the Reynolds Adolescent Depression Scale.* Odessa, FL: Psychological Assessment Resources.

Reynolds, W. M. (1989). *Professional manual for the Reynolds Child Depression Scale.* Odessa, FL: Psychological Assessment Resources.

Roberts, M. W., & Powers, S. W. (1988). The compliance test. *Behavioral Assessment, 10,* 375–397.

Robin A. L., & Foster, S. L. (1989). *Negotiating parent–adolescent conflict: A behavioral–family systems approach.* New York: Guilford Press.

Sasso, G. M., Reimers, T. M., Cooper, L. J., Wacker, D., Berg, W., Steege, M., Kelly, L., & Allaire, A. (1992). Use of descriptive and experimental analysis to identify the functional properties of aberrant behavior in school settings. *Journal of Applied Behavior Analysis, 25,* 809–821.

Semrud-Clikeman, M. (1990). Assessment of childhood depression. In C. R. Reynolds & R. W. Kamphaus (Eds.), *Handbook of psychological and educational assessment of children: Personality, behavior, and context* (pp. 279–297). New York: Guilford Press.

Shapiro, E. S., & Kratochwill, T. R. (1988). Analogue assessment: Methods for assessing emotional and behavioral problems. In E. S. Shapiro & T. R. Kratochwill (Eds.), *Behavioral assessment in schools: Conceptual foundations and practical applications* (pp. 290–321). New York: Guilford Press.

Sheridan, S. M., & Walker, D. (1999). Social skills in context: Considerations for assessment, intervention, and generalization. In C. R. Reynolds & T. B. Gutkin (Eds.), *The handbook of school psychology* (3rd ed., pp. 686–708). New York: Wiley.

Spielberger, C. D. (1973). *Manual for the state–trait anxiety inventory for children.* Palo Alto, CA: Consulting Psychologists Press.

Stark, K. (1990). *Childhood depression: School-based intervention.* New York: Guilford Press.

Stephens, T. M. (1992). *Social skills in the classroom.* Columbus, OH: Cedars Press.

Stephens, T. M., & Arnold, K. D. (1992). *Social Behavior Assessment Inventory: Professional Manual.* Odessa, FL: Psychological Assessment Resources.

Stokes, T. F., & Baer, D. M. (1977). An implicit technology of generalization. *Journal of Applied Behavior Analysis, 10,* 349–367.

Sulzer-Azaroff, B., & Mayer, G. R. (1991). *Behavior analysis for lasting change.* Fort Worth, TX: Harcourt Brace.

Van Hasselt, V. B., Hersen, M., & Bellack, A. S. (1981). The validity of role play tests for assessing social skills in children. *Behavior Therapy, 12,* 202–216.

Van Hasselt, V. B, Hersen, M., Bellack, A. S., Rosenblum, N. D., & Lamparski, D. (1979). Tripartite assessment of the effects of systematic desensitization in a multi-phobic child: An experimental analysis. *Journal of Behavior Therapy and Experimental Psychiatry, 10,* 51–55.

Waksman, S. A. (1985). *The Waksman Social Skills Rating Scale.* Portland, OR: ASIEP Education.

Walker, H. M., & McConnell, S. R. (1988). *The Walker–McConnell Scale of Social Competence and School Adjustment.* Austin, TX: Pro-Ed.

Walker, H. M., McConnell, S. R., Holmes, D., Todis, B., Walker, J., & Golden, H. (1983). *The Walker social skills curriculum: The ACCEPTS program.* Austin, TX: Pro-Ed.

Walker, H., & Severson H. (1992). *Systematic screening for behavior disorders.* Longmont, CO: Sopris West.

Wolchik, S. A., Beals, J., & Sandler, I. N. (1989). Mapping children's social support networks: Conceptual and methodological issues. In D. Belle (Ed.), *Children's social networks and social support* (pp. 191–220). New York: Wiley.

Wolf, M. M. (1978). The case for subjective measurement or how applied behavior analysis is finding its heart. *Journal of Applied Behavior Analysis, 11,* 203–214.

Zatz, S., & Chassin, L. (1983). Cognitions of test-anxious children. *Journal of Consulting and Clinical Psychology, 51,* 526–534.

CHAPTER 6

Analogue Assessment

Research and Practice in Evaluating Academic Skills Problems

MARIBETH GETTINGER
JILL K. SEIBERT
University of Wisconsin–Madison

Assessment is fundamental to promoting academic competence and improving academic performance for all children. Many researchers and educators have argued that information derived from conventional psychometric approaches may not be adequate for enhancing achievement among all learners, in particular, children from diverse cultural, social, economic, and educational backgrounds (Reschly, 1996). Test-based assessment of academic skills often does not reflect the goals, instructional content, and teaching practices of classrooms in which children learn. Most concerns with standardized testing practices focus specifically on the limited authenticity of both assessment tasks (e.g., To what extent do assessment tasks reflect the child's actual curriculum?) and assessment contexts (e.g., To what extent does the assessment context simulate the child's classroom instruction?). These concerns have contributed to the development of alternate assessment approaches.

The focus of this book is on behavioral assessment in schools. A behavioral perspective provides an alternate framework for academic skill assessment that circumvents many problems inherent in standardized achievement testing. The use of behavioral assessment procedures in schools has evolved from applying a behavior–analytic perspective to academic concerns. A behavioral approach to academic skills assessment recognizes that children's learning is a function of the relationship between individual student characteristics and dimensions of the task, as well as aspects of the instructional environment in which students are expected to perform. Thus a major objective of academic assessment is to evaluate multiple learner, task, and setting variables that either promote or interfere with academic skill acquisition.

The use of behavioral assessment methods for evaluating school-based problems is becoming more widespread. The behavioral assessment procedures addressed in this volume have been used successfully in both school and nonschool settings for evaluating social and emotional behaviors in children. Considerably less attention, however, has been given to the use of behavioral assessment in the evaluation of academic skills. The purpose of this chapter is to address one type of behavioral approach that is appropriate for the assessment of academic abilities and learning behaviors in school settings. This assessment approach, referred to as *analogue assessment*, requires the child to respond to stimuli that simulate as closely as possible those found in the natural classroom environment.

In this chapter, analogue assessment is a term used to characterize a number of different methods which, although having evolved from diverse orientations, share two important procedural characteristics. First, the role of examiners in analogue assessment is interactive. Analogue assessment typically involves some type of interaction (e.g., teaching, prompting, questioning, etc.) between the examiner and student. This assessment approach places a heavy emphasis on how children learn and how they can profit from either modifications in instructional strategies or changes in the level and content of curriculum materials. Second, with analogue assessment, a deliberate effort is made to change or improve performance of the skill being evaluated, or to arrive at a better understanding of why the student is experiencing problems. This requires taking environmental factors into consideration when evaluating academic performance. The value of analogue assessment is that it prescribes teaching procedures or instructional tasks, rather than describes student performance. Analogue measurement is designed to provide teachers with relevant information regarding instructional planning. As such, there is a direct link to classroom instruction.

RATIONALE FOR ANALOGUE ASSESSMENT

In recent years there has been a shift in the way educators and psychologists think about the teaching–learning process and, in turn, about assessing academic skills among school-age children (Gettinger & Stoiber, 1999). Behavioral and cognitive theories alike have contributed to several new directions for the assessment of academic skill problems. Cognitive theorists, for example, advocate the use of assessment tasks that emphasize higher-order thinking and provide an understanding of students' thinking and problem solving (Tittle, 1991). Behavioral theories advocate the use of functional assessment in which relationships between environmental events (instruction) and target behaviors (academic skills) are identified (Horner, 1994).

Analogue assessment approaches reflect a trend away from the exclusive use of standardized testing approaches and paper-and-pencil formats toward more dynamic and interactive approaches. Failure to answer questions correctly on a test is an indicator of what students do not know. Although students may lack the requisite knowledge at the time of testing, there is no direct assessment of (1) the extent to which the student might benefit from instruction, or (2) the nature of teaching that will promote skill acquisition. Some children, for example, may not have acquired the skills being assessed because of inadequate or ineffective teaching but nonetheless, may be able to so if given the opportunity or appropriate instruction.

Current best-practice recommendations emphasize that educational assessment should generate functional statements about a child's academic competence (statements that articulate a child's academic performance functions in relation to key environmental and task variables), and should demonstrate a strong link to interventions for academic success (Fuchs, 1994). Furthermore, good assessment practices are based on the notion that children's learning must be examined in the context of what they know, what they can do, and where they are in their learning. Thus assessment should incorporate tasks that require actual performance of skills as well as observation of children's performance during authentic learning situations.

The fundamental principles and procedures associated with analogue assessment are highly consistent with current thinking about academic assessment. With analogue assessment an evaluation of academic skills is linked to the curriculum and the instructional context in which the student has learned. This process of linking an evaluation of academic skills to classroom instruction requires several unique features of assessment that characterize an analogue approach. First, assessment occurs as part the actual teaching–learning process. Rather than removing the student from a learning context to participate in assessment activities, both teaching and testing are incorporated into the assessment process. Second, the conditions surrounding assessment are as similar as possible to the conditions for learning in a child's classroom. Children's performance is evaluated on meaningful and authentic tasks that closely match the curriculum or expected outcomes. For example, during analogue assessment students may be given variable and sufficient time to complete an assessment activity; they may be allowed to use appropriate tools (calculator, manipulatives, etc.); or they may have an opportunity to revise or edit their work, depending on what is done in their regular classrooms. Finally, analogue assessment methods provide useful information to teachers and parents in order to promote student learning and achievement. In sum, analogue assessment of academic skills is designed to focus on what a learner knows, incorporates authentic or natural learning activities, relies on familiar learning contexts, and generates information to plan appropriate academic interventions.

KEY DIMENSIONS OF ANALOGUE ASSESSMENT

Theoretically, analogue assessment approaches are linked to both cognitive and behavioral perspectives of children's learning. First, analogue assessment has been greatly influenced by Vygotsky's view of learning and development, which emphasizes the critical role that interactions with adults play in children's learning (Meltzer, 1994; Minick, 1987).

Traditional tests assess a child's unaided success and failure. That is, the child either answers a test item correctly (without instruction or prompts from the examiner) or the child fails the item. From a Vygotskian perspective, this child may be somewhere between "failure" and "unaided success," for example, unable to perform a math problem independently, but still able to perform the task with minimal assistance such as pointing out that addition is required rather than subtraction. As Vygotsky noted, "If I know arithmetic, but run into difficulty with the solution of a complex problem, a demonstration will immediately lead to my own resolution of the problem. If, on the other hand, I do not know higher mathematics, a demonstration of the resolution of a differential equation will not move my thought in that direction by a single step" (Vygotsky, 1935/1978, p. 204). This in-between state is referred to as the *zone of proximal development*; it is "the distance between the actual developmental level as determined by independent problem-solving and the level of potential development as determined through problem solving under adult guidance or in collaboration with more capable peers" (Vygotsky, 1935/1978, p. 85). In effect, analogue assessment focuses on a child's zone of proximal development. Assessment activities seek to answer such questions as "What are a student's strengths, and what does the student do in the process of performing a task or solving a problem?" or "What instruction will foster the advancement of the student's learning and thinking?" According to Wansart (1990), analogue approaches are examples of "microanalytic assessment," which delineate trial-by-trial interactions between student variables (such as prior knowledge or motivation) and performance on an academic task. A microanalytic assessment approach, such as analogue assessment, is able to document changes in learners over a brief period of intervention or structured teaching.

Analogue assessment of academic skill problems is equally rooted in a behavioral perspective. When academic skill problems are assessed through the use of analogue methods, the assessment questions are conceptualized and operationalized in concrete, behavioral terms. Analogue assessment requires two preliminary steps: (1) an analysis of what is already known or theorized about the academic skill to be assessed, and (2) an analysis of hypothesized functional linkages between the performance of interest and specific instructional variables (Gettinger, 1995). Because academic responding occurs within the context of an instructional environment, literacy skills lend themselves to systematic, functional analysis. Determining how acquisition of a skill functions in relation to specified characteristics of the instructional environment constitutes the analysis component of analogue assessment and evolves from the use of a test–teach–test paradigm. Within a behavior analytic framework, skill acquisition is analyzed by measuring variability in performance as a function of planned variations in the instructional environment or task during an experimental "teaching" phase.

Analogue assessment provides controlled situations in which the academic performance of interest is likely to occur. Using analogue assessment, an evaluation of academic skills is made under conditions similar to the learning environment in which skills are taught. As such, analogue assessment provides an evaluation of a child's academic skills within an environmental context that simulates classroom learning, including similar instructional materials, teaching strategies, or reinforcement contingencies. Because the child is asked to respond to learning situations or curriculum materials that are analogous to those found in the classroom, the use of analogue assessment allows for a direct observation of the learning behaviors of interest. Furthermore, because all data are generated under simulated teaching conditions, analogue methods also yield information that has a high degree of instructional utility.

Campione (1989) compared analogue measures of academic skills on the basis of three key dimensions: (1) focus, (2) interaction, and (3) target. *Focus* is the manner in which the outcomes of analogue assessment are operationalized and how the child's performance is quantified. Although most analogue assessment methods involve some type of test–teach–test paradigm, the specific focus of measurement may be one or more of three types: (1) change in academic skill performance from pretraining to posttraining; (2) level of academic skill performance at posttraining only; or (3) quality of performance during the analogue teaching or training phase of the assessment process.

The second dimension, *interaction*, describes the nature of the interaction between the examiner and the student during the assessment process. In analogue assessment, some type of interaction or teaching usually occurs during a training phase. The interaction, or simulated instruction, may be either standardized or individualized. With a standardized training phase, examinees receive a scripted brief teaching intervention, such as highlighting relevant information in math word problems. When the interaction is individualized, the analogue teaching intervention is dynamic and clinical in nature and matched to each student's individual needs, such as providing increasingly directive instruction or prompts as needed. There is some evidence to suggest that an individualized approach may yield assessment information that is more useful for instructional planning than a standardized approach. For example, Day and Cordon (1993) trained third-graders to a mastery level of performance on a math task dealing with weights and measures using analogue assessment. Children were trained through either an individualized, scaffolded instructional method, in which the amount of help they received decreased as their proficiency increased, or with a standardized, nonscaffolded method, in which the amount of help was constant, scripted, and did not vary according to children's performance. These researchers found that children who received scaffolded instruction during the simulated teaching task performed better on maintenance and transfer tasks. Furthermore, a measure of their responsiveness to scaffolded instruction (i.e., number of instructional prompts required to reach mastery) was a better predictor of performance on math tasks than their level of performance following the standardized procedure. Similar to Day and Cordon, other researchers have also found that noncontingent, nonscaffolded, nonindividualized instruction during analogue mini-lessons, although beneficial for some children, does not produce significant pre–post change for either beginning learners or learners with special needs (Day, Engelhardt, & Maxwell, 1997; Missiuna & Samuels, 1989; Tzuriel & Klein, 1985).

Another way in which the interaction dimension of analogue assessment may vary is the actual type of teaching that is simulated during either a standardized or individualized interaction. In some models, examiners provide children with a graduated series of increasingly explicit cognitive hints until they reach mastery-level performance (Spector, 1992); in others, examiners provide direct and complete instruction of the material to be learned first, and then follow-up with varying assistance matched to the needs of the child (Day & Zajakowski, 1991). Some researchers have simply increased the amount and explicitness of feedback about performance to children during testing (Carlson, 1989). Still other researchers have compared different content and instructional methods during an analogue testing situation, for example, direct word teaching versus invented spelling approach (Gettinger, 1993).

To date, the precise nature of instruction needed to bring about change in performance during analogue assessment has not been clearly established. Therefore, a review of what is known about effective teaching and the development of academic skills should be used to guide the conceptualization and design of instruction during analogue assessment. A major challenge to proceeding with analogue assessment is to operationalize and differentiate instructional variables in behavior–analytic terms. For example, instruction may vary with respect to the nature of responding, the type of instructional stimuli or task, and the type or frequency of feedback. In analogue assessment, the simulated instruction must be operationalized to incorporate the major conceptual elements of the experimental method, while also preserving common instructional elements that are similar to the natural learning environment.

The third dimension of analogue academic assessment is *target*. This refers to the type of skills that are tested. Early models of dynamic assessment (e.g., Budoff, 1987; Feuerstein, 1979) focused on domain-general skills associated with cognitive ability, such as performance on block design tasks. More recently, however, researchers have advocated the use of academically relevant tasks, either teaching skills that influence achievement in a specific domain, for example, teaching phonemic awareness to enhance reading skill acquisition (Good & Kaminski, 1996), or using tasks that sample the curriculum directly, for example, curriculum-based probes of reading ability (Campione & Brown, 1987).

Increasingly, researchers have been investigating the utility of analogue assessment in the context of domain-specific skills embodied by instructional classroom activities. Research support for targeting domain-specific knowledge and skills has significant implications for the types of tasks used in analogue assessment. It is important to understand that the process of analogue assessment is *not* synonymous with the use of a particular set of tasks or procedures, such as Feuerstein's Learning Potential Assessment Device (LPAD; Feuerstein, 1979). In fact, the LPAD may not be the most appropriate analogue assessment procedure when the purpose of assessment is to develop teaching recommendations that are useful for classroom teachers. The reason is that the targets or tasks used in the LPAD tend to be far removed from academic content such as reading, science, or math. The LPAD is just one example of analogue assessment that relies on broad cognitively oriented, domain-general abilities.

For much academic assessment, however, it is important to use assessment tasks that provide information about the domain-specific knowledge and skills being taught. For example, Campione and Brown (1987) described an analogue assessment approach for evaluating reading comprehension. The interaction or brief instruction they provided during the diagnostic teaching phase was reciprocal teaching (Palincsar & Brown, 1984); the skills they targeted for assessment were directly related to reading comprehension (e.g., prediction, summarization, etc.).

Bransford, Delclos, Vye, Burns, and Hasselbring (1987) described another example of domain-specific analogue assessment in the area of mathematics. They found that an analysis of errors committed during math problem-solving tasks enabled them to identify specific teaching strategies. Overall, it appears that restricting analogue assessment targets to inductive reasoning tasks may limit the extent to which appropriate interventions for classroom instruction can be identified. On the other hand, when the targets of analogue assessment are exclusively skill oriented, the resulting teaching recommendations may be too task related, with limited emphasis on general principles of cognitive mediation or general strategies. For example, Hasselbring, Goin, and Bransford (1988) used an analogue-assessment paradigm to test the effects of reinforcement on the speed and accuracy of math computation skills among fifth- and sixth-graders who had significant math delays. Although students' speed and accuracy improved, there was no improvement in strategy utilization for enhancing their overall computation skills. Hasselbring and colleagues found that the analogue teaching actually reinforced the use of an inefficient strategy, that is, counting on fingers, which led to correct responding on posttraining measures, but failed to promote the development and use of effective computation strategies.

ANALOGUE ASSESSMENT METHODS

In recent years, practitioners have turned to a variety of analogue assessment approaches to gain useful information during assessment and to avoid problems often associated with standardized testing. Despite the strong rationale and growing popularity of analogue assessment, few efforts have been made to formalize these methods for the assessment of academic skill problems. A variety of analogue assessment strategies can be used to obtain information about what to teach and how to teach academic skills. Analogue assessment is aimed at improving educational practice by monitoring the outcomes of learning under assessment conditions that simulate classroom instruction. Furthermore, analogue assessment is concerned with generating meaningful descriptions of strengths and weaknesses among learners who experience academic skill problems, and providing valid information for developing effective interventions. A review of the assessment literature reveals that analogue approaches utilize diverse formats which vary in terms of either their technique or purpose. First, different techniques can be used to provide some form of instruction or help to the examinee during the assessment process, such as modifying the format in which the test is administered, providing direct instruction in strategies for solving problems, or relying on curriculum-based materials for assessment tasks. Similarly, the specific purpose of analogue assessment can vary, such as maximizing performance on the test, measuring the extent to which examinees are responsive to instruction, or evaluating the effectiveness of specific instructional approaches and modifications.

There are several assessment procedures that can be considered analogue measures. Because of the diverse types of analogue assessment procedures, it is helpful to devise a categorization scheme for drawing distinctions and making comparisons among the various approaches. In the section that follows, analogue procedures are described on the basis of the particular dimension of the natural environment that is simulated during assessment. Specifically, one or more of three key dimensions of classroom learning may be simulated during analogue assessment: (1) treatment, (2) content, or (3) response. (See Table 6.1.) In *treatment* analogues, brief interventions that are analogous to or simulate teaching procedures during classroom instruction are administered during the actual assessment process. Two assessment approaches

TABLE 6.1   Analogue Assessment Methods for Evaluating Academic Skills

Analogue type	Description of procedure	Example of procedure
Treatment analogue	Brief interventions that simulate classroom teaching are administered during the assessment process.	Dynamic assessment Functional assessment
Content analogue	Assessment materials/tasks are directly related to the curriculum materials used during classroom teaching.	Curriculum-based assessment
Response analogue	Responses during assessment are analogous to responding that occurs during classroom instruction.	Think-aloud assessment Performance assessment

are described below, dynamic assessment and functional assessment, which are both examples of a treatment analogue approach for academic skills assessment. With *content* analogues, the assessment materials used during the controlled assessment situations are equivalent to or directly related to the curriculum materials used in classroom instruction. Curriculum-based assessment is described as an example of a content analogue assessment approach. Finally, with *response* analogue assessment, the child's response that is prompted and observed during assessment is analogous to the type of processing or responding (overt as well as covert) that occurs during actual instruction. In this chapter, think-aloud approaches and performance-based assessment are presented as examples of response analogue assessment. The last approach that is described, computer-assisted assessment, has the potential to simulate all three dimensions of classroom learning, including (1) instruction, (2) curricular materials, and (3) responding or processing during classroom learning. It is an approach that illustrates all three types of analogues.

Dynamic or Assisted Assessment

Dynamic assessment is an example of a treatment or teaching analogue approach. Dynamic assessment incorporates a teaching component into the testing situation and allows the examiner to observe a learner's responsiveness to teaching. Dynamic assessment relies on a pretest–teach–posttest paradigm to evaluate students' potential for change and to determine the nature and type of instruction that promotes change. By examining learners' responses to a series of brief, experimental "instructional episodes," diagnosticians are able to predict and recommend appropriate interventions (Kirshenbaum, 1998).

Dynamic assessment methods differ from static assessment methods in several important ways. First, static assessment methods measure academic skills by presenting tasks that require students to access previously acquired knowledge or skills, and to respond to test items without any assistance. Dynamic assessment, on the other hand, starts with a static baseline measurement, but then allows the examiner to guide the student to a solution or correct answer through specific instruction. Within a dynamic approach, assessment occurs while learners are in the process of learning, rather than after they have completed a task. Second, the goal of static assessment is to obtain a highly reliable, quantitative measure of academic skills. The child's test performance is compared with a norm or with the performance of other learners. The goal of dynamic assessment, however, is to arrive at a description of the child's problem solving and performance, and to examine the effect of a brief intervention on his or her learning. A child's performance on targeted tasks is compared before and after a simulated teaching session, rather than to a norm.

A third distinction between static and dynamic assessment is that static assessment methods fail to examine the extent of learners' understanding of procedures needed to perform academic tasks, such as algorithms to solve mathematical problems or strategies to enhance reading comprehension. Dynamic assessment focuses on evaluating the cognitive processes involved in learning and change. Although there are significant differences among the various dynamic assessment procedures, a common element is the provision of some form of assistance to the learner. Hence, dynamic assessment is often referred to as "assisted assessment."

Feuerstein, the primary developer of a dynamic assessment approach, based his approach to assessment on a theory of cognitive functioning in which a lack of mediated learning experiences results in cognitive deficiencies (1979). Feuerstein's original model of cognitive modifiability and dynamic assessment was the result of his frustration with traditional assessment devices that focused on what students failed to learn, not on how students learned or what they were capable of learning. Feuerstein developed a dynamic assessment procedure, called the Learning Potential Assessment Device (LPAD), which is a content-free instrument that provides interactive materials for assessing children's potential for cognitive growth, as measured by change in performance on domain-general tasks, such as matrices (Haywood, Brown, & Wingenfeld, 1990).

Campione and Brown's (1987) assisted assessment approach for mathematics differs from that of Feuerstein in that it relies on instructional content and procedures that are more authentic in nature. Ecologically valid learning tasks related to actual school tasks provide the context for their assessment procedures. Campione and Brown's approach incorporates a test–teach–test format that includes a description of initial or baseline level of skill performance. During assisted assessment, the student is introduced to a learning task that is specific to a content domain (math) and linked with classroom demands (independent math problem solving). The goal is to assess the amount of instruction required by the student not only to learn a set of rules for doing the task (acquisition), but also to apply the rules to a related, transfer task (generalization). The nature of the analogue teaching is referred to as "titrated instruction," which is instruction that begins with general prompts from the evaluator and then proceeds to more detailed instruction (Brown, Campione, Webber, & McGilly, 1992). Using an assisted assessment approach, a variety of instructional techniques, such as varying the teaching materials, methods of presentation, or types of feedback, are systematically implemented and evaluated within a brief assessment period. Assisted assessment attempts to define the instructional conditions that encourage more effective performance as well as to specify obstacles to effective learning. The assessment outcome is an evaluation of performance over a brief period of time, where the unit of comparison is the learner's initial performance before teaching rather than performance of a normative group.

Jitendra and Kameenui (1993) characterize a "testing-the-limits" approach to assessment as another type of dynamic assessment, in that specific interventions are integrated directly within the testing process. Testing-the-limits approaches are used to assess the limits of children's abilities by incorporating into a testing situation various procedures that have been documented as leading to higher levels of test performance. Procedures may include, for example, providing immediate and corrective performance feedback, providing the child with reinforcement for completing items correctly, or prompting the child to verbalize a self-guiding strategy for monitoring performance and solving problems.

Several examples of dynamic assessment methods can be found in the literature focusing on a range of academic skills. Jitendra, Kameenui, and Carnine (1994) demonstrated the utility of a dynamic assessment approach for evaluating third-grade students' understanding of the concept of "borrowing" in solving two-digit subtraction problems and ability to solve multi-step word problems. The dynamic- or assisted-assessment component in their research followed a standard, three-step approach. First, students were given a set of two-digit subtraction problems to solve on their own (unaided). Next, they were given a second set of problems to solve using manipulatives, as a way to observe students' problem-solving strategies directly. Finally, students solved a third set of problems with assistance or prompts from the examiner to determine the amount and type of assistance necessary to facilitate problem solving. Jitendra and colleagues (1994) found that dynamic assessment provided important information concerning the nature of students' understanding of the concept of "borrowing," their strategies for solving problems and, most importantly, the reasons for students' failure or success in solving word problems. The manipulatives and prompts enabled researchers to discern students who arrived at correct answers but lacked an understanding of the underlying concept of "borrowing," and to identify students who lacked the mechanical or computation skills to complete problems correctly, but understood the process conceptually.

Carney and Cioffi (1990) described the application of a dynamic assessment approach for evaluating word-reading abilities. Their basic procedure for the dynamic assessment of word recognition was to present words through different formats and different instructional approaches until the student was able to identify the word. Correct identification of words shown in flash presentation was the targeted response in their assessment approach. If the student failed to respond correctly, the examiner proceeded to present words in an untimed mode to ascertain the degree to which word-reading problems were attributable to limited automaticity. If word reading continued to be incorrect, the examiner presented the words in a variety of different ways, selecting strategies based on the student's initial attempts to read the word, knowledge of effective teaching, or through collaboration with the classroom teacher.

Coleman (1994) examined a program for disadvantaged children in kindergarten through third grade that used portfolio assessment combined with dynamic assessment. Sample or mini-lessons focusing on inquiry and problem solving were taught to children during brief diagnostic teaching or assisted-assessment sessions. Examiners observed target behaviors during the analogue teaching–learning process. The assessment information derived from this approach included: (1) indicators of learning potential based on observations during the treatment analogue, and (2) recommendations for individualized instruction, again based on observations during the assessment process of techniques that facilitated task performance.

The majority of research using dynamic assessment has involved children of average or below-average intelligence, although a few studies have documented the utility of dynamic assessment for children with exceptional abilities (Bolig & Day, 1993). Overall, researchers have concluded that dynamic assessment provides information that can be used in the design of effective classroom interventions to promote children's learning. In particular, dynamic assessment allows for the fact that children with similar competencies on static tests may profit differentially from instruction (Haywood, Tzuriel, & Vaught, 1992).

Functional Assessment

Although functional assessment has been researched primarily as an approach to address behavior problems, in recent years researchers and clinicians have begun to apply this method to academic issues as well. Functional assessment is designed to identify contingencies that may be maintaining a child's academic performance. To identify these contingencies, the diagnostician must seek to understand the purpose or function a behavior serves. Although children may exhibit similar academic problems, very different contingencies might be operating to maintain them. Once contingencies have been identified, educational interventions can be developed to alter or modify them.

Similar to dynamic assessment, functional assessment is an example of a treatment analogue approach. The goal of functional assessment is to identify variables in the instructional environment that are related to a student's academic performance, and to identify teaching procedures that are most effective for circumventing problems and promoting academic learning. Researchers have delineated three key steps in conducting a functional assessment of academic behavior: (1) Observe and describe the educational environment in which the student's academic difficulty occurs; (2) generate hypotheses about possible contingencies maintaining the academic behaviors; and (3) test hypotheses by conducting a functional analysis (Belfiore & Hutchinson, 1998; Daly, Witt, Martens, & Dool, 1997). The first step is to identify functional relations between students' instructional environments and their academic functioning. During the second step hypotheses are generated about the function of behavior, on the basis of observed relations. The final step allows for the experimental manipulation of specific instructional interventions and variables to test their effect on the academic behavior of interest (Gresham & Lambros, 1998). In conducting an experimental or functional analysis, there are certain conditions that should be met. For example, the experimental instructional episodes should be brief, easy to implement, and lead to immediate and measurable change in performance. In addition, performance measures must be sensitive to short-term gains in academic skills (Daly et al., 1997).

Daly and colleagues (1997) proposed that students' academic problems fall into two categories, lack of skills or failure to perform skills. In conducting a functional analysis, the effects of different instructional strategies on performance are evaluated to ascertain whether students possess the requisite skills needed to perform an academic task, or whether there are problems in their performance or demonstration of skills. Based on a review of the literature and observations of children with academic problems, Daly and co-workers (1997) identified five common hypotheses or reasons underlying academic skill problems: (1) Students do not want to do the academic task or perform the skill (lack of motivation); (2) They have not spent enough time working on it (insufficient learning time); (3) They have not had enough help (inadequate assistance or feedback); (4) They have not been required to perform the task or demonstrate the skill in the manner or format required; or (5) The work is too difficult. Although Daly and colleagues offer support for each of these hypotheses, it is important to remember that other hypotheses may warrant consideration during a functional analysis, depending on the individual characteristics of both the learner and his or her educational environment.

Whereas Daly and colleagues (1997) focused on the functional assessment of specific academic behaviors, Belfiore and Hutchinson (1998) suggested that functional assessment can be used to evaluate and improve academic routines and strategies to enhance learning and achievement, such as note taking, study skills, time management, and homework completion. According to Belfiore and Hutchinson, a functional assessment of academically related routines allows researchers and practitioners to examine closely the match between school-related variables and students' academic achievement.

Linehan and Brady (1995) conducted a study that examined the effects of functional assessment information on teachers' decisions about instructional objectives and recommendations for service delivery. A total of 86 teachers of students with mental retardation were provided with either developmental assessment reports containing standardized assessment information, or functional assessment reports. Although the researchers found no significant differences in the quality of Individualized Education Program (IEP) objectives, they did find that the actual content of the IEPs differed significantly between groups. Specifically, the IEPs of the group that received reports containing functional information included a larger number of objectives related to social skills (79% vs. 36%), interaction skills (82% vs. 54%), vocational skills (33% vs. 13%), domestic skills (76% vs. 67%), and community performance (48% vs. 38%).

A difference was also found in placement recommendations between the two groups. Educators who read functional reports recommended less restrictive placements than those who read developmental reports. This difference is both significant and meaningful, especially for students with cognitive disabilities. Recommendations for students' placement can have a strong impact on their educational outcomes. In more restrictive school environments, students with mental retardation have limited access to age-appropriate educational experiences, social interactions, and opportunities to experience real-life situations. Lack of access to natural settings, both vocational and educational, can result in a significant disadvantage in acquiring skills for independent living. In addition, students with severe mental retardation have particular difficulty with transfer and generalization of learning experiences; this difficulty is exacerbated when students are taught in restrictive, self-contained environments. (Horner, McDonnell, & Bellamy, 1984). The results of Linehan and Brady suggest that placement decisions should be made based on reports of performance by students with mental retardation in authentic learning situations, rather than the results of standardized tests, which are often normed on students without mental retardation.

There are several benefits to using functional assessment. First, functional assessment provides information that promotes the individualization of instruction and educational environments. Greer (1994) noted that for education to be effective, there must be a shift away from a group-oriented model toward an individualized education model. Functional assessment facilitates this shift toward greater individualization. Knowing what function a behavior serves for a student allows for the development of interventions designed to match that student's individual needs. The use of functional assessment procedures also provides for greater individualization by identifying which interventions are most effective. The experimental analysis component of functional assessment allows teachers to be certain they are using an effective intervention that is well suited to students in their classroom.

Curriculum-Based Assessment

Curriculum-based assessment (CBA) is any testing approach that uses "assessment materials and procedures that mirror instruction in order to ascertain whether specific instructional objectives have been accomplished and to monitor progress directly in the curriculum being taught" (Salvia & Ysseldyke, 1991, p. 652). Because assessment materials and tasks are based on the student's actual curriculum, CBA is an example of a content analogue assessment approach. During CBA, the primary dimension of the natural learning environment that is simulated is the student's curriculum. CBA allows a teacher to identify a student's strengths and weakness in the context of the actual curriculum content and objectives. Once that assessment information has been collected, it can be used to make curriculum changes that will promote the student's academic growth.

CBA encompasses a wide range of assessment techniques, including informal reading and math inventories, an analysis of class assignments, end-of-the-unit mastery tests, or the use of short probes measuring fluency or skill performance (Shinn, 1995). CBA is a systematic process that can be used (1) to identify an individual's current performance or skill level, (2) to measure change in performance or skill level on a continuing basis, and (3) to make informed instructional decisions. Although a variety of different assessment tools and procedures can be used in a curriculum-based assessment, five standard models of CBA have been described in the literature.

The first model focuses on the design and modification of instructional environments (Gickling & Rosenfield, 1995). This model is used to design instruction that is appropriately matched to a student's skill level (Shinn, Rosenfield, & Knutson, 1989). The initial assessment in this model focuses on determining what the student knows and does not know. Based on this initial assessment, a teacher develops instructional materials that match the student's "instructional level." Instructional match is achieved when lessons are designed to challenge students while providing them with sufficient opportunities to experience success. Within this model, assessment of student progress involves the use of brief probes to monitor the "instructional match" on a continuous basis. "CBA is structured to help teachers build on entry-level skills of students, thus maximizing on-task time during learning activities" (Gickling & Rosenfield, 1995, p. 588).

A second model of CBA has been described as the use of "teacher-constructed criterion-referenced tests" (Blankenship, 1985; Marston, 1989). The objective of this model is to evaluate student performance relative to current instructional objectives. Like Gickling's approach, this model is also useful in instructional planning. The information provided by this model is intended to help teachers determine specific content to include in their teaching. In the initial assessment, a test is constructed for each curricular objective, and cut-off scores are established to determine mastery and nonmastery (Shinn et al., 1989). Teachers use initial assessment information to develop instructional materials that teach curriculum objectives that have not yet been mastered. Continued assessment of student progress includes the use of probes of varying length designed to determine when instructional objectives have been met.

Curriculum-based measurement, developed by Deno (1985) and his collogues, is the third model of CBA. This model focuses on (1) evaluating a student's progress in his or her current curriculum, and (2) evaluating the effects of instructional interventions (Shinn et al., 1989). In this model, an initial assessment is used to determine where a student is relative to the curriculum in which he or she is being taught, and to signal when instructional changes are in order. Assessment of student progress over time relies on standardized, short-term fluency measures that are sensitive to detect small changes in student performance.

Curriculum-based evaluation, another form of CBA, is the fourth model (Howell, Fox, & Morehead, 1993). In this model, the focus is on determining student achievement of short-term instructional objectives. The purpose of assessment is to test what is being taught and to guide teaching of the skills being tested (Howell et al., 1993). In this model, assessment information is used to develop hypotheses about why a student's academic performance is less than expected, and to monitor progress toward skill acquisition. An initial assessment is designed to collect general information about the student's current skill level. A wide range of measures may be used in the initial assessment, including norm-referenced achievement tests, teacher-developed tests, direct observations, teacher interviews, and classroom assignments (Shinn et al., 1989). Based on these data, teachers develop instructional interventions to address skill deficiencies. Assessment of student progress uses short probes tailored to the specific objectives or skills a student is being taught.

Finally, Shapiro (1996) designed an integrated curriculum-based assessment model that incorporates features of the models described by Gickling and Rosenfield (1995), Blankenship (1985), Deno (1985), and Howell, Fox, and Morehead (1993). This integrated model includes both an assessment of the instructional ecology of the classroom as well as a determination of student progress relative to both short-term and long-term goals. Assessment information is used to make decisions about changes in the instructional environment. The initial assessment evaluates a student's academic environment and determines the student's instructional level on curriculum materials (Shapiro, 1990). Ongoing collection and graphing of assessment data are used to monitor a student's progress toward both short-term objectives and end-of-year goals.

Curriculum-based assessment has a high degree of utility for treatment planning because the assessment tasks are linked directly to curriculum content or objectives. CBA relies on a curriculum analogue for both evaluating academic skills and for monitoring progress toward targeted outcomes. In recent years the popularity of curriculum-based assessments has grown among school psychologists, teachers, and students. Shapiro and Eckert (1993), for example, reported that school psychologists found CBA to be more acceptable than norm-referenced measures for identifying academic skill problems and for communicating information about academic performance to teachers and parents. In this study, school psychologists also indicated they believed CBA is less biased than most norm-referenced tests, particularly for assessing children from culturally diverse backgrounds. Eckert and Shapiro (1995) also examined teachers' beliefs about CBA and found that both regular and special education teachers rated CBA as being highly acceptable. Finally, Davis and Fuchs (1995) found that CBA is highly acceptable to students as well, and has the positive effect of increasing student involvement in the learning process.

Think-Aloud Assessment

We know that students with comparable scores on tests may have taken different paths to obtain their scores. A consideration of these differences provides information of additional diagnostic value and has led to the development of think-aloud assessment approaches. Whereas dynamic assessment and functional analysis are examples of treatment/teaching analogue approaches and curriculum-based assessment is an example of a content analogue approach, think-aloud assessment is an example of a response analogue approach, where the underlying processes that are implicated during classroom learning and the performance of classroom tasks are simulated during assessment.

Reading research has emphasized the importance of comprehension monitoring and text-processing strategies for good comprehension (Jacobs & Paris, 1987). During reading tasks, good comprehenders monitor their understanding of text and use appropriate strategies to enhance their comprehension (predicting, questioning, clarifying, and summarizing what they read). Parallel research on mathematical problem solving has also underscored the importance of cognitive processes in successful problem solving (Montague & Bos, 1990). Good math problem solvers organize their knowledge, employ systematic problem solving steps, and engage in self-monitoring while they perform tasks. Although it is impossible to know the exact type of thinking that occurs as children perform reading or math tasks, there is a growing consensus among researchers that think-aloud assessment can provide a rich source of information about children's comprehension processes and problem-solving strategies during the performance of academic tasks (Ericsson & Simon, 1993; Moats, 1994; Pressley & Afflerbach, 1995). Thus reading comprehension or math problem solving are often the focus of think-aloud assessment.

Using an analogue think-aloud approach, a child is exposed to a problem or learning situation and asked to respond as naturally as possible. The think-aloud component requires children to report overtly and continuously what they are thinking while engaged in the academic activity. Assessment of cognitive processing during analogue learning situations relies on simultaneous verbalizations of thought processes and performance of the task to identify strategies and processes individuals use as they solve problems or engage in reading-comprehension activities (Garner, 1988). This information is used to develop remedial methods to enhance children's effective use of strategies during classroom learning. As an alternative to assessment procedures that rely on standardized tests, think-aloud measures provide valuable information about learners' cognitive and metacognitive strategies which can lead to better interventions for strategy training in reading or mathematics.

Think-aloud techniques have been used effectively to evaluate reading comprehension processes (Crain-Thoreson, Lippman, & McClendon-Magnuson, 1997; Pressley & Afflerbach, 1995) as well as mathematical problem-solving approaches (Montague & Applegate, 1993; Swanson, 1996). Critics of think-aloud assessment have questioned whether the reading comprehension or math problem-solving process is significantly altered by the requirement to stop and report what one is thinking, thereby posing a threat to the validity of the information derived from this approach. In fact, research has shown that the additional cognitive load imposed by the directive to verbalize thoughts while performing a task is actually quite negligible (Crain-Thoreson et al., 1997; Fletcher, 1986; Ericsson & Simon, 1993; Montague & Applegate, 1993).

Ward and Traweek (1993) described three different methods to obtain information about children's thinking during their performance of academic tasks. The first method is *concurrent thinking aloud*. In this approach, the examiner instructs children to verbalize continuously all thoughts that come to mind while they are engaged in an academic activity. If children are capable of doing this, concurrent thinking aloud provides the most comprehensive sample of children's mediational or thinking processes. Many children over the age of 8 years, however, have learned to inhibit vocalizations during task performance, or their thinking associated with task performance has become so habitual that thoughts may go unreported. A *concurrent interview procedure* may be easier for older children. In this procedure the examiner stops the task periodically and asks specific questions to probe children's strategies and thinking at the time. Although there are limitations to this procedure (e.g., interruptions may interfere with task performance), it is a productive approach for many learners. The third method is a *reconstruction procedure*, in which the analogue problem-solving or comprehension activity is videotaped, and children are asked to review the tape and reveal their thinking at various times (either signaled or spontaneously) while they were engaged in the task. Across all three procedures, think-aloud assessment has been shown to provide valuable information about learners' cognitive and metacognitive strategies that can lead to better interventions in strategy training.

Performance-Based Measurement

Although definitions of performance-based assessment vary, most include an emphasis on tasks that require students to use or demonstrate the knowledge and skills they have (Poteet, Choate, & Stewart, 1993). Similar to think-aloud approaches, performance assessment can be viewed as analogue assessment in that it incorporates a response analogue that simulates responding or performance on authentic or "real-world" tasks (Guskey, 1994). Unlike think-aloud assessment, however, the response of interest is overt performance rather than verbal reports of covert processing. Performance assessment goes beyond measuring isolated skills or single facts to evaluating directly what students can do with their knowledge in relation to curriculum goals.

With performance assessment, examiners observe students while they are performing an analogue task, or they examine products created as a result of completing a task. According to Stiggins (1997), performance assessment requires three steps: (1) clarifying and specifying the performance to be evaluated; (2) devising assessment tasks to elicit the desired performance; and (3) developing a system for making and recording observations and judgements. Within these broad guidelines, performance assessment includes any procedure in which children demonstrate or perform behaviors and skills specified by the evaluator. Performance assessment includes several different assessment methods that have been developed as alternatives to standardized, norm-referenced testing (Herman, Aschbacher, & Winter, 1992).

One type of performance assessment, play-based assessment, has been researched and developed specifically for use with young children and/or children with disabilities and developmental delays (Linder, 1993). There are several learning and developmental characteristics of children's play which hold significance for intervention with young children. As such, play is an appropriate response analogue for young children because it is spontaneous and voluntary and requires active engagement of children. Moreover, the motivation for play is highly intrinsic. Play is systematically related to important areas of development among young children, including cognitive understanding, social-emotional development, language usage, and physical-motor development. Play-based assessment is the observation of one or more children engaged in play activities specifically for the purpose of understanding their developmental, sensorimotor, cognitive, social, and communicative functioning. This assessment approach relies on several different formats for observing and evaluating children's play behavior, including unstructured play facilitated by the evaluator, structured play activities, activities involving child–child interactions, activities involving parent–child interactions, and motor play activities. Because play is the primary means through which children learn and develop, an evaluation of play skills in analogue situations should constitute a major component of assessment with young children.

Computer-Assisted Assessment

The use of computers in analogue assessment is becoming increasingly widespread. Computer-assisted assessment is capable of simulating all three dimensions of classroom learning: (1) treatment, (2) content, and (3) response. Advances in computer technology have supported the development and dissemination of computer-assisted assessment programs that are able to deliver instructional interventions, evaluate the effectiveness of interventions, determine where a student is in the curriculum, analyze patterns of errors made during assessment, and provide immediate feedback and reinforcement to students.

Two examples of a dynamic assessment procedure that relies on the use of a computer program are Sherlock I and II (Lajoie & Lesgold, 1992). These programs were developed for the purposes of both assessing and teaching academic skills to students in the context of having them solve a problem that requires them to use the new skills. First, students are presented with a problem. As they work through the problem the computer provides individual tutoring and prompts by modifying the information provided to students. Next, students are assessed to determine if they have acquired the basic knowledge underlying skill performance and, furthermore, if they understand when and where to apply that knowledge. If they have acquired the necessary skill knowledge, then they move on to the next skill. If not, the computer provides additional instruction or prompting. One stated purpose of this type of dynamic computer-assisted assessment procedure is "to improve instruction by identifying when learners are at an impasse so that appropriate remediation can be provided" (Lajoie & Lesgold, 1992, p. 366).

In addition to evaluating and teaching academic skills, the Sherlock programs also focus on students' metacognitive skills. Once students have been presented with a problem, the program assesses and monitors how students plan to solve the problem. If there is no plan or if an ineffective plan is used, the program provides students with a model of appropriate planning. Assessing and teaching metacognative skills in this manner was found to be highly effective; over time the researchers found that students' need for assistance with metacognitive strategies decreased significantly (Lajoie & Lesgold, 1992).

Researchers have also developed methods to use computers to enhance curriculum-based measurement (CBM). In a series of studies, researchers have examined the extent to which CBM software can be used effectively and efficiently for collecting and managing data, analyzing student skills, and making decisions about instructional programming. In particular, several studies have evaluated the effects of computer-based assessment on time requirements, teacher satisfaction, level or degree of implementation of CBM, and student achievement (Fuchs & Fuchs, 1989; Fuchs, Fuchs, & Hamlett, 1989; Fuchs, Fuchs, Hamlett, & Ferguson, 1992; Fuchs, Fuchs, & Stecker, 1989). The results consistently demonstrate that using CBM software can help teachers use their time more efficiently, encourages teachers to implement CBM procedures more frequently and more accurately, and can improve student achievement. Research has also found that teachers have a preference for using CBM software over paper-and-pencil recording of CBM information.

Computer-assisted analogue assessment provides users with many additional benefits. The most recent computer-assisted assessment programs are highly interactive and can be adapted to the individual ability level of the student. Thus much of the clinical decision making that rests with the diagnostician during analogue assessment is done by a computer. Computer-assisted dynamic assessment programs can be used to tailor both assessment and "trial" instructional approaches to the needs of an individual student. For example, a pretest is used to determine a student's entry-level skills. If the student has not yet achieved mastery of a targeted skill, the computer presents a lesson that provides instruction of the skill. If, however, the student has demonstrated mastery of the skill, he or she may move on to the pretest for the next level. When instruction is matched to the skill level of a student in this manner, the student is always working at an appropriate instructional level. "Matching learners' prior achievement with the appropriate instruction reduces learner frustration from instruction that is too difficult, while avoiding the tedium and lack of challenge that can accompany instruction that is too simplistic" (Dalton & Goodrum, 1991, p. 205). Computer programs can also provide more consistent, immediate feedback. Students generally like to use computers, so using computers for analogue assessment is a source of intrinsic motivation and reinforcement.

Computer-assisted analogue assessment is precise and efficient. The use of computers reduces the amount of time needed for conducting an analogue assessment session and for scoring performance during the assessment process. Computers have the capability to continuously and simultaneously monitor, record, and preserve changes in the knowledge and skills of multiple students. Unlike most analogue assessment methods, the use of computers allows for multiple assessments to be conducted at the same time. Computers can also analyze errors in students' responding quickly and accurately (Lajoie & Lesgold, 1992; Watkins & Kush, 1988).

Although computer-based analogue assessment has many benefits, concerns have been raised about the appropriateness of this format for all students. Varnhagen and Gerber (1984), for example, found that while students preferred completing *The Test of Written Spelling* (Larsen & Hammill, 1976) on the computer, they made more errors and took more time to complete the test than when they completed it in a standard paper-and-pencil format. Upon closer examination, the researchers found that many errors were typographical and that students required a significant amount of time to locate letters on the keyboard. The use of a computer keyboard for recording answers may be very different from the way that students are asked to record their answers in their regular learning environment. Thus it remains questionable whether responding on a computer is an appropriate response analogue for all students.

Watkins and Kush (1988) examined both accuracy and satisfaction among students who participated in computerized assessment. For their assessment, they incorporated modifications that allowed the program to alter the difficulty level of items presented and to make mastery decisions, unlike the computerized approach used by Varnhagen and Gerber (1984). Their results showed no difference in accuracy between students who used the computer and students who used paper and pencil. In addition, students showed a stronger preference for the computerized format. Watkins and Kush concluded that the capability to adapt to individual ability levels is a critical component of any computer-based assessment program. They also concluded, however, that it is possible that students' familiarity with computers affects the overall validity of the analogue task.

LIMITATIONS OF ANALOGUE ASSESSMENT

Although there are many advantages associated with using analogue assessment procedures, it is important to keep some limitations in mind. One important limitation lies in the extent to which it is possible for diagnosticians to generalize from what they observe during an analogue assessment situation to the actual classroom environment. There are methods to minimize concerns about generalizability, such as developing analogue procedures on the basis of collaboration with classroom teachers, observing learners in their natural learning environments, and working to gain an understanding of effective teaching and the nature of the academic skill problem. These best-practice guidelines, however, do not eliminate the concerns about generalizability. Analogue assessment uses controlled situations to evaluate a target behavior or skill, and to assess the effects of experimental interventions on academic performance. Controlled analogue situations, however, will never be able to duplicate exactly the complex nature of instruction and classroom environments. For example, the teacher–student ratio in an analogue situation differs from the typical school learning environment. Furthermore, the teaching styles of examiners may be different from those of teachers in students' actual classrooms.

Another limitation surrounds the lack of empirical data regarding the psychometric properties of analogue assessment methods. Little has been done to examine the reliability and validity of these assessment procedures. In fact, CBM is the only analogue assessment procedure to be standardized with documented reliability. With the exception of research by Vellutino and colleagues (Vellutino, Scanlon, & Tanzman, 1998), few studies have looked at the long-term outcomes of interventions derived from analogue assessment procedures. Furthermore, the individualized nature inherent in treatment analogue procedures (dynamic assessment and functional assessment) makes them difficult to standardize.

The limitation of having minimal information on the reliability of analogue assessment for evaluating academic skills is compounded by the lack of training many professionals have obtained toward developing and implementing analogue assessment procedures (Jitendra & Kameenui, 1995). A primary concern in utilizing most analogue assessment approaches is the extensive amount of time involved. Analogue assessment procedures require greater time and skills to administer than static, standardized, paper-and-pencil measures. Furthermore, to design appropriate analogue assessment procedures, a diagnostician must have knowledge about assessment design, academic skills, instruction, curriculum, and classroom practices.

IMPLICATIONS AND FUTURE DIRECTIONS IN ANALOGUE ASSESSMENT OF ACADEMIC SKILLS

The need to align assessment with instruction to provide information for planning interventions provides a strong rationale for research and further development of analogue assessment methods. Analogue assessment is a viable approach for evaluating academic skills that has yet to be fully utilized in education. Although a call for instruction-oriented assessment has been in the literature for decades, only recently has serious attention been given to analogue assessment (Haywood & Wingenfeld, 1992). Despite a limited research base, several implications for assessment practices and directions for future research can be offered.

One potential application of analogue assessment is the development of screening measures to identify young children who may be at risk for experiencing academic problems. Spector (1992) found that kindergarten children's performance on a dynamic measure of phonemic awareness was a stronger predictor of their reading achievement at the end of the school year than static measures of phonemic awareness skills. In this study, children participated in one 15-minute analogue testing session during which they were given corrective feedback and supportive prompts (cueing, modeling, etc.) to enable them to segment 12 words correctly into component sounds. The analogue assessment procedure required minimal training on the part of examiners and was administered during one brief session. Scores derived from this assessment approach reflected the degree of independence children achieved in performing the segmentation task (i.e., number of prompts), and proved to be good predictors of end-of-year standardized reading test scores. Furthermore, by observing children's responsiveness to instruction during the analogue "teaching" situation, examiners were able to identify appropriate instructional approaches to promote the development of phonemic awareness skills in each child.

As research continues to pinpoint skills that underlie the development of academic abilities, such as the relationship between phonemic awareness and reading acquisition, there is greater potential for developing analogue assessments of children's prerequisite skills and for evaluating children's responsiveness to the teaching of those skills. Thus both early identification and early intervention designed to prevent academic skill problems can be enhanced.

Another implication of analogue approaches lies in their potential for developing direct assessments of children's strategy use. Kletzien and Bednar (1990) developed an analogue reading assessment procedure to determine readers' knowledge and use of effective reading-comprehension strategies. Their assessment model included three steps: (1) an initial or baseline assessment of reading ability and strategy use; (2) presentation of a brief, structured mini-lesson for teaching deficient strategies using direct instruction, guided practice, and independent practice; and (3) postassessment of strategy use and comprehension on alternative forms of the initial baseline measures. Kletzien and Bednar have used their procedure with a range of at-risk readers and a variety of curriculum materials for identifying deficient reading strategies. The total assessment time is similar to what is required for standardized, individual reading assessments. For example, the initial baseline assessment is completed in 20 minutes; the mini-lesson takes 15 to 20 minutes; and the postassessment requires another 20 minutes. Thus even a relatively brief session of analogue teaching can provide useful prescriptive information.

To use Kletzien and Bednar's analogue assessment approach effectively, examiners must have a firm understanding of validated reading strategies and an ability to infer strategy use from students' responses during baseline assessment. Furthermore, examiners need a requisite level of expertise in using instructional techniques to teach strategies during the analogue teaching phase. Kletzien and Bednar (1990) recommended that analogue interventions should be developed based on an understanding of effective teaching as well as knowledge of specific learner characteristics (e.g., task persistence, organizational strategies, error patterns, kinds of stimuli attended to, speed of performing, etc.). Lidz (1991) also emphasized the need to align analogue assessment tasks and procedures closely with actual instruction and instructional goals. Thus analogue assessment tasks must be carefully selected from the curriculum in which the child is experiencing problems.

Despite this recommendation for a strong foundation in curriculum and instruction, many school psychologists report limited expertise in designing and implementing instructional programs (Fish & Margolis, 1988). Furthermore, teachers often indicate that assessment reports from psychologists incorporate limited information about the type of instruction that might be used effectively with children. Therefore, a review of educational literature and collaboration with classroom teachers are important for diagnosticians to develop and simulate instruction that is both effective and typical of instructional approaches used in classroom settings. Professionals who conduct academic assessments must form partnerships with teachers to gather information about the effects of different approaches to instruction with different types of learners. Such a partnership permits the alignment of the curriculum, assessment, educational goals, and instruction necessary to support analogue assessment.

Paris, Calfee, Filby, Hiebert, Pearson, Valencia, and Wolf (1992) described a useful framework for analogue literacy assessment they developed in consultation with teachers, parents, and district administrators to best meet the assessment needs of a particular school district. What began as a researcher–teacher collaboration to evaluate a school's whole language curriculum evolved into the development of an analogue approach for overall literacy assessment. The framework of Paris and colleagues involves five decision-making phases in which decisions were shared among teachers, administrators, support staff, and parents. The phases include (1) identifying the dimensions of literacy to reflect daily classroom practices and goals; (2) identifying measurable and observable attributes of literacy dimensions; (3) developing analogue methods for collecting evidence about literacy proficiency (treatment, content, and response analogues); (4) scoring children's performance on samples derived from analogue assessments; and (5) interpreting and using the data. This project underscores the importance of partnerships between teachers and evaluators and illustrates the feasibility of a large-scale analogue approach for enhancing assessment of literacy skills.

Another direction for analogue assessment lies in the potential for identification of learners with special education needs. Pointing to the substantial increase in the number of children classified as having learning disabilities (LD) in the past 20 years, many researchers have advocated for the use of a dynamic analogue assessment approach to identifying children with LD (Berninger & Abbott, 1994; Johnsen, 1997; Swanson, 1996). These individuals have proposed that learning disability be conceptualized as resistance to intervention or failure to respond to intervention. An analogue approach can be useful for identifying students with learning disabilities within this new conceptualization. Using an analogue model, static, test-based assessment might flag at-risk students, however, a label of LD is deferred, pending the outcome of dynamic assessment. Within this approach students are presented with a valid treatment protocol and their responsiveness to the treatment is measured over time. If students fail to respond adequately to the treatment, their resistance to intervention is used to identify them as having a learning disability.

Berninger and Abbott (1994) described such a dynamic assessment model for defining learning disability as a "failure to respond over time to validated intervention protocols" (p. 163). They recommend basing a diagnosis of learning disability on the outcomes of dynamic assessment. Children who show measurable gains during analogue assessment using within-subject data analysis techniques are considered "treatment responders." These students do not have a true learning disability, but are able to learn when given sufficient opportunities and an appropriate instructional approach. Those who fail to demonstrate measurable gains are "treatment non-responders," and are likely to have a true learning disability. The key to the success of this approach lies in the development of treatment protocols that research has shown to be effective with children exhibiting similar learning problems as the target child.

Vellutino and colleagues (Vellutino, Scanlon, & Tanzman, 1998) have adopted this analogue approach for identifying children with learning disabilities and have implemented it successfully on a longitudinal basis. Specifically, they track children from kindergarten through first grade, providing intensive tutoring and instructional assistance to children who experience reading difficulty. At the end of first grade, children who do not make adequate progress in reading, despite intensive, individualized assistance, are candidates for being classified as having a learning disability. Recent research has demonstrated the utility and feasibility of implementing analogue assessment over an extended period of time (Abbott, Reed, Abbott, & Berninger, 1997; Vellutino et al., 1998). Vellutino and colleagues (1998) make the case that test-based assessment should not be the sole vehicle for diagnosing reading disability. They recommend, instead, that assessment should be conducted using an analogue assessment framework. Specifically, in their research program, early and intensive remediation is provided to young at-risk children, and children's responsiveness and progress are evaluated over time. A child's ability to profit from such intervention is the most important piece of diagnostic information in determining learning or reading disability. These authors advocate the use of labor-intensive intervention as a primary vehicle for diagnosing learning disabilities. In their research, analogue assessment data (treatment outcome data), in conjunction with test data, provided the best diagnostic information. Vellutino and colleagues caution, however, that redefining learning disability in terms of whether a child responds to instruction in an analogue situation raises certain methodological and measurement issues. For example, an important question is how long it would take to detect a treatment effect in an analogue assessment situation. The measurement of change linked to treatment effects is complex and standard models for evaluating change may be limited in their ability to evaluate this. Experts suggest that measurement of change requires, at minimum, three assessment points.

A strong case has also been made for greater use of analogue assessment in the identification of gifted-and-talented learners (Bolig & Day, 1993; Kirshenbaum, 1998). According to Borland and Wright (1994), observation should play a large role in identifying young, potentially gifted, economically disadvantaged students. The advantage of analogue assessment over objective, static tests is that it is flexible to allow an examiner to observe children's performance and to explore ways of encouraging children to demonstrate their ability. In Coleman's (1994) study, for example, examiners were trained to observe children's behaviors during experimental lessons as signs of potential and to individualize the mini-instruction to capitalize on students' ability. An interesting outcome in Coleman's research was the positive effect of analogue assessment on teachers' thinking about students. Teachers who received assessment information commented at the conclusion of the study that their perceptions and expectations of students had changed. Many teachers noticed that what they had regarded previously as indications of negative behavior in children were actually signs of exceptional potential.

The positive impact of analogue assessment on teacher perceptions represents another implication and area for future research. In addition to Coleman, other researchers have documented a positive effect of analogue assessment on teachers' perceptions of students. For example, Delclos, Burns, and Kulewicz (1987) found that teachers who observed students during an analogue assessment situation rated students as more competent and more knowledgeable than teachers who viewed the same students in a static testing situation. In a follow-up study, Vye, Delclos, and McGoldrick (1988) examined the effects of having teachers view a videotape of an analogue assessment session in which three types of instruction being "tested" by the examiner were explained. Before and after viewing the videotape, participants were asked to teach an academic task to a child who was experiencing difficulty in the same content domain as the child depicted on the video. The video presentation changed teachers' instructional methods in important ways. For example, teachers demonstrated a significant increase in their use of corrective feedback, a strategy which had been shown to enhance children's performance during the videotaped analogue assessment.

Other research has documented similar effects (Kirshenbaum, 1998; Shaklee, 1993; Wright & Borland, 1993). In these studies, after viewing analogue assessment situations or receiving information derived from analogue assessment sessions, teachers' perceptions of students changed from one in which they judged students as being academically deficient to a perception of students as being more capable than expected on certain types of tasks. Teachers learned to recognize students' strengths and to alter their own teaching practices to develop these strengths rather than focus on academic deficits and direct most of their efforts toward skill remediation.

According to Nichols (1994), decisions requiring instructional adaptation require a different approach toward assessment than decisions regarding selection, labeling, or identification. "There is a current emphasis on helping individuals to succeed in educational opportunities, in contrast to selecting individuals for those opportunities" (p. 578). Analogue assessment fits well with this current movement toward "assessment of enablement." Information derived from analogue assessment enables educators to draw conclusions about students' instructional needs and to develop effective instructional interventions. Analogue assessment of academic skills clearly merits continued research and development, as well as greater implementation in schools.

References

Abbott, S. P., Reed, E., Abbott, R. D., & Berninger, V. W. (1997). Year-long balanced reading/writing tutorial: A design experiment used for dynamic assessment. *Learning Disability Quarterly, 20,* 249–263.

Belfiore, P. J., & Hutchinson, J. M. (1998). Enhancing academic achievement through related routines: A functional approach. In T. S. Watson & F. M. Gresham (Eds.), *Handbook of child behavior therapy* (pp. 83–97). New York: Plenum Press.

Berninger, V. W., & Abbott, R. D. (1994). Redefining learning disabilities: Moving beyond aptitude-achievement discrepancies to failure to respond to validated treatment protocols. In G. R. Lyon (Ed.), *Frames of reference for the assessment of learning disabilities: New views on measurement issues* (pp. 163–183). Baltimore: Paul H. Brookes.

Blankenship, C. S. (1985). Using curriculum-based assessment data to make instructional management decisions. *Exceptional Children, 42,* 233–238.

Bolig, E. E., & Day, J. D. (1993). Dynamic assessment and giftedness: The promise of assessing training responsiveness. *Roeper Review, 16,* 110–113.

Borland, J. H., & Wright, L. (1994). Identifying young, potentially gifted, economically disadvantaged children. *Gifted Child Quarterly, 38,* 65–69.

Bransford, J. D., Delclos, V. R., Vye, N. J., Burns, M. S., & Hasselbring, T. S. (1987). State of the art and future directions. In C. S. Lidz (Ed.), *Dynamic assessment: An interactional approach to evaluating learning potential* (pp. 470–496). New York: Guilford Press.

Brown, A., Campione, J. C., Webber, L. S., & McGilly, K. (1992). Interactive learning environment: A new look at assessment and instruction. In B. Gifford & M. C. O'Connor (Eds.), *Changing assessments: Alternative view of aptitude, achievements and instruction* (pp. 121–211). Boston: Kluwer Academic Publishers.

Budoff, M. (1987). Measures for assessing learning potential. In C. S. Lidz (Ed.), *Dynamic assessment: An interactional approach to evaluating learning potential* (pp. 173–195). New York: Guilford Press.

Campione, J. C. (1989). Assisted assessment: A taxonomy of approaches and an outline of strengths and weaknesses. *Journal of Learning Disabilities, 22,* 151–165.

Campione, J. C., & Brown, A. L. (1987). Linking dynamic assessment with school achievement. In C. S. Lidz (Ed.), *Dynamic assessment: An interactional approach to evaluating learning potential* (pp. 82–115). New York: Guilford Press.

Carlson. J. S. (1989). Advances in research on intelligence: The dynamic assessment approach. *Mental Retardation and Learning Disability Bulletin, 17*, 1–20.

Carney, J. J., & Cioffi, G. (1990). Extending traditional diagnosis: The dynamic assessment of reading abilities. *Reading Psychology, 11*, 177–192.

Coleman, L. J. (1994). Portfolio assessment: A key to identifying hidden talents and empowering teachers of young children. *Gifted Child Quarterly, 38*, 65–69.

Crain-Thoreson, C., Lippman, M. Z., & McClendon-Magnuson, D. (1997). Windows on comprehension: Reading comprehension processes as revealed by two think-aloud procedures. *Journal of Educational Psychology, 89*, 579–591.

Dalton, D. W., & Goodrum, D. A. (1991). The effects of computer based pretesting strategies on learning and continuing motivation. *Journal of Research on Computing in Education, 24*, 204–214.

Daly, E. J., Witt, J. C., Martens, B. K, & Dool, E. J. (1997). A model for conducting a functional analysis of academic performance problems. *School Psychology Review, 26*, 554–574.

Davis, L. B., & Fuchs, L. S. (1995). 'Will CBM help me learn?' Students' perception of the benefits of curriculum-based measurement. *Education and Treatment of Children, 18*, 19–33.

Day, J. D., & Cordon, L. A. (1993). Static and dynamic measures of ability: An experimental comparison. *Journal of Educational Psychology, 85*, 75–82.

Day, J. D., Engelhardt, J. L., & Maxwell, S. E. (1997). Comparison of static and dynamic assessment procedures and their relation to independent performance. *Journal of Educational Psychology, 89*, 358–368.

Day, J. D., & Zajakowski, A. (1991). Comparisons of learning ease and transfer propensity in poor and average readers. *Journal of Learning Disabilities, 24*, 421–426.

Delclos, V. R., Burns, M. S., & Kulewicz, S. (1987). Effects of dynamic assessment on teachers' expectations of handicapped children. *American Educational Research Journal, 24*, 325–336.

Deno, S. (1985). Curriculum-based measurement: The emerging alternative. *Exceptional Children, 52*, 219–232.

Eckert, T. L., & Shapiro, E. S. (1995). Teachers' ratings of the acceptability of curriculum-based assessment methods. *School Psychology Review, 24*, 497–508.

Ericsson, K. A., & Simon, H. A. (1993). *Protocol analysis: Verbal reports as data.* Cambridge, MA: MIT Press. (Original work published 1984)

Feuerstein, R. (1979). *The dynamic assessment of retarded performers: The Learning Potential Assessment Device, theory, instruments, and techniques.* Baltimore: University Park Press.

Fish, M. C., & Margolis, H. (1988). Training and practice of school psychologists in reading assessment and intervention. *Journal of School Psychology, 26*, 399–404.

Fletcher, C. R. (1986). Strategies for the allocation of short-term memory during comprehension. *Journal of Memory and Language, 25*, 43–58.

Fuchs, L. S. (1994). *Connecting performance assessment to instruction.* Reston, VA: Council for Exceptional Children.

Fuchs, L. S., & Fuchs, D. (1989). Enhancing curriculum-based measurement through computer applications: review of research and practice. *School Psychology Review, 18*, 317–327.

Fuchs, L. S., Fuchs, D., & Hamlett, C. L. (1989). Computers and curriculum-based measurement: Effects of teacher feedback systems. *School Psychology Review, 18*, 112–125.

Fuchs, L. S., Fuchs, D., Hamlett, C. L., & Ferguson, C. (1992). Effects of expert system consultation within curriculum-based measurement, using a reading maze task. *Exceptional Children, 58*, 436–450.

Fuchs, L. S., Fuchs, D., & Stecker, P. M. (1989). Effects of curriculum-based measurement on teachers' instructional planning. *Journal of Learning Disabilities, 22*, 51–59.

Garner, R. (1988). Verbal-report data on cognitive and metacognitive strategies. In C. Weinstein, E. Goetz, & P. Alexander (Eds.), *Learning and study strategies: Issues in assessment, instruction, and evaluation* (pp. 53–67). San Diego: Academic Press.

Gettinger, M. (1993). Effects of invented spelling and direct instruction approaches on spelling performance of second-grade boys. *Journal of Applied Behavior Analysis, 26*, 281–291.

Gettinger, M. (1995). Evaluating spelling treatment effects: A tutorial in the application of single-case methodology. In K. A. Hinchman, D. J. Leu, & C. K. Kinzer (Eds.), *Perspectives on literacy* research and practice: Forty-fourth yearbook of the National Reading Conference (pp. 374–383). Chicago: National Reading Conference.

Gettinger, M, & Stoiber, K. C. (1999). Excellence in teaching: A review of instructional and environmental variables. In C. R. Reynolds & T. B. Gutkin (Eds.), *Handbook of school psychology* (3rd ed., pp. 933–958). New York: Wiley.

Gickling, E. E., & Rosenfield, S. (1995). Best practices in curriculum-based assessment. In A. Thomas & J. Grimes (Eds.), *Best practices in school psychology–III* (pp. 587–595). Washington, DC: National Association of School Psychologists.

Good, R. H., & Kaminski, R. A. (1996). Assessment for instructional decisions: Toward a proactive/prevention model of decision-making for early literacy skills. *School Psychology Quarterly, 11,* 326–336.

Greer, R. D. (1994). A systems analysis of the behaviors of schooling. *Journal of Behavioral Education, 4,* 255–263.

Gresham, F. M., & Lambros, K. M. (1998). Behavioral and functional assessment. In T. S. Watson & F. M. Gresham (Eds.), *Handbook of child behavior therapy* (pp. 3–22). New York: Plenum Press.

Guskey, T. R. (1994). What you assess may not be what you get. *Educational Leadership, 51*(6), 51–54.

Hasselbring, T. S., Goin, L. I., & Bransford, J. D. (1988). Developing math automaticity in learning handicapped children: The role of drill and practice. *Focus on Exceptional Children, 20*(6), 1–7.

Haywood, H. C., Brown, A. L., & Wingenfeld, S. (1990). Dynamic approaches to psychoeducational assessment. *School Psychology Review, 19,* 411–422.

Haywood, H. C., Tzuriel, D., & Vaught, S. (1992). Psychoeducational assessment from a transactional perspective. In H. C. Haywood & D. Tzuriel (Eds.), *Interactive assessment* (pp. 38–63). New York: Springer.

Haywood, H. C., & Wingenfeld, S. A. (1992). Interactive assessment as a research tool. *Journal of Special Education, 26,* 253–268.

Herman, J. L., Aschbacher, P. R., & Winter, L. (1992). *A practical guide to alternative assessment.* Alexandria, VA: Association for Supervision and Curriculum Development.

Horner, R. H. (1994). Functional assessment: Contributions and future directions. *Journal of Applied Behavior Analysis, 27,* 401–404

Horner, R. H., McDonnell, J. J., & Bellamy, T. (1984). Efficient instruction of generalized behaviors: General case programming in simulation and natural settings. In R. H. Horner, L. H. Meyer, & H. D. Fredericks (Eds.), *Education of learners with severe handicaps: Exemplary service strategies* (pp. 289–314). Baltimore: Paul H. Brookes.

Howell, K. W., Fox, S. L., & Morehead, M. K. (1993). *Curriculum-based evaluation: Teaching and decision making* (2nd ed.). Pacific Grove, CA: Brooks/Cole.

Jacobs, J. E., & Paris, S. G. (1987). Children's metacognition about reading: Issues in definition, measurement, and instruction. *Educational Psychologist, 22,* 255–278.

Jitendra, A. K., & Kameenui, E. J. (1993). Dynamic assessment as a compensatory assessment approach: A description and analysis. *Remedial and Special Education, 14*(5), 6–18.

Jitendra, A. K., Kameenui, E. J., & Carnine, D. W. (1994). An exploratory evaluation of dynamic assessment and the role of basals on comprehension of mathematical operations. *Education and Treatment of Children, 17,* 139–162.

Johnsen, S. K. (1997). Assessment beyond definitions. *Peabody Journal of Education, 72*(3), 136–152.

Kirschenbaum, R. J. (1998). Dynamic assessment and its use with underserved gifted and talented populations. *Gifted Child Quarterly, 42,* 140–147.

Kletzien, S. B., & Bednar, M. R. (1990). Dynamic assessment for at-risk readers. *Journal of Reading, 33,* 528–533.

Lajoie, S. P., & Lesgold, A. M. (1992). Dynamic assessment of proficiency for solving procedural knowledge tasks. *Educational Psychologist, 23,* 365–384.

Larsen, S., & Hammill, D. (1976). *The test of written spelling.* Austin, TX: Pro-Ed.

Lidz, C. S. (1991). *Practitioner's guide to dynamic assessment.* New York: Guilford Press.

Linder, T. W. (1993). *Transdisciplinary play-based assessment: A functional approach to working with young children.* Baltimore: Paul H. Brookes.

Linehan, S. L., & Brady, M. P. (1995). Functional versus developmental assessment: Influences on instructional planning decisions. *Journal of Special Education, 29,* 295–310.

Marston, D. (1989). A curriculum-based measurement approach to assessing academic performance: What is it and why do it? In M. Shinn (Ed.), *Curriculum-based measurement: Assessing special children* (pp. 18–78). New York: Guilford Press.

Meltzer, L. J. (1994). Assessment and learning disabilities: The challenge of evaluating the cognitive strategies and processes underlying learning. In G. R. Lyon (Ed.), *Frames of reference for the assessment of learning disabilities: New views on measurement issues* (pp. 403–425). New York: Guilford Press.

Minick, N. (1987). Implications of Vygotsky's theories for dynamic assessment. In C. S. Lidz (Ed.), *Dynamic assessment: An interactional approach to evaluating learning potential* (pp. 116–140). New York: Guilford Press.

Missiuna, C., & Samuels, M. T. (1989). Dynamic assessment of preschool children with special needs: Comparison of mediation and instruction. *Remedial and Special Education, 10*(2), 53–62.

Moats, L. C. (1994). Strategy assessment in perspective. In G. R. Lyon (Ed.), *Frames of reference for the assessment of learning disabilities: New views on measurement issues* (pp. 607–626). New York: Guilford Press.

Montague, M., & Applegate, B. (1993). Middle school students' mathematical problem solving: An analysis of think-aloud protocols. *Learning Disability Quarterly, 16,* 19–32.

Montague, M., & Bos, C. (1990). Cognitive and metacognitive characteristics of eighth-grade students' mathematical problem solving. *Learning and Individual Differences, 2,* 109–127.

Nichols, P. D. (1994). A framework for developing cognitively diagnostic assessments. *Review of Educational Research, 64,* 575–603.

Palincsar, A. S., & Brown, A. L. (1984). Reciprocal teaching of comprehension-fostering and monitoring activities. *Cognition and Instruction, 1,* 117–175.

Paris, S. G., Calfee, R. C., Filby, N., Hiebert, E. H., Pearson, D. P., Valencia, S. W., & Wolf, K. P. (1992). A framework for authentic literacy assessment. *Reading Teacher, 46*(2), 88–98.

Poteet, J. A., Choate, J. S., & Stewart, S. C. (1993). Performance assessment and special education: Practices and prospects. *Focus on Exceptional Children, 26*(1), 1–20.

Pressley, M., & Afflerbach, P. (1995). *Verbal protocols of reading: The nature of constructively responsive reading.* Hillsdale, NJ: Erlbaum.

Reschly, D. J. (1996). Functional assessment and special education decision making. In W. Stainback & S. Stainback (Eds.), *Controversial issues confronting special education: Divergent perspectives* (pp. 115–128). Boston: Allyn and Bacon.

Salvia, J., & Ysseldyke, J. S. (1991). *Assessment* (5th ed.). Boston: Houghton Mifflin.

Shaklee, B. (1993). Preliminary findings of the early assessment for exceptional potential project. *Roeper Review, 16,* 105–109.

Shapiro, E. S. (1990). An integrated model for curriculum-based assessment. *School Psychology Review, 19,* 331–349.

Shapiro, E. S. (1996). *Academic skills problems: Direct assessment and intervention* (2nd ed.). New York: Guilford Press.

Shapiro, E. S., & Eckert, T. L. (1993). Curriculum-based assessment among school psychologists: Knowledge, use, and attitudes. *Journal of School Psychology, 31,* 357–383.

Shinn, M. R. (1995). Best practices in curriculum-based measurement and its use in a problem-solving model. In A. Thomas & J. Grimes (Eds.), *Best practices in school psychology–III* (pp. 547–567). Washington, DC: National Association of School Psychologists.

Shinn, M. R., Rosenfield, S., & Knutson, N. (1989). Curriculum-based assessment: A comparison of models. *School Psychology Review, 18,* 299–316.

Spector, J. E. (1992). Predicting progress in beginning reading: Dynamic assessment of phonemic awareness. *Journal of Educational Psychology, 84,* 353–363.

Stiggins, R. J. (1997). *Student-centered classroom assessment* (2nd ed.). Upper Saddle River, NJ: Merrill.

Swanson, H. L. (1996). Classification and dynamic assessment of children with learning disabilities. *Focus on Exceptional Children, 28*(9), 1–20.

Tittle, C. K. (1991). Changing models of student and teacher assessment. *Educational Psychologist*, 26, 157–165.

Tzuriel, D., & Klein, P. S. (1985). The assessment of analogical thinking modifiability among regular, special education, disadvantaged and mentally retarded children. *Journal of Abnormal Child Psychology*, 13, 539–553.

Varnhagen, S., & Gerber, M. M. (1984). Use of microcomputers for spelling assessment: Reasons to be cautious. *Learning Disability Quarterly*, 7, 266–270.

Vellutino, F. R., Scanlon, D. M., & Tanzman, M. S. (1998). The case for early intervention in diagnosing specific reading disability. *Journal of School Psychology*, 36, 367–397.

Vye, N. J., Delclos, V. R., & McGoldrick, J. A. (1988). *Effects of dynamic assessment on teacher instruction and child performance.* Paper presented at the annual meeting of the American Educational Research Association, New Orleans, April.

Vygotsky, L. S. (1978). Interaction between learning and development. In M. Cole, V. John-Steiner, S. Scribner, & E. Souberman (Eds. and Trans.), *Mind in society: The development of higher psychological processes* (pp. 79–91). Cambridge, MA: Harvard University Press. (Original work published 1935)

Wansart, W. L. (1990). Learning to solve a problem: A microanalysis of the solution strategies of learning disabled children. *Journal of Learning Disabilities*, 23, 164–170.

Ward, L., & Traweek, D. (1993). Application of a metacognitive strategy to assessment, intervention, and consultation: A think-aloud technique. *Journal of School Psychology*, 31, 469–485.

Watkins, M. W., & Kush, J. C. (1988). Assessment of academic skills of learning disabled students with classroom microcomputers. *School Psychology Review*, 17, 81–88.

Wright, L., & Borland, J. H. (1993). Using early childhood developmental portfolios in the identification and education of young, economically disadvantaged, potentially gifted students. *Roeper Review*, 15, 205–210.

CHAPTER 7

Analogue Assessment of Academic Skills

Curriculum-Based Measurement and Performance Assessment

LYNN S. FUCHS
DOUGLAS FUCHS
Peabody College, Vanderbilt University

Most academic assessment is analogue in nature. School settings rarely afford data-collection opportunities in which children perform academic skills within naturally occurring situations. Even systematic observation of students completing classroom worksheets or exercises fails to mirror the natural contexts within which authentic skill application is required. In light of the pervasive transfer problems many students with learning problems demonstrate, a disparity may exist between students' demonstration of competence on classroom exercises and students' application of that competence within authentic situations. Nevertheless, some analogue forms of academic assessment are more authentic and are more strongly linked to the goals teachers hold for their students than are other forms of academic assessment.

The most widely used form of assessment for indexing students' academic competence and learning is the traditional commercial achievement test. Unfortunately, in recent years, traditional commercial achievement tests have increasingly been criticized for at least three problems. First, because they are time consuming and expensive and because they provide few, if any, alternate forms, these tests are administered annually; such infrequent testing limits its utility for instructional planning.

Second, because traditional commercial achievement tests are designed to maximize differences between students, these tests sample information broadly, across multiple years of potential learning. Such broad behavior-sampling precludes highly detailed analyses of student performance and makes it difficult to formulate decisions about the extent to which students have learned the school's annual curriculum.

Finally, because of efficiency concerns, traditional commercial achievement tests tend to rely on multiple-choice response formats of basic, factual content. Such a sampling plan ignores much of the schools' curriculum, and some argue that traditional commercial achievement tests omit the more important, challenging, and authentic segments of the school curriculum (Darling-Hammond, 1992; Mory & Salisbury, 1992).

Curriculum-based measurement and performance assessment are two alternatives designed to avoid many of the weaknesses inherent in traditional commercial tests. In this chapter we first provide an overview of curriculum-based measurement (CBM). We discuss the CBM model. We briefly review the research documenting CBM's utility and, we highlight CBM's limitations. Then we discuss our recent attempts to expand CBM to higher-order academic domains of learning by integrating CBM with performance assessment.

CURRICULUM-BASED MEASUREMENT

CBM (Deno, 1985) is a set of methods for indexing academic competence and progress. Based on a program of research conducted at multiple sites since 1977 (Deno, 1985; Fuchs, 1995; Shinn, 1989), CBM specifies procedures for sampling test stimuli from local curricula, for administering and scoring those assessments, and for summarizing and interpreting the resulting database (Deno & Fuchs, 1987). Research has documented that CBM produces reliable and valid information about a student's academic standing at a given point in time (Marston, 1989) and that when performance is measured routinely on alternate forms of the assessment, CBM models academic progress reasonably well (Good, Deno, & Fuchs, 1995).

Because the same datum, aggregated in different ways, can be used to index standing as well as growth, and because a longstanding research program (Fuchs, 1995) documents CBM's capacity to inform, foster, and document treatment effectiveness, CBM can be used in flexible ways. In fact, over the years CBM has been incorporated into unified assessment systems to address a variety of psychoeducational decisions. These decisions include identifying students for special services (Marston & Magnusson, 1988; Shinn, 1995), as well as developing intervention plans (Wesson, 1989), monitoring the effectiveness of and formatively improving those plans over time (Fuchs, Deno, & Mirkin, 1984; Fuchs, Fuchs, Hamlett, & Stecker, 1991; Jones & Krouse, 1988; Wesson, 1991), decertifying and reintegrating students into general education (Allen, 1989; Fuchs, Fuchs, & Fernstrom, 1993), and evaluating the effectiveness of school programs (Germann & Tindal, 1985; Marston, 1987–1988).

In this discussion of CBM, we first explain the research-and-development process underlying CBM and explain how CBM combines conventional with innovative approaches to assessment. Second, we use a case study to illustrate how practitioners use CBM for a variety of decision-making purposes. Next, we provide an overview of CBM research, which provides the basis for using CBM for multidimensional decision making. Finally, we discuss some key limitations associated with CBM.

Development

In developing CBM, Deno and colleagues (see Deno, 1985) sought to establish a measurement system that (1) teachers could use efficiently; (2) would produce accurate, meaningful information with which to index growth; (3) could answer questions about the effectiveness of programs in producing academic growth; and (4) would provide information to help teachers plan better instructional programs. To accomplish this goal, a systematic program of research, conceptualized as a 3 × 3 matrix (Deno & Fuchs, 1987), was undertaken. The rows in this matrix specified three essential questions for the development of a measurement system: (1)what to measure, (2) how to measure, and (3) how to use the resulting database; the columns provided three criteria against which decisions could be formulated: (1) technical adequacy, (2) treatment validity, and (3) feasibility. A 15-year research program has addressed each of the nine cells in this matrix with multiple studies.

CBM deliberately integrates key concepts from traditional measurement theory and from the conventions of classroom-based observational methodology to forge an innovative approach to assessment. As with traditional measurement, every CBM assessment samples a relatively broad range of skills: Each dimension of the annual curriculum is represented on each weekly test. Consequently, each repeated measurement is an alternate form, of equivalent difficulty, assessing the same constructs. This principle is illustrated in CBM's spelling assessment, which samples the same relatively large domain of spelling words in the same way, to include multiple phonetic patterns and irregular spellings and to represent the same constructs and difficulty level (Fuchs, Allinder, Hamlett, & Fuchs, 1990). This sampling strategy differs markedly from typical classroom-based assessment methods, where teachers assess mastery on a list of 10–20 words and, after mastery is demonstrated, move on to a different set of words (see Fuchs & Deno, 1991). CBM also relies on a traditional psychometric framework by incorporating conventional notions of reliability and validity so that the standardized test administration and scoring methods yield accurate and meaningful information (Deno, Mirkin, Lowry, & Kuehnle, 1980).

By sampling broadly and relying on standardized administration and scoring procedures, the total CBM score can be viewed as a "performance indicator": It produces a broad dispersion of scores across individuals of the same age (i.e., when measuring spelling, scores typically range from 15 to 180 letter sequences correct), with rank orderings that correspond to important external criteria, and it represents an individual's global level of competence in the domain (e.g., Deno et al., 1980). Practitioners can use this performance indicator to identify discrepancies in performance levels between individuals and peer groups, which can inform decisions about the need for special services or the point at which decertification and reintegration of students with disabilities might occur.

At the same time, however, CBM departs from conventional psychometric applications by integrating the concepts of standardized measurement and traditional reliability and validity with key features from classroom-based observational methodology: repeated performance sampling, fixed time recording, graphic displays of time-series data, and qualitative descriptions of student performance. Reliance on these classroom-based observational methods permits estimates of slope for different time periods and alternative interventions for the same individual; this creates the necessary data for testing the effectiveness of different treatments for a given student. Research also suggests that, when combined with prescriptive decision rules, these time-series analytic methods result in better instruction and learning: Teachers raise goals more often and develop higher expectations (Fuchs, Fuchs, & Hamlett, 1989a), introduce more revisions to their instructional programs (Fuchs, Fuchs, & Hamlett, 1989b), and effect better achievement (Fuchs, Fuchs, Hamlett, & Stecker, 1991).

In addition, because each assessment simultaneously samples the multiple skills embedded in the annual curriculum, CBM can yield rich, qualitative descriptions of student performance to supplement the graphed, quantitative analysis of performance. These diagnostic profiles demonstrate adequate reliability and validity (see Fuchs, Fuchs, Hamlett, & Allinder, 1989; Fuchs, Fuchs, Hamlett, Thompson, Roberts, Kubec, & Stecker, 1994), offer the advantage of being rooted in the local curriculum, provide a framework for determining strategies for improving student programs (see Fuchs, Fuchs, & Hamlett, 1994), and result in teachers planning more varied, specific, and responsive instruction to meet individual student needs (Fuchs, Fuchs, Hamlett, & Allinder, 1991).

Consequently, CBM bridges traditional psychometric and classroom-based observational assessment paradigms to forge an innovative approach to measurement. Through this bridging of frameworks CBM simultaneously yields information about relative standing as well as change; about global competence as well as skill-by-skill mastery. It can, therefore, be used to answer questions about interindividual differences (e.g., How different is Henry's academic level from that of other students in the class, school, or district?); questions about intraindividual improvement (e.g., How successful is an adapted regular classroom in producing better academic growth for Henry?); and questions about how to strengthen an individual student's program (e.g., On which skills in the annual curriculum does Henry require instruction?).

Case Study Illustrating CBM's Application

We illustrate the multifaceted application of CBM with a fictitious fourth-grader, Margie, in the area of mathematics. Each week, Margie's teacher administered to the entire class one alternate form of the CBM math computation test and the CBM concepts/applications test. Sample tests are shown in Figure 7.1. These CBMs are constructed so that each assessment samples the entire year's curriculum in the same way, with different problems presented in different order across tests. Each test is brief, lasting between 1 and 8 minutes, depending on grade level.

In September and October, as shown in Figure 7.2, the mean CBM performance of Margie's classroom peers was 24 problems answered correctly (standard deviation (SD) = 9); their slope averaged .37 problems increased per week (SD = .14). These data verified an acceptable instructional environment, as demonstrated by a classroom growth rate that conforms well with normative fourth-grade data (Fuchs, Fuchs, Hamlett, Walz, & Germann, 1993). Margie's CBM performance, by contrast, aver-

Sheet #1   Computation 4

Password: ARM

Name: _____ Date: _____

A $\frac{3}{7} - \frac{2}{7} =$	B $1\frac{6}{7} + 3 =$	C $4\overline{)6}$	D $6\overline{)78}$	E $\begin{array}{r} 875 \\ \times\ \ 7 \end{array}$
F $\begin{array}{r} 6 \\ \times 3 \end{array}$	G $\begin{array}{r} 9 \\ \times 0 \end{array}$	H $\begin{array}{r} 244 \\ \times\ \ 7 \end{array}$	I $6\overline{)48}$	J $5\overline{)20}$
K $2\overline{)50}$	L $\begin{array}{r} 6144 \\ -\ 4420 \end{array}$	M $\begin{array}{r} 33 \\ \times 10 \end{array}$	N $\begin{array}{r} 6 \\ \times 0 \end{array}$	O $7\overline{)30}$
P $\begin{array}{r} 95225 \\ +\ 75268 \end{array}$	Q $8\overline{)32}$	R $\begin{array}{r} 1156 \\ 2824 \\ +\ \ \ 83 \end{array}$	S $7\frac{4}{7} - 2 =$	T $\begin{array}{r} 38 \\ \times 33 \end{array}$
U $\frac{3}{5} + \frac{1}{5} =$	V $\begin{array}{r} 982 \\ -\ 97 \end{array}$	W $\begin{array}{r} 9 \\ \times 5 \end{array}$	X $\begin{array}{r} 4 \\ \times 1 \end{array}$	Y $7\overline{)56}$

FIGURE 7.1   A sample fourth-grade CBM computation test and a sample fourth-grade CBM concepts/applications test.

Name _____ Date _____ Test 2 Page 1

Column A **Applications 4** Column B

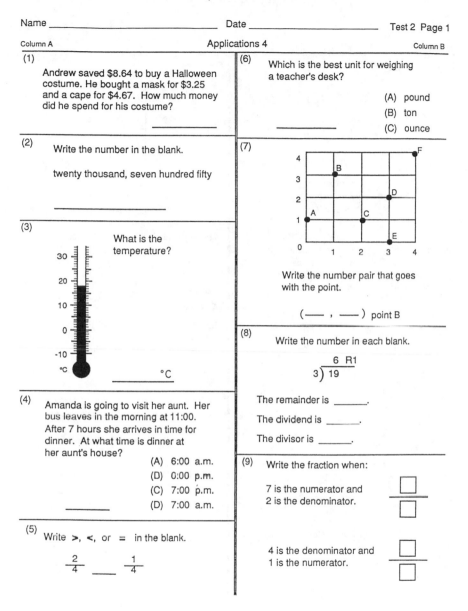

(1) Andrew saved $8.64 to buy a Halloween costume. He bought a mask for $3.25 and a cape for $4.67. How much money did he spend for his costume?

_____

(2) Write the number in the blank.

twenty thousand, seven hundred fifty

_____

(3) What is the temperature?

30
20
10
0
-10
°C

_____ °C

(4) Amanda is going to visit her aunt. Her bus leaves in the morning at 11:00. After 7 hours she arrives in time for dinner. At what time is dinner at her aunt's house?

(A) 6:00 a.m.
(D) 0:00 p.m.
(C) 7:00 p.m.
(D) 7:00 a.m.

_____

(5) Write >, <, or = in the blank.

$\frac{2}{4}$ ____ $\frac{1}{4}$

(6) Which is the best unit for weighing a teacher's desk?

(A) pound
(B) ton
(C) ounce

_____

(7)

4
3   B
2   A   C
1

0   1   2   3   4

D
E
F

Write the number pair that goes with the point.

(____ , ____) point B

(8) Write the number in each blank.

6 R1
3) 19

The remainder is _____.

The dividend is _____.

The divisor is _____.

(9) Write the fraction when:

7 is the numerator and 2 is the denominator.

☐
—
☐

4 is the denominator and 1 is the numerator.

☐
—
☐

(continued)

Name _____   Date _____   Test 2 Page 2

Column C   Applications 4   Column D

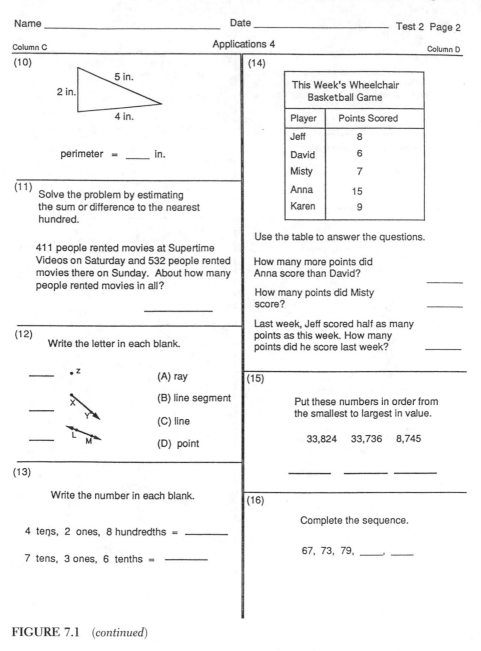

(10)

5 in.

2 in.

4 in.

perimeter = _____ in.

(11)   Solve the problem by estimating
the sum or difference to the nearest
hundred.

411 people rented movies at Supertime
Videos on Saturday and 532 people rented
movies there on Sunday. About how many
people rented movies in all?

_____

(12)   Write the letter in each blank.

_____   • Z   (A) ray

_____   X   (B) line segment
            Y
                                (C) line
_____   L
            M   (D) point

(13)

Write the number in each blank.

4 tens, 2 ones, 8 hundredths = _____

7 tens, 3 ones, 6 tenths = _____

(14)

This Week's Wheelchair Basketball Game	
Player	Points Scored
Jeff	8
David	6
Misty	7
Anna	15
Karen	9

Use the table to answer the questions.

How many more points did
Anna score than David?   _____

How many points did Misty
score?   _____

Last week, Jeff scored half as many
points as this week. How many
points did he score last week? _____

(15)

Put these numbers in order from
the smallest to largest in value.

33,824   33,736   8,745

_____   _____   _____

(16)

Complete the sequence.

67, 73, 79, ____, ____

FIGURE 7.1   (continued)

Name _____ Date _____ Test 2 Page 3

Column E · Applications 4 · Column F

(17)

The 126 children who are on a field trip to the zoo are divided among 6 groups. How many children are in each group? _____

(18)

Look at the number:

147.23

Which digit is in the hundredths place? _____

(19)

Area = _____ sq. units

(20)

Write the number in each blank.

8 ten thousands, 5 hundreds, 1 ones

_____

8 thousands, 7 hundreds, 7 tens, 6 ones

_____

(21)

Look at the number.

54.2

Which digit is in the tenths place? _____

(22)

Write a number in the blank.

_____ days = 1 week

(23)

Rewrite as a decimal.

(A) $\dfrac{9}{100}$ = _____

(B) $\dfrac{72}{100}$ = _____

(24)

Number of Birds Observed at Sanibel Sanctuary

Each 🐦 stands for 4 birds.

Use the pictograph to answer the questions.

How many more birds did David see than Ayesh? _____

Natalie saw 4 times as many birds in her back yard as in the sanctuary. How many birds did she see in her back yard? _____

How many birds did Erin see? _____

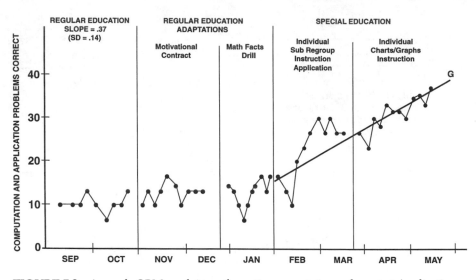

FIGURE 7.2 A sample CBM graph in mathematics computation and concepts/applications.

aged only 10 problems correct, with a slope of .14 increase in correct answers per week. This dual discrepancy, in both level and growth, placed Margie one standard deviation below the classroom mean both in terms of performance level and slope. The classroom teacher, then, in consultation with the school psychologist, conducted a prereferral assessment by developing and testing two preferral interventions: a motivational contract (with which Margie monitored her completion of classroom work during math instruction and received a negotiated reward for work completion) and math facts drill using a computer. When it became clear, based on the CBM data, that neither prereferral intervention had improved Margie's rate of math growth, special education services were employed for 25 minutes of daily individual math instruction.

The special education teacher first established a goal of 1.5 weekly increase in problems correct for Margie. This desired rate of improvement appears on Margie's graph as a diagonal line (with "G" showing the end-of-year goal). Then, based on a diagnostic skills analysis of Margie's current CBM math errors (see Figure 7.3), the special education teacher identified subtraction with regrouping as problematic. Therefore, during an initial special education intervention, the teacher provided instruction in subtraction with regrouping and incorporated systematic, explicit teaching to help Margie apply this skill in problem-solving situations. With this intervention, Margie's rate of growth increased to 1.72 problems per week—a level higher than the teacher's stated goal.

After several weeks of this intervention, however, the special educator noted a leveling-off in Margie's CBM scores. At that time, the teacher conducted another diagnostic analysis of Margie's CBM database, this time identifying charts and graphs as a problematic skill. Consequently, the special educator designed the next intervention to address this skill. As shown in Figure 7.2, with this intervention, Margie maintained a strong and acceptable rate of growth in mathematics.

Margie — Computation 4

Sep	Oct	Nov	Dec	Jan	Feb	Mar	Apr	May

A1 Adding
S1 Subtracting
M1 Multiplying basic facts
M2 Multiplying by 1 digit
M3 Multiplying by 2 digits
D1 Dividing basic facts
D2 One-step dividing
D3 Two-step dividing
F1 Add/subtract simple fractions
F2 Add/subtract mixed fractions

■ HOT. You've got it!
◨ VERY WARM. Almost have it.
▦ WARM. Starting to get it.
▢ COOL. Trying these.
□ COLD. Not tried

Margie — Applications 4

Sep	Oct	Nov	Dec	Jan	Feb	Mar	Apr	May

NC Number concepts
NN Names of numbers and vocabulary
Me Measurement
GR Grid reading
CG Charts and graphs
AP Area and perimeter
Fr Fractions
De Decimals
WP Word Problems

■ HOT. You've got it!
◨ VERY WARM. Almost have it.
▦ WARM. Starting to get it.
▢ COOL. Trying these.
□ COLD. Not tried

FIGURE 7.3 A sample CBM skills profile for mathematics computation and for concepts/applications.

How CBM Meets the Technical Requirements
for Multifaceted Decision Making

To meet the technical requirements associated with a variety of psychoeducational decisions (e.g., screening, prereferral intervention, instructional planning), CBM must demonstrate technical adequacy for modeling academic growth, distinguishing between ineffective general education environments and unacceptable individual student learning, informing instructional planning, and evaluating relative treatment effectiveness.

Requirement 1: Modeling Academic Growth

For longitudinally modeling individual change, instruments must demonstrate certain technical features, all found in CBM. First, the instrument must produce data with interval scale properties, free from ceiling or floor effects. With CBM, a common test framework is administered to children within a fixed age range; so, it is possible to judge performance over an academic year on the same raw score metric. When performance is measured on the appropriate instructional level of the curriculum, floor and ceiling effects do not occur.

Second, the construct and the difficulty level measured over time must remain constant: The construct tapped by CBM over the course of an academic year is qualitatively constant, and the difficulty level remains the same.

The third technical requirement for the modeling of growth is that a sufficient number of alternate forms be available to obtain accurate estimates of the parameters of change. With CBM, one can sample the curriculum repeatedly to create as many alternate forms as necessary.

Given an appropriate instrument or set of measurement methods, current techniques for measuring change reconceptualize growth as a continuous, rather than an incremental process. The goal is to describe trajectories, or continuous time-dependent curves, which reflect the change process. An initial step in such a process is to formulate a model for change at the individual level. Fuchs and colleagues (1993), for example, examined students' academic growth rates when CBM was conducted for one school year in reading, spelling, and math. For many students on each CBM measure, a linear relationship adequately modeled student progress within one academic year. These findings, in combination with corroborating evidence (Good et al., 1995; Good & Shinn, 1990), support a conceptualization of CBM growth characterized by a linear relationship, where slope is a primary parameter describing the change process.

Requirement 2: Distinguishing Between Ineffective Instruction
and Unacceptable Individual Learning

To determine whether a student's individual growth rate may indicate a serious learning problem requiring special intervention, it is necessary to interpret that growth rate relative to the growth of other students receiving the same instruction. The effectiveness of regular classroom instructional settings is not constant. In our work using CBM in math, for example, we have found that the effectiveness of most and least effective teachers working with comparable groups of children varies dramatically (Fuchs & Fuchs, 1999). Because lack of responsiveness and potential learning problems therefore must be judged situationally, a database that generates classwide growth rates must be collected in general education classrooms.

Even with the availability of such classwide databases, it is necessary to determine whether CBM dual discrepancies identify appropriate pools of students. To begin to address this question, we have examined groups of students for whom CBM data have been collected classwide (e.g., Fuchs & Fuchs, 1999). These analyses have lent empirical support for using CBM within a dual-discrepancy model of initial identification, which simultaneously examines discrepancies in students' levels of performance and growth over time relative to classroom peers.

Requirement 3: Informing Instructional Planning

A longstanding research program documents how CBM enhances teacher planning and student outcomes in three ways: (1) by helping teachers maintain appropriately ambitious student goals (Fuchs, Fuchs, & Hamlett, 1989a), (2) by assisting teachers in determining when revisions to their instructional programs are necessary to prompt better student growth (Fuchs, Fuchs, & Hamlett, 1989b; Stecker, 1994; Wesson, Skiba, Sevcik, King, & Deno, 1984), and by stimulating ideas for potentially effective instructional adjustments (Fuchs, Fuchs, Hamlett, & Allinder, 1991; Fuchs, Fuchs, & Hamlett, 1989c; Fuchs, Fuchs, Hamlett, & Stecker, 1991).

Research also has examined the overall efficacy and treatment validity of CBM methods. Studies (Fuchs, Deno, & Mirkin, 1984; Fuchs, Fuchs, Hamlett, & Allinder, 1991; Fuchs, Fuchs, Hamlett, & Ferguson, 1992; Jones & Krouse, 1988; Stecker, 1994; Wesson et al., 1984; Wesson, 1991) conducted over the past two decades provide corroborating evidence of dramatic effects on student outcomes in reading, spelling, and mathematics when special and general educators rely on CBM to inform their instructional planning.

Requirement 4: Evaluating Treatment Effectiveness

The fourth requirement is that CBM must provide an adequate database for judging treatment effectiveness; that is, the assessment must demonstrate sensitivity to student growth and to relative treatment effects and must permit comparisons of the effectiveness of alternative service-delivery options.

With respect to sensitivity to change and relative treatment effects, in an early study devoted to the issue of sensitivity to academic change, Marston and colleagues (1986) tested students on traditional, commercial achievement tests and on curriculum-based reading and written language measures early in October and 10 weeks later in

December. CBM registered more student growth than did the traditional tests, suggesting greater sensitivity to student growth. In an operational replication, published as a second study in the same article, Marston and colleagues pre- and posttested students 16 weeks apart on traditional, commercial reading achievement tests; assessed these students weekly on CBM for 16 weeks; and had teachers rate student progress in reading over this 16-week period. As with the first study, results demonstrated CBM's greater sensitivity to student growth compared to the traditional, commercial measures of reading achievement. In addition, CBM produced the largest correlation with teachers' judgments of learning; there was also a statistically significant difference between the correlation based on CBM and the one based on a traditional test.

Studies have also demonstrated that CBM slopes reflect treatment effects more sensitively than traditional measures administered on a pre/post basis. Fuchs, Fuchs, and Hamlett (1989b) showed that on the Stanford Achievement Test—Reading Comprehension Subtest, administered to detect incremental change between two points in time, change scores of the treatment groups were not significantly different. By contrast, on CBM slope data, differences between groups achieved statistical significance and were associated with a much larger effect size. This pattern showing substantially larger effect sizes for CBM slope data has been corroborated by other treatment effectiveness research (Fuchs, Fuchs, Hamlett, & Stecker, 1991; Fuchs, Fuchs, Hamlett, Phillips, & Bentz, 1994).

In terms of comparisons of alternative service-delivery options, Marston (1987–1988) compared the relative effectiveness of regular and special education by analyzing slopes on weekly CBM reading scores. An initial pool of 272 fourth-, fifth-, and sixth-graders were selected for the year-long study on the basis of performance at or below the 15th percentile on the Minneapolis Benchmark Test. The CBM reading performance of these 272 children was measured weekly. The 11 students who (1) spent at least 10 weeks in regular education, (2) were referred to and placed in special education, and (3) spent at least 10 weeks in special education were the focus of the analysis.

To determine the relative treatment effects of the two service-delivery arrangements, a repeated measures analysis of variance was applied to the CBM slope data. Slopes were statistically significantly greater in special than in regular education, with the average slopes increasing from .60 to 1.15 words across the two service-delivery settings. For 10 of 11 students the slopes were larger in special education; in 7 of the 10 cases the difference was dramatic.

In a similar way, Fuchs, Fuchs, and Fernstrom (1993) used slope to examine the relative effectiveness of special and regular education for individual students as they moved in the opposite direction—as they reintegrated into general education. Twenty-one special-education students had been randomly assigned to a condition designed to facilitate successful reintegration into regular classroom math instruction. Special educators used CBM to inform and strengthen planning in the area of mathematics; at the same time they monitored the target student's CBM growth and that of three low-performing members of the general education setting. When the target student's performance level approached that of the low-performing peers, reintegration occurred, and the onus for instruction was transferred to the regular classroom teacher. After reintegration, CBM data continued to be collected for the target student and for the low-performing peers in the regular classroom. Within special education, the experimental students' slopes were significantly greater than those of the low-performing peers. However, after reintegration, the slopes of the target students plunged and were significantly lower than that of the comparison students. As with the Marston (1987–1988) study, this database clearly revealed the effectiveness of the special, over the general education setting for many (although not all) students. Both studies demonstrate CBM's capacity to document the effects of service-delivery options.

Limitations of the CBM Model

As discussed, the empirical basis for CBM's technical adequacy for describing students' academic competence at one point in time, for modeling student growth over time, and for identifying pools of students appropriate for further assessment is promising. Moreover, a strong body of research clearly documents how CBM can simultaneously inform, strengthen, and document the effects of academic interventions. Despite this strong technical basis supporting CBM, at least two limitations associated with CBM exist. The first limitation concerns feasibility questions; the second concerns CBM's narrow focus on skill acquisition.

Feasibility

Feasibility questions address schools' capacity to conduct routine CBM data collection on large numbers of students. When individually administered by teachers, CBM can be time consuming. Observations of teachers conducting CBM indicate that to prepare, provide directions for, administer, and score one assessment, and to graph and analyze data for one student in one academic area, a teacher devotes approximately 2.5 minutes (Fuchs, Fuchs, Hamlett, & Hasselbring, 1987; Wesson, Fuchs, Tindal, Mirkin, & Deno, 1986). Multiplied over a class of 25 pupils and over two academic areas, weekly assessment demands a substantial allocation of teacher time.

Despite these figures, some school districts have demonstrated the capacity to conduct weekly, schoolwide CBM data collection. Hiawatha Elementary School in Minneapolis, for example, has employed support staff, aides, and volunteers to collect CBM reading data on every student in the school, every week of the year (Self, Benning, Marston, & Magnusson, 1991). Clearly, however, such an effort requires systemic support at the school level.

In an effort to address the time required to collect and manage an ongoing assessment database, we have developed computer applications over the past decade (Fuchs, Fuchs, & Hamlett, 1993; Fuchs, Fuchs, & Hamlett, 1994, for summaries of the related research programs). This software automatically (1) administers and scores the assessments as students work at computers; (2) provides performance feedback to students; (3) graphs performance over time and calculates slopes of growth; (4) applies decision rules to the graphed data and makes recommendations to raise goals or change programs accordingly; (5) summarizes students' strengths and weaknesses in the curriculum; (6) analyzes the assessment profile and interacts with the teacher to formulate recommendations about how to adjust the teaching program for individual students; and (7) produces classwide reports that summarize the performance of the class, make large- and small-group teaching recommendations, and automatically identify students with dual discrepancies from their classmates in performance level and slope. With this software, the time teachers devote to the mechanics of implementing CBM is eliminated, and satisfaction with the process increases (Fuchs, Hamlett, Fuchs, Stecker, & Ferguson, 1988). Over the past five years, numerous school systems have relied on these computer programs to facilitate CBM data collection.

Limited Focus on Skill Acquisition

CBM represents a well-developed measurement system that teachers can implement, having confidence that the assessment information is accurate and meaningful. It represents student progress well, and informs their instructional decision making in important ways that enhance student progress. A major limitation associated with CBM, however, is its failure to base the assessment process in real-life problem-solving contexts. Instead, CBM, especially in the area of mathematics, traditionally has focused on the acquisition of skills without attention to students' capacity to integrate and apply those skills in authentic situations. (It is important to note that this is less true for reading than for math; see Fuchs & Fuchs, 1999 for discussion.) Because of this shortcoming, especially in the area of math, over the past 5 years we have invested considerable effort in extending CBM to a problem-solving mathematics assessment framework. This framework is known as performance assessment.

EXTENDING CBM WITH PERFORMANCE ASSESSMENT

Performance assessment (PA) provides students with real-life problem-solving situations and requires them to develop solutions that involve the application and integration of multiple skills and strategies. The goal of PA is to inform teachers about students' strategies and processes, rather than about isolated skill deficiencies, and to redirect teachers' instructional efforts to incorporate learning activities with greater generalizability to real-life dilemmas (see Archbald & Newmann, 1988; Fuchs, 1994; Shepard, 1989; Wiggins, 1989).

Despite this lofty goal, serious questions remain about how PAs can be designed to enhance teachers' capacity to monitor the effects of their instruction and to improve their teaching so that student learning increases. In this section, we review some of the problems and challenges presented by PA for classroom assessment purposes. We then describe our recent activities designed to expand CBM into the mathematics problem-solving domain using PA. Finally, we discuss early findings related to the technical adequacy of that CBM system designed to track students' development of mathematical problem-solving capacity.

Strengths, Problems, and Challenges of PA

PA demonstrates three key features: (1) The assessment tasks require students to construct, rather than select, responses; (2) the assessment formats create opportunities for teachers to observe student behavior on tasks reflecting real-world requirements; and (3) the scoring methods reveal patterns in students' learning and thinking in addition to the correctness of the students' answers. The major purposes of PA are to direct teachers and students toward important, well-integrated learning outcomes and to enhance teachers' capacity to design superior instructional plans and effect better student learning.

Many varieties of PA are described in the literature, and a wide range of methods are implemented today in classrooms (Baker, O'Neil, & Linn, 1993). Because PA is relatively new, underdeveloped, and yet to be studied systematically, practitioners are often in the undesirable position of interpreting vague design features and operationalizing those features into specific assessments on their own (see Baker, 1991; Brewer, 1991; Sammons, Kobett, Heiss, & Fennell, 1992). These operationalizations take a variety of forms, some of which are closer than others in approximating PA's conceptual and theoretical underpinnings (Baker et al., 1993; Fuchs, 1994).

PA, therefore, exists more as a vision of what classroom assessment methods might strive to achieve, rather than as a clearly defined, readily useable assessment technology. Difficult issues in operationalizing these assessments remain. Relatedly, although rhetoric suggests PA's potential contribution to instructional planning (e.g., Archbald & Newmann, 1988), research examining that contribution is only beginning to emerge. Nevertheless, in this section, we provide a *conceptual* analysis of PA's potential strengths and limitations, while relying to the greatest extent possible on available empirical evidence to determine whether, and if so how, PA might achieve its intended goals.

Strengths

PA's major advantages include (1) measuring skill application and integration, (2) yielding rich analyses that correspond to instructional decisions, and (3) serving as a communication vehicle. With respect to measuring skill application and integration, a major, distinctive advantage of PA is its deliberate focus on authentic performances that require students to integrate many skills within age-appropriate, real-world situations. As with all assessment methods (see Fuchs, 1994), however, tension exists between (1) designing an assessment strategy that mirrors valued, authentic, real-world performances in a world where those values may change rapidly and (2) developing a measurement system that can focus teachers and learners on an appropriately sized instructional domain (i.e., a small enough chunk for students to learn). One clear challenge for PA is to resolve this dilemma. At the present time it is unclear whether PA provides teachers and diagnosticians with a small enough chunk to preclude floors on student performance and to facilitate specific links to instructional strategies. To resolve this dilemma, core sets of outcomes need to be identified, which avoid unmanageably long lists of assessment domains and avoid short ones with only tangential relation to truly critical outcomes (Baker, 1991).

With respect to communicating the goals of learning to teachers and students, a much discussed advantage of PA is that the assessments closely reflect the desired instructional goals. Therefore, teachers should be able to use performance assessments to direct their instruction. Moreover, to the extent that the scoring rubrics are clear, concrete, and visible to students, pupils should be able to use performance assessments to establish personal learning goals and to seek assistance in achieving those goals. Communicating clearly about what is important for teachers to teach and students to learn is a highly valued emphasis of PA. Consequently, as methods are defined we should expect to see clearly articulated goals and scoring criteria to assist teachers and students in translating the assessments into everyday learning activities.

In terms of instructional decision making, given that providing insights into students' strategies is a major tenet of PA, we assume that useful diagnostic planning decisions can be formulated on the basis of the assessments. PAs should permit teachers to identify the strategies students employ in addressing complicated problems. Ideally, this focus on strategies should yield rich descriptions of student performance with clear connections to specific instructional ideas. As with any assessment method, however, teachers' capacities vary considerably in the extent to which they can identify insights into students' strategic behavior and relate those descriptions to specific instructional techniques. Research suggests that teachers typically experience difficulty in both dimensions of diagnostic planning—even when the assessment method and the conceptual framework for learning are more simple than with PA. With CBM, for example, research suggests that teachers experience difficulty in generating accurate skills profiles on the basis of assessments that incorporate multiple skills (e.g., Fuchs, Fuchs, Hamlett, & Stecker, 1990). Because of this difficulty, we eventually moved to computerized strategies for generating reliable profiles of student competence based on CBM. In addition, teachers sometime find it difficult to connect student problems with corrective instructional strategies (e.g., Fuchs, Fuchs, Hamlett, & Stecker, 1991). Because of this difficulty, CBM typically is used in conjunction with human or computerized instructional consultation methods. Consequently, despite PA's potential for yielding rich, detailed analyses of student performance that connect to instructional methods, work is still required to identify the means by which this can be achieved.

Problems

Despite these three important, potential strengths associated with PA, major concerns exist about PA's capacity to measure skill acquisition, to index growth and provide the basis for formative evaluation decisions, to produce technically viable information, and to be implemented feasibly within the constraints of ordinary classroom life. With respect to measuring skill acquisition, when a child fails to demonstrate skill application and integration within the context of a complex, rich task, it is not possible to identify whether the failure to apply knowledge is a function of poor strategies for generalizing acquired skills or whether the child has not mastered the skill in isolation.

Moreover, assessment methods should provide the basis for formative evaluation decisions. Unfortunately, the methods by which formative evaluation decisions might be derived are unclear. Such decisions require scoring methods that can be used to describe progress as well as procedures for designing alternate forms of relatively complex problems. Initial work suggests the potential difficulty in achieving assessment comparability when different, complex problems are involved (Baxter, Shavelson, Goldman, & Pine, 1992; Shavelson, Baxter, & Pine, 1992).

With respect to feasibility, PAs require large amounts of teacher time for (1) the design and administration of assessments and (2) the careful scrutiny of student performances to identify accurate learning patterns and to connect those patterns to corrective teaching strategies. Therefore, constraints on teacher time need to be addressed, especially in light of increasing student caseloads in both general and special education settings and increasing diversity of student skills in public school settings (Stallings, 1995).

In addition, planning decisions formulated on the basis of PAs can lead to a complicated instructional setting, where different students need to be working on different content in different ways. It is easy to imagine, for example, how developing plans to address simultaneously the needs of 20 to 30 students can lead some teachers quickly to reject the assessment paradigm—unless we address the issue of how to feasibly implement performance assessment-based plans within the constraints of everyday classroom life. With CBM, for example, a similar problem exists. The assessment system often leads teachers to introduce different intervention strategies for different students at different times (see Fuchs, Fuchs, Hamlett, Phillips, & Bentz, 1994). Over the years it became evident that unless we could identify feasible ways for teachers to implement the variety of instructional decisions based on the assessment, teachers would reject the assessment method. In response to this problem within general education, we designed peer-assisted teaching methods to facilitate implementation of the instructional decisions produced via CBM (e.g., Fuchs, Fuchs, Hamlett, Phillips, & Bentz, 1994). PA developers inevitably will have to face this issue.

In terms of generating accurate, meaningful information, at this time little is known about the extent to which PA systems satisfy technical criteria (Baker et al., 1993; Elliott, 1998). Early evidence from a large-scale state accountability assessment program does, however, raise concern. For example, a comprehensive evaluation (Hambleton, Jaeger, Koretz, Linn, Millman, & Phillips, 1995) of Kentucky's Instructional Results Information System, which relies strongly on PA, concluded that the large improvement registered on this statewide assessment program did not correspond to results on another, better developed assessment instrument; the setting of performance standards was seriously flawed; and the assessment information resulted in high rates of misclassification in the state's reward program. With respect to students with learning difficulties, Fuchs, Fuchs, Karns, Hamlett, Katzaroff, and Dutka (1998) studied fourth-graders who completed three measures representing three points on a traditional-alternative mathematics assessment continuum: a traditional, commercial multiple-choice achievement test; computation and application CBMs; and a PA. The traditional test and CBM demonstrated the capacity to discriminate individuals with and without serious learning problems; the PA did not.

These preliminary investigations, conducted within the context of large-scale testing programs rather than classroom-based assessment, indicate that substantial work remains to develop technically acceptable PAs, especially for students at the lower end of the achievement continuum. If experienced test developers with substantial measurement expertise have difficulty creating PAs that yield accurate, meaningful information, then it seems probable that classroom teachers will experience problems in developing sound assessments to match their classroom curricula. Clearly, additional work that defines PA features and test-development methods is required.

Over the past five years we have been developing a model that bridges CBM with PA in the area of mathematics problem solving. Our goal in developing a problem-solving assessment system was to extend the general outcome measurement model (Fuchs & Deno, 1991) beyond CBM's focus on basic skills acquisition to complex problem-solving situations. In preserving the general outcome measurement model, we strove to satisfy four key features associated with CBM: (1) to generate alternate forms that permit repeated measurement of long-term goal mastery, (2) to specify standardized methods that demonstrate traditional reliability and validity, (3) to provide a system with the capacity to model student growth, and (4) to provide a system with the capacity to inform instructional planning. Below, we describe the CBM problem-solving assessment system and provide an overview of research to date, which has examined the system's capacity to fulfill these four features.

Description of the CBM Problem-Solving Assessment System

Development

At each grade level, for grades 2 through 6, we developed six alternate forms of a PA using the following procedure. First, we selected a "massed concepts" PA framework (Sammons et al., 1992), designed to assess students' application of a "core" set of skills considered essential for successful entry to the next grade. Because the same core set of skills is incorporated into each PA at a given grade, massed concepts PAs can be considered alternate forms that are administered over the course of an academic year to track students' development of mathematical problem-solving competence toward the long-term (i.e., annual) goal. In this way our PA system is conceptually consistent with CBM's general outcome measurement model.

Having identified a conceptualization for our PA system, we developed one fourth-grade massed concepts PA. This illustrative PA, adapted from Sammons et al.

(1992), was piloted with 131 fourth-graders, for whom correlations between PA scores and the Comprehensive Test of Basic Skills Total Mathematics Battery ranged between .22 and .52 (Fuchs, Fuchs, Karns, Hamlett, Katzanoff, & Dutka, 1998).

The next step in the development process required a one-day teacher meeting. One week prior to the meeting, teachers had read a paper providing background information about PA (Fuchs & Fuchs, 1996). At the meeting, in grade-level groups, teachers reviewed the statewide mathematics curriculum to identify (1) 10 core skills most essential for successful entry to the next grade and (2) a list of important mathematics skills with which they expect students to enter the grade they teach. Then, in the large group, the teachers compared (1) the skills they specified as important for entering the next higher grade with (2) the skills identified by teachers in that next higher grade as critical for successful entry. With this input, teachers returned to grade-level teams to finalize lists of core skills. Teachers also identified and rank-ordered 20 themes that represented real-life situations students might face now or in the next few years, were interesting, could incorporate all 10 core skills, and were age appropriate. Finally, teachers individually completed the illustrative PA, were taught in the large group to use a PA scoring rubric, and split off into grade-level teams to score five sample PAs and to make suggestions for modifying the scoring rubric and the basic structure of the illustrative PA.

Working with this input, we collectively developed five PAs, one at each grade level. We piloted each PA with three students who were entering and three who were exiting the target grade. Based on the range of performances and the students' input about what they liked, disliked, and found confusing, we modified these initial PAs. We next developed a framework for developing the remaining five alternate PA forms at each grade level and then developed those remaining PAs.

The following sequence then recurred three times. At each grade level, five experienced teachers completed each of the six PAs. These adults, who were unfamiliar with the development process, identified every skill they applied in solving the PA; described inconsistencies in difficulty level and skills applications requirements across alternate forms; and noted potential sources of confusion within the narrative and questions. Based on this input, we revised the PAs.

Finally, four students (two exiting and two entering the target grade level) completed all six PAs at each grade. Based on their responses and input, we made a final set of revisions. See Figure 7.4 for one fourth-grade PA.

Format

Each two- to three-page PA begins with a multiparagraph narrative describing the problem situation. Each dilemma also presents students with tabular and graphic information for potential application in the PA. The problem includes questions that provide students opportunities to (1) apply the core set of skills, (2) discriminate relevant from irrelevant information in the narrative, (3) generate information not contained in the narrative, (4) explain their mathematical work, and (5) generate written communication related to the mathematics. At fourth grade, be-

Name _____   Date _____

Teacher _____   Grade   4   PA#   F

Garage Sale

Three families, the Hamletts, the Thompsons, and the Nelsons, are plannng a garage sale to sell clothes, toys, and books. The garage sale takes place in the Thompsons's garage, which is 20 feet long and 30 feet wide. Each family pitched in $35.00 to cover expenses. You figure at least 525 people will come to the garage sale if you hold it at a good time.

The families are renting tables for the sale. Each family needs its own table or set of tables. Each table costs 1/2 the price listed on the chart to rent. Each table is 5 feet long and 3 feet wide and can hold up to 15 items.

The families also need a price sticker for every item. Stickers come in packs of 40, but the families can share packs of stickers. Each pack costs 79¢.

Number of Items For Sale by Families	
Hamlets	🐻🐻
Nelsons	🐻🐻🐻
Thompsons	🐻🐻🐻🐻🐻

Key: Each 🐻 means 10 items.

Prices of Expenses for Garage Sale	
Renting 1 Table	$12.00
1 Pack of Stickers (40 in 1 Pack)	79¢
Running a Newspaper Advertisement	$27.00

**Table is 1/2 the price listed on the chart.

FIGURE 7.4 A sample fourth-grade CBM problem-solving test (i.e., performance assessment).

Name _____   Date _____

(1) The families are getting together to put an advertisement in the newspaper. Write the advertisement. Be sure to include everything customers need to know.

(2) How much will stickers cost?

(3) How many tables will the families need? Show all your work.

(4) Is there enough money to cover all of the expenses? If no, how much more money do they need? If yes, how much money do they have left and what other things for the garage sale might they buy? How much might each of these things cost?

(*continued*)

Name _____   Date _____

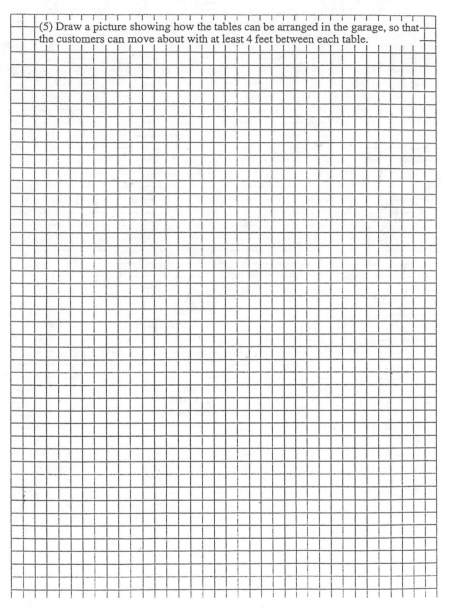

(5) Draw a picture showing how the tables can be arranged in the garage, so that the customers can move about with at least 4 feet between each table.

FIGURE 7.4   (*continued*)

cause one question on each PA requires use of graph paper, every page of the PA is superimposed onto graph paper. Between each question, ample space for response is provided.

Performance is scored according to the rubric shown in Figure 7.5, which we adapted from the Kansas Quality Performance Assessment (Kansas State Board of Education, 1991). In studies we have conducted (e.g., Fuchs, Fuchs, Karns, Hamlett, Katzaroff, & Dutka, 1998; Fuchs, Fuchs, Kazdan, Karns, Calhoon, Hamlett, & Hewlett, 2000), scorers have independently used this rubric with high levels of agreement (e.g., greater than 95%).

Initial Information about the PA System's Capacity to Meet Features of the General Outcome Measurement Model

In a series of studies, we have examined the technical features of this PA system in terms of its capacity to estimate students' levels of performance as well as their growth over time. We have also begun to explore teachers' use of this system for instructional decision making.

Repeated Measurement of Long-Term Goals

As discussed, in the development process, we attempted to conceptualize and operationalize a PA framework that tracks students' development of competence with respect to the long-term, or annual, goal for instruction. Therefore, through a careful specification process, we attempted to design alternate PA forms within grade levels. To test empirically our success in framing alternate forms, we examined alternate form/test–retest reliability among a sample of 350 students (Fuchs, Fuchs, Karns, Hamlett, Katzaroff, & Dutka, 1998). Coefficients ranged from .66 to .76. These figures, although lower than for conventional forms of assessment, exceed those demonstrated in prior work with other types of PAs (e.g., Baxter et al., 1992). Of course, given that we relied on a massed model of PA, we anticipated greater alternate form reliability.

Standardized Methods with Reliability and Validity for Describing Performance Levels

Among these 350 pupils, correlations with the more traditional Comprehensive Test of Basic Skills and the Mathematics Operations and Applications Test ranged from .62 to .68. Correlations with the Performance Assessments of the Iowa Test of Basic Skills ranged from .60 to .67. Therefore, by conventional standards, our PAs demonstrate respectable criterion validity with other measures of overall mathematical competence.

Score

Dimension	0	1	2	3	4	5
Conceptual underpinnings	No response or relevant information.	Responses show no understanding of ideas/concepts; misconceptions are evident.		Responses lack clarity, but show some, but incomplete, understanding of the mathematical concepts and ideas addressed.		Responses are clear and reflect indepth understanding of the mathematical concepts and ideas addressed.
Computational application	No response or relevant information.	Computations contain many errors.		Computations contain some errors.		Computations are completely correct.
Problem-solving strategies	No response or relevant information.	Problem-solving strategies incorporate few pieces of relevant data and simplistic reasoning.		Problem-solving strategies incorporate some relevant data and a defensible, although faulty, reasoning.		Problem-solving strategies incorporate all relevant pieces of data and are defensible, logical correct reasoning.
Communication	No response or relevant information.	Communication is poor with no viable rationale for decisions, methods, conclusions; mathematical terminology is missing or incorrect.		Communication is clear in places and ambiguous in other places; explains rationale for many steps of the problem-solving strategy; incorporates some correct mathematical terminology.		Communication is clear, complete, effective, and unambiguous; incorporates correct mathematical terminology.

FIGURE 7.5 CBM problem-solving scoring rubric.

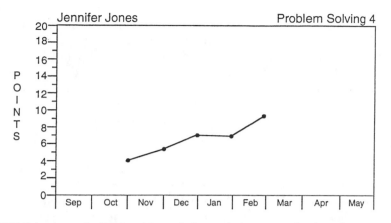

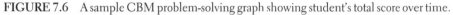

FIGURE 7.6   A sample CBM problem-solving graph showing student's total score over time.

Capacity to Index Growth

In a study involving more than 400 students, we administered five alternate-form PAs over a four-month interval to examine slopes of performance, or growth over time. Each student's total score across the four scoring dimensions was graphed against time (see Figure 7.6). For students with and without disabilities, respectively, PA slopes were .09 (SD = .17) and .32 (SD = .23). Slopes for students without disabilities were statistically significantly greater than for students with disabilities. In addition, students who were classified by teachers at the beginning of the study as high-, mid-, and low-achieving in mathematics earned PA slopes that were statistically significantly ordered as would be predicted: high, .54 (SD = .20); mid, .28 (SD = .20), and low, .11 (SD = .12). Consequently, PA slopes demonstrated discriminative validity.

Utility for Instructional Planning

Fuchs, Fuchs, Karns, Hamlett, and Katzaroff (in press) conducted a year-long investigation to examine instructional planning and student improvement as a function of the introduction of our PA system to classrooms. In this project we provided eight general educators with ongoing support for understanding PAs and for integrating this assessment information into their instructional plans.

   Between September and April, teachers administered the six alternate-form PAs within their grade level. In September, students received one 45-minute lesson on how PAs are structured, strategies for approaching PAs, and scoring methods. Following each PA administration, we provided each teacher with a release day. During each release day, teachers first scored: They reviewed procedures for scoring the PAs and providing written feedback to students; they then worked with fellow teachers at their grade level to achieve interscorer agreement of at least 80% on five protocols from their classrooms and to discuss their written comments back to students; they then scored the performances of all their own students. During lunch, research assistants entered the teachers' scores into software that managed the student's PA and CBM database. After lunch, teachers received a computerized summary report describing each student's performance on the PA. This report listed the teacher's scores on the four PA scoring dimensions and the teacher's scores reflecting the student's performance on each of the core skills in terms of (1) application of that skill (as demonstrated on the PA) and (2) acquisition of that skill (as demonstrated on the student's traditional CBM). See Figure 7.7 for a sample PA report. In addition to these individual student reports, the computer also summarized the performance of the class (see Figure 7.8).

During the afternoon of each release day, teachers reviewed a scripted lesson for teaching their students how to interpret PA feedback; brainstormed in the large group about how to modify their instruction to enhance student performance on the PAs; and completed instructional plan sheets on which they described their plans to modify instructional programs before the next PA administration. Within two days

Individualized Report

Teacher: CHAN Grade 2

Name: Danyale Blackwell

Date: January 22, 1996

TEACHER'S BIRTHDAY PARTY

Making Sense	0	1	[2]	3	4	5
Computation	0	[1]	2	3	4	5
Problem Solving	0	1	[2]	3	4	5
Communication	0	1	[2]	3	4	5

	Weekly Math Test	Problem Solving Test
Adding--Basic Facts	■	▥
Adding--Regrouping	□	□
Subtract--Basic Facts	▦	□
Subtract--No Regrouping	□	□
Subtract--Regrouping	▥	□
Money	▥	▥
Names of Numbers	▥	▤
Charts/Graphs	▥	□
Calendar		□

FIGURE 7.7   A sample CBM problem-solving skills profile.

after this session, teachers delivered the lesson explaining to students how to interpret PA feedback and distributed the scored PAs.

As reported on the instructional plan sheets across the release days, teachers modified instructional programs to address the PA content by teaching (1) computational skills (cited 5 times); (2) application skills (cited 11 times); (3) word problems (cited 9 times); (4) problem-solving strategies (cited 28 times); (5) methods for labeling and showing work (cited 23 times); and (6) content aligned directly to the PA activities (cited 27 times). If we combine the last two categories, methods for labeling/showing work and directly aligned content, we see that teachers allocated much of their revised instructional activity to methods that might be considered test preparation or practice. This pattern of findings echoes those of Koretz and colleagues (1996), who examined teachers' curricular modifications in response to participation in a Maryland high-stakes assessment program that incorporated PA.

Importantly, however, we also measured student learning as a function of students' prior learning histories. We found an interaction between learning and students' prior learning histories on all three types of outcome measures we indexed: an acquisition task (a PA structured in parallel fashion to the alternate forms students took in their classrooms), a near-transfer task (a PA structured similarly but assessing a different, easier set of skills), and far-transfer task (a commercial PA, The Performance Assessments of the Iowa Test of Basic Skills, which was structured differently and assessed different skills). On the acquisition and near-transfer measures, high-achieving and average-achieving pupils grew more than comparable sets of students in "control" classrooms, who received the same mathematics curriculum without use of the PAs. In contrast to the high- and average-achieving students, low-achieving pupils failed to demonstrate more learning than comparable sets of control students. On the far-transfer task, only the high-achieving students demonstrated superior learning compared to their control peers.

Consequently, teachers attempted to teach the computation skills, applications skills, word problem skills, and problem-solving strategies represented on these assessments. They also provided direct practice on and exposure to similar activities during their classroom activities where the teachers were free to mediate their learners' experiences with these PA tasks. Nevertheless, students who had demonstrated persistent and serious problems in the past failed to profit. It is important also to note that our participating teachers were highly motivated and earnest in their attempts to help their students master these authentic, complex mathematical tasks. Clearly, difficult challenges remain for teachers and researchers alike to develop methods that can help practitioners capitalize on PA potential to refocus effort on teaching for skill application and generalization within complex, authentic problem-solving contexts.

Limitations

The research base exploring the tenability of this problem-solving CBM system is exploratory; it clearly warrants further work. In addition to exploring the technical features of PA, a systematic program of research is required to identify strategies for

Class Report

PERFORMANCE ASSESSMENT CLASS PROFILE

Teacher: CHAN

Title: TEACHER'S BIRTHDAY PARTY

Date: January 22, 1996

	A1	A3	S1	S2	S3	Mn	NN	CG	Ca
Danyale Blackwell									
Lauren Bright									
Terrance Brown									
Dan Burger									
Andre Cooper									
Beth Dunning									
MuyLee Ear									
Cody Evans									
Will Fairhurst									
Kristy Gastiger									
Adam Gregg									
Jennifer Hardin									
Samara Hopkins									
Rokeya Jones									
Jordan McConnell									
Katie McDonald									
John Miller									
Beth Stewart									
Meggie Tucker									
Paige Watson									
Caroline Wilkey									
Sharita Winston									

	A1	A3	S1	S2	S3	Mn	NN	CG	Ca
☐ Not Attempted	5	9	5	7	10	3	8	6	3
⊞ Not Mastered	3	1	1	0	5	4	0	0	11
◩ Mastered in Isolation	2	1	2	1	2	0	0	0	1
■ Mastered in Context	9	8	11	11	2	12	11	13	4

FIGURE 7.8   A sample CBM problem-solving class report.

enhancing the feasibility of scoring PA and for improving teachers' capacity to connect PA information to instructional planning.

In terms of feasibility, the task of scoring PAs for a classroom of many students is formidable. With respect to instructional planning, our preliminary work suggests that it is insufficient to supply teachers with rich assessment feedback about their students' performance. Rather, teachers require consultation about how to connect this assessment feedback with their instructional programs. This need for consultation surrounding the provision of assessment feedback has been demonstrated with more simple forms of assessment, such as CBM. For the more challenging, complex curriculum addressed with PA, this need may be even more pressing.

In light of these concerns, we have recently begun to develop software that conducts functions similar to those performed by our CBM software. This PA software,

PERFORMANCE ASSESSMENT CLASS PROFILE

Teacher: CHAN

Title: TEACHER'S BIRTHDAY PARTY

Date: January 22, 1996

	Making Sense	Computation	Problem Solving	Communication
Danyale Blackwell	2	1	2	2
Lauren Bright	3	3	3	3
Terrance Brown	0	0	0	0
Dan Burger	5	4	5	5
Andre Cooper	2	2	1	2
Beth Dunning	5	4	5	4
MuyLee Ear	1	1	1	1
Cody Evans	3	3	4	3
Will Fairhurst	4	3	3	3
Kristy Gastiger	2	2	3	2
Adam Gregg	3	3	2	2
Jennifer Hardin	3	3	4	3
Samara Hopkins	3	3	3	3
Hokeya Jones	2	1	1	1
Jordan McConnell	0	0	0	0
Katie McDonald	4	5	5	4
John Miller	4	3	4	3
Beth Stewart	5	4	5	5
Meggie Tucker	3	3	4	3
Paige Watson	3	3	3	3
Caroline Wilkey	3	2	3	3
Sharita Winston	0	0	0	0
Number scoring 0	3	3	3	3
Number scoring 1	1	3	3	2
Number scoring 2	4	3	2	4
Number scoring 3	8	9	6	9
Number scoring 4	3	3	4	2
Number scoring 5	3	1	4	2
Mean score:	2.73	2.41	2.77	2.5

called Monitoring Authentic Problem Solving (MAPS), automatically performs the following tasks: (1) It presents the problem situation, via video or text, to the student; (2) It facilitates the student's response construction, permitting the student to avoid many of the writing demands associated with mathematics PAs; (3) It scores the student's response and provides the student with his or her scores as well as tips for increasing those scores; (4) It organizes a classroom's worth of feedback into teacher reports; and (5) It provides teachers with specific instructional recommendations for enhancing student performance. This software, although still in a field-testing phase of development, looks promising for helping make PA a classroom reality, which improves teachers' capacity for helping students achieve mathematical problem-solving competence. As product development occurs we will use the software as a framework for conducting a systematic line of inquiry addressing the feasibility and treatment validity of this PA system.

CONCLUSIONS

CBM and PA are two forms of classroom-based assessment, designed to assess student competence, track the development of competence over time, and assist teachers with their instructional planning. CBM is a well-established form of alternative, classroom-based, academic assessment; practitioners can have confidence that CBM provides accurate, meaningful information and helps them plan more effective instructional programs. Despite this utility, CBM research and development has focused almost exclusively on the acquisition of basic academic skills. Over the past five years we have begun to extend the CBM general outcome measurement model to a mathematics problem-solving domain. Despite some progress, additional work is needed to establish the technical features of this extended system, to enhance the feasibility of scoring the protocols, and to improve teachers' capacity to connect the assessment information in the service of instruction.

References

Allen, D. (1989). Periodic and annual reviews and decision to terminate special education services. In M. R. Shinn (Ed.), *Curriculum-based measurement: Assessing special children* (pp. 182–201). New York: Guilford Press.

Archbald, D. A., & Newmann, F. M. (1988). *Beyond standardized testing: Assessing academic achievement in the secondary school.* Reston, VA: National Association of Secondary School Principals.

Baker, E. L. (1991). *Expectations and evidence for alternative assessment.* Paper presented at the annual meeting of the American Educational Research Association, Chicago, April.

Baker, E. L., O'Neil, H. F., & Linn, R. L. (1993). Policy and validity propects for performance-based assessment. *American Psychologist, 48,* 1210–1218.

Baxter, G. P., Shavelson, R. J., Goldman, S. R., & Pine, J. (1992). Evaluation of procedure-based scoring for hands-on science assessment. *Journal of Educational Measurement, 29,* 1–17.

Brewer, R. (1991). *Authentic assessment: The rhetoric and the reality.* Paper presented at the annual meeting of the American Educational Research Association, Chicago, April.

Darling-Hammond, L. (1992). *Reframing the school reform agenda: Developing capacity for school transformation.* Paper presented at the annual meeting of the American Educational Research Association, San Francisco, April.

Deno, S. L. (1985). Curriculum-based measurement: The emerging alternative. *Exceptional Children, 52,* 219–232.

Deno, S. L., & Fuchs, L. S. (1987). Developing curriculum-based measurement systems for data-based special education problem solving. *Focus on Exceptional Children, 19*(8), 1–16.

Deno, S. L., Mirkin, P., & Chiang, B. (1982). Identifying valid measures of reading. *Exceptional Children, 49,* 36–45.

Deno, S. L., Mirkin, P., Lowry, L., & Kuehnle, K. (1980). *Relationships among simple measures of spelling and performance on standardized achievement tests* (Research Report No. 22). Minneapolis: University of Minnesota Institute for Research on Learning Disabilities.

Elliott, S. N. (1998). Performance assessment of students' achievement: Research and practice. *Learning Disabilities Research and Practice, 13,* 253–262.

Fuchs, D., Fuchs, L. S., & Fernstrom, P. J. (1993). A conservative approach to special education reform: Mainstreaming through transenvironmental programming and curriculum-based measurement. *American Educational Research Journal, 30,* 149–178.

Fuchs, L. S. (1994). *Connecting performance assessment to instruction.* Reston, VA: Council for Exceptional Children.

Fuchs, L. S. (1995). *Curriculum-based measurement and eligibility decision making: An emphasis on treatment validity and growth.* Washington, DC: National Academy of Sciences.

Fuchs, L. S., Allinder, R. M., Hamlett, C. L., & Fuchs, D. (1990). An analysis of spelling curriculua and teachers' skills in identifying errors. *Remedial and Special Education, 11*(1), 42–53.

Fuchs, L. S., & Deno, S. L. (1991). Paradigmatic distinctions between instructionally relevant measurement models. *Exceptional Children, 57*, 488–501.

Fuchs, L. S., Deno, S. L., & Marston, D. (1983). Improving the reliability of curriculum-based measures of academic skills for psychoeducational decision making. *Diagnostique, 8*, 135–149.

Fuchs, L. S., Deno, S. L., & Marston, D. (1997). *Alternative measures for predicting performance on graduation standards.* Paper presented at the fifth annual Pacific Coast Research Conference, La Jolla, CA.

Fuchs, L. S., Deno, S. L., & Mirkin, P. K. (1984). The effects of frequent curriculum-based measurement and evaluation on student achievement, pedagogy, and student awareness of learning. *American Educational Research Journal, 21*, 449–460.

Fuchs, L. S., & Fuchs, D. (1996). Connecting performance assessment and curriculum-based measurement. *Learning Disabilities Research and Practice, 11*, 182–192.

Fuchs, L. S., & Fuchs, D. (1999). Monitoring student progress toward the development of reading competence. *School Psychology Review, 28*, 659–671.

Fuchs, L. S., & Fuchs, D. (1999). Treatment validity: A unifying concept for reconceptualizing the identification of learning disabilities. *Learning Disabilities Research and Practice, 13*, 204–219.

Fuchs, L. S., Fuchs, D., & Deno, S. L. (1982). Reliability and validity of curriculum-based informal reading inventories. *Reading Research Quarterly, 18*, 6–26.

Fuchs, L. S., Fuchs, D., & Hamlett, C. L. (1989a). Effects of alternative goal structures within curriculum-based measurement. *Exceptional Children, 55*, 429–438.

Fuchs, L. S., Fuchs, D., & Hamlett, C. L. (1989b). Effects of instrumental use of curriculum-based measurement to enhance instructional programs. *Remedial and Special Education, 10*(2), 43–52.

Fuchs, L. S., Fuchs, D., & Hamlett, C. L. (1989c). Monitoring reading growth using student recalls: Effects of two teacher feedback systems. *Journal of Educational Research, 83*, 103–111.

Fuchs, L. S., Fuchs, D., & Hamlett, C. L. (1993). Technological advances linking the assessment of students' academic proficiency to instructional planning. *Journal of Special Education Technology, 12*, 49–62.

Fuchs, L. S., Fuchs, D., & Hamlett, C. L. (1994). Strengthening the connection between assessment and instructional planning with expert systems. *Exceptional Children, 61*, 138–146.

Fuchs, L. S., Fuchs, D., Hamlett, C. L., & Allinder, R. M. (1989). The reliability and validity of skills analysis within curriculum-based measurement. *Diagnostique, 14*, 203–221.

Fuchs, L. S., Fuchs, D., Hamlett, C. L., & Allinder, R. M. (1991). Effects of expert system advice within curriculum-based measurement on teacher planning and student achievement in spelling. *School Psychology Review, 20*, 49–66.

Fuchs, L. S., Fuchs, D., Hamlett, C. L., & Ferguson, C. (1992). Effects of expert system consultation within curriculum-based measurement using a reading maze task. *Exceptional Children, 58*, 436–450.

Fuchs, L. S., Fuchs, D., Hamlett, C., & Hasselbring, T. S. (1987). Using computers with curriculum-based progress monitoring. *Journal of Special Education Technology, 8*(4), 14–27.

Fuchs, L. S., Fuchs, D., Hamlett, C. L., Phillips, N. B., & Bentz, J. (1994). Classwide curriculum-based measurement: Helping general educators meet the challenge of student diversity. *Exceptional Children, 60*, 518–537.

Fuchs, L. S., Fuchs, D., Hamlett, C. L., Phillips, N., Karns, K., & Dutka, S. (1997). Enhancing students' helping behavior during peer-mediated instruction with conceptual mathematics explanations. *Elementary School Journal, 97*, 223–250.

Fuchs, L. S., Fuchs, D., Hamlett, C. L., & Stecker, P. M. (1990). The role of skills analysis in curriculum-based measurement in math. *School Psychology Review, 19*, 6–22.

Fuchs, L. S., Fuchs, D., Hamlett, C. L., & Stecker, P. M. (1991). Effects of curriculum-based measurement and consultation on teacher planning and student achievement in mathematics operations. *American Educational Research Journal, 28*, 617–641.

Fuchs, L. S., Fuchs, D., Hamlett, C. L., Thompson, A., Roberts, P. H., Kubec, P., & Stecker, P. M. (1994). Technical features of a mathematics concepts and applications curriculum-based measurement system. *Diagnostique*, 19(4), 23–49.

Fuchs, L. S., Fuchs, D., Hamlett, C. L., Walz, L., & Germann, G. (1993). Formative evaluation of academic progress: How much growth can we expect? *School Psychology Review*, 22, 27–48.

Fuchs, L. S., Fuchs, D., Karns, K., Hamlett, C. L., & Katzaroff, M. (in press). Mathematics performance assessment in the classroom: Effects on teacher planning and student learning. *American Educational Research Journal*.

Fuchs, L. S., Fuchs, D., Karns, K., Hamlett, C. L., Katzaroff, K., & Dutka, S. (1998). Comparisons among individual and cooperative performance assessments and other measures of mathematics competence. *Elementary School Journal*, 98, 3–22.

Fuchs, L. S., Fuchs, D., Kazdan, S., Karns, K., Calhoon, M. B., Hamlett, C. L., & Hewlett, S. (2000). The effects of workgroup structure and size on student productivity during collaborative work on complex tasks. *Elementary School Journal*, 100, 83–212.

Fuchs, L. S., Hamlett, C. L., Fuchs, D., Stecker, P. M., & Ferguson, C. (1988). Conducting curriculum-based measurement with computerized data collection: Effects on efficiency and teacher satisfaction. *Journal of Special Education Technology*, 9(2), 73–86.

Germann, G., & Tindal, G. (1985). An application of curriculum-based assessment: The use of direct and repeated measurement. *Exceptional Children*, 52, 244–265.

Good, R. H., Deno, S. L., & Fuchs, L. S. (1995). *Modeling academic growth for students with and without disabilities*. Paper presented at the third annual Pacific Coast Research Conference, Laguna Beach, CA, February.

Good, R. H., & Shinn, M. R. (1990). Forecasting accuracy of slope estimates for reading curriculum-based measurement: Empirical evidence. *Behavioral Assessment*, 12, 179–194.

Goodman, J. (1995). Change without difference: School restructuring in historical perspective. *Harvard Educational Review*, 65, 1–28.

Hambleton, R. K., Jaeger, R. M., Koretz, D., Linn, R. L., Millman, J., & Phillips, S. E. (1995). *Review of the measurement quality of the Kentucky Instructional Results Information System* (Final Report). Prepared for the Office of Educational Accountability, Kentucky General Assembly.

Jones, E. D., & Krouse, J. P. (1988). The effectiveness of data-based instruction by student teachers in classrooms for pupils with mild learning handicaps. *Teacher Education and Special Education*, 11, 9–19.

Kansas State Board of Education (1991). *Kansas Quality Performance Accreditation*. Topeka: Author.

Koretz, D., Mitchell, K., Barron, S., & Keith, S. (1996). *Final report*: Perceived effects of the Maryland School Performance Assessment Programs. National Center for Research on Evaluation, Standards, and Student Testing (CRESST). Los Angeles: University of California.

Linn, R. L., Baker, E. L., & Dunbar, S. B. (1991). Complex, performance-based assessment: Expectations and validation criteria. *Educational Researcher*, November, 15–21.

Marston, D. (1987–1988). The effectiveness of special education: A time-series analysis of reading performance in regular and special education settings. *Journal of Special Education*, 21(4), 13–26.

Marston, D. (1989). Curriculum-based measurement: What is it and why do it? In M. R. Shinn (Ed.), *Curriculum-based measurement: Assessing special children* (pp. 18–78). New York: Guilford Press.

Marston, D., Fuchs, L. S., & Deno, S. L. (1986). Measuring pupil progress: A comparison of standardized achievement tests and curriculum-related measures. *Diagnostique*, 11, 71–90.

Marston, D., & Magnusson, D. (1988). Curriculum-based assessment: District-level implementation. In J. Graden, J. Zins, & M. Curtis (Eds.), *Alternative educational delivery systems: Enhancing instructional options for all students* (pp. 137–172). Washington, DC: National Association of School Psychologists.

Mory, E., & Salisbury, D. (1992). *School restructuring: The critical element of total system design*. Paper presented at the annual meeting of the American Educational Research Association, San Francisco, April.

Sammons, K. B., Kobett, B., Heiss, J., & Fennell, F. S. (1992). Linking instruction and assessment in the mathematics classroom. *Arithmetic Teacher*, February, 11–15.

Self, H., Benning, A., Marston, D., & Magnusson, D. (1991). Cooperative teacher project: A model for students at risk. *Exceptional Children, 58,* 26–35.

Shavelson, R. J., Baxter, G. P., & Pine, J. (1992). Performance assessments: Political rhetoric and measurement reality. *Educational Researcher, 21*(4), 22–27.

Shepard, L. A. (1989). Why we need better assessments. *Educational Leadership, 46,* April.

Shinn, M. R. (Ed.). (1989) *Curriculum-based measurement: Assessing special children.* New York: Guilford Press.

Shinn, M. R. (1995). Best practices in curriculum-based measurement and its use in a problem-solving model. In A. Thomas & J. Grimes (Eds.), *Best practices in school psychology* (Vol. III, pp. 547–567). Washington, DC: National Association of School Psychologists.

Stallings, J. A. (1995). Ensuring teaching and learning in the 21st century. *Educational Researchers, 24*(6), 4–8.

Stecker, P. M. (1994). *Effects of instructional modifications with and without curriculum-based measurement on the mathematics achievement of students with mild disabilities.* Unpublished doctoral dissertation, Vanderbilt University, Nashville, TN.

Stiggins, R. J., Griswald, M., & Green, K. R. (1988). *Measuring thinking skills through classroom assessment.* Paper presented at the 1988 annual meeting of the National Council on Measurement in Education, New Orleans, April.

Wesson, C. L. (1989). An efficient technique for establishing reading groups. *Reading Teacher,* 466–469.

Wesson, C. L. (1991). Curriculum-based measurement and two models of follow-up consultation. *Exceptional Children, 57,* 246–257.

Wesson, C. L., Fuchs, L. S., Tindal, G., Mirkin, P. K., & Deno, S. L. (1986). Facilitating the efficiency of ongoing curriculum-based measurement. *Teacher Education and Special Education, 9,* 166–172.

Wesson, C. L., Skiba, R., Sevcik, B., King, R., & Deno, S. (1984). The effects of technically adequate instructional data on achievement. *Remedial and Special Education, 5,* 17–22.

Wiggins, G. (1989). A true test: Toward more authentic and equitable assessment. *Phi Delta Kappan, 70,* May, 703–713.

CHAPTER 8

Self-Monitoring

Theory and Practice

CHRISTINE L. COLE
LINDA M. BAMBARA
Lehigh University

Self-monitoring is a well-established technique that has been used in school settings for well over two decades (Broden, Hall, & Mitts, 1971; Nelson, 1977; Shapiro & Cole, 1994). In self-monitoring, students are instructed to observe and record specific aspects of their behavior. Self-monitoring includes the two activities of self-observation and self-recording. *Self-observation* involves being aware of one's actions and knowing whether or not the behavior of interest has occurred. *Self-recording* refers to the activity of noting the occurrence of the observed behavior, typically using a paper-and-pencil method. For example, a student who engages in disruptive talking during independent seatwork may be asked to notice each time he talks to a peer during this period. Following each self-observation, the child records the talking-out behavior by placing a check mark on an index card taped to his desk. Also included in the broad framework of self-monitoring processes are self-report, self-graphing, and verbal and written self-assessment activities.

Self-monitoring is considered both an assessment and intervention technique. When self-monitoring is used for assessment purposes, a student may be asked to collect data on the frequency of a particular targeted behavior. This activity may be part of a functional assessment process designed to obtain an initial behavior level or determine specific antecedents and consequences of behavior. Self-monitoring can also be used for more extended periods as an outcome measure to determine the effects of intervention procedures or instructional activities over time. The most obvious benefit of using a self-monitoring approach for data collection is that child-collected data are more convenient to obtain than data collected by adult observers. Self-monitoring may allow teachers and other adults to successfully track targeted behaviors without the presence of independent observers (Reid, 1996). Students can record data even when these adults are not present or are busy with other instructional activities. A self-monitoring approach that shifts responsibility for data collection from the teacher to the student may ultimately reduce time demands on teachers.

In addition to its potential usefulness as an assessment tool, self-monitoring may also be a valuable means for behavior change. Numerous studies have demonstrated that activities of observing and recording one's behavior often result in reactive effects, or positive changes in the behavior being self-monitored (Gardner & Cole, 1988; Mace & Kratochwill, 1985; Reid, 1996; Shapiro & Cole, 1994). Simply the act of engaging in self-monitoring without any additional intervention components can lead to changes in the targeted behavior. Although reactivity does not always result from self-monitoring (e.g., Howell, Rueda, & Rutherford, 1983), it does occur frequently enough to support its usefulness as an intervention. In fact, self-monitoring has most often been used for intervention purposes with children and adolescents in school settings.

Although there is strong empirical support for the use of self-monitoring as an intervention in school settings (e.g., Gardner & Cole, 1988; Shapiro & Cole, 1994), the use of self-monitoring for assessment purposes is not typical with the school-age population (Shapiro & Cole, 1999). Even though self-monitoring as an assessment tool is conceptually sensible, the use of self-monitoring for purposes of assessment with children introduces substantial problems. As noted by La Greca (1990) and Stone and Lemanek (1990), the accuracy of any type of child self-report may vary widely, depending on a child's developmental level and the nature of the behavior being reported. For example, young children can be influenced substantially through suggestion to falsely report events that never actually occurred (Bruck, Ceci, & Hembrooke, 1998). The host of potential biases in data that are self-monitored by children with no independent verification are clear.

As a result, most of the self-monitoring literature with children has examined the use of self-monitoring as an intervention strategy, rather than an assessment tool. These studies demonstrate the potential reactive effects of self-monitoring and measure the outcomes of the self-monitoring procedure, but rarely use self-monitoring as a means to assess the effects of another intervention on student behavior. Two exceptions are use of self-monitoring for internalizing problems such as anxiety and depression, and use of self-monitoring as one component in multicomponent self-regulation packages. Each of these applications will be discussed in more detail later in the chapter.

It is also important to note that the developmental literature has conceptualized self-monitoring somewhat differently (Shapiro & Cole, 1999). Although the clinical and behavior change literature has focused on the "monitoring" process within self-monitoring, the developmental literature has focused on the "self." From the developmental perspective, self-monitoring is viewed as a cognitive construct or personality trait that reflects the extent to which individuals monitor their expressive behavior and self-presentation through the processes of self-observation and self-control (Snyder, 1979).

The focus of this chapter is on the techniques and strategies used in empirical research on self-monitoring in school settings. Given the theme of the text, our primary emphasis is on the assessment methodology of self-monitoring, rather than the outcomes of the studies in which these techniques are used. The descriptions of empirical studies are representative of the procedural, conceptual, and practical concerns relating to self-monitoring. For more detail, the interested reader may refer to studies cited in this chapter and to recent reviews of the self-monitoring literature by Shapiro and Cole (1999), Reid (1996), and Webber, Scheuerman, McCall, and Coleman (1993).

We begin with an initial description of the methodology of self-monitoring, and a discussion of the issues of accuracy and reactivity in self-monitoring for assessment. Next, specific school-based applications of self-monitoring are examined including self-monitoring of on-task behavior, academic performance (academic productivity and academic accuracy), independent student behaviors, and problem behaviors involved in both externalizing and internalizing disorders in children. In the final section we discuss some of the emerging applications of self-monitoring within a self-regulatory framework, and offer recommendations for future research and practice.

METHODOLOGY OF SELF-MONITORING

Student Characteristics

The empirical literature has demonstrated the feasibility of self-monitoring procedures with children and adolescents presenting a variety of individual differences. Students in general and special education classes, schools, or residential settings who have a range of behavioral, social, and academic difficulties have successfully assessed their behavior using self-monitoring. These include students with developmental disabilities (Hughes, Korinek, & Gorman, 1991), learning disabilities (Dunlap & Dunlap, 1989), autism (Koegel & Koegel, 1990), and emotional/behavioral disorders (Hughes, Ruhl, & Misra, 1989), as well as students with no exceptionality who are in non-special-education settings (e.g., Wood, Murdock, Cronin, Dawson, & Kirby, 1998). Children of all ages, from preschool to high school, can learn to use self-monitoring. It is evident that this procedure may be useful with the entire range of children served in school settings.

Self-Monitoring by Individuals and Groups

Self-monitoring typically has been used by an individual child to observe and record target behaviors that occur in one or more settings (e.g., Kern, Marder, Boyajian, Elliot, & McElhattan, 1997). However, self-monitoring has also been used successfully with groups of students in both special and general education classes. For example, Kern, Dunlap, Childs, and Clarke (1994) successfully used self-monitoring with an entire class of adolescent boys with emotional and behavioral disorders. Each student in the class was able to self-monitor his on-task and one additional target behavior throughout a 45-minute math period. Miller, Strain, Boyd, Jarzynka, and McFetridge (1993) also successfully used a self-assessment strategy with a group of preschoolers during transition, free play, and small group instruction activities. Self-assessment entailed using a poster that visually depicted the target behaviors and asking the students to indicate by a thumbs-up or thumbs-down signal if they felt they had performed each behavior during the activity.

It is clear that self-monitoring procedures are adaptable for use with individual members of a group, multiple members of a group, or an entire class. The relatively unobtrusive nature of self-monitoring contributes to its potential for use as an assessment procedure in schools.

Types of Behaviors Self-Monitored

The types of behaviors that can be self-monitored by children and adolescents range from objective behaviors that are readily observable by the student and others (e.g., getting out of seat, math problems completed) to subjective behaviors that are observable only to the person (e.g., negative thoughts, urges to talk during class). Recent examples include self-monitoring teachers' expectancies by middle-school students with learning disabilities (Clees, 1994), self-monitoring in-class transition behaviors by preschoolers with developmental delays (Connell, Carta, Lutz, Randall, & Wilson, 1993), self-monitoring spelling study behavior by elementary-school students with severe behavior disorders (McDougall & Brady, 1995), and self-monitoring attending behavior by elementary students with attention-deficit/hyperactivity disorder (ADHD) (Mathes & Bender, 1997). Almost any relevant target behavior may be successfully self-monitored by children and adolescents in school settings.

Self-Monitoring Procedures

In selecting a procedure for self-monitoring, several factors should be considered to ensure that students will, in fact, self-record behavior and that this recording will be accurate. Initially, a procedure should be selected that is appropriate for the behaviors being recorded and that is relatively easy to use. For example, a procedure that requires students to self-monitor following specified time intervals would be appropriate for high-rate or ongoing behaviors such as on-task behavior. To be feasible for use in school settings the procedure should be inexpensive and relatively unobtrusive. Although, as discussed later in this chapter, an obtrusive recording device may serve as a cue for self-monitoring and therefore potentially enhance the accuracy of self-monitoring, a balance is needed between the obtrusiveness of the recording device and one that is feasible and acceptable to the student, the teacher, and for the classroom setting.

Types of Data Collected

Most often, self-monitoring in school settings involves data collected using time sampling. With time sampling, a target behavior is self-monitored at the end of each specified time interval. Wood and colleagues (1998) used a time-sampling procedure with four at-risk middle-school students. At the end of each 50-minute experimental class period, the adolescents assessed whether they had remained in seat, used materials appropriately, worked on the assigned task, followed teacher directions, and accepted teacher feedback appropriately.

A popular variation of this procedure used with self-monitoring on-task behavior is that of momentary time sampling, or spot-checking, (e.g., Prater, Hogan, & Miller, 1992). Using this procedure, children are signaled by an auditory tone to self-monitor several times throughout a class period following short intervals of time, such as every 1–5 minutes. At the tone, children are instructed to decide whether they were attending or not attending at the sound of the tone, and mark a + or – on their recording sheet. These self-monitored data are summarized as the percentage on-task, which is calculated by dividing the number of on-task occurrences by the total number of times the signal was given, and then multiplying by 100. Although most often used with on-task behavior, momentary time sampling can be used to self-monitor other behaviors. In one example by McDougall and Brady (1995), three elementary-school students with severe behavior disorders were taught to self-monitor their use of a study strategy during a spelling study period.

Another commonly used data-collection procedure involves having students self-monitor each occurrence of the target behavior, usually at the time of occurrence. This procedure is most useful when frequency of the target behavior is relatively low, when the occurrence is of short duration, and when the behavior is discrete. Two examples include self-monitoring completion of homework assignments by adolescents with learning disabilities (Trammel, Schloss, & Alper, 1994) and self-monitoring negative statements by an adolescent with mild mental retardation (Martella, Leonard, Marchand-Martella, & Agran, 1993). These types of data are summarized as total frequency during each period or, if self-monitoring sessions vary in length, as rate of occurrence. Behavior rate is calculated by dividing the total number of occurrences by the total observation time.

With academic performance behaviors such as the completion of math problems, students may be asked to record the number of problems completed and/or number of problems completed correctly at the end of each independent work period. In this case, data are summarized as percentage of problems completed and/or percentage completed correctly. In one example, Lam, Cole, Shapiro, and Bambara (1994) had 13- and 14-year-old students with emotional and behavioral disorders record their accuracy in math problems each time they heard an audible tone played at random intervals. Students were taught to compare their responses to those on an answer sheet, mark those that were correct, record this on their worksheets, and then graph the results at the end of the work session.

Self-monitoring may also be useful in the initial functional behavioral assessment stages of selecting a target behavior and developing hypotheses about possible factors involved in its occurrence. This type of preliminary data may be provided by a student in the form of narrative descriptions in a behavioral log or diary, and may be structured or unstructured. For example, the child could be asked to record occurrences of a specified behavior and the circumstances involved, such as the setting or situation in which the behavior occurred (e.g., classroom, hallway), or antecedents and consequences.

Recording Devices

A variety of recording devices is available for use in self-monitoring. The most popular recording devices in school settings are paper-and-pencil procedures (e.g., Harris, Graham, Reid, McElroy, & Hamby, 1994). Paper-and-pencil recording forms may vary, from an index card or a slip of paper on which the child makes a tally mark at each cue, to a more detailed individualized form. The recording form may be placed on the child's desk (e.g., Wood et al., 1998), taped to the table (DeHaas-Warner, 1992), placed on the wall next to the child's desk (e.g., Workman, Helton, & Watson, 1982), included in the child's packet of work materials (e.g., Schunk, 1982), or carried by the adolescent throughout the day (e.g., Clees, 1994). Examples of the use of mechanical devices such as hand-held, belt-worn, or wrist counters for self-monitoring also appear in the literature (e.g., Nelson, Lipinski, & Boykin, 1978; Ollendick, 1981).

Recently, other more unconventional strategies have been used to replace paper-and-pencil recording following children's self-monitoring. One example was the study involving preschoolers who used a thumbs-up or thumbs-down signal when teachers asked them to monitor their behavior following transition, free play, and small group instruction times (Miller et al., 1993). A similar procedure involved having preschoolers raise their hands to indicate they had engaged in in-class transition behaviors (Connell et al., 1993). In another example, teenagers with autism removed a token from their back pocket and placed it in their front pocket to self-monitor each transition to a new activity (Newman, Buffington, O'Grady, McDonald, Poulson, & Hemmes, 1995).

A number of factors should be considered in designing a recording procedure. First, to increase the accuracy of self-monitoring, the device should be available for recording the target behavior as it occurs. If it is to be used in more than one setting, obviously the recording device must be portable. Second, the recording device should be easy to use and not distracting. If the child continues to manipulate or attend to the device following self-monitoring, other task requirements may not be met. Third, the device should be sufficiently obtrusive so the child is aware of it and will use it for recording, but should not be excessively conspicuous to attract attention from others. This is a particular concern in inclusive school-based and community-based settings. A final consideration in selecting a recording device is its cost. For example, although wrist counters may be ideal to use with a large class because the device is portable and serves as a reminder for self-monitoring, the cost to the school, teacher, or family may be prohibitive.

Prompts to Self-Monitor

A number of different types of prompts may be used to signal students to self-monitor their behavior. In school settings, this tactic has most often involved the use of external prompts. *External prompts* can be either verbal or nonverbal, and can be delivered by another person (e.g., teacher, aide, support person) or by a mechanical device (e.g., tone on a prerecorded tape, kitchen timer). Verbal prompts may be useful when an entire class is self-monitoring and can involve a simple reminder from the teacher to self-monitor at the end of each class period. In other cases in which only one or a few students are self-monitoring, it may be more feasible to use nonverbal prompts such as having the teacher periodically signal or tap the individual student(s) on the shoulder when it is time to self-monitor their behavior. One of the most commonly used prompts is a prerecorded tone because it requires limited teacher time and can be used with an individual or an entire class.

Another type of prompting that has been used successfully in school settings is self-prompting (e.g., Heins, Lloyd, & Hallahan, 1986; Hertz & McLaughlin, 1990). With *self-prompting*, or noncued self-monitoring, students are typically instructed to note on their own, from time to time during the designated self-monitoring period, whether or not they were engaging in the target behavior. No external prompting is provided. This type of self-prompting procedure has been used most often with self-monitoring on-task behavior and will be described in more detailed in an upcoming section.

Self-Monitoring Training

The methods used in training children to self-monitor their behavior are related to the complexity of the data collected and of the self-monitoring procedure itself, as well as student characteristics such as age, cognitive level, and presence of competing behaviors. The training procedures selected may range from simple verbal instructions to detailed training programs involving instruction, modeling, behavior rehearsal, performance feedback, and reinforcement. Direct instruction combined with behavior rehearsal of simulated scenes, or videotaped scenes of actual behaviors and situations, may be used. Training may occur in the natural setting or in a separate training location.

For very young children or students with more severe disabilities, other novel approaches to self-monitoring training may be used. For example, in two studies with preschoolers, DeHaas-Warner (1991, 1992) used a story as the vehicle for training children to self-monitor their on-task behavior. Individual training sessions outside the classroom involved reading a story to each child about a preschooler who had difficulty completing tasks without talking, looking around the room, or getting out of his seat. Drawings that depicted appropriate and inappropriate on-task behavior and corresponded to the story were also used.

The specific training procedures selected should ensure that the child understands what is expected and has the skills to implement the self-monitoring procedure. To increase the probability of accurate self-monitoring by children, training programs should include (1) explicit definition of the target behavior; (2) simplified behavior counting and recording procedures; (3) specific and relatively short time periods in which self-monitoring occurs; (4) teacher reliability checks and student feedback; and (5) sufficient practice to ensure that fluency in self-monitoring is attained (Frith & Armstrong, 1985).

ISSUES OF ACCURACY AND REACTIVITY
IN SELF-MONITORING FOR ASSESSMENT

Accuracy of Self-Monitoring

The usefulness of self-monitoring as an assessment strategy during target behavior selection, functional behavioral assessment, or outcome evaluation activities depends to a great extent on the accuracy with which students are able to monitor their behavior. In most self-monitoring studies, accuracy of self-monitored data is determined by comparing self-recordings made by the child with those made simultaneously by another observer, usually an adult such as the teacher (e.g., Dunlap & Dunlap, 1989). The extent to which a student is able to match an observer's recordings of a particular behavior will determine the accuracy of self-monitoring. Although logic would suggest that adult observers' recordings are more accurate than children's self-recordings and therefore should be used as the standard of comparison, there currently are insufficient data to support that assumption.

Many studies have demonstrated that children and adolescents, varying widely in cognitive, social, emotional, and behavioral characteristics, are capable of accurately self-monitoring a variety of target behaviors (e.g., Carr & Punzo, 1993; Kern et al., 1997; Wood et al., 1998). Many of these studies have reported child–observer agreement levels of at least 80%, which is the generally established minimum for acceptable levels of agreement (e.g., Wood et al., 1998).

Although children's accuracy has been found to be acceptable in most instances, some studies have reported low or inconsistent accuracy. For example, in the previously mentioned study in which preschoolers self-monitored on-task behavior, De Haas-Warner (1992) found accuracy levels ranging from 61 to 100%, from minimally acceptable to excellent. McDougall and Brady (1995) also found large variations between individual participants in their study of self-monitoring with students with severe behavior disorders. Accuracy levels ranged from an average of 30 to 83%, with large day-to-day discrepancies in individuals' accuracy levels, ranging from 0 to 100%.

A large number of early studies in self-monitoring investigated factors that may influence the accuracy of self-monitoring. Specific variables found to influence self-monitoring accuracy of children and adolescents include students' awareness of accuracy assessment (e.g., Nelson, Lipinski, & Black, 1975), reinforcement for accurate self-monitoring (e.g., Lloyd & Hilliard, 1989), training in accurate self-monitoring (e.g., Shapiro, McGonigle, & Ollendick, 1980), the valence of the target behavior (e.g., Nelson, Hay, Devany, & Koslow-Green, 1980), and the nature of the recording device (e.g., Nelson et al., 1978). Generally, this literature would suggest targeting desired appropriate behaviors for self-monitoring and using a simple, but relatively obtrusive, recording device to enhance student accuracy. In addition, students should be provided initial training in accurate self-monitoring, should be aware that their accuracy will be checked using a random teacher matching procedure, and should be reinforced whenever they do match with the teacher. Each of these issues should be considered whenever self-monitoring procedures are used for assessment purposes to increase the likelihood of accurate assessment by children and adolescents.

Reactivity of Self-Monitoring

Even though positive change in student behavior is usually welcomed by practitioners, behavior change may create difficulties when self-monitoring is used primarily for assessment purposes. In instances where practical or financial constraints prevent the use of an independent observer, the child may be the sole data collector. In these cases, self-monitoring is actually being used simultaneously as both an assessment and an intervention procedure. Because of potential reactivity, it may be impossible to obtain a clear picture of initial behavioral levels. The reactive effects would potentially begin with the initiation of self-monitoring and, as a result, would confound data interpretation.

Reactivity would be an even greater concern if self-monitoring were used in research investigations as a data collection procedure to assess the effects of other variables. For example, in research evaluating the effects of self-monitoring by children who vary in age or type of problem, or in studies investigating the potential reactivity of other specific variables such as intrusiveness of the self-recording device, the use of independent observers to collect both baseline and intervention data obviously would be needed. Independent data-collection procedures also would be required when self-monitored data are used to assess the effects of other independent behavior-change variables. For example, a study evaluating the effects of different levels of academic task difficulty on the on-task behavior of children with learning disabilities could use self-monitoring as the data-collection procedure. However, any changes in on-task behavior following the manipulation of task difficulty may reflect the joint or interactive effects of self-monitoring and task difficulty.

The specific mechanisms responsible for the reactivity of self-monitoring remain a matter of speculation. Two basic theoretical explanations, one emphasizing covert, mediational variables (Kanfer, 1970, 1977), and the other focusing on external controlling variables (Rachlin, 1974) have been offered. The latter position has been expanded by Nelson and Hayes (1981) to include a wider range of controlling influences. Although there is empirical support for each of these positions, it is possible that both cognitive and environmental influences interact to produce reactive effects (Gardner & Cole, 1988). Obviously, additional research is needed to evaluate these theoretical positions further.

COMMON SCHOOL-BASED APPLICATIONS
OF SELF-MONITORING

Common school-based applications of self-monitoring include self-monitoring on-task behavior, self-monitoring academic performance, self-monitoring to promote student independence, and self-monitoring problem behaviors. Table 8.1 provides a summary of recent self-monitoring studies in each of these areas.

Self-Monitoring On-Task Behavior

Paying attention to tasks is generally assumed to be a prerequisite for learning, and problems of attention have been associated with poor academic performance (Barkley,

1990; DuPaul & Stoner, 1994). Because paying attention is an important classroom behavior for children and adolescents, attending to tasks, or on-task behavior, has been the focus of many school-based self-monitoring investigations. However, self-monitoring on-task has typically been used as an intervention strategy to increase on-task behavior, and its use as an assessment strategy with children and adolescents has seldom been isolated (Shapiro & Cole, 1999).

The prototypical procedure for self-monitoring on-task behavior in the classroom was developed by Hallahan, Lloyd, and Stoller (1982) and involves recording self-observations using momentary time sampling. At the sound of a tone played on a variable-interval schedule, students are taught to ask themselves the question, "Was I paying attention when I heard the tone?" and record "yes" or "no." For example, McCarl, Svobodny, and Beare (1991) had three highly distractible girls with mild to moderate mental handicaps, ages 9 to 11, place a "Y" or an "N" in one square, on a sheet of paper with 3 rows of 10 squares, to indicate whether they were working at the sound of the tone.

As previously described, there may be some instances in which children are distracted by the cue and so a noncued self-monitoring procedure (i.e., students self-monitor "whenever they think of it") may be beneficial. In a study by Heins and colleagues (1986), cued and noncued self-recording of attention to task were compared. Four boys with learning disabilities were trained to self-monitor under each condition—cued self-monitoring and noncued self-monitoring. One condition was in effect for the first half of each period and the other for the second half, with the order randomly determined. Although students did learn to self-monitor under both conditions, results suggested their self-recording was inconsistent under the noncued condition and fewer reactive effects were reported than with cued self-monitoring.

There is no set standard length of intervals for self-monitoring on-task behavior and intervals have varied widely in the literature, from self-monitoring every few seconds to every few hours. Typically the interval will depend on characteristics of the students involved, such as their age, extent of disability, and severity of attentional difficulties. In some cases, self-monitoring intervals are variable. This precludes students being able to predict the point at which the self-monitoring cue will be delivered so that they might only pay attention at that time. For example, DiGangi, Maag, and Rutherford (1991) used a tape-recorded tone that was randomly spaced from 30 to 90 seconds apart with elementary-aged students with learning disabilties.

In other cases, increasingly longer self-monitoring intervals have been used with students in an effort to reduce their reliance on external cueing over time. Boyle and Hughes (1994) found that the use of two different audiotapes was effective at improving the on-task behavior of elementary students with moderate mental retardation who self-monitored during prevocational workshop sessions. Tones on the first audiotape were emitted, on average, every 45 seconds and children were to ask themselves, "Am I working?" During fading conditions a second tape was used, which emitted tones at consecutive intervals of 2 minutes, 4 minutes, and 6 minutes during the work period.

In another example, Blick and Test (1987) used a series of four different 40-minute audio tapes with a group of 12 high-school students with mild disabili-

TABLE 8.1 Recent Examples of Common School-Based Applications of Self-Monitoring

Reference	Participants	Setting	Monitored behavior	Accuracy	Reactivity
Self-monitoring on-task behavior					
Boyle & Hughes (1994)	5 elementary students with moderate mental retardation (CA 10–11)	Special education classroom	On-task behavior	Individual student means 76–92%	Increased on-task
De Haas-Warner (1992)	4 preschoolers with attentional difficulties (CA 4–6)	Integrated preschool classroom	On-task behavior	Individual student mean kappa coefficients .61–1.0	Increased on-task
Hughes & Boyle (1991)	3 elementary students with moderate mental retardation (CA 9–10)	Special education classroom	On-task behavior	Individual student means 87–91%	Increased on-task and academic performance
Maag, Rutherford, & DiGangi (1992)	6 elementary students with learning disabilities (CA 7–11)	General education classroom	On-task behavior	No data	Increased on-task behavior and academic performance
Marshall, Lloyd, & Hallahan (1993)	4 males with learning disabilities (CA 9–10)	Special education classroom	On-task behavior	Initial individual student means 39–53%; following accuracy training 78–97%	Increased on-task
Mathes & Bender (1997)	3 males with Attention-deficit/hyperactivity disorder (CA 8–11)	Resource classroom	On-task behavior	No data	Increased on-task
McCarl, Svobodny, & Beare (1991)	3 highly distractible females (CA 9–11)	Special education classroom	On-task behavior	No data	Increased on-task and academic performance
Prater, Hogan, & Miller (1992)	1 9th-grade male with learning and behavior difficulties (CA 14)	Resource classroom	On-task behavior	No data	Increased on-task and academic performance
Stewart & McLaughlin (1992)	1 secondary-age male with ADHD (CA 15)	Special education classroom	On-task and off-task behavior	No data	Decreased off-task behavior
Wood, Murdock, Cronin, Dawson, & Kirby (1998)	4 at-risk middle school students (CA 13–15)	Charter school classroom	On-task behavior	Mean range 80–100%	Increased on-task and academic performance

Self-monitoring academic performance

Carr & Punzo (1993)	3 male middle school students with emotional and behavioral difficulties (CA 13–15)	Special education classroom	Academic productivity & accuracy	Mean range 75–100%	Increased academic performance and on-task
Dunlap & Dunlap (1989)	3 students with learning disabilities (CA 10–13)	Resource classroom	Steps of an academic task	No data	Increased academic performance
Harris, Graham, Reid, McElroy, & Hamby (1994)	8 elementary students with learning disabilities (CA 9–12)	Special education classroom	Academic productivity, accuracy, & on-task behavior	No data	Increased academic performance in two students
Lam, Cole, Shapiro, & Bambara (1994)	3 male students with emotional and behavior disorders (CA 13–14)	Private school classroom	Academic accuracy, on-task behavior, & disruptive behavior	Individual student range 40–100%	Increased academic performance and on-task; decreased disruptive behavior
Maag, Reid, & DiGangi (1993)	6 elementary-age students with learning disabilities (mean CA 9–11)	General education and resource classrooms	Academic productivity, accuracy, and on-task behavior	No data	Increased academic performance and on-task
McDougall & Brady (1995)	3 males with behavior disorders (CA 5–8)	Special education classroom	Study method	Individual student means 30–83%	Increased academic performance and on-task

Self-monitoring to promote student independence

Clees (1994)	4 middle school students with learning disabilities (CA 12)	General education classrooms	Teachers' daily expectancies	No data	Increased completion of daily expectancies
Connell, Carta, Lutz, Randall, & Wilson (1993)	3 preschoolers with mild to moderate delays (CA 4)	Early intervention preschool	Transition behaviors	No data	Increased active engagement and independent responding
Flores, Schloss, & Alper (1995)	8 secondary students with mild to moderate mental retardation or severe learning disabilities (CA 17–18)	Special education classroom	Completion of responsibilities	No data	Increased completion of responsibilities

(continued)

TABLE 8.1 *(Continued)*

Reference	Participants	Setting	Monitored behavior	Accuracy	Reactivity
Kern, Marder, Boyajian, Elliot, & McElhattan (1997)	2 males with emotional and behavioral difficulties (CA 7 & 14)	Hospital-based settings (classroom, living area, cafeteria, outdoor playground)	Inappropriate vocalizations	Mean 89 & 100%	Decreased inappropriate vocalizations and independent initiations
Newman, Buffington, O'Grady, McDonald, Poulson, & Hemmes (1995)	3 males with autism (CA 14–17)	After-school classroom	Activity changes (transitions)	Range 0–100% (increasing trend)	Increased accurate and independent identification of activity changes
Trammel, Schloss, & Alper (1994)	8 secondary students with learning disabilities (CA 13–16)	Resource classroom	Homework assignments	Mean 95%	Increased homework completion
Self-monitoring problem behaviors					
Fitzgerald & Werner (1996)	2 male students with learning and behavior difficulties (CA 9 & 12)	Resource and general education classroom	Disruptive classroom behaviors (aggression & inappropriate talk-outs)	No data	Decreased aggression; no change in talk-outs

Authors (year)	Participants	Setting	Target behavior	Data	Outcome
Kern, Dunlap, Childs, & Clarke (1994)	6 male students with emotional and behavioral disorders (CA 11–13)	Special education classroom	Disruptive and on-task behavior	Individual student range 84–100%	Decreased disruptive behavior for 1 student; increased on-task for all students
Martella, Leonard, Marchand-Martella, & Agran (1993)	1 male student with mild mental retardation (CA 21)	Special education classroom	Negative statements	52–100%	Decreased disruptive behavior
Ninness, Ellis, Miller, Baker, & Rutherford (1995)	4 male junior high students with emotional and behavioral difficulties (CA 14–15)	Special education classroom	Socially appropriate behavior	No data	Decreased aggressive behavior with multi-component package
Ninness, Fuerst, & Rutherford (1995)	2 male junior high students with emotional and behavioral difficulties (CA 13 & 14)	Special education classroom & hallway to/from cafeteria	On-task & socially appropriate behavior	No data	Decreased off-task/disruptive behavior with multicomponent package
Storey, Lawry, Ashworth, Danko, & Strain (1994)	1 male kindergarten student with disruptive behavior (CA 6)	General education classroom	Socially appropriate behavior	No data (teacher-prompted)	Decreased disruptive behavior
Strain, Kohler, Storey, & Danko (1994)	3 preschool boys with autism (CA 3–5)	Preschool & home	Appropriate social interactions	No data	Increased social interactions with peers and/or siblings

ties. Two different cues could be heard on each of these tapes—one signaling the teacher to record student behavior (*chime*) and the other cueing students to self-monitor (verbal "*record*"). Initially students were cued to self-monitor every 5 minutes, but this was increased to every 10 minutes, and then every 20 minutes in subsequent tapes. In the final phase, students were no longer required to self-record their behavior so their cue was eliminated, although the audiotape continued to chime every 5 minutes to prompt teacher recording. Results showed that cues to both the teacher and student were effective in improving the on-task behavior of all children, and changes were maintained as the audible cues were faded.

Some education personnel may find the use of multiple tapes too cumbersome and it may not be necessary to increase the self-monitoring interval gradually. Rather, some students may be able to self-monitor on-task behavior following rather lengthy intervals (e.g., at the end of the class period) at the outset. The previously described study by Wood and colleagues (1998), involving middle-school students who were considered at-risk for school failure showed students successfully self-monitored five specific on-task behaviors at the end of each of these 50-minute class periods. The authors reported that this self-monitoring procedure was easy to use and the lengthy self-monitoring intervals required no extra teacher time, effort, or prompting. They also noted that this strategy could easily be implemented by teachers or other school personnel without assistance from outside consultants

Self-Monitoring Academic Performance

Self-monitoring of academic performance typically has involved the simple observation and recording of discrete behaviors such as the completion of problems on a worksheet, number of words written in an essay, or number of words spelled correctly on a spelling test. In some cases students are asked to record only that problems are completed (i.e., productivity), whereas in other cases they record whether or not the problems are completed accurately (i.e., accuracy). Like self-monitoring on-task behavior, self-monitoring academic performance typically uses paper-and-pencil recording devices (e.g., Dunlap & Dunlap, 1989; Hallahan, Lloyd, Kneedler, & Marshall, 1982; Reid & Harris, 1993).

When the strategies of self-monitoring academic productivity is used, production of the response is defined as evidence that the student has completed the required academic performance irrespective of its accuracy. For example, Harris and colleagues (1994) had students record the number of words written in an essay regardless of spelling accuracy as a measure of performance. In their study, students were instructed to count the number of words read and graph these after completing their writing assignments. Maag, Reid, and DiGangi (1993), working with fourth-grade students with learning disabilities on math assignments, had students in one condition record the number of problems completed at the moment that audible tones were heard. These tones were played on a variable interval schedule and students were instructed to count the number of problems completed since the last tone and record this on their self-monitoring sheets. McCarl and colleagues (1991) had

9- to 11-year-old students with mild mental retardation record the number of movements made during an independent math worksheet assignment. Independent movements were defined as numerals written in answer spaces or as part of a regrouping problem in arithmetic. In each of these examples a specific academic behavior was identified (such as completed math problems or answering questions on an answer sheet), and the student was instructed to count and record the production of their response, without regard to accuracy.

Frequently, self-monitoring academic performance involves the recording of the accuracy of a response, not just its production. With this procedure students are instructed to record the number of correct responses. For example, Harris and co-workers (1994) had fourth- to sixth-grade students with learning disabilities record and graph the number of words written correctly from weekly spelling lists during practice sessions. In another example, Maag and colleagues (1993) had students under one condition record not only that they had completed the problems, but also whether the problem was completed accurately. Again, these results were displayed graphically by the students. Many other studies exist where self-monitoring of accurate academic responding was used (e.g., Carr & Punzo, 1993; Maag, Rutherford, & DiGangi, 1992; Prater et al., 1992).

One other form of self-monitoring of academic performance involves the monitoring of the processes required to successfully reach the outcome of the academic task. For example, Miller, Miller, Wheeler, and Selinger (1989) had students self-monitor whether they had completed each step of a self-instruction procedure designed to teach the steps in regrouping in the solution of math problems. Two students with behavior disorders were taught to record their use of each step of the procedure. In a similar example, Dunlap and Dunlap (1989) used an error analysis to develop individualized self-monitoring checklists that students with learning disabilities used as they completed their subtraction assignments. The checklists contained specific reminders that students would refer to and check-off after each problem (e.g., "I regrouped when I needed to." "I borrowed correctly.").

Consistent across almost all studies of self-monitoring academic performance, students show improvements in their behaviors. At the same time, there is evidence that the reactive effects of self-monitoring may be quite idiosyncratic. For example, Shapiro, Browder, and D'Huyvetters (1984) noted substantial differences in effects across four students with severe disabilities when these students self-monitored their academic productivity. Harris and coworkers (1994) noted that self-monitoring of academic performance improved performance in two of four students. In addition to individual participant variability, investigations comparing the reactive effects of self-monitoring on-task and academic performance behaviors have produced inconclusive results. For example, several studies reported increased on-task behavior for both self-monitoring approaches, with neither emerging as clearly superior (e.g., Harris, 1986; Lloyd, Bateman, Landrum, & Hallahan, 1989; Roberts & Nelson, 1981). Others have found self-monitoring academic performance (i.e., productivity or accuracy) to be slightly superior (e.g., Lam et al., 1994; Maag et al., 1993). Thus, while reactivity is not a universal phenomenon and the most optimal academic target remains uncertain, the frequent reactivity reports in the literature have made self-monitoring a generally accepted method for improving children's academic performance (Shapiro & Cole, 1999).

Self-Monitoring to Promote Student Independence

Although a degree of control and responsibility is given to children and adolescents who self-monitor, generally students are still subject to a great deal of adult regulation. Most self-monitoring programs are, in fact, designed by adults, trained by adults, and monitored, evaluated, and modified by adults. However, a few investigators have looked at ways of promoting student independence. For example, Kern and colleagues (1997) increased the participants' independence by teaching students to self-initiate their implementation of self-monitoring across settings and activities. Two boys who engaged in inappropriate vocalizations were first taught to self-monitor appropriate and inappropriate vocalizations during didactic instruction and practice sessions. One child was also taught to operate a cassette recorder and the other boy was taught to use a hand-held timer. During the second training phase, the children received instruction in independent initiation of the self-monitoring procedures. This involved instruction in discriminating situations when particular types of vocalizations were inappropriate, gathering the self-monitoring materials, and independently initiating the procedures. Results indicated that one child successfully initiated the procedures 40% of the sessions, while the other child self-initiated 95% of the time.

Other studies have focused on having students self-monitor their independent completion of daily responsibilities. For example, Clees (1994) successfully taught four middle-school students with learning or behavior problems to self-monitor completion of their general and special education teachers' daily expectancies (bringing necessary materials to class, writing homework assignments in the assignment book, completing all class work) prior to and following each academic period throughout the day. Trammel and colleagues (1994) had adolescents with learning disabilities self-monitor homework assignments to increase assignments completed. Flores, Schloss, and Alper (1995) successfully taught eight secondary students with special needs to use a daily calendar to self-monitor personal responsibilities such as completing chores, practicing for the Special Olympics, and completing homework.

Self-Monitoring Problem Behaviors

Self-Monitoring Externalizing Problems

A variety of methods have been used by children and adolescents to self-monitor problem behaviors. However, it is obvious that self-monitoring of externalizing problems is always used as an intervention strategy, rather than for assessment purposes. The method selected may depend on the specific behavior and how easily the procedure can be implemented in the target setting. In school-based and community-based settings in particular, self-monitoring procedures are designed to be unobtrusive, practical, and socially acceptable to those involved. With free operant behaviors such as social or interpersonal interactions, event recording is common. For example, Martella and coworkers (1993) taught a 12-year-old student with mild mental retardation to put a mark in the box on his recording sheet whenever he emitted a negative statement during class. If his frequency data were in agreement with the trainer (i.e., 80% or higher) and the number of negative statements was at or below a preset criterion level, he received a small reward of his choice. Minner (1990) had three third-grade students with behavior disorders self-monitor the time it took them to walk to classes. Prior to leaving for the resource room, the students were asked to press a button located near the door of their general education classroom that activated a stopwatch. Upon arriving at the resource room, they pressed another button to stop the stopwatch. Students then self-recorded whether they had taken 58 seconds or less (i.e., average number of seconds for a nondisabled peer) to get to their special class by placing a "+" or "0" on the recording sheet for that day. Accuracy checks indicated perfect agreement between the teacher and one of the students throughout the study, and only three discrepancies between the teacher and the other two students.

An obvious consideration when self-monitoring problem behaviors with children and adolescents is that they must be clear about the behavior being targeted for recording. With young children, and children with more severe disabilities, ongoing visual reminders of the target behaviors may be necessary. Kunzelmann (1970) recommended using simple stick-figure drawings that demonstrate the correct behaviors to be self-monitored. These "countoons" can provide ongoing reminders to children of the behaviors that are supposed to be self-monitored. An example was provided by Houghton (1991) in a study with a young child with an intellectual impairment who was engaging in inappropriate classroom behaviors that were preventing his full integration into mainstream classes. Prior to the start of each daily lesson in the special education class, the teacher reviewed three rules specifically relating to his behavior (i.e., "Put your hand up to speak." "Sit up nicely." and "Fold your arms."). As a cue, the child was provided a brightly colored card taped to his desk depicting, in simple picture form, a boy engaging in each of the three rules. Next to each picture was a series of squares drawn in the shape of a grid. Every 5 minutes the teacher pointed to each of the pictures in turn and asked the child if he had engaged in that behavior. All positive responses resulted in the child placing a sticker on a square next to the appropriate picture. As the child learned the procedure the teacher no longer pointed to the pictures and only stated, "Five minutes have passed."

Fitzgerald and Werner (1996) described a computerized self-monitoring program designed for a 12-year-old male with mild mental retardation and autistic-like behaviors. A computer consultant worked with the curriculum development team to design behavior-training materials to support the student in integrated education environments. The team targeted humming and talk-outs as the first step in preparing this student for entry into an inclusion classroom. Computer-based instruction was combined with a multicomponent self-monitoring strategy called "STAR" (Stop–Think–Act–Results) (Morris, 1980). This cognitive–behavioral procedure focused on building impulse control, making choices, following through with action plans, and self-monitoring outcomes. In this case, computer software was developed so that the student could create his plan and self-monitoring card. The program was designed to guide him through a series of three choices to identify (1) a target behavior to focus on that day, (2) a covert direction to say to himself as a self-control cue, and (3) a specific appropriate behavior to practice. After his third choice, the computer assembled a personal card that was printed for use at his work site. A grid at the bottom of the card instructed the student to "Mark + for Yes, – for No" when the teacher periodically cued him to self-monitor his behavior. After he self-monitored his behavior during the independent work period, the student returned to the computer program to enter his results. Although this student never progressed to a level of independent use with his self-monitoring procedure (i.e., an aide was needed to interrupt talk-outs that occurred as he worked), the team believed the process increased his awareness of his talk-outs and held promise as a tool for use with other students in less restrictive, integrated settings.

Self-Monitoring Internalizing Problems

Self-monitoring has been used less frequently with internalizing disorders such as childhood anxiety and depression (Beidel, Neal, & Lederer, 1991; King, Ollendick, & Murphy, 1997). However, self-monitoring offers some distinct advantages over the more traditional assessment methods that rely on interviews or self-report inventories. With self-monitoring, specific information concerning covert thoughts and feelings, levels of anxious or depressed feelings, and conditions surrounding the problem situations may be reported. This information is critical to treating the internalizing disorder, yet inaccessible through more traditional assessment methods.

When self-monitoring is used to assess internalizing disorders, children or adolescents are typically instructed to record specific behaviors that occur prior to, during, or immediately following problem situations. For example, commonly self-monitored responses for assessment of social anxiety include frequency and duration of contacts, number of social interactions, and rate of speech dysfluencies (Donohue, Van Hasselt, & Hersen, 1994). In general, methods that have been used for self-monitoring childhood anxiety and depression include the behavioral diary and counting devices (e.g., wrist counters).

As might be expected, self-monitoring for assessment of internalizing disorders is typically used with older children and adolescents, because very young children may not be able to accurately identify and report anxious or depressed thoughts, feelings, or situational events (King et al., 1997). Obviously, whenever self-monitoring is selected as an assessment strategy for use with older children or adolescents, the behaviors should be clearly specified and the recording procedures uncomplicated (Shapiro, 1984).

Self-monitoring has been used to assess several different types of anxiety in school-age children. In one investigation by Beidel and colleagues (1991), test-anxious elementary-school children were selected for study based on prior research that demonstrated these children actually express a broad range of fears, particularly in the social-evaluative realm. The authors examined the use of a daily diary to assess the range and frequency of anxious events in children. A total of 57 children (32 test anxious and 25 non-test anxious) in third through sixth grade participated in the study. Children were given a diary that consisted of 50 formatted pages (printed version or picture version) bound in a spiral notebook, and were instructed to complete one diary page each time something happened that made them feel anxious. Children were also provided with a sample of a correctly completed diary page, and each step in the entry was reviewed verbally as well as illustrated in the sample. The diary itself assessed, in checklist format, situational parameters related to the occurrence of anxious events including time of day, location, specific anxiety-producing event, and behavioral responses to the event. The specific items included on the checklist were based on prior research and were intended to present a range of potentially anxiety-producing situations across classrooms, school cafeteria, home, outside, or with friends.

Results indicated that, overall, children complied with the self-monitoring instructions at an acceptable level and the self-monitored data appeared to be reliable. Although the specific format appeared to make no difference in compliance or mean number of events recorded for fifth- and sixth-grade children, the third- and fourth-grade children who completed the written version of the diary were less likely to adhere to the diary format than the other groups. An additional finding was that children who met DSM diagnostic criteria for overanxious disorder or social phobia reported significantly more emotional distress and more negative behaviors (e.g., crying, somatic complaints, or behavioral avoidance) surrounding the occurrence of self-monitored events than the matched normal control participants. This provided some initial validity for the use of self-monitoring as a tool for the assessment of specific anxious behaviors in children with anxiety disorders.

Ollendick (1995) used self-monitoring successfully in the assessment and treatment of four adolescents diagnosed with panic disorder with agoraphobia. These adolescents were instructed to monitor the date, time, duration, location, circumstance, and symptoms experienced (the 13 DSM symptoms) during their panic attacks. They were asked to record this information on a daily basis for the upcoming week and the information was reviewed at the beginning of each subsequent session. In addition to ongoing self-monitoring, participants were asked during each session to provide self-efficacy ratings for coping with panic and ratings of the extent to which they had actually avoided each of three problematic agoraphobic situations. Results indicated panic attacks were eliminated, agoraphobic avoidance was reduced, and self-efficacy for coping with attacks was enhanced as a function of cognitive–behavioral treatment. In addition, heightened levels of anxiety sensitivity, trait anxiety, fear, and depression were reduced to normative levels for these adolescents.

In treatment of childhood and adolescent depression, self-monitoring has been employed as both an assessment and intervention procedure (Lewinsohn & Clarke, 1999). With depression, self-monitoring typically involves the child self-recording the occurrence of a targeted response in either an unstructured journal format or a checklist of predetermined behaviors. As depressed children and adolescents, like depressed adults, tend to focus on negative rather than positive events (Kaslow, Rehm,

& Siegel, 1984), they may need to be taught to self-monitor pleasant events. Reynolds and Stark (1985) developed a procedure for creating a pleasant events schedule for children that ensures an up-to-date representation of pleasant activities. The procedure involves initial schoolwide administration of a short questionnaire to identify positive and current age-appropriate activities. From this list, the most frequently identified activities can be constructed and placed into the child's self-monitoring diary. Children can then be asked to self-monitor with a check mark every time they participate in an enjoyable activity or have a pleasant thought. This way, students are likely to pay more attention to, and perhaps participate more in, the positive activities in their lives (Reynolds & Stark, 1987).

In general, self-monitoring has been used as an effective mechanism for monitoring the private events of children and adolescents with various types of internalizing disorders. Studies have typically used diaries or data-recording devices that simplify the procedures. What is unclear in these studies is whether the outcomes reported through self-monitoring are related to the implementation of the specific treatment programs, or are simply a result of repeated exposure to the assessment process itself. If used as the sole data-collection method in research, the veracity of the self-monitored data may be questionable and studies need to provide additional indices of effectiveness beyond self-monitored data alone.

APPLICATION OF SELF-MONITORING WITHIN A SELF-REGULATORY FRAMEWORK

Other applications of self-monitoring have included multiple processes that go far beyond the simple recording of discrete behaviors. These applications have emerged more recently and are related to the effort to enhance student, or *self-regulated*, learning. Within this framework, emphasis is placed on teaching students a process that will promote self-initiated and sustained learning, as well the application of skills across new settings and problem situations.

Kanfer and Karoly (1982) were among the first to define self-regulation as an integrated and organized series of "component processes that serve to achieve the person's objectives" (p. 577). Two phrases are important in this definition. First, *component processes* underscores the concept that self-regulation involves multiple, interrelated strategies or components, of which self-monitoring is one. The second phrase, *to achieve the person's objectives*, emphasizes the importance of maintaining a focus on the learner's own goals. In general, in the context of self-regulation, self-monitoring is viewed as a form of self-assessment in which students gather information about themselves and their behavior, and then use this information to modify their own learning and subsequent actions.

An example of a self-regulation model is provided by Zimmerman, Bonner, and Kovach (1996), who describe self-regulation as a continuous learning cycle consisting of four major components: (1) self-evaluation and self-monitoring—students judge their personal effectiveness, often from observations and recording of their own behavior; (2) goal setting and strategic planning—students analyze the learning task, set goals, and plan and refine their strategy to obtain their goal; (3) strategy implementation and monitoring—students execute a strategy and monitor their accuracy implementation; and (4) strategic-outcome monitoring—students draw a link between learning outcomes and the strategic process to determine the strategy's effectiveness.

An interesting feature of Zimmerman's model is the way self-monitoring is applied in the self-regulatory process. Going beyond the simple recording of behavior, self-monitoring is used at several junctures—students monitor their baseline performance, their success in implementing their learning strategy, and the strategy's effectiveness in meeting their goals. According to the authors, self-monitoring provides essential information that can change the student's subsequent goals, use of particular strategies, or performance efforts. When self-monitoring is embedded within other self-regulatory components, emphasis is placed on the learning process, not just on the learning outcomes, as is the case when self-monitoring is used in isolation.

Thus, according to self-regulation theory, self-monitoring for the purpose of self-assessment requires the skillful combination of multiple cognitive processes. This implies that, when teaching students to self-monitor, the role of the teacher is greater than ensuring that students accurately record their behavior. It requires that teachers carefully model all steps of the self-regulatory process, so that students can see the connection between assessment of their own behavior and evaluation of their learning strategies with their achievement of self-selected goals (Zimmerman et al., 1996).

Emerging Applications

Strategy Instruction

The Zimmerman and colleagues (1996) model represents application of self-monitoring for academic strategy instruction, which is gaining increasing recognition. In their book *Developing Self-Regulated Learners*, Zimmerman and coauthors (1996) describe how a self-regulatory process can be used with middle- and high-school students to enhance summarization of text materials, note taking, exam preparation, and writing skills. For example, students may be asked to set goals based upon their assessment of their baseline performance, determine if their performance on a desired academic task is moving along lines consistent with attaining these goals, use a rubric to score their performance against an established criterion, and evaluate whether their approach or strategy to the problem is successful in helping them to solve the problem. As described, self-monitoring in this model is used to assess the effectiveness of the learning strategy as well as student performance.

Efforts to develop procedures to improve the written language skills of students with learning disabilities represent another example of how self-monitoring is included within a complex process for teaching higher-order thinking. Graham and colleagues have developed a procedure called self-regulated strategy development (SRSD). The technique involves teaching students to self-monitor productivity, frame and plan text, generate content, edit, revise, and write sentences. In one study, Harris and Graham (1985) taught two sixth-grade students with learning disabilities to brainstorm as part of a larger strategy to improve composition skills. In another study (Graham, Harris, MacArthur, & Schwartz, 1991), students were taught strategies for framing by posing and answering questions involving different parts of stories. As part of the SRSD strategy, students were taught how to use scoring rubrics that examine stories for specific elements of story grammar (main character, locale, time, starter event, goal action, ending, and reaction). Still another part of the process involved goal setting. Graham and coauthors (1991) taught a specific goal-setting prewriting strategy to students by having students pick goals, list ways to meet their goals, make notes, sequence their notes, and test whether they met their goals.

Results showed that students improved their writing skills in terms of the number of story elements, as well as the quality of their writing. Prior to the learning strategy, students spent less than 5 seconds of prewriting time on their stories. This increased to approximately 8 minutes following instruction. Total composing time increased from 12 minutes in baseline to 20 minutes after intervention. In addition, generalization to other story areas not discussed as part of the intervention showed improvements as well. Similar findings have been reported by Sexton, Harris, and Graham (1998). In that study, the full SRSD strategy included self-graphing of outcomes at different phases of the strategy-learning process.

There is some research that has attempted to separate the impact of self-monitoring alone from that of the self-regulatory strategies. Malone and Mastropieri (1992) found that students who were trained in a summarization strategy with self-monitoring performed better than those who were taught the summarization strategy alone. Graham and colleagues (Graham & Harris, 1989; Sawyer, Graham, & Harris, 1992) reported, in a component analysis of SRSD for teaching story grammar, no differences between SRSD with or without a self-regulation (i.e., self-monitoring) condition. Sawyer and colleagues (1992), however, found that the full SRSD procedure led to better generalization.

Inclusion Settings

With the growing emphasis on inclusion, strategies that can enhance the performance of students with disabilities in general education classrooms are valuable tools. A small number of studies have shown that, when used as an intervention technique, self-monitoring can improve the on-task and academic performance of students with mild learning and behavior problems in inclusive classroom settings (e.g., Maag, DiGangi, & Rutherford, 1992; Maag et al., 1993; Prater et al., 1992). Snyder and Bambara (1997) illustrated the combined use of self-monitoring with other self-regulatory strategies to teach three middle-school students with learning disabilities a process for self-managing their daily preparation for class. Specifically, the focus of the study was on improving several classroom survival skills considered necessary for academic success in general education settings such as arriving to class on time, coming to class with all necessary materials (e.g, books, pen, paper), being ready to participate at the start of class, and completing and submitting all homework assignments. Students were taught a five-step self-regulatory process involving problem identification (students identified problem areas in their current classroom preparation), goal setting (students identified objectives to improve their performance), self-monitoring (students recorded the completion of seven targeted class preparation behaviors), self-evaluation (students noted what they did or did not do, and what they could do better), and self-reinforcement (students assessed their satisfaction with their performance). Completion of the last two steps set the stage for repeating the entire self-regulatory process. For example, if the students assessed their performance to be poor, they were guided to identify contributing problem factors, set new goals, and identify strategies for improving classroom readiness.

Through guided practice and feedback, the self-regulation skills were taught to students by their learning support teacher in a self-contained classroom where they were specifically instructed to apply the process in both their learning support and general education social studies classes. Dramatic improvements in students' classroom preparation skills in both classroom settings were seen following intervention. These results were maintained as the learning support teacher faded her involvement. Moreover, social validity measures indicated that the students performance was on par with their peers in the general education class and that marked improvements were noted by the social studies teachers in their routine progress reports. The latter outcomes are especially noteworthy in that the social studies teachers were not involved in any aspect of the training, nor were they aware that the students were self-monitoring their performance during the social studies class. As in the studies of academic strategy instruction, this study illustrates the potential use of self-monitoring as one component in a self-regulatory intervention to promote generalization, in this case across settings.

Self-Determination Models

Broader applications of self-monitoring within a self-regulatory framework can be found within the growing self-determination movement for students with disabilities. Despite its varied definitions, self-determination can be described as the opportunities, attitudes, and skills necessary for directing one's life (Bambara, Cole, & Koger, 1998). As such, self-determination may be viewed as the ultimate outcome of self-regulation for young learners. The emphasis on self-determination is a natural outgrowth of the student-rights and disability movements.

However, recent language in the Individuals with Disabilities Education Act (IDEA) is credited for creating the primary impetus for promoting self-determination in the schools (Wehmeyer, 1998). IDEA requires that IEP transition plans for post-school life be based on students' individual needs and take into account student preferences and interests. Because self-determination is viewed as a lifelong learning process, this IDEA requirement has been interpreted to mean that students must be actively involved in planning for their transition and has resulted in numerous model demonstration programs funded by the Office of Special Education Programs (OSEP), aimed at enhancing educational decision making and empowerment for students with and without disabilities (see Wehmeyer & Sands, 1998).

Two such curriculum programs are the *Choicemaker Series* (Martin & Huber, 1998) and *The Self-Determined Learning Model of Instruction* (Mithaug, Wehmeyer, Agran, Martin, & Powers, 1998). In these programs, self-monitoring plays a small, yet integral role in the overall curriculum for developing self-determination. The *Choicemaker Series* features three instructional sections designed to foster long-range educational planning and decision making: (1) choosing goals (e.g, personal, educational, career, and daily living), (2) expressing goals at IEP meetings, and (3 taking action. In teaching students to take action, self-monitoring is used to guide students to monitor their task performance, evaluate their success and the effectiveness of their self-selected management strategies, and change their goals, strategy, or standards on the basis of their self-assessments. Similarly, in the *Self-Determined Learning Model of Instruction*, three curriculum components are emphasized including (1) setting goals, (2) taking action, and (3) adjusting. Self-monitoring in this curriculum is used as an assessment strategy for students to self-evaluate their progress and revise their goals or action plan as needed (Mithaug et al., 1998).

CONCLUSIONS

Self-monitoring has been used infrequently as a strategy for assessment in children and adolescents (Shapiro & Cole, 1999). Rather, self-monitoring has been consistently viewed by researchers and practitioners as an intervention technique, aimed at producing reactive effects in a variety of student target behaviors. Among the many studies that have included self-monitoring as a behavior-change mechanism, self-monitoring frequently has been found to result in reactivity across age groups, for both academic and nonacademic problems, and across many different types of disabilities.

Despite the acceptance and impact of using self-monitoring as a behavior-change process, its use as an assessment tool alone with children remains largely uninvestigated. It is possible that such a direction for self-monitoring research has not been pursued because it may be inconsistent with the expectation that children and adolescents will self-report accurately. The problem may be simply that it does not make sense to use self-monitoring as an assessment tool alone, given its potential for reactivity. Certainly, from a practical standpoint, it may be much more useful as an intervention than an assessment procedure. Additionally, if the reliability of data collected through self-monitoring processes is questionable, the likelihood for acceptance of self-monitoring for assessment purposes is lower (Shapiro & Cole, 1999).

However, this is not to say that self-monitoring should be restricted to a simple behavior-change strategy. In fact, the brightest future for self-monitoring may be in its application within a self-regulatory framework. When self-monitoring is embedded among other components in a self-regulatory process, emphasis is placed on assessment for the self. That is, students are taught a particular strategy for achieving learning goals and a strategy for monitoring and evaluating their success. Each component informs the other, with the ultimate goal of promoting student-directed learning that is readily transferable across new problem situations. Contrast this with the use of self-monitoring in isolation, where the focus is on the mechanical aspects of data collection and the emphasis on assessment may be distorted or lost.

The degree to which self-monitoring as a single component of this self-regulation process is critical or can be isolated is yet unknown. While researchers may be encouraged to examine how the self-monitoring component impacts overall learning in a self-regulatory strategy, it may be impossible to isolate this component from the overall procedures embedded within the process. For example, how would one remove self-monitoring without removing self-evaluation and goal planning, or remove self-monitoring without removing planning? Indeed, many researchers may not see this as a fruitful line of research. Zimmerman and Kitsantas (1996) found that the premature concentration on outcomes before a skill was fully developed and fully internalized increases the cognitive complexity of the task and makes interpreting outcomes difficult. In some cases it may make sense to use self-monitoring to influence the acquisition and fluency of a skill first, and then apply the process more broadly to focus on the assessment of learning outcomes. This is similar to the views that self-monitoring may be a successful strategy for achieving long-term maintenance of behavior change once fundamental skills are acquired (e.g., Shapiro & Cole, 1994). However, one implication from the self-regulatory literature is clear: The long-term isolation of self-monitoring from other cognitive processes is neither prudent nor wise when the eventual goal is to teach students how to independently self-assess their own actions.

References

Bambara, L. M., Cole, C. L., & Koger, F. (1998). Translating self-determination concepts into support for adults with severe disabilities. *Journal of the Association for Persons with Severe Handicaps, 23*, 27–37.

Barkley, R. A. (1990). *Attention-deficit hyperactivity disorder: A handbook for diagnosis and treatment.* New York: Guilford Press.

Beidel, D. C., Neal, A. M., & Lederer, A. S. (1991). The feasibility and validity of a daily diary for the assessment of anxiety in children. *Behavior Therapy, 22*, 505–517.

Blick, D. W., & Test, D. W. (1987). Effects of self-recording on high-school students' on-task behavior. *Learning Disability Quarterly, 10*, 203–213.

Boyle, J. R., & Hughes, C. A. (1994). Effects of self-monitoring and subsequent fading of external prompts on the on-task behavior and task productivity of elementary students with moderate mental retardation. *Journal of Behavioral Education, 4*, 439–457.

Broden, M., Hall, R. V., & Mitts, B. (1971). The effects of self-recording on the classroom behavior of two eighth-grade students. *Journal of Applied Behavior Analysis, 4*, 191–199.

Bruck, M., Ceci, S. J., & Hembrooke, H. (1998). Reliability and credibility of young children's reports: From research to policy to practice. *American Psychologist, 53*, 136–151.

Carr, S. C., & Punzo, R. P. (1993). The effects of self-monitoring of academic accuracy and productivity on the performance of students with behavior disorders. *Behavioral Disorders, 18*, 241–250.

Clees, T. J. (1994). Self-recording of students' daily schedules of teachers' expectancies: Perspectives on reactivity, stimulus control, and generalization. *Exceptionality, 5*, 113–129.

Connell, M. C., Carta, J. J., Lutz, S., Randall, C., & Wilson, J. (1993). Building independence during in-class transitions: Teaching in-class transition skills to preschoolers with developmental delays through choral-response-based self-assessment and contingent praise. *Education and Treatment of Children, 16*, 160–174.

DeHaas-Warner, S. (1991). Effects of self-monitoring on preschoolers' on-task behavior: A pilot study. *Topics in Early Childhood Special Education*, 11, 59–73.

DeHaas-Warner, S. (1992). The utility of self-monitoring for preschool on-task behavior. *Topics in Early Childhood Special Education*, 12, 478–495.

DiGangi, S. M., Maag, J. W., & Rutherford, R. B. (1991). Self-graphing of on-task behavior: Enhancing the reactive effects of self-monitoring on on-task behavior and academic performance. *Learning Disabilities Quarterly*, 14, 221–230.

Donohue, B. C., Van Hasselt, V. B., & Hersen, M. (1994). Behavioral assessment and treatment of social phobia. *Behavior Modification*, 18, 262–288.

Dunlap, L. K., & Dunlap, G. (1989). A self-monitoring package for teaching subtraction with regrouping to students with learning disabilities. *Journal of Applied Behavior Analysis*, 22, 309–314.

DuPaul, G. J., & Stoner, G. (1994). *ADHD in the schools: Assessment and intervention strategies*. New York: Guilford Press.

Fitzgerald, G. E., & Werner, J. G. (1996). The use of the computer to support cognitive–behavioral interventions for students with behavioral disorders. *Journal of Computing in Childhood Education*, 7, 127–148.

Flores, D. M., Schloss, P. J., & Alper, S. (1995). The use of a daily calendar to increase responsibilities fulfilled by secondary students with special needs. *Remedial and Special Education*, 16, 38–43.

Frith, G. H., & Armstrong, S. W. (1985). Self-monitoring for behavior disordered students. *Teaching Exceptional Children*, 18, 144–148.

Gardner, W. I., & Cole, C. L. (1988). Self-monitoring procedures. In E. S. Shapiro & T. R. Kratochwill (Eds.), *Behavioral assessment in schools: Conceptual foundations and practical applications* (pp. 106–146). New York: Guilford Press.

Graham, S., & Harris, K. R. (1989). Component analysis of cognitive strategy instruction: Effects on learning disabled students' compositions and self-efficacy. *Journal of Educational Psychology*, 81, 353–361.

Graham, S., Harris, K. R., MacArthur, C. A., & Schwartz, S. (1991). Writing and writing instruction for students with learning disabilities. Review of a research program. *Learning Disabilities Quarterly*, 14, 89–114.

Hallahan, D. P., Lloyd, J. W., Kneedler, R. D., & Marshall, K. G. (1982). A comparison of the effects of self versus teacher-assessment of on-task behavior. *Behavior Therapy*, 13, 715–723.

Hallahan, D. P., Lloyd, J. W., & Stoller, L. (1982). *Improving attention with self monitoring: A manual for teachers*. Charlottesville: University of Virginia.

Harris, K. R. (1986). Self-monitoring of attentional behavior versus self-monitoring of productivity: Effects on on-task behavior and academic response rate among learning disabled children. *Journal of Applied Behavior Analysis*, 19, 417–423.

Harris, K. R., & Graham, S. (1985). Improving learning disabled students' composite skills: Self-control strategy training. *Learning Disability Quarterly*, 8, 27–36.

Harris, K. R., Graham, S., Reid, R., McElroy, K., & Hamby, R. S. (1994). Self-monitoring of attention versus self-monitoring of performance: Replication and cross-task comparison studies. *Learning Disability Quarterly*, 17, 121–139.

Heins, E. D., Lloyd, J. W., & Hallahan, D. (1986). Cued and noncued self-recording of attention to task. *Behavior Modification*, 10, 235–254.

Hertz, V., & McLaughlin, T. F. (1990). Self-recording: Effects for on-task behavior of mildly handicapped adolescents. *Child & Family Behavior Therapy*, 12, 1–11.

Houghton, S. J. (1991). Promoting generalization of appropriate behavior across special and mainstream settings: A case study. *Educational Psychology*, 7, 49–54.

Howell, K. W., Rueda, R., & Rutherford, R. B. (1983). A procedure for teaching self-recording to moderately retarded students. *Psychology in the Schools*, 20, 202–209.

Hughes, C. A., & Boyle, J. R. (1991). Effects of self-monitoring for on-task behavior and task productivity on elementary students with moderate mental retardation. *Education and Treatment of Children*, 14, 96–111.

Hughes, C. A., Korinek, L., & Gorman, J. (1991). Self-management for students with mental retardation in public school settings: A research review. *Education and Training in Mental Retardation, 26,* 271–291.

Hughes, C. A., Ruhl, K. L., & Misra, A. (1989). Self-management with behaviorally disordered students in school settings: A promise unfulfilled? *Behavioral Disorders, 14,* 250–262.

Kanfer, F. H. (1970). Self-monitoring: Methodological limitations and clinical applications. *Journal of Consulting and Clinical Psychology, 35,* 143–152.

Kanfer, F. H. (1977). The many faces of self-control. In R. B. Stuart (Ed.), *Behavioral self-management: Strategies, techniques, and outcomes.* New York: Brunner/Mazel.

Kanfer, F. H., & Karoly, P. (1982). The psychology of self-management: Abiding issues and tentative directions. In *Self-management and behavior change: From theory to practice* (pp. 571–599). New York: Pergamon Press.

Kaslow, N. J., Rehm, L. P., & Siegel, A. W. (1984). Social-cognitive and cognitive correlates of depression in children. *Journal of Abnormal Child Psychology, 12,* 605–620.

Kern, L., Dunlap, G., Childs, K. E., & Clarke, S. (1994). Use of a classwide self-management program to improve the behavior of students with emotional and behavioral disorders. *Education and Treatment of Children, 17,* 445–458.

Kern, L., Marder, T. J., Boyajian, A. E., Elliot, C. M., & McElhattan, D. (1997). Augmenting the independence of self-management procedures by teaching self-initiation across settings and activities. *School Psychology Quarterly, 12,* 23–32.

King, N. J., Ollendick, T. H., & Murphy, G. C. (1997). Assessment of childhood phobias. *Clinical Psychology Review, 17,* 667–687.

Koegel, R. L., & Koegel, L. K. (1990). Extended reductions in stereotypic behavior of students with autism through a self-management treatment package. *Journal of Applied Behavior Analysis, 23,* 119–127.

Kunzelmann, H. D. (Ed.). (1970). *Precision teaching.* Seattle: Child Publications.

La Greca, A. M. (1990). Issues and perspective on the child assessment process. In A. M. La Greca (Ed.), *Through the eyes of the child: Obtaining self-reports from children and adolescents* (pp. 3–17). Boston: Allyn and Bacon.

Lam, A. L., Cole, C. L., Shapiro, E. S., & Bambara, L. M. (1994). Relative effects of self-monitoring on-task behavior, academic accuracy, and disruptive behavior in students with behavior disorders. *School Psychology Review, 23,* 44–58.

Lewinsohn, P. M., & Clarke, G. N. (1999). Psychosocial treatment for adolescent depression. *Clinical Psychology Review, 19,* 329–342.

Lloyd, J. W., Bateman, D. F., Landrum, T. J., & Hallahan, D. P. (1989). Self-recording of attention versus productivity. *Journal of Applied Behavior Analysis, 22,* 315–323.

Lloyd, M. E., & Hilliard, A. M. (1989). Accuracy of self-recording as a function of repeated experience with different self-control contingencies. *Child and Family Behavior Therapy, 11(2),* 1–14.

Maag, J. W., DiGangi, S. A., & Rutherford, R. B. (1992). Effects of self-monitoring and contingent reinforcement on on-task behavior and academic productivity of learning-disabled students. A social validation study. *Psychology in the Schools, 29,* 157–172.

Maag, J. W., Reid, R., & DiGangi, S. A. (1993). Differential effects of self-monitoring attention, accuracy, and productivity. *Journal of Applied Behavior Analysis, 26,* 329–344.

Maag, J. W., Rutherford, A. B., & DiGangi, S. A. (1992). Effects of self-monitoring and contingent reinforcement on on-task behavior and academic productivity of learning-disabled students: A social validation study. *Psychology in the Schools, 29,* 157–172.

Mace, F. C., & Kratochwill, T. R. (1985). Theories of reactivity in self-monitoring: A comparison of cognitive–behavioral and operant models. *Behavior Modification, 9,* 323–344.

Malone, L. D., & Mastropieri, M. (1992). Reading comprehension instruction: Summarization and self-monitoring training for students with learning disabilities. *Exceptional Children, 58,* 270–279.

Marshall, K. J., Lloyd, J. W., & Hallahan, D. P. (1993). Effects of training to increase self-monitoring accuracy. *Journal of Behavioral Education, 3,* 445–459.

Martella, R. C., Leonard, I. J., Marchand-Martella, N. E., & Agran, M. (1993). Self-monitoring negative statements. *Journal of Behavioral Education, 3,* 77–86.

Martin, J. E., & Marshall, L. H. (1998). Choicemaker. In M. L. Wehmeyer & D. J. Sands (Eds.), *Making it happen: Student involvement in educational planning and decision making* (pp. 211–240). Baltimore: Paul H. Brookes.

Mathes, M. Y., & Bender, W. N. (1997). The effects of self-monitoring on children with attention-deficit/hyperactivity disorder who are receiving pharmacological interventions. *Remedial and Special Education, 18*, 121–128.

McCarl, J. J., Svobodny, L., & Beare, P. L. (1991). Self-recording in a classroom for students with mild to moderate mental handicaps: Effects on productivity and on-task behavior. *Education and Training in Mental Retardation, 26*, 79–88.

McDougall, D., & Brady, M. P. (1995). Using audio-cued self-monitoring for students with severe behavior disorders. *Journal of Educational Research, 88*, 309–317.

Miller, M., Miller, S. R., Wheeler, J., & Selinger, J. (1989). Can a single-classroom treatment approach change academic performance and behavioral characteristics in severely behaviorally disordered adolescents: An experimental inquiry. *Behavioral Disorders, 14*, 215–225.

Miller, L. J., Strain, P. S., Boyd, K., Jarzynka, J., & McFetridge, M. (1993). The effects of classwide self-assessment on preschool children's engagement in transition, free play, and small group instruction. *Early Education and Development, 4*, 162–181.

Minner, S. (1990). Use of a self-recording procedure to decrease the time taken by behaviorally disordered students to walk to special classes. *Behavioral Disorders, 15*, 210–216.

Mithaug, D. E., Wehmeyer, M. L., Agran, M., Martin, J. E., & Powers, S. (1998). The self-determined learning model of instruction: Engaging students to solve their learning problems. In M. L. Wehmeyer & D. J. Sands (Eds.), *Making it happen: Student involvement in educational planning and decision making* (pp. 299–328). Baltimore: Paul H. Brookes.

Morris, N. (1980). *Star control: Super problem solving*. Unpublished manuscript. The University of Iowa, Child Psychiatry Service, Iowa City.

Nelson, R. O. (1977). Assessment and therapeutic functions of self-monitoring. In J. D. Cone & R. P. Hawkins (Eds.), *Progress in behavior modification* (Vol. 5, pp. 263–308). New York: Academic Press.

Nelson, R. O., Hay, L. R., Devany, J., & Koslow-Green, L. (1980). The reactivity and accuracy of children's self-monitoring: Three experiments. *Child Behavior Therapy, 2*(3), 1–24.

Nelson, R. O., & Hayes, S. C. (1981). Theoretical explanations of reactivity in self-monitoring. *Behavior Modification, 5*, 3–14.

Nelson, R. O., Lipinski, D. P., & Black, J. L. (1975). The effects of expectancy on the reactivity of self-recording. *Behavior Therapy, 6*, 337–349.

Nelson, R. O., Lipinski, D. P., & Boykin, R. A. (1978). The effects of self-recorders' training and the obtrusiveness of the self-monitoring device on the accuracy and reactivity of self-monitoring. *Behavior Therapy, 9*, 200–208.

Newman, B., Buffington, D. M., O'Grady, M. A., McDonald, M. E., Poulson, C. L., & Hemmes, N. S. (1995). Self-management of schedule following in three teenagers with autism. *Behavioral Disorders, 20*, 190–196.

Ninness, H. A. C., Ellis, J., Miller, W. B., Baker, D., & Rutherford, R. (1995). The effect of a self-management training package on the transfer of aggression control procedures in the absence of supervision. *Behavior Modification, 19*, 464–490.

Ninness, H. A. C., Fuerst, J., & Rutherford, R. (1995). A descriptive analysis of disruptive behavior during pre- and post-unsupervised self-management by students with serious emotional disturbance. *Journal of Emotional and Behavioral Disorders, 3*, 230–240.

Ollendick, T. H. (1981). Self-monitoring and self-administered overcorrection: The modification of nervous tics in children. *Behavior Modification, 5*, 75–84.

Ollendick, T. H. (1995). Cognitive behavioral treatment of panic disorder with agoraphobia in adolescents: A multiple baseline design analysis. *Behavior Therapy, 26*, 517–531.

Prater, M. A., Hogan, S., & Miller, S. R. (1992). Using self-monitoring to improve on-task behavior and academic skills of an adolescent with mild handicaps across special and regular education settings. *Education and Treatment of Children, 15*, 43–55.

Rachlin, H. (1974). Self-control. *Behaviorism, 2*, 94–107.

Reid, R. (1996). Research in self-monitoring with students with learning disabilities: The present, the prospects, the pitfalls. *Journal of Learning Disabilities, 29,* 317–331.

Reid, R., & Harris, K. R. (1993). Self-monitoring of attention versus self-monitoring of performance: Effects on attention and academic performance. *Exceptional Children, 60,* 29–40.

Reynolds, W. M., & Stark, K. D. (1985). *Procedures for the development of pleasant activity schedules for children.* Unpublished manuscript.

Reynolds, W. M., & Stark, K. D. (1987). School-based intervention strategies for the treatment of depression in children and adolescents. *Special Services in the Schools, 3*(3–4), 69–88.

Roberts, R. N., & Nelson, R. O. (1981). The effects of self-monitoring on children's classroom behavior. *Child Behavior Therapy, 3,* 105–120.

Sawyer, R. J., Graham, S., & Harris, K. R. (1992). Direct teaching, strategy instruction, and strategy instruction with explicit self-regulation: Effects on the composition skills and self-efficacy of students with learning disabilities. *Journal of Educational Psychology, 84,* 340–352.

Schunk, D. H. (1982). Progress self-monitoring: Effects on children's self-efficacy and achievement. *Journal of Experimental Education, 51,* 89–93.

Sexton, M., Harris, K. R., & Graham, S. (1998). Self-regulated strategy development and the writing process: Effects on essay writing and attributions. *Exceptional Children, 64,* 295–311.

Shapiro, E. S. (1984). Self-monitoring procedures. In T. H. Ollendick & M. Hersen (Eds.), *Child behavioral assessment: Principles and procedures.* (pp. 148–165). New York: Pergamon Press.

Shapiro, E. S., Browder, D. M., & D'Huyvetters, K. K. (1984). Increasing academic productivity of severely multi-handicapped children with self-management: Idiosyncratic effects. *Analysis and Intervention in Developmental Disabilities, 4,* 171–188.

Shapiro, E. S., & Cole, C. L. (1994). *Behavior change in the classroom: Self-management interventions.* New York: Guilford Press.

Shapiro, E. S., & Cole, C. L. (1999). Self-monitoring in assessing children's problems. *Psychological Assessment, 11,* 448–457.

Shapiro, E. S., McGonigle, J. J., & Ollendick, T. H. (1980). An analysis of self-assessment and self-reinforcement in a self-managed token economy with mentally retarded children. *Applied Research in Mental Retardation, 1,* 227–240.

Snyder, M. (1979). Self-monitoring processes. In L. Berkowitz (Ed.), *Advances in experimental social psychology* (Vol. 12, pp. 85–128). New York: Academic Press.

Snyder, M. C., & Bambara, L. M. (1997). Teaching secondary students with learning disabilities to self-management classroom survival skills. *Journal of Learning Disabilities, 30,* 534–543.

Stewart, K. G., & McLaughlin, T. F. (1992). Self-recording: Effects of reducing off task behavior with a high school student with an attention deficit hyperactivity disorder. *Child and Family Behavior Therapy, 14,* 53–59.

Storey, K., Lawry, J. R., Ashworth, R., & Danko, C. D. (1994). Functional analysis and intervention for disruptive behaviors of a kindergarten student. *Journal of Educational Research, 87,* 361–370.

Strain, P. S., Kohler, F. w., Storey, K., & Danko, C. D. (1994). Teaching pre-schoolers with autism to self-monitor their social interactions: An analysis of results in home and school settings. *Journal of Emotional and Behavioral Disorders, 2,* 78–88.

Sugai, G., & Rowe, P. (1984). The effect of self-recording on out-of-seat behavior of an EMR student. *Education and Training of the Mentally Retarded, 19,* 23–38.

Trammel, D. L., Schloss, P. J., & Alper, S. (1994). Using self-recording, evaluation, and graphing to increase completion of homework assignments. *Journal of Learning Disabilities, 27,* 75–81.

Webber, J., Scheuermann, B., McCall, C., & Coleman, M. (1993). Research on self-monitoring as a behavior management technique in special education classrooms: A descriptive review. *RASE: Remedial and Special Education, 14*(2), 38–56.

Wehmeyer, M. L. (1998). Student involvement in education planning, decision making, and instruction: An idea whose time has arrived. In M. L. Wehmeyer & D. J. Sands (Eds.), *Making it happen: Student involvement in educational planning and decision making* (pp. 3–23). Baltimore: Paul H. Brookes.

Wehmeyer, M. L., & Sands, D. J. (1998). *Making it happen: Student involvement in educational planning and decision making.* Baltimore: Paul H. Brookes.

Wood, S. J., Murdock, J. Y., Cronin, M. E., Dawson, N. M., & Kirby, P. C. (1998). Effects of self-monitoring on on-task behaviors of at-risk middle school students. *Journal of Behavioral Education*, 8, 263–279.

Workman, E. A., Helton, G. B., & Watson, P. J. (1982). Self-monitoring effects in a four-year-old child: An ecological behavior analysis. *Journal of School Psychology*, 20, 57–64.

Zimmerman, B. J., Bonner, S., & Kovach, R. (1996). *Developing self-regulated learners: Beyond achievement to self-efficacy*. Washington, DC: American Psychological Association.

Zimmerman, B. J., & Kitsantas, A. (1996). Self-regulated learning of a motoric skill: The role of goal setting and self-monitoring. *Journal of Applied Sport Psychology*, 8, 60–75.

CHAPTER 9

Informant Reports

Theory and Research in Using Child Behavior Rating Scales in School Settings

KENNETH W. MERRELL

The University of Iowa

The use of behavior rating scales, once avoided by many behaviorally oriented practitioners and researchers because of concerns about unreliability and validity, have emerged as one of the most popular methods of assessing social-emotional behavior of children and youth (Wilson & Reschly, 1996). Today, school and clinical child psychologists and other education/mental health professionals routinely utilize child behavior rating scales as either a primary component of an assessment design or as a key means of obtaining behavioral information prior to, during, and following interventions. One explanation for the increased acceptance of behavior rating scales is that numerous advances in rating scale technology during the latter two or three decades of the 20th century enhanced the psychometric properties and empirical support for this form of assessment, thus making it more acceptable to consumers (Elliott, Busse, & Gresham, 1993; Merrell, 1999). Now, rating scales are considered to be one important component of a functional assessment of child and adolescent behavior problems in school settings (Alberto & Troutman, 1996).

The purpose of this chapter is to discuss and analyze selected issues related to theoretical, research, and clinical applications of child behavior rating scales, with a particular emphasis on their use in school settings. Three major areas are the focus of this chapter. First, issues related to rater and instrument differences in behavior rating scale scores are discussed. Specifically, issues involving cross-informant correlations, error variance, and situational factors are addressed. Second, issues regarding group differences in rating scales are analyzed. This section includes a focus on gender, ethnicity, optimal norm sampling techniques, and practical considerations in determining when the use of separate norms for specific groups might be justified. Third, some potential clinical applications of behavior rating scales are overviewed, including screening, diagnosis, treatment selection, and progress monitoring/outcome measurement. Because the number of possible topics related to behavior rating scales are so large, this chapter necessarily focuses on only these three areas. Readers who desire to consult other sources on scientific and practical aspects of using child behavior rating scales are referred to other chapters by this author (e.g., Merrell, 1994a, 1994b, 1999, 2000).

CROSS-INFORMANT CORRELATIONS,
ERROR VARIANCE, AND SITUATIONAL FACTORS

When behavior rating scales began to become more widely used in child behavior assessment in the 1960s and 1970s, one of the perplexing issues that became associated with their use was the typically modest to low correlations of scores produced by differing raters who evaluated the same child. Unlike direct behavioral observation, where systematic observer training practices and objective coding procedures could easily result in interrater reliability coefficients of .80 or higher (e.g., Reid, 1982), interrater reliability among rating scale users was typically at a much lower level. Clinicians were quick to notice that rating scales completed on the same student by two teachers in differing classrooms often yielded score patterns that were only slightly similar. Parent ratings of students, based on their observations of the child in the home environment, were typically even more dissimilar to teacher's ratings than were ratings produced by differing teachers.

Early efforts to understand why differing raters, instruments, settings, and time periods produced such varying rating scale results often led to the conclusion that rating scales were lacking in most types of reliability and validity. However, as rating scale use and the resulting empirical base for it increased, new ideas and conclusions emerged regarding the reliability issue, and various forms of validity were demonstrated. This section overviews the yield of research from the previous two decades regarding cross-informant reliability issues, as well as theoretical aspects of rating scale error variance. In addition, some of the practical clinical issues surrounding situational variables in rating scale use are presented.

Cross-Informant Correlations

One of the most thoroughly detailed efforts to understand cross-informant correlations of informant reports of behavioral and emotional problems was a meta-analytic review study conducted by Achenbach, McConaughy, and Howell (1987). In this investigation, 269 samples across 119 studies were examined to produce meta-analyses of Pearson r product–moment correlations of behavioral/emotional ratings of children and adolescents. These comparisons were made using ratings provided by teachers, parents, mental health workers, observers, peers, and child/adolescent self-reports.

The results of this widely influential study provided a standard by which subsequent research efforts have often been compared. Achenbach and colleagues (1987) found that the average cross-informant correlation (the weighted mean r) among all types of informants was .28. However, this very modest to low average r camouflages the complexity of the other related findings. One major finding was that agreement among pairs of informants with similar roles (such as two parents, pairs of teachers) was higher than agreement among informant pairs with differing roles (such as a parent and a teacher). The range of weighted mean r's for raters with similar roles was .54 (pairs of mental health workers) to .64 (pairs of teachers), whereas the range of weighted mean *r*'s for differing types of informants was .24 (parents and mental health workers) to .42 (teachers and observers). Another key finding was that correlations between child/adolescent self-reports of behavior and all other informant reports were exceptionally low, with an average *r* of .22, and a range from .20 to .27. This level of average association is high enough to be considered meaningful (or not occurring by chance alone), but barely, indicating that child/adolescent subjects of behavioral assessment and those informants who observe them in a variety of settings tend to see things in a substantially differing manner.

Some other findings from this meta-analysis are also worth noting. For example, it was found that there was a slightly higher average cross-informant *r* for ratings of younger children (ages 6–11) than for adolescents, and there tended to be significantly higher agreement on ratings of externalizing (undercontrolled) problems, as opposed to internalizing (overcontrolled) problems, which tended to produce the lowest average *r*'s. Finally, the authors of this study argued that the issue of correlations among differing informants should be separated from the issue of reliability. In other words, the modest to low average correlations found in this meta-analysis should not necessarily be interpreted as an indication of unreliability of behavior rating scales. Because many of the rating scales that were used in the various studies had exceptionally high levels of internal consistency reliability as well as strong test–retest reliability, the differences among various informants might be best attributed to other factors, such as situational specificity of behavior.

In the intervening several years since the publication of Achenbach and colleagues' (1987) meta-analysis, this investigation has come to represent a general standard for understanding cross-informant correlations of ratings of child and adolescent socialemotional behaviors. Numerous studies published since this meta-analysis have generally produced findings consistent with the conclusions reached by Achenbach and colleagues, even when more recent assessment instruments have been used.

However, there have been some exceptions to this general agreement that are worth noting. One of the exceptions concerns the range of cross-informant correlations for various age groups. Whereas Achenbach and colleagues found somewhat higher average correlations with elementary-age children (ages 6–11) than with adolescents (ages 12–19), other individual studies have produced the opposite finding. For example, Verhulst and Akkerhuis (1989) found that agreement between parent and teacher ratings of behavioral/emotional problems (using Achenbach's Child Behavior Checklist and Teacher's Report Form) was slightly higher for older than for younger children.

Additionally, Merrell and Caldarella (1999), and Robbins and Merrell (in press) found agreement between parents and teacher ratings of social behavior of early adolescent students who were considered to be at-risk for school dropout and substance abuse to be considerably less than would be expected based on Achenbach and colleagues' meta-analysis. Also, in the Robbins and Merrell study, correlations between ratings of student behavior (using the School Social Behavior Scales) provided by at-risk program teachers and regular education teachers were in the .17 to .46 range, substantially lower than the predicted .60 range indicated by Achenbach and coworkers. Interestingly, ratings of antisocial behavior produced higher cross-informant

TABLE 9.1   Summary of Major Findings Regarding Cross-Informant Correlations with Child and Adolescent Behavior Rating Scales

- In general, correlations of behavior ratings made by all types of informants are statistically significant but modest.
- Agreement among pairs of informants in similar roles (e.g., two parents, two teachers) is higher than agreement among informants in dissimilar roles (e.g., a parent and a teacher).
- Cross-informant agreement for ratings of externalizing problems is higher than for ratings of internalizing problems.
- Correlations between child/adolescent self-report and informant report are typically low (.20s range) but statistically significant.
- Gender of rater or child/adolescent assessment subject does not appear to be an important factor in cross-informant correlation.
- Age of child/adolescent assessment subject may influence the association of cross-informant ratings, but the specific influence of age level is not yet fully understood.
- Modest correlations of rating scale scores provided by differing informants cannot generally be attributed to unreliability of the measures.
- "It is clear that no one type of informant typically provides the same data as any other type of informant" (Achenbach, McConaughy, & Howell, 1987, p. 227).

correlations than ratings of social skills in the Robbins and Merrell study. Perhaps specific age ranges, specific behavioral risk factors, and specific types of classroom environments play important roles in situational specificity of child behavior problems. These issues certainly are in need of clarification through further research.

In sum, although some specific issues related to cross-informant correlations with behavior rating scales still need to be clarified, research conducted during the previous two decades has provided a fairly consistent series of findings in this area. A summary of the most consistently replicated findings regarding cross-informant correlations with behavior rating scales is found in Table 9.1.

Response Bias and Error Variance

Having explored the evidence regarding cross-informant correlations of behavior rating scale scores, it is now worthwhile to consider some theoretical issues that may play an important role in shaping differences among informants in the way they rate the behavior of a given child. Prior to doing so, it may be useful to examine briefly the common and technical meaning of error. The common or colloquial meaning of this word is "to make a mistake," or "deviate from what is true or correct." The mathematical or statistical meaning of error is somewhat different. In this use, error indicates a deviation from the true value not caused by mistakes of observation or measurement, or the difference between the observed value of an entity and its true magnitude. When discussing error variance in connection with behavior rating scales, the mathematical or statistical meaning of this term is more appropriate.

More than two decades ago, the basic measurement problems of rating scales in general were formally articulated by Saal, Downey, and Lahey (1980). Later, these issues were specifically applied to the kinds of rating scales used by school and clinical child psychologists (Martin, Hooper, & Snow, 1986; Merrell, 1994a, 1999). These issues or problems are generally divided into two classes of measurement bias or error: *bias of response,* and *error variance.*

Bias of Response

Bias of response refers to the way that informants who complete rating scales may produce measurement error because of the way in which the scales are used. Three specific types of response bias are generally discussed: (1) *Halo effects* are said to involve rating a student in a decidedly positive or negative manner just because that student may possess positive or negative characteristics unrelated to the rating scale task that somehow influences the rater. (2) *Leniency or severity* effects are said to involve the tendency of some raters to have an overly generous or overly critical response set. Such raters might produce rating scores that are consistently higher or lower than is warranted. (3) *Central tendency effects* are said to exist when some informants demonstrate a tendency to consistently select midpoint ratings, thus avoiding endpoints of the scale.

Error Variance

In contrast to bias of response, error variance has less to do with the way in which particular informants approach the task of completing the rating scale measure, and more to do with some of the problems encountered because of the nature of this assessment method. Four particular types of error variance relevant to child behavior rating scale measures were listed by Martin and co-workers (1986). These four types were consistent with the earlier work of Saal and co-workers (1980), but placed it specifically within the context of child behavior assessment.

Source variance involves subjectivity of the rater. For example, some raters may evaluate child behavior in a very unique or idiosyncratic manner as complete behavior rating scales. Source variance is therefore closely related to bias of response.

Setting variance results from the fact that individuals behave somewhat differently in each setting in which they must respond, assumably because of the differing stimulus/antecedent conditions and reinforcing or punishing properties that are specific to those settings. In other words, some child behavioral or emotional characteristics are not highly stable traits: they may differ markedly from setting to setting, depending on the environmental properties present to elicit and maintain them. Setting variance is closely related to a phenomenon known as situational specificity of behavior. Within each situation or setting, child behavior is likely to be exhibited in a differing manner because of the properties of that situation, in combination with the notion that few child behaviors reflect highly stable traits. Although situational specificity may be accurately thought of as a form of variance, it does not necessarily involve error in the common sense, but may accurately reflect the fact that behavior varies from place to place because of differing conditions.

Temporal variance involves inconsistency of behavior ratings over time. Like setting variance, temporal variance is thought to exist because most child behavioral characteristics are not entirely stable traits. In other words, child behavior is likely to change over time, somewhat independent from changes in the environment. It is also possible that temporal variance may occur because of changes or inconsistency in a rater's approach to the measurement task over time. Thus temporal variance is probably related to the construct that is measured, as well as bias of response.

Finally, *instrument variance* is a theoretical type of error variance that is thought to exist because rating scales (even those purported to measure similar constructs), might actually measure slightly differing hypothetical constructs. Because of differences between child behavior rating scales in item content, item wording, or rating scale format, such variation is likely to occur when differing instruments are included in an assessment battery. For example, the Teacher's Report Form and the Behavioral Assessment System for Children teacher form are generally purported to measure similar constructs. Though strong, correlations between these measures reflect a moderate degree of variability among the two instruments and the constructs they measure. Another reason for instrument variance is that each rating scale is developed with a unique normative sample. If norm samples are not randomly selected and entirely representative of the population as a whole, then variance among instruments might be expected because of these sampling differences.

In sum, there are various types of error that may influence consistency and stability of child behavior ratings, whether these ratings are provided by the same rater or by differing raters. Fergusson and Horwood (1986), through a study of variation in maternal and teacher ratings of child behavior, concluded that up to two-thirds of observation variation may be caused by method or random variation, as opposed to variation in the actual trait or characteristic that is measured. Although no percentages within categories have been demonstrated convincingly, it is at least useful to consider this possibility when designing child behavior assessments for research and clinical purposes. Table 9.2 provides a listing and brief description of each type of response bias and error variance.

Situational Specificity of Behavior: Some Additional Comments

Much of what has been written in this section relates to the concept of *situational specificity* in behavior assessment. This section concludes with a brief discussion on some of the key points relating to this important idea. Several years ago, Kazdin (e.g., 1979, 1981, 1982) and other researchers (e.g., Stokes, Baer, & Jackson, 1974; Wahler, 1975) first wrote on the topic of situational specificity of behavior from both the theoretical and applied perspectives. There has been additional research during the past

TABLE 9.2 Summary of Bias of Response and Error Variance Components in Behavior Rating Scales

Component	Description
Bias of response	
Halo	Rater evaluates a student in a wholly positive or negative manner because that student has positive or negative characteristics unrelated to the rating scale task that influence rater.
Leniency/severity	Rater has an overly generous or overly critical response set; obtained ratings are consistently higher or lower than warranted.
Central tendency	Rater has tendency to consistently select midpoint ratings, thus avoiding end points of scale.
Error variance	
Source	Differences in ratings provided by various persons; related to bias of response.
Setting	Differences in ratings across settings; related to situational specificity of behavior.
Temporal	Differences in ratings over time; related to lack of stability of underlying construct that is measured.
Instrument	Differences in ratings gathered using various instruments; related to slight differences in constructs measured by instruments, and possibly due to variations across normative samples.

two decades to help refine the topic, but the basic understanding of situational specificity has been relatively consistent.

Essentially, behavioral and emotional characteristics exhibited by children and adolescents in one particular setting may or may not be similar to these characteristics exhibited in other settings. In most cases there appears to be substantial variation in how behavioral and emotional problems are exhibited across settings. The exception to this general rule may be children and youth who exhibit *extremely* high rates and intensity of deviant behavior (Loeber & Dishion, 1984). In the case of such children, deviant behavioral and emotional characteristics may be a relatively stable trait.

Theoretically, variations in child behavior across settings may be caused by a combination of factors, such as the strength and stability of the trait in question, the specific eliciting and reinforcing properties of differing environments, and various types of response bias and rater/informant error variance. In reality it is probably not that important for clinicians to be concerned with which particular force is accounting for such variation. Thus "assessment of most children must take account of variance in the situations and informants on which assessment depends. This renders moot the theoretical question of whether children's behavioral and emotional problems are truly situation specific" (Achenbach et al. 1987, p. 227).

The practical implication of these notions is that it is important to conduct behavior assessments using rating scales across settings, and using multiple informants whenever possible. This type of assessment practice is likely to yield a composite picture that helps to overcome the limitations inherent in making judgments based on information provided by single raters in specific settings. Such an assessment design has been referred to as "multiaxial empircally based assessment" (McConaughy, 1993), and "multimethod, multisource, multisetting assessement" (Merrell, 1994a, 1994b, 1999). This type of broad assessment practice is preferred for many reasons. However, there are times when practical considerations make such an elaborate assessment design extremely difficult, if not impossible. In such cases, the use of a single behavior rating scale based on observations from only one setting might provide, with limitations, "a reasonable sample of what would be provided by other informants of the same type who see the child under generally similar conditions" (Achenbach et al., 1987, p. 227). More comments regarding the practical or clinical applications of behavior rating scales are presented in the concluding section of this chapter.

ISSUES REGARDING GROUP DIFFERENCES

An issue that has received surprisingly little attention among researchers and developers of behavior rating scales is group differences in and differential prediction of assessment scores. Much of what seems to have evolved in this area as standard practice in developing and using child behavior rating scales seems to have been extrapolated from research and practice with cognitive assessment (e.g., intelligence and achievement tests). For the most part, cognitive assessment instruments have been shown to yield consistent mean score differences between specific racial/ethnic groups, and also to be susceptible to assessment bias when used with some individuals from racial/ethnic minority groups (Reynolds & Kaiser, 1990). However, gender differences in performance on cognitive assessment instruments tend to be negligible when total scores or overall ability is considered, and generally are limited to specific domains, such as verbal ability and visual–spatial reasoning (Halpern, 1992). Age of the examinee or subject is also a variable that has been analyzed extensively. However, age as a group difference issue in behavior rating scales will not be dealt with extensively in this section. Rather, the focus will be more specifically on gender and race/ethnicity issues.

Because of the fairly consistent findings with regard to race/ethnicity and gender in cognitive assessment, it might seem logical to make the same set of assumptions for research-and-development efforts with behavior rating scales. Yet, group differences in behavior rating scale and other social-emotional assessment data may follow quite a different pattern than with cognitive assessment instruments, and some of the generalizations based on cognitive assessment findings may be misleading. This section provides a structured exploration of some of the relevant issues related to potential group differences and differential prediction with child behavior rating scales.

Group differences in mean scores on behavior rating scales are important to examine and evaluate. Another important concern relates to *differential prediction*. As defined in the *Standards for Educational and Psychological Testing* (1985) "differential prediction is a broad concept that includes the possibility that different prediction equations may be obtained for different demographic groups, for groups that differ in their prior experiences, or for groups that receive different treatments or are involved in different instructional programs" (1985, p. 12). Of course, just because different prediction equations with rating scale data may be found for various groups does not mean that the instruments are necessarily biased. For example, one might expect that students with behavioral and emotional disorders should receive behavior rating scale scores that differ significantly from typical students. But this issue is actually much more complicated than identification of significant mean score differences between various groups. As the *Standards* indicate, the larger issue involves the accuracy of predictive relationships:

> The accepted technical definition of predictive bias implies that no bias exists if the predictive relationship of two groups being compared can be adequately described by a common algorithm (e.g., regression line). In the simple regression analysis for selection using one predictor, selection bias is investigated by judging whether the regressions differ among identifiable groups in the population. If different regression slopes, intercepts, or standard errors of estimate are found among different groups, selection decisions will be biased when the same interpretation is made of a given score without regard to the group from which a person comes. Differing regression slopes or intercepts are taken to indicate that a test is differentially predictive for the groups at hand. (1985, pp. 12–13)

Gender

The issue of gender and behavior rating scale data provides a good example of how group differences should not necessarily be construed as evidence of bias, or as evidence of differential prediction patterns. Numerous behavioral and emotional disorders are known to exist at substantially different levels across gender lines. For example, according to the *Diagnostic and Statistical Manual of Mental Disorders* (DSM-IV; American Psychiatric Association, 1994) and various epidemiologic studies, the prevalence rate for attention-deficit/hyperactivity disorder (ADHD) and conduct disorder is significantly higher for males than for females. In contrast to these figures there are other disorders, such as depression and eating disorders, where the prevalence rates are clearly higher for females, particularly after the onset of adolescence. Therefore, behavior rating scales, unlike cognitive assessment instruments, should be expected to yield significantly different mean scores for samples of males and females, particularly when these scales include constructs that are known to have differing ratios across gender lines.

An examination of the technical manuals of some of the most popular child behavior rating scales currently in use provides some interesting corroborating evidence regarding the issue of gender differences. In general, most nationally standardized behavior rating scales designed to measure either problem behaviors or positive social skills evidence substantial differences in mean scores based on gender. The manual for the Conners Rating Scales—Revised (CRS-R; Conners, 1997) is one of the most thorough in terms of evaluation of gender differences. Because ADHD characteristics and covarying behavior problems (the main emphasis of the CRS-R) are known to be sensitive to changes across age span, the CRS-R rightly divides the standardization data into five different age groupings. But within each age level and across each subscale of the several instruments in the CRS-R system, significant mean score differences based on gender are apparent. The size of these differences varies, but mean score differences in the range of one-half to one standard deviation (SD) (or effect sizes of .50 to 1.00) are typical. Gender differences on child behavior rating scale scores are not limited to problem behavior scales. In the manual for the Social Skills Rating System (SSRS; Gresham & Elliott, 1990) the authors state, regarding social skills, "teachers, parents, and students consistently gave higher ratings to female students at almost every grade level from preschool through tenth grade" (p. 125). A careful inspection of the descriptive statistics provided in the SSRS manual reveals that standard mean score differences for social skills, based on gender, tend to range from one-third to one-half standard deviations (effect sizes of .30 to .50). Therefore, users of rating scales designed to measure problem behaviors or social skills might expect that, as a group, females will consistently receive more positive ratings than males.

Ethnicity

Unlike the area of cognitive assessment, where there has been substantial research, best-selling books and, at times, bitter controversy regarding racial/ethnic effects and issues, the area of social-emotional and behavioral assessment has seen relatively little activity. When only child behavior rating scales are considered the amount of activity is even more limited. Readers should understand that the comments in this section are focused exclusively on the use of child behavior rating scales, because there has indeed been criticism of the cross-ethnic validity of standardized social-emotional assessment procedures in general (e.g., Dana, 1995).

Because there is little theoretical basis upon which to build a priori predictions regarding racial/ethnic differences in rating scale results, and because this area generally lacks the controversial politically charged implications manifest in the cognitive assessment arena, researchers and instrument developers have had little reason to explore such differences. However, the yield of what little work there has been in this area indicates that race/ethnicity probably plays a very minor role in terms of group differences and differential prediction with child behavior rating scales. Based on previous examinations of this topic by this author (Merrell, 1999; Merrell & Gimpel, 1998), the covarying influence of socioeconomic status may account for most of the small racial/ethnic group differences that are found. In other words, if a large nationwide data set containing behavior rating scale scores of children and youth were analyzed carefully, some minimal effects for race and ethnicity might be found. But, if socioeconomic status (such as family income and/or parents' education level) were used as a covariate in the analysis, or if cases were matched by race/ethnicity and socioeconomic status using a randomized block design, then it is very likely that any score differences between groups would be negligible or insignificant.

Nonetheless, despite the apparent weak influence of race/ethnicity in behavior rating scale scores, there are a few interesting (and sometimes conflicting) pieces of evidence that are worth examining. First, it is possible that an individual's race/ethnicity may influence the way that she or he values particular child behaviors, if not actually influencing their objective ratings of behavior. For example, a study conducted by O'Reilly, Tokuno, and Ebata (1986) found significant differences in the way that European American and Asian American mothers ranked the relative importance of eight common social skills. Second, research conducted by V. R. Lethermon and colleagues (Lethermon et al., 1984; Lethermon, et al., 1986) found that child behavior ratings may be influenced by the amount of similarity between the rater and the subject of the rating. Although this research area does not appear to have been carried out by any other researchers, the findings by Lethermon and colleagues are interesting because they indicated that raters were more likely to positively evaluate the social behavior of children who were similar to them in terms of race/ethnicity, yet the most socially valid ratings appeared to be obtained from rater/ratee pairs who were *dissimilar* in race/ethnicity. This line of research raises some interesting questions regarding the effect of race/ethnicity on child behavior ratings provided by teachers in school settings, but there is simply not enough evidence to speculate further.

Of the child behavior rating scales currently in widespread use in public schools, some have been carefully analyzed to study the possibility of racial/ethnic effects in their normative samples. The results of such investigations generally support the notion that race/ethnicity tends to exert only a minor influence on scores. One of the earlier investigations in this regard was conducted by Achenbach and Edelbrock (1981), who analyzed parent ratings of social competence and problem behavior of 2,600 referred and nonreferred children, half of whom where Caucasian, and half of whom were African American. These cases were selected from the normative samples of the first published version of the Child Behavior Checklist. The authors found only minimal differences in problem behavior and social competence scores when race was used as an independent variable. These differences were even smaller, and almost negligible, when socioeconomic status of the parent raters was controlled in the analyses.

In the process of developing both the School Social Behavior Scales (Merrell, 1993) and the Preschool and Kindergarten Behavior Scales (Merrell, 1994b), I analyzed race/ethnicity of children and their parents as an independent variable, using a somewhat different methodologic strategy than was employed by Achenbach and Edelbrock (1981). Using the national norm samples for each measure (1,852 and 2,855, respectively) bivariate correlations were computed between SSBS and PKBS scores, and various race/ethnicity categories. Because the numbers of some ethnic minority participants in the normative samples were quite small and not randomly selected, specific minority group categories were combined and collapsed into larger categories in some instances. In all cases, the obtained coefficients were small (ranging from .08 to .15), with many resulting coefficients near zero. In these analyses, socioeconomic status was not used as a covariate because of limitations in how the data were coded. It should probably be assumed that the obtained range of coefficients was probably inflated in this regard.

The Conners Rating Scales—Revised (CRS-R; Conners, 1997), includes in the technical manual extensive evidence regarding race/ethnicity effects on parent and teacher ratings of child behavior. Using data collected from more than 8,000 cases across several forms within the CRS-R system, a series of analyses of covariance (ANCOVAs) were computed on the various scale and subscale scores, using race/ethnicity of children as an independent variable, with age level used as a covariate. Because the sample sizes for Caucasian and African American participants were so much larger than for other groups, random subsets of 125 cases from each these groups were generated for comparison with other groups. In most instances, the ANCOVA did not result in significant effects for race/ethnicity, or if it did, follow-up multiple comparison procedures often did not identify significant differences between particular groups. Of the instances where significant differences between groups were detected, there did not appear to be any consistent pattern to these differences. Further inspection of the means and standard deviations of CRS-R scores by racial/ethnic group, based on the tables presented in the technical manual, indicates that where the occasional statistically significant difference was found, these differences were, for the most part, minimally important in practical terms, often producing an effect size of less than .30. Aside from the lack of a clear trend among group differences, some more important issues regarding the few significant differences found based on race/ethnicity are that socioeconomic status was not controlled in the analyses, and that the size of some of the subgroups was particularly limited (e.g., as few as 25 Native Americans). Presumably, the use of socioeconomic status as a covariate or matching variable, coupled with sufficently large numbers of randomly selected cases for each group, would result in ever fewer (if any) significant differences between racial/ethnic groups. Unfortunately, such detailed analyses are seldom possible with standardization data sets for behavior rating scales, even with extremely large and exemplary standardization samples such as were gathered for the CRS-R. In sum, the available evidence with child behavior rating scales indicates that although race/ethnicity effects may exist, such effects tend to be unsystematic and not particularly strong.

Optimal Norm Sampling

The way in which instrument norm samples are gathered and analyzed may be one of the most important issues regarding whether significant group differences are found with rating scales scores. This issue particularly appears to be relevant for race/ethnicity and socioeconomic status, which are both much more difficult to stratify adequately than gender when developing instrument norms. Because gender is a dichotomous variable and numbers will be essentially equal no matter where a sample is obtained, instrument developers generally do not need to be concerned about obtaining adequate sampling by gender. Rather, the more important issues regarding gender tend to be whether the scale yields similar results for males and females, and whether or not separate norm groups are justified.

Although race/ethnicity generally produces much smaller effects than gender in terms of behavior rating scale scores, it is actually a more complicated matter when developing a rating scale normative sample. As has already been discussed, race/ethnic group effects on psychological or educational assessment instruments are often confounded by socioeconomic status. Because of this potential confound, it is desirable (but often quite difficult) to stratify norm samples by ethnicity and socioeconomic status. Short of this lofty ideal, another strategy is to use socioeconomic status as a covariate with race/ethnicity when analyzing rating scale data for racial/ethnic group effects.

Another race/ethnicity-based problem that tends to occur when developing normative samples is that members of American minority groups tend to be clustered geographically, which can easily cause over- or underrepresentation of specific subgroups, depending on where the instrument developer is able to obtain norm samples. For example, populations of Asian Americans tend to be highly concentrated in the west coast region, particularly in urban areas. Hispanics, the most rapidly growing ethnic minority group in the United States, are found in greater numbers in the southwest region, in the northeast, and in the extreme southeast (e.g., Florida). African Americans, currently the largest racial/ethnic minority group, tend to be particularly populous in the southern states, and in urban areas of the midwest and northeast. A large percentage of Native Americans live in rural reservation areas of the southwest and plains regions. Therefore, geographical representation may also be an important issue in the development of norm samples for behavior rating scales. Ideally, norm samples for behavior rating scales should include adequate representation of all U.S. geographical regions, as well as an appropriate sampling of urban, suburban, and rural locales. Such sampling representation may indirectly result in a more proportional distribution of the norm group based on race/ethnicity.

With regard to representation of students in rating scale norm samples based on race/ethnicity, the current most common practice is for instrument developers to compare group representation with that of the general U.S. population (assuming the instrument is developed in and for the United States), based on the most current data available from the Bureau of the Census. In some cases, instrument developers have attempted to stratify the racial/ethnic group representation of norm samples based on the census data, and in other cases, have simply attempted to approximate it as closely as is feasible. In fact, these conventions seem to have emerged as a supposed best practice. However, in reality, the assumptions behind such proportional representation do not certify or warrant that an instrument so developed is equally valid for all groups.

The issue of optimal ethnic representation in norm samples is actually much more complex than current common practices might suggest, as demonstrated by a quick analysis of U.S. racial/ethnic group membership data from the 1990 census (Bureau of the Census, 1990). For purposes of illustrating this point, assume that an instrument developer has created a new general-purpose problem behavior rating scale for use by teachers of students in grades K–6. Let's also assume that the scale developer has carefully created a norm sample of 1,500 cases that is designed to be exactly the same as the census data in terms of race/ethnicity percentages of student cases. Using the figures from the 1990 census, Table 9.3 shows how many cases of the 1,500 total would be members of the six primary categories for proportional representation.

Although almost no one would criticize a sample of 1,500 as being too small to be representative of the K–6 population, a quick look at the data in Table 9.3 reveals that for certain racial/ethnic groups, the actual numbers of cases yielded from using such a methodology are unsettling in certain cases. For example, are the 10 cases that would be yielded in the American Indian, Eskimo, or Aleut category sufficiently representative of all Native American children to warrant confidence in the use of the instrument with this group? Or, taking a closer look at the 42 hypothesized cases from the Asian or Pacific Islander category, would members of this group consider this level of representation to be sufficient to warrant confidence in using the instrument? What if 35 of these 42 Asian cases were gathered from ratings of students who are first-generation Cambodian and Laotian immigrants in one school in the State of Washington? Should one have confidence in the notion that such norm sampling should generalize adequately to Chinese American and Japanese American students from across the United States?

As can easily be seen through such an exercise, there are no easy answers to these questions, and the current accepted practices for group representation in norm samples can be neither vindicated nor vilified in the absence of more compelling evidence. However, an interesting study conducted by Fan, Wilson, and Kapes (1996) provides some possible clues on this issue. These researchers systematically examined the issue of whether or not an ethnic group's representation in test construction normative samples (with cognitive measures) would have an impact on the item selection process in such a way that systematic test bias would be built into the test. Using random sampling procedures to artificially create varying percentages of representation for each group, their findings indicated that there was no bias detected against any of the groups, even those with 0% representation in the test construction

TABLE 9.3   Representation of Six Race/Ethnicity Categories in a Hypothesized Behavior Rating Scale Norm Sample of 1,500 Cases, Based on Percentages from the 1990 U.S. Census

Race/ethnicity	Percentages from 1990 census	Proportional sample
White/Caucasian	75.6%	1,134
African American	11.8%	177
Hispanic	9.0%	135
American Indian, Eskimo, Aleut	0.7%	10
Asian or Pacific Islander	2.8%	42
Other	0.1%	2
Total	100%	1,500

sample, *as long as random sampling procedures were used*. It should be understood, of course, that these findings were not based on behavior rating scale data, and that they would only apply to instruments that had strong validity in the first place. However, they do indicate that the degree of racial/ethnic group proportionality in an instrument standardization sample may be less important than the overall validity of the instrument and the sampling procedures used to develop the norm group.

Evidence to date indicates that race/ethnicity tends to be a relatively weak variable, by itself, in influencing rating scale scores. In the absence of more compelling evidence to the contrary, users of behavior rating scales should proceed conservatively but with some confidence in using reliable and valid measures with children of diverse racial/ethnic background, so long as there is evidence of acceptable general sampling and stratification procedures in development of norm samples.

When Are Separate Norm Groups Justified?

Because behavior rating scales may produce differing results for groups of subjects, based on age and gender groups (and, to a lesser extent, racial/ethnic groups), test developers and users often struggle with the issue of using separate norm samples based on such divisions. It is common practice, for example, for behavior rating scales to include separate norm samples (and sometimes separate forms) for elementary- and secondary-age students. It is not uncommon for instruments to use separate norm samples for male and female students. However, there is no clear standard in this regard. The use of separate norm samples or score conversion tables based on demographic breakdowns of the normative sample should not necessarily be construed as the best practice, and the absence of such separate interpretive strategies should not necessarily be thought to reflect poor test development practices. Although we do lack a specific rigid standard in this regard, the necessity for using separate normative groups really depends on whether such practice maximizes the validity of the scale, and whether the lack of separate norms minimizes the validity of the scale for use with specific groups or for specific purposes.

The *Standards for Educational and Psychological Testing* provide some guidance on this issue without setting forth specific rules or conventions. For example, standard 4.3 states: "Norms that are presented should refer to clearly described groups. These groups should be the ones with whom users of the test will ordinarily wish to compare the people who are tested. Test publishers should also encourage the development of local norms by test users when the published norms are insufficient for particular test users" (p. 33). Furthermore, the comment regarding this standard provides some additional guidance: "Differentiated norms or summary information about differences between gender, ethnic, grade, or age groups, for example, may be useful. Users also need to be made alert to situations in which norms are less appropriate for one group than for another" (p. 33).

As the *Standards* rightly indicate, the necessity of reporting separate summary information or using separate norm groups based on group divisions depends on whether or not such practices are warranted by the evidence gathered during the instrument development process. As a practical matter, developers of behavior rating scales should address the issue within technical manuals and users guides, because most developmentally sensitive test users will be interested in issues regarding age, gender, and ethnicity. However, specific expectations for separate norm groups do not seem warranted at the present time, but should be driven by the evidence regarding the particular rating scale and normative sample.

To illustrate the complexities involved in using separate norm groups based on group divisions, even when large differences in mean scores are expected, it is interesting to examine the issue of gender in assessment of attention-deficit/hyperactivity disorder (ADHD). As has previously been demonstrated in this section, it is well known that large gender differences exist in the prevalence of ADHD, with males exhibiting the disorder at a substantially higher rate than females. In fact, the DSM-IV indicates that ADHD may exist in a 6:1 male/female ratio. Such clear evidence of gender differences in this construct would presumably result in significant group differences in mean scores in behavior rating scales designed to measure ADHD. Therefore, is this a clear case where separate norms are needed for male and female students? Not necessarily. The DSM-IV criteria for diagnosis of ADHD do not indicate that males and females should be evaluated according to differing standards. The practical impact of using separate norm groups for an ADHD rating scale is complex, and not necessarily beneficial to either gender group. Because it is known that males are substantially more likely to exhibit ADHD than females, comparing the rating scale scores of a boy to only those of other boys might lead to an increased chance of a false-negative error, and comparing the rating scale scores of a girl to only those scores of other girls might lead to an increased chance of a false-positive error. The exception to this potential problem would happen only if separate empirically derived clinical cutoff points had been developed for males and females, using specificity, sensitivity, and "hit rates" of various score configurations to derive optimal score levels associated with a diagnosis of ADHD. This practice essentially involves obtaining separate criterion-related validity data based on gender, which is a rather difficult challenge for instrument developers.

Recommendations

Given what is known regarding the potential influences of age, gender, race/ethnicity, and social class, developers of behavior rating scales and researchers who use these instruments should describe clearly their participant samples with as much detail as is reasonable. Where it appears to be theoretically important, appropriate demographic variables should be included as an independent variable in statistical analyses. For example, suppose that a researcher had developed a behavior rating scale designed specifically to assess ADHD and, in the process, developed an empirically based criterion for a "clinical range" cutoff score. In a situation such as this, it should be expected that the test developer would, at a minimum, report the percentages of males and females in the normative sample who met or exceeded this clinical criterion. Where it is feasible (where numbers of participants are large enough and sampling procedures are adequate to warrant confidence in generalization), researchers and test developers should also consider reporting supplementary norms, by specific subgroups, for comparison purposes.

Because group differences in rating scale scores do not singularly equate to differential prediction patterns, instrument developers and researchers should begin to aim for a higher standard in providing appropriate evidence in this domain. For example, normative samples gathered in the development of behavior rating scales could easily be analyzed by specific subgroups to provide evidence that the instrument performs similarly (or not) across groups. Internal consistency coefficients of scale and subscale scores might be considered a minimum requirement in this respect, and such evidence would go far toward helping consumers evaluate the validity of purported uses for the instrument with specific groups. If the total score internal consistency of a behavior rating scale yielded an alpha coefficient of .95 for the total sample, then it might be expected that alpha coefficients for specific subgroups within the sample should not deviate too far from this level. There is no absolute standard to follow in this regard, but common sense should dictate that, assuming there is a reasonable n for each subsample, differential prediction might be a possibility of the internal consistency for any one group that appears to be noticeably lower than for the total sample. Using the example of a .95 total sample coefficient, one might become legitimately concerned if the alpha coefficient for a specific racial/ethnic group deviated below, say, .80. If the numbers within subsample cells are sufficiently large, then it would also be helpful if test developers and researchers reported other forms of reliability, such as test–retest, and interrater, by specific subgroup, to provide evidence regarding whether the instrument performs similarly with persons of differing demographic background. These practices are consistent with recommendations from experts regarding the evidence needed to detect the presence or absence of test bias (e.g., Jensen, 1980; Reynolds & Kaiser, 1990; Witt, Elliott, Gresham, & Kramer, 1988).

Aside from reporting reliability evidence by demographic subgroups, there are other important types of evidence that would be useful in analyzing behavior rating scale scores for differential prediction patterns. Although criterion-related validity coefficients are unfortunately not often reported in behavior rating scale technical manuals, such information might be very helpful in not only helping to ascertain whether differential prediction patterns exist, but also whether purported validity claims are justified. For example, using our previous example of a behavior rating scale designed to assess ADHD, the test developer could calculate a Spearman point-biserial correlation coefficient between participants' rating scale scores and whether or not (in a yes/no manner) they independently had been found to have ADHD, based on standard diagnostic criteria. Although we would naturally assume that there should be significant gender differences in mean scores for such a scale, there is probably no a priori reason to believe that the instrument should yield differing validity coefficients based on gender. These examples are merely some basic suggestions. Many more effective ways of dealing with group differences and differential prediction with rating scale data are possible, most of which are well beyond the scope of this chapter. Essentially, the purpose of this section was to provoke thought and discussion among rating scale developers, researchers, and users regarding these important issues, and to begin to take the state of the art to a higher level.

CLINICAL APPLICATIONS

Although the primary purpose of this chapter is to discuss and analyze some current issues related to theory and research with child behavior rating scales, there are certainly some important clinical applications of these instruments that should be considered. Detailed discussion of the practical uses and clinical applications of child behavior rating scales is provided in other sources by this author (e.g., Merrell, 1999, 2000). Readers are referred to these sources for more information on this topic, as well as for reviews of some of the most widely used rating instruments. Rather than replication of the detailed specific information presented in these sources, this section includes a brief discussion of some of the general clinical applications of behavior rating scales that have emerged during the past three decades as rating scale technology has been refined.

Screening

Because of their relatively low cost in terms of professional time and training, and because of their generally strong psychometric properties, child behavior rating scales are a potentially excellent tool for use in screening. In school settings, screening activities of this nature would generally be for the purpose of identifying out of a larger population (such as a classroom, grade level, or entire school population) a smaller group of students who may have moderate to serious behavioral and emotional problems, and thus potentially benefit from additional assessment and intervention programming. Because the purpose of screening is to determine who is a "good suspicion" to meet the stated screening criteria (Kauffman, 1997), it is best initially to use fairly liberal screening criteria.

During the screening process, *false-positive* errors (identifying a student who really does not have significant behavioral or emotional problems) should not be a major concern, because these students can easily be eliminated from the screening pool later on in the process. Rather, avoiding *false-negative* errors (failing to identify a student who truly does have significant problems) should be a more important consideration. The way to minimize false-negative errors when screening with behavior rating scales is to set the initial screening criterion fairly loose. I (Merrell, 1994, 1999) have previously suggested that a criterion of one standard deviation above the normative group in terms of problem behavior scores (or 1 SD below the normative group mean in terms of social skills scores) is a reasonable standard for screening with behavior rating scales. This criterion will result in some false-positive errors that can be corrected easily later in the process, but it should produce few, if any, false-negative errors, depending on the size and other characteristics of the screening group.

More sophisticated uses of behavior ratings in screening processes are also possible, particularly when they are used in conjunction with other assessment methods in a standardized or systematic screening procedure. The Systematic Screening for Behavior Disorders (SSBD; Walker & Severson, 1992) and the Early Screening Project (ESP; Walker, Severson, & Feil, 1995) are perhaps the most exemplary multimethod behavioral screening tools currently in use. These systems, which are both bolstered by extensive empirical support, utilize behavior rating scales early in the screening process. After an initial population of "at-risk" students are identified through low-cost means such as rating scales, the size of the population is systematically reduced through the use of more time-intensive assessment methods such as direct behavioral observation. Each step in the screening process constitutes a "gate" that can only be passed through if specific behavioral criterion are met. At the end of the multiple gating process, a small population of students remain in the pool. These students should be those who are truly at-risk for developing serious conduct and emotional problems.

Diagnosis/Classification

Behavior rating scales, like any other assessment method, should never be used as the sole basis for making a diagnostic or classification decision. However, if used correctly, they may be helpful for this purpose. The most widely used diagnosis or classification systems likely to be used by school, pediatric, and clinical child psychologists are the DSM-IV (American Psychiatric Association, 1994) and for school psychologists, federal and state special education eligibility category systems. Although the two types of systems have little in common, they both share the primary characteristic of requiring yes/no judgments for the presence or absence of characteristics of particular disorders or disability conditions (Achenbach et al, 1987). Because the vast majority of rating scales used today have abandoned the older checklist (yes/no) format in favor of a more sophisticated rating format that may include as many as five rating points, a simple yes/ no decision is not always possible. Therefore, best practice for using rating scales should dictate that for diagnostic decisions, rating scales from multiple informants should be obtained, and consistency across settings should be indicated for key behaviors of concern if they are to be judged as present. For example, behaviors such as stealing, fighting, and coercing others to get what one wants are all key characteristics of conduct disorder. These specific behavioral problems are commonly listed as individual items on most broad-spectrum problem behavior rating scales, such as the Behavior Assessment System for Children, Child Behavior Checklist/Teacher's Report Form, and School Social Behavior Scales. If more than one rater across more than one setting indicates that one of these behaviors occurs "sometimes," "often," or "frequently," then an analysis of individual items may provide strong confidence that the specific yes/no criterion in question has been met.

In contrast to the relatively straightforward practice of examining individual items on rating scales, examiners should use great caution when interpreting subscale or factor scores that bear the name of specific disorders. It is not uncommon for broad-spectrum problem behavior rating scales to include a subscale labeled "attention problems," "hyperactivity," or some combination of the two terms. However, an elevated score on one of these scales should not necessarily be construed as indicative of the presence of attention-deficit/hyperactivity disorder. Because subscales or factors on rating scales are arbitrarily named by instrument developers, and because some of the items within a particular subscale are likely to bear little overt similarity to the characteristics of a particular similarly titled disorder, such scales should be used cautiously, primarily as a means of generating hypotheses. Diagnostic or classification criteria should be clearly indicated by the presence of specific evidence before such criteria are assumed to be met.

Treatment Selection/Intervention Planning

An obvious and relatively straightforward clinical application of child behavior rating scales is to use them for treatment selection or intervention planning. One example of this type of use is to carefully analyze rating scales completed on the same student across settings, to determine in which settings specific problems are exhibited (McMahon, 1984). Because child behavior problems are situation specific in many cases, the particular settings in which they are exhibited can be targeted for additional functional analysis, hypothesis generation, and intervention.

Another example of using behavior rating scales in treatment selection or intervention planning is to match the intervention to a specific set of problems (Peacock Hill Working Group, 1991). A simple way to link rating scale data to intervention in this manner is to review carefully the completed rating scales and make a list of the items or clusters of items that are rated as the most significant concerns. If any of these items are rated as consistently problematic across raters and settings, then they should be targeted in the intervention. After a narrowed list of key behaviors has been identified and targeted, specific intervention techniques that precisely match those behaviors can be selected. This method of treatment selection is similar to the *Keystone Behavior Strategy*, which has been touted as a promising way to effectively link assessment data to intervention planning (Nelson & Hayes, 1986; Shapiro, 1996).

Admittedly, there is actually very little empirical evidence to support specific techniques for using behavior rating scales for treatment selection/intervention planning. The suggestions offered in this section, as well as many other practical suggestions that have been offered in other sources (e.g., Merrell, 1999, 2000) tend to be based more on theory and common sense than on specific empirical findings. This void in supporting evidence is an important area to be targeted by future research efforts.

Progress Monitoring and Outcome Evaluation

Successful implementation of interventions for behavioral problems may be enhanced greatly by continuous assessment and monitoring of student progress following the initial assessment and during treatment (Kerr & Nelson, 1989). Progress toward behavioral intervention goals may be monitored with behavior rating scales by obtaining weekly or biweekly ratings, and this type of continuous measurement may be useful in modifying the intervention if it proves to be less effective than desired (Merrell & Gimpel, 1998). However, full-length rating scale measures (many of which contain over 100 items) may be too long and time consuming for frequent and repeated use in school settings. In these situations, one might select a few critical items from the rating scales that were targeted for intervention following the initial assessment, and use the resulting short scale as a brief informal measure of intervention progress. An additional set of behavior rating scales completed *following* the intervention may also be useful. Such follow-up assessment is primarily conducted to determine how well treatment effects have been maintained over time (e.g., after 3 months), and how well the behavioral changes have generalized to other settings (e.g., other classrooms). Information gathered from a follow-up assessment using cross-informant behavior rating scales may help to determine whether or not additional interventions or "booster sessions" are needed.

CONCLUSIONS

Behavior rating scales, which only three decades ago were seldom used in school settings and were plagued by concerns regarding technical issues, have become a behavioral assessment staple among practitioners and researchers alike. Significant advances in research and the development of new instruments and analysis technologies have enhanced tremendously the acceptance of rating scales.

Despite these relatively recent gains and advances, there are still several areas of concern. Although research such as the influential meta-analysis conducted by Achenbach and colleagues (1987) has bettered our understanding of the problems of modest cross-informant correlations, and helped to separate the issues of association and reliability, much work remains to be done in order for the field to fully understand associations among raters and various forms of error variance with rating scales.

An area that is even more vague in terms of our understanding of its implications for behavioral assessment is group differences in rating scale scores. Many of the assumptions developed from group differences research on cognitive assessment simply do not appear to generalize well to behavior rating scale assessment. Although gender may exhibit a substantial impact on average group scores, it is not clear that such differences signify a pattern of differential prediction for rating scale scores of boys and girls. Aside from gender issues in group differences, even less is clearly known regarding the influences of ethnicity and socioeconomic status, which, although apparently smaller than gender differences, may potentially impact interpretation of rating scale scores. Instrument developers, researchers, and practitioners should all aim for a higher standard in development and use of child behavior rating scales and, perhaps more importantly, should not hold to assumptions about best practices in scale development that are not truly warranted and supported by strong evidence.

Although there is not a great deal of current empirical support for some clinical applications of behavior rating scales, there seems to be a very strong potential in this area. Screening, diagnosis/classification, treatment selection/intervention planning, and progress monitoring/outcome evaluation all appear to be appropriate clinical uses. However, these uses certainly need to be more clearly articulated and validated through future research and practical efforts.

The future of using behavior rating scales for assessing child and adolescent behavior in school settings seems to be assured for the next several decades. Such assurance should not provide a "rationale" for keeping the field static. New effort is required to enhance the application of behavior rating scales for specific purposes and with specific populations.

References

Achenbach, T. M., & Edelbrock, C. S. (1981). Behavioral problems and competencies reported by parents of normal and disturbed children aged four through sixteen. *Monographs of the Society for Research in Child Development, 46*(1 Serial, No. 88).

Achenbach, T. M., McConaughy, S. H., & Howell, C. T. (1987). Child/adolescent behavioral and emotional problems: Implications of cross-informant correlations for situational specificity. *Psychological Bulletin, 101,* 213–232.

Alberto, P. A., & Troutman, A. C. (1996). *Applied behavior analysis for teachers* (4th ed.). Columbus, OH: Merrill.

American Psychiatric Association. (1994). *Diagnostic and statistical manual of mental disorders* (4th ed.) (DSM-IV). Washington, DC: Author.

Conners, C. K. (1997). *Conners Rating Scales—Revised*. North Tonowanda, NY: Multi-Health Systems.

Dana, R. H. (1995). Impact of the use of standard psychological assessment on the assessment and treatment of ethnic minorities. In J. F. Aponte, R. Y. Rivers, & J. Wohl (Eds.), *Psychological interventions and cultural diversity* (pp. 57–72). Boston: Allyn & Bacon.

Elliott, S. N., Busse, R. T., & Gresham, F. M. (1993). Behavior rating scales: Issues of use and development. *School Psychology Review, 22,* 313–321.

Fan, X., Wilson, V. L., & Kapes, J. T. (1996). Ethnic group representation in test construction samples and test bias: The standardization fallacy revisited. *Educational and Psychological Measurement, 56,* 365–381.

Fergusson, D. M., & Horwood, L. J. (1986). The trait and method components of ratings of conduct disorder: Part I. Maternal and teacher evaluations of conduct disorder in young children. *Journal of Child Psychology and Psychiatry, 28,* 249–260.

Gresham, F. M., & Elliott, S. N. (1990). *Social Skills Rating System*. Circle Pines, MN: American Guidance Service.

Halpern, D. F. (1992). *Sex differences in cognitive abilities* (2nd ed.). Hillsdale, NJ: Erlbaum.

Jensen, A. R. (1980). *Bias in mental testing*. New York: Free Press.

Kauffman, J. M. (1997). *Characteristics of behavior disorders of children and youth* (6th ed.). Upper Saddle River, NJ: Prentice-Hall.

Kazdin, A. E. (1979). Situational specificity: The two-edged sword of behavioral assessment. *Behavioral Assessment, 1,* 57–55.

Kazdin, A. E. (1981). Behavioral observation. In M. Hersen & A. S. Bellack (Eds.), *Behavioral assessment: A practical handbook* (pp. 101–124). New York: Pergamon Press.

Kazdin, A. E. (1982). *Single-case research designs: Methods for clinical and applied settings*. New York: Oxford University Press.

Kerr, M. M., & Nelson, C. M. (1989). *Strategies for managing behavior problems in the classroom* (2nd ed.). Columbus, OH: Merrill.

Lethermon, V. R., Williamson, D. A., Moody, S. C., Granberry, S. W., Lenauer, K. L., & Bodiford, C. B. (1984). Factors affecting the social validity of a role-play test of children's social skills. *Journal of Behavioral Assessment, 6,* 231–245.

Lethermon, V. R., Williamson, D. A., Moody, S. C., & Wozniak, P. (1986). Racial bias in behavioral assessment of children's social skills. *Journal of Psychopathology and Behavioral Assessment, 8,* 329–337.

Loeber, R., & Dishion, T. J. (1984). Boys who fight at home and school: Family conditions influencing cross-setting consistency. *Journal of Consulting and Clinical Psychology, 52,* 759–768.

Martin, R. P., Hooper, S., & Snow, J. (1986). Behavior rating scale approaches to personality assessment in children and adolescents. In H. Knoff (Ed.), *The assessment of child and adolescent personality* (pp. 309–351). New York: Guilford Press.

McConaughy, S. H. (1993). Advances in empirically based assessment of children's behavioral and emotional problems. *School Psychology Review, 22,* 285–307.

McMahon, R. J. (1984). Behavior checklists and rating scales. In T. H. Ollendick & M. Hersen (Eds.), *Child behavior assessment; Principles and practices* (pp. 80–105). New York: Pergamon Press.

Merrell, K. W. (1993). *School Social Behavior Scales.* Austin, TX: Pro-Ed.

Merrell, K. W. (1994a). *Assessment of behavioral, social, and emotional problems: Direct and objective methods for use with children and adolescents.* White Plains, NY: Longman.

Merrell, K. W. (1994b). *Preschool and Kindergarten Behavior Scales.* Austin, TX: Pro-Ed.

Merrell, K. W. (1999). *Behavioral, social, and emotional assessment of children and adolescents.* Mahwah, NJ: Erlbaum.

Merrell, K. W. (2000). Using child behavior rating scales in school settings· Considerations, tools, and best practices for effective assessment. In E. S. Shapiro & T. R. Kratochwill (Eds.), *Conducting school-based assessments of child and adolescent behavior.* New York: Guilford Press.

Merrell, K. W., & Caldarella, P. (1999). Social-behavioral assessment of at-risk early adolescent students: Psychometric characteristics and validity of a parent report form of the School Social Behavior Scales. *Journal of Psychoeducational Assessment, 17,* 36–49.

Merrell, K. W., & Gimpel, G. A. (1998). *Social skills of children and adolescents· Conceptualization, assessment, treatment.* Mahwah, NJ: Erlbaum.

Nelson, R. O., & Hayes, S. C. (Eds.) (1986). *Conceptual foundations of behavioral assessment.* New York: Guilford Press.

O'Reilly, J. P., Tokuno, K. A., & Ebata, A. T. (1986). Cultural differences between Americans of Japanese and European ancestry in parental valuing of social competence. *Journal of Comparative Family Studies, 17,* 87–97.

Peacock Hill Working Group (1991). Problems and promised in special education and related services for children and youth with emotional or behavioral disorders. *Behavioral Disorders, 16,* 299 313.

Reid, J. B. (1982). Observer training in naturalistic research. In D. P. Hartmann (Ed.), *Using observers to study behavior* (pp. 37–50). San Francisco: Jossey-Bass.

Reynolds, C. R., & Kaiser, S. M. (1990). Bias in assessment of aptitude. In C. R. Reynolds & R. W. Kamphaus (Eds.), *Handbook of psychological and educational assessment of children: Intelligence and achievement* (pp. 611–653). New York: Guilford Press.

Robbins, R., & Merrell, K. W. (in press). *Cross informant comparisons of the Home and Community Social Behavior Scales and the School Social Behavior Scales.* Diagnostique submitted for publication.

Saal, F. E., Downey, R. G., & Lahey, M. A. (1980). Rating the ratings: Assessing the psychometric quality of rating data. *Psychological Bulletin, 88,* 413–428.

Shapiro, E. S. (1996). *Academic skills problems: Direct assessment and intervention* (2nd ed.). New York: Guilford Press.

Standards for educational and psychological testing (1985). Washington, DC: American Psychological Association.

Stokes, T. F., Baer, D. M., & Jackson, R. L. (1974). Programming among the generalization of a greeting response in four retarded children. *Journal of Applied Behavior Analysis, 7,* 599–610.

U.S. Bureau of the Census. (1990). *Dicenniel Census of the United States*. Washington, DC: U.S. Government Printing Office.

Verhulst, F. C., & Akkerhuis, G. W. (1989). Agreement between parents' and teachers' ratings of behavioral/emotional problems of children aged 4–12. *Journal of Child Psychology and Psychiatry, 30*, 123–136.

Wahler, R. G. (1975). Some structural aspects of deviant child behavior. *Journal of Applied Behavior Analysis, 8*, 27–42.

Walker, H. M., & Severson, H. (1992). *Systematic Screening for Behavior Disorders* (2nd ed.). Longmont, CO: Sopris West.

Walker, H. M., Severson, H., & Feil, E. G. (1995). *The Early Screening Project: A proven child find process*. Longmont, CO: Sopris West.

Wilson, M. S., & Reschly, D. J. (1996). Assessment in school psychology training and practice. *School Psychology Review, 25*, 9–23.

Witt, J. C., Elliott, S. N., Gresham, F. M., & Kramer, J. J. (1988). *Assessment of special children*. Boston: Scott Foresman.

CHAPTER 10

Informant Reports

Conceptual and Research Bases of Interviews with Parents and Teachers

BARBARA RYBSKI BEAVER
R. T. BUSSE
University of Wisconsin–Whitewater

When evaluating children and adolescents the need for information from other sources is unquestionable. As a practical concern, children often are unable, or unwilling, to report their own behaviors and symptoms; therefore it is necessary to seek information from other sources — most often parents or parent surrogates and teachers. This does not mean, however, that informant reports may take the place of child assessment. Self-report and informant reports are not interchangeable in assessing children's behavior problems. Lack of agreement between children, parents, and other informants often is observed, with agreement varying with the behaviors or disorder being assessed (e.g., Achenbach, McConaughy, & Howell, 1987; Hodges, Gorden, & Lennon, 1990). Informant reports should not be taken as a standard against which to compare child reports; rather, they contribute essential information to the assessment process.

The essential nature of informant reports is underscored by the recognition that children do not exist in isolation from their environments. Rather, many interconnections exist among the various systems in the child's life. Ecological-systems theories address systemic influences (home, school, other) and as such, view the child's "problems" as a function of the interaction of the child (such as internal factors) with the different systems of which he or she is a part. Because the different systems are seen as interconnected, change in one system is associated with change in other systems. Therefore, an assessment process that considers only the school environment would be viewed as incomplete and less likely to lead to a successful intervention plan.

Obtaining information from a range of informants allows the psychologist to be aware of the child's difficulties and strengths in different systems as well as the interrelationships among various individuals and environments in the child's life (Apter, 1982). Although little specific information has been provided regarding how to utilize an ecological-systems approach in interviewing, the theoretical model may be integrated with other therapeutic approaches, such as behavioral models (e.g., Gutkin & Curtis, 1999; Sheridan, 1997). Additional questions remain regarding how to combine data derived from different sources of information and the explicit methods used to obtain that information.

Informant reports may be obtained through a variety of methods. One of the most common and economical methods is through the use of behavior rating scales and checklists completed by parents and/or teachers. As discussed by Edelbrock (1988), these measures have several advantages, including ease of administration and the ability to provide a great deal of information quickly with minimal need for the professional's involvement. A major drawback to these measures is that it may not always be certain how the informant interpreted various items or responses (e.g., seldom, often). Similarly, the psychologist or evaluator may be unable to interpret some of the responses or obtain additional information relevant to the specific case. These limitations can be readily addressed by the use of informant interviews. Interviews allow the psychologist to assess behaviors of concern while obtaining information about the individual child that can be relevant to intervention planning.

In this chapter we briefly explore the historical and theoretical premises of interviewing parents and teachers, followed by an overview of interview methods and formats. We then turn to an analysis of the current state of research on behavioral interviews, and suggestions for future directions toward advancing knowledge and use of behavioral interviews. As the title of the chapter and this overview imply, we are examining concepts and research regarding interviews with parents and teachers rather than providing information on specific interviewing skills. The interested reader is directed to the companion to this volume (Shapiro & Kratochwill, in press), and other useful works that provide practical information on interviewing skills and techniques (e.g., Ivey, 1994; Kratochwill & Bergan, 1990; Lentz & Wehmann, 1995; Sattler, 1998; Sheridan, Kratochwill, & Bergan, 1996).

HISTORICAL AND THEORETICAL ISSUES

Historically, many interviewers were influenced by psychodynamic models, typically resulting in an open-ended, free-flowing type of interview style. In other cases, interviews were more structured and goal-oriented with a focus on diagnostic assessment. In the 1960s, interviewers often were influenced by Rogers' nondirective style and emphasis on developing an optimal therapeutic relationship (Groth-Marnat, 1997). At that time child assessment was usually conducted via parent interviews. In the 1970s, however, there was an increase in child involvement in the assessment process as well as greater interest in more structured interviews for both adults and children. This interest was largely attributable to the plethora of criticisms toward the less structured, more dynamically oriented interviews that were seen as possessing questionable reliability and validity, and lacking in cost-effectiveness.

Behavioral theories and strategies changed the focus of the interviews from a concern with history and diagnosis to a more objective assessment of behaviors. Kanfer and Grimm (1977) described the necessary interview components as being assessments of behavioral excesses and deficiencies, inappropriate stimulus control in the environment or individual, and examination of contingencies for positive reinforcement. Although these trends continued into the 1980s, there was a concomitant increased emphasis on developing measures to be consistent with the *Diagnostic and Statistical Manual of Mental Disorders* system (DSM-III-R; American Psychiatric Association, 1987). At the end of the 1990s, an emphasis on more brief interventions increased the need for interview methods that would allow for thorough, accurate, but also concise assessment of client needs (Groth-Marnat, 1997). This is no less true in school settings, where school psychologists must respond to the needs of an increasingly diverse student population.

As seen above, interview formats tend to be related to the theoretical model or approach of the interviewer. Interviewers who subscribe to a person-centered model will tend to utilize more open-ended and nondirective interview formats consistent with the belief that the individual and relationship are the best sources of information and change. In contrast, behaviorally oriented interviewers who conceptualize problems in terms of specific behavioral and environmental factors are likely to use more structured interviews intended to gain information about specific behaviors and maintaining variables. In addition to theoretical influences, interview formats also are related to the goal or intent of the interview. When a formal diagnosis is required, a structured, diagnostic format is likely to be the best fit; however, in many cases a clinical diagnosis may be neither desirable nor appropriate. Instead, the focus may be on developing intervention plans to address behavioral problems such as those observed in the classroom. In this situation a different interview format may be more effective, such as a structured behavioral interview. Interviewers also may utilize a combination of interview methods which vary in format and style. Researchers have found that most interviewers tend to utilize a combination of more traditional and behavior assessment methods (Haynes & Uchigakuichi, 1993; Piotrowski & Keller, 1984). We will discuss interviews in terms of the level of information the interview is designed to obtain: omnibus, behavior specific, and problem-solving levels of content (Busse & Beaver, in press), and in terms of the type of format: unstructured, structured, or semi-structured.

INTERVIEW FORMATS

Omnibus formats are designed for gathering a wide range of information. The "traditional" clinical interview typically utilized an omnibus format in that it obtained a wide range of information about a patient's symptom history, such as current functioning, family and social relationships, mental status, and vocational/educational history. The main advantage of an omnibus format is that the interviewer can gather information on a variety of issues and behaviors to aid in diagnostic evaluations and intervention planning. Relatedly, their greatest disadvantage is the amount of time such a comprehensive interview can take to administer.

Behavior-specific interviews are more narrow in scope and focus on the assessment of a limited number of specific problem areas. A behavior-specific format is useful when the presenting problem has been generally identified and the goal is to obtain a more detailed assessment of specific behaviors. The advantage of this format lies in its efficiency for obtaining specific information with regard to a behavior of concern. The disadvantage is apparent in cases where the initial referral issue was incorrect or only a portion of the problem was identified, which necessitates that the interviewer change to a different format or behavior focus.

Problem-solving interviews focus on presenting concerns with the goal of developing an intervention plan. Problem-solving interviews differ from the behavior-specific interviews in that they have a more exploratory focus and involve defining the problem situation rather than narrowly assessing specific behaviors. Interviewers are likely to include behavior-specific interviewing as a component of a problem-solving interview (Busse & Beaver, 2000). Depending upon interviewer needs, these levels of content may be present in different types of interview formats. For example, a "problem-solving" interview in which the interviewer focuses specifically on a presenting problem and potential intervention strategies may be conducted in a very structured, almost scripted format, or may be done in a more free-flowing unstructured style. As explained below, there are advantages and disadvantages to each approach.

Unstructured Interviews

Unstructured interviews, such as the "traditional" clinical interview, vary greatly in content, but generally are at the omnibus level. Typically, they will focus on historical information, providing developmental information about the child, history of the problem behaviors, and family background. Academic and social issues relevant to the problem also are likely to be addressed. Although this format provides great flexibility to the interviewer, it tends to lack standardization, which leaves this type of interview vulnerable to concerns about the reliability and validity of information gathered in this manner (Edelbrock & Costello, 1990). One of the greatest concerns here is the possibility of interviewer bias, including halo effects and confirmatory bias. Additionally, specific behavioral information needed to define problem behaviors and plan an intervention may not be gathered. It also can be difficult to compare information obtained from unstructured interviews with different informants or interviewers, because very different content areas may have been addressed. Because of these concerns, several standardized interviews for use with children and their parents have been developed. These interviews often focus on diagnostic criteria with the goal of reaching a diagnosis consistent with the DSM system.

Structured Interviews

Structured interviews provide a standardized method for asking questions and following-up on informant responses. Several structured interviews for use with children, adolescents, and parents have been developed for research and, more recently, for clinical use (Kamphaus & Frick, 1996). Structured interviews have the advantage of increased reliability through the use of clear and standardized formats for the interview and explicit guidelines for scoring the information that is obtained. Structured interviews typically are updated to stay consistent with current diagnostic criteria and research. Many of the available structured diagnostic interviews assess for disruptive behavior disorders, affective disorders, and anxiety disorders in children and adolescents. Depending upon the specific measures, assessment of schizophrenia, eating disorders, or substance use may also be possible. Several of the standardized structured interviews utilize an omnibus format. As noted by Hodges (1993), allowing the psychologist to assess for more than one diagnosis is a great advantage of structured interviews, given the high comorbidity rates observed in most childhood disorders. Major structured interview schedules that include parent formats are the Diagnostic Interview for Children and Adolescents—Revised (DICA-R; Reich, 1996), the NIMH Diagnostic Interview Schedule for Children (DISC-2.3; Shaffer et al., 1996) and the Child Assessment Schedule (CAS; Hodges, 1997). Although these interviews were developed for use with children and adolescents, parallel parent formats are used to provide additional assessment information. The interviews typically take 60–90 minutes to complete, with interviews with parents of more symptomatic children requiring longer time periods because of the need to ask more follow-up questions. In addition to parent versions, the DISC-2.3 has an available experimental teacher version (Frick, Silverthorn, & Evans, 1994).

The NIMH Diagnostic Interview Schedule for Children was developed for use in large-scale epidemiological studies and has undergone several revisions. It is a highly structured measure originally intended for use by lay interviewers to make diagnoses consistent with the DSM system. Its authors suggested it may be useful in clinical research and service settings where availability of a qualified clinician for assessments is limited (Shaffer et al., 1996). The parent version is used for parents or knowledgeable caregivers of children between the ages of 6 and 17 years. One of the unique aspects of the DISC is that, in addition to examining symptoms for diagnostic classification, it also assesses age of onset and level of impairment. Responses to DISC questions typically consist of "yes," "no," and "sometimes" or "somewhat," although a few open-ended questions are also included. Computerized versions also have been developed (see Shafer et al., 1996). Test–retest reliabilities of impairment are acceptable (kappa greater than or equal to .4) for all diagnoses but social phobia and avoidant disorder (Shaffer et al., 1996). Test–retest reliabilities of the symptoms and criterion scales were also reported to be good to excellent for the parent scales, and generally good for the child versions. Reports of concurrent validity vary depending on the specific diagnosis. In general, agreement is good for the externalizing disorders (ADHD and conduct disorder kappas > .70) and fair to good levels of agreement for composite internalizing categories (Schwab-Stone et al., 1996). The dysthymic disorder and anxiety disorders categories may require additional revision because of relatively lower levels of reliability and validity. Acceptable reliability has been reported for French (Breton et al., 1998) and Spanish (Ribera et al., 1996) versions of the DISC.

In addition to the general diagnostic interviews, behavior-specific or disorder-specific measures also have been developed. For example, adaptive and maladaptive behaviors may be assessed via the Scales of Independent Behavior—Revised (SIB-R; Bruininks, Woodcock, Weatherman, & Hill, 1996). A particular advantage of the SIB-R is the inclusion of an Individual Plan Recommendation form that is used to plan and track the person's needs for support and services. As such, this interview may be easily related to intervention planning and evaluation. The strength of the various structured interview measures lies in their ability to obtain information relevant to making a diagnostic assessment; however, in their emphasis on categorization a true behavioral assessment may not be obtained, thereby limiting the information usable for intervention planning.

In general, structured interviews may not be a desirable way to begin an assessment process with parents or teachers. The structured format is unlikely to facilitate rapport with parents or teachers and may frustrate parents who have difficulty fitting the complexity of their child's behavior into the confines of the interview questions (Kamphaus & Frick, 1996). An alternative interview format that provides more options to the interviewer and informant, greater opportunities to obtain detailed information about the problem behaviors, and is not limited by categorization needs is the semistructured interview.

Semistructured Interviews

This format maximizes the benefits while minimizing the weaknesses of the other two formats. Semistructured interviews allow for greater flexibility for the interviewer than more structured formats. At the same time, they have stronger psychometric properties than unstructured interviews. A semistructured interview typically provides the interviewer with a framework and specific questions while allowing for more variability in follow-up. At the diagnosis-specific level is the Autism Diagnostic Interview—Revised (ADI-R; Lord, Rutter, & Le Couteur, 1994), a semistructured interview for caregivers of children or adults who may have a pervasive developmental disorder. Through the ADI-R the interviewer obtains information on the child's history and behavioral profile. In addition, through the application of strict scoring procedures and diagnostic algorithms, interviewers may make a DSM-IV or ICD-10 diagnosis. Research findings indicate that the ADI-R is a valid and reliable instrument for diagnosing autistic disorder in young children. Kappa coefficients for interrater reliability range from .62 to .89. Actual percent agreement for the items was over 90% with the range of the kappas restricted because of low frequency of some items. Validity evidence also is positive with the diagnostic algorithms with significant differences obtained for the scores of children with autistic disorder and those with nonautistic cognitive or language impairments (Lord et al., 1994). It should be noted that the research described above was conducted with preschool-age children; more research with older children and adults is needed to establish the reliability and validity of the measure with a broader population.

A behaviorally based example of a semistructured interview is the Vineland Adaptive Behavior Scales (Sparrow, Balla, & Cicchetti, 1984). The Vineland Scales are one of the most widely used measures of adaptive behavior. The current version is a revision and expansion of the Vineland Social Maturity Scale. The Vineland Scales Interview Edition has both Expanded (577 items) and Survey (297 items) forms that allow for assessment of several domains of personal and social skills. Additionally, there is a Classroom Edition, which consists of a questionnaire that is independently completed by the teacher to obtain information about adaptive behavior in the classroom. In general, the Vineland Scales have shown good evidence of reliability with median composite scores split-half reliability coefficients ranging from .83 to .94 for the Survey Form on the behavioral Domains (Sparrow et al., 1984). Median internal consistency coefficient alphas for the Classroom Edition range from .80 to .95 for the Domains (Sparrow, Balla, & Cicchetti, 1985). Validity studies also have shown correlations between the Vineland Scales and other measures of adaptive behavior, such as the AAMD Adaptive Behavior Scale, to be in the moderate to moderately high range (Sparrow et al., 1984).

The Vineland Scales have been found to be useful in school settings in that they provide a systematic assessment of nonacademic skill deficits that may then be translated into educational objectives (Harrison, 1984). One disadvantage of the Vineland Scales is the length of the measure, particularly if one uses the Expanded Interview and/or the companion 244-item Classroom Edition, which is significantly longer than many teacher rating scales. Other concerns include using the scales to evaluate infants and toddlers for eligibility for special services. Raggio and Massingale (1990) reported that in children between birth and 2 years the overall adaptive functioning scores on the Survey Form of the scales are significantly higher than those obtained with the original Vineland scales, thereby resulting in the exclusion of some children from services. In a second study to examine the scores of infants being evaluated for developmental delay, the correlation between the current Vineland Survey Form and the original Vineland Social Maturity Scale was reported at .39. Vineland Survey Form scores also were found to be significantly higher than scores on the Bayley Mental Development Index ($r = .59$), whereas no significant difference was obtained between scores on the Bayley Index and the Vineland Social Maturity Scale (Raggio & Massingale, 1993).

Other omnibus level semistructured interviews have been developed to assist in psychiatric diagnosis. The Schedule for Affective Disorders and Schizophrenia for School-Age Children is available in a number of current versions that may be regarded as semistructured, omnibus level interviews. These interviews are intended to be used by experienced clinicians familiar with DSM diagnostic criteria. (For comparison of the different K-SADS versions, see Kaufman et al., 1997.) We will focus on the Kiddie-SADS—Present and Lifetime Version (K-SADS-PL; Kaufman et al., 1997), which was developed from the Present Episode version of the K-SADS (Chambers et al., 1985) to address several limitations of previous versions of the K-SADS. The K-SADS-PL is designed to assess both current and past episodes of psychopathology in children and adolescents with regard to both DSM-III-R and DSM-IV criteria. Unlike the DISC, as a semistructured interview the probes for the K-SADS are not intended to be recited verbatim. In addition to symptom assessment, the K-SADS-PL allows for diagnostic-specific impairment ratings. Diagnoses are typically reached by integrating parent and child data, usually giving greater weight to the parent information, although this is an issue of clinical judgment. Reliability and validity data for the K-SADS-PL are positive, but limited. Test–retest reliability for diagnoses obtained with the K-SADS-PL range from excellent (most depressive disorders, generalized anxiety disorder, conduct disorder, oppositional defiant disorder) to good (PTSD, anxiety disorders) for lifetime diagnoses (Kaufman et al., 1997). Kaufman and colleagues (1997) also reported preliminary support for diagnoses generated by the K-SADS-PL.

It is apparent that many of the available structured and semistructured interviews focus on DSM diagnoses and, as such, may be of limited use in school settings. Interviews that focus on school-related problems and IDEA placement criteria are more likely to be of benefit to school professionals. For example, the SIB-R, Vineland, and ADI-R provide data that are directly linked to school-based assessment of adaptive and autistic behavior. There also are other interviews that, although at present are not as well studied with regard to psychometric properties, can be useful in school settings. One example that is useful for assessing academic problems is the Teacher Interview Form for Academic Problems (Shapiro, 1996), which is a semistructured format that focuses on academic difficulties and provides an efficient method for gathering information that is directly pertinent to behavior of concern. Another useful measure is found in The Instructional Environment System–II (TIES-II; Ysseldyke & Christensen, 1993), which provides child, teacher, and parent semistructured interviews that can be integrated with observational data to evaluate home and school learning environments, and are linked to potential interventions. For descriptive information regarding a child's bio-psycho-social history, a useful measure that can be used in either a semistructured interview or self-completed format is the parent Structured Developmental History of the Behavior Assessment System for Children (BASC; Reynolds & Kamphaus, 1992).

BEHAVIORAL INTERVIEWING

Conceptual Bases

The majority of interview formats we have addressed, whether structured or unstructured, have tended to focus on "traditional" interview concerns such as history and diagnosis. Indeed, many of the more recent standardized interview formats have the assessment goal of reaching a specific diagnostic conclusion. Although in many circumstances this goal may be useful, even required, diagnostic interviewing often does not provide the behavioral information necessary to develop and implement an intervention plan, particularly in school settings. Interviews that focus on both problem assessment and development of intervention plans may be accomplished through a behavioral format. (Table 10.1 provides a comparison of traditional and behavioral interview models.)

In contrast to other interview formats, behavioral interviews focus on current behaviors and environmental conditions with the goal of determining the specific situations and factors that generate and maintain problematic behaviors. Given that

TABLE 10.1   A Comparison of Behavioral and Traditional Interview Approaches

	Behavioral interviews	Traditional interviews
Interview goals	Identification of problem behaviors and related maintaining factors Development of an intervention plan Evaluation of the effectiveness of the intervention plan	Formulation of a diagnosis based on symptom profile Identification of etiological factors To guide thinking on prognosis and treatment
Assumptions	Behavior problems are caused by situational factors and/or an interaction of person and situation Present-oriented	Behavior problems are symptoms of a broader "disorder" Intrapsychic explanations are likely to be emphasized over the interpersonal or environmental Historical orientation
Interview skills	Problem specification Low inference Basic empathic listening and attending skills	Same High inference Same

the major foci of behavioral interviews are the specification of target behaviors and aiding in the assessment of manipulable variables, these types of interviews may readily lead to intervention planning. Gresham and Davis (1988) identified several advantages of behavioral interviews, including their flexibility in relation to other behavioral assessment methods, and facilitating obtainment of both general and specific information about the problem situation. Additionally, the interviewer may assess the teacher's or parent's receptiveness to intervention ideas as well as evaluate the assumptions that the informants may hold about the child's difficulties.

Behavioral interviews provide a method for engaging in a functional assessment of the behaviors of concern. In conducting the interview, the psychologist obtains data regarding behavioral deficits that may contribute to the problem, behavioral excesses, problems with environmental stimulus control, and inappropriate self-control of stimuli as well as inappropriate use of contingency management methods (Kanfer & Grimm, 1977). The specific format for a behavioral interview may vary. In school settings a consultation model of service delivery often is utilized that employs a problem-solving interview format. Bergan and Kratochwill (Bergan, 1977; Bergan & Kratochwill, 1990; Kratochwill & Bergan, 1990) have developed the best-known system for conducting behavioral interviews within consultation. Within this model, three standardized, semistructured problem-solving interviews are conducted to identify the problem (Problem Identification Interview; PII), to develop a plan for implementation (Problem Analysis Interview; PAI), and to evaluate the treatment plan (Treatment Evaluation Interview; TEI). The standard interview objectives are summarized in Table 10.2.

TABLE 10.2   Behavioral Consultation Interview Objectives

Problem identification interview	Problem analysis interview	Treatment evaluation interview
Opening salutation	Opening salutation	Opening salutation
General problem statement	General opening statement	Outcome questions
Behavior specification	Examine behavior strength	Goal-attainment questions
1. Specify examples	Examine behavior conditions	Internal validity
2. Specify priorities	1. Antecedent	External validity
Behavior setting	2. Sequential	Plan continuation
1. Specify examples	3. Consequent	Plan modification
2. Specify priorities	Summarize and validate	Generalization and
Identify antecedents	Interpretation of behavior	maintenance
Identify sequential	Plan statement	Follow-up assessment
conditions	Summarize and validate	Future interviews
Identify consequences	Continuing data collection	Termination
Summarize and validate	Establish next meeting	Closing salutation
Identify behavior strength	Closing salutation	
Summarize and validate		
Tentative definition of goal		
Identify child's assets		
Existing procedures		
Summarize and validate		
Data-collection procedures		
1. Directional statement		
2. Procedure		
Summarize and validate		
Date to begin data collection		
Establish next meeting		
Closing salutation		

A recent modification of this system is the development of conjoint behavioral consultation interviews in which parents and teachers are interviewed together (see Sheridan, Kratochwill, & Bergan, 1996). This variation of behavioral consultation is defined as

> a systematic, indirect form of service delivery, in which parents and teachers are joined to work together to address the academic, social, or behavioral needs of an individual for whom both parties bear some responsibility. It is designed to engage parents and teachers in a collaborative problem-solving process with the assistance of a consultant, wherein the interconnections between home and school systems are considered crucially important. (Sheridan & Kratochwill, 1992, p. 122)

In conjoint behavioral consultation the emphasis is on the collaboration between home and school in the problem-solving process (Sheridan & Steck, 1995). This problem-solving process involves four stages drawn from the behavioral consultation model of Bergan and Kratochwill. The first stage is termed *problem identification*, in which the consultants work with the parent(s) and teacher(s) to specifically identify the problematic behaviors and situations. As part of this stage, the participants agree on how to collect baseline data. In the *problem analysis* stage, the baseline data are reviewed and the functional properties of the behavior are considered. The outcome of this stage is a *plan* for addressing the problem, which is then carried out in the *treatment implementation* stage. The fourth stage is the *treatment evaluation* stage, in which the consultant, parent(s), and teacher(s) evaluate the effectiveness of the intervention plans in resolving the problem.

Prior to the advent of the standardized interview objectives, most behavioral interviewing was unstructured, relying on conceptual goals rather than incorporating specific interview content likely to be meaningful in a behavioral assessment (Mash & Terdal, 1981). The use of a standardized, semistructured interview framework coupled with the flexibility of a problem-solving interview format represents a significant advance in the behavioral literature by providing for integrity for the interview and consultation processes. Moreover, the standardized format allows for replication of the general content of the interviews, thereby facilitating research and practice through a consistent methodology.

An adjunct to the behavioral interview objectives is the Consultation Analysis Record, which was developed as a research and training tool by Bergan and Tombari (1975; see also Bergan & Kratochwill, 1990). The CAR is a verbal interaction coding scheme designed specifically for behavioral interviews within consultation. The measure is intended to articulate with the behavioral consultation problem-solving model developed by Bergan (1977) and expanded by Bergan and Kratochwill (Bergan & Kratochwill, 1990; Kratochwill & Bergan 1990).

The CAR consists of various message classification categories and subcategories designed to provide indices of verbalizations deemed important in behavioral interviews (Bergan & Kratochwill, 1990). Four classification categories are used in analyzing interviews: (1) source, (2) content, (3) process, and (4) control. *Source* refers to the person speaking (i.e., consultant or consultee). The *content* dimension of the CAR is used to code the topics that a consultant and consultee discuss in the behavioral interview, including background environment, behavior setting, behavior, individual characteristics, observation, plan, and other. The *process* category refers to the functions performed by the verbal messages, including negative evaluation, positive evaluation, inference, specification, summarization, negative validation, and positive validation. Finally, the *control* category separates all statements into two subcategories depending on whether they request action or information (elicitor) or provide information (emitter). Data provided by the CAR include single category (e.g., specification) and combined category (e.g., behavior setting/specification) percentages. Thus the data provide percentages within and across categories.

Bergan and Tombari (1975) offered *suggested guidelines* (see Table 10.3) for message effectiveness that should occur in each of the problem-solving interviews. These guidelines were based on the rationale that "consultant verbalizations ought to articulate to the purposes of the consultation process" (p. 219). During the problem-identification interview the majority of verbalizations should occur in the message-content areas of behavior, behavior setting, and observation. The message-process

TABLE 10.3   Guidelines for Effective Occurrences of Consultant Verbalizations

Interview	Content	Process	Control
Problem identification	Behavior Behavior setting Observation	Specification Summarization Validation	Elicitor
Problem analysis	Behavior Observation Plan	Specification Summarization Validation	Elicitor
Treatment evaluation	Behavior Plan Observation	Specification Summarization Validation	Elicitor

Note. The general guidelines do not provide specifics regarding the number of statements that should occur in each subcategory; rather, they should be focused upon and occur frequently.

area requires emphases on specification, summarization, and validation. In the message-control domain, elicitors should be used "frequently" to guide the consultation process. In the problem-analysis interview, important message-content verbalizations are concerned with behavior, observation, and plan. The important message-process categories are specification, summarization, and validation. In message-control, elicitors should be used frequently. In the treatment evaluation interview, message-content should be more frequent for behavior, plan, and observation. Message-process areas should focus on specification, summarization, and validation. Finally, as in problem identification and analysis, elicitors should be used to guide the TEI process.

Based on these guidelines, four measures of interviewing skill can be computed from the CAR: (1) content relevancy, (2) content focus, (3) verbal effectiveness, and (4) message control. Content relevancy during problem identification includes behavior, behavior setting, and recording/observation procedures. During problem analysis, content relevancy includes behavior, behavior setting, and plan categories. Content relevancy during treatment evaluation includes behavior, observation, and plan categories. Content focus refers to maintaining a topic during sets of five statements. Verbal effectiveness is defined as the average verbal information expressed in specification, summarization, and validation over long sets of 25 verbalizations. The last index of interviewing skill, message-control, is computed by the overall proportion of consultant elicitors.

The CAR is based on the premises of behavioral assessment and clinical aspects of interviewing and has been used in several research studies on behavioral consultation interviews to explore verbalization patterns and their relations to consultation outcomes such as child outcomes, and teacher perceptions and skills. The CAR, however, remains more of a conceptual tool that is in need of further empirical evaluation, particularly regarding the suggested interview guidelines and indices of effective interviewing.

Research Bases

The general conceptual bases of behavioral interviewing are relatively well established. Compared to other methods of behavioral assessment, however, behavioral interviews are lacking a solid, cohesive research base. In the previous edition of this volume, Gresham and Davis (1988) discussed research regarding the psychometric properties of behavioral interviews with parents and teachers. Since then, several authors have attempted to strengthen and clarify the research base of behavioral interviews, many of whom have used interviews conducted within a behavioral consultation approach. In the following sections, we discuss research on behavioral problem-solving interviews, drawing from the excellent discussion and review provided by Gresham and Davis (1988), coupled with an overview of the current research base.

Before continuing, we should point out that we have taken a psychometric approach to examining the use of behavioral interviews. We use this approach for a variety of reasons. First, most research on behavioral interviews lacks cohesion, that is, there are many research studies that have included behavioral interviews, but few works that have attempted to examine in a systematic manner interviews as a method of assessment. Second, we believe a reductive–inductive approach best helps us examine the multiple variables and aspects of behavioral interviewing. Third, we hope to model a positivistic method for empirically examining the application of behavioral interviews in practice and research. Finally, from a practical vantage, using a psychometric approach allows for a commonly used method for examining assessment procedures, and provides for a coherent method of presentation.

RELIABILITY AND VALIDITY OF BEHAVIORAL INTERVIEWS

Behavioral interviewing is a method of assessment and, as such, needs to be subjected to criteria that allow for establishing its appropriate use for children. Some authors have argued, however, that because a behavioral model involves the direct measurement of behaviors that are situation specific, traditional test applications of psychometric properties are inconsistent with the theoretical underpinnings of behavioral assessment (e.g., Nelson, Hay, & Hay, 1977). Others argued that the data derived from behavioral assessment methods should be subjected to psychometric scrutiny (e.g., Cone, 1977; Gresham, 1984; Gresham & Davis, 1988; Linehan, 1980).

One issue in the debate relates to the use of traditional psychometric methods in establishing the validity of behavioral assessment. Traditional psychometric methods are based on normative samples and comparisons, which, from a behavioral standpoint, may be obviated because the sample of behavior in essence stands alone as an idiographic, situation-specific phenomenon. The question arises whether the assessment method reliably and validly measures the behavior of concern. One may directly sample a behavior, however, what are the assurances that the behavior is adequately measured? The issue may be based in differing perceptions of psychometrics and measurement theory. For example, if we draw from "classic" measurement theory and consider that all measurements contain error (E), and a "true" score (T) or observation is a sum of the observed score (O) plus error (i.e., $T = O + E$), one must provide a method for minimizing that error. Moreover, although a direct measurement of a behavior may increase the likelihood that an observation of a true behavior occurs (i.e., there is minimal error), the target behavior may be incorrectly or inadequately identified and/or the measure may not be adequately related to important assessment outcomes (i.e., lacking validity). Finally, problem behaviors are social phenomena wherein, from a behavioral standpoint, a problem is defined as a discrepancy between actual and desired behavior. Thus the behavior is judged problematic in relation to a social criterion. If one makes the analogy that desired behavior is a comparison of current behavior to a norm (social criterion), then the concept of normative comparison can be readily applied to behavioral assessment.

Although the traditional psychometric approach typically is used to examine the validity of assessment methods, alternative frameworks exist. For example, Gresham and Davis (1988) discussed the applications of social behaviorism psychometrics and generalizability theory to behavioral assessment. In essence, rather than supplanting the traditional psychometric approach, these frameworks provide a method for extending the concepts of reliability and validity to include behavioral concepts such as response class and behavior generality. Thus the *logic* of the psychometric approach can and, in our opinion, should be applied to behavioral assessment. The application of the logic of psychometrics is of even greater importance for behavioral interviews, which are an indirect method of assessment. Interviews in general, and informant interviews in particular, further complicate this issue in that they may be viewed as an assessment of the informant's perceptions of a behavior or event rather than a direct assessment of the behavior itself. (At the same time it should be noted that an informant interview does provide a direct assessment of those perceptions and the accompanying attitudes and behaviors of the informant.)

As with any assessment method, there is no single test to establish the reliable and valid use of behavioral interviews; rather, one must examine evidence from multiple sources and methods from which a convergent decision can be made. As noted, one of the major obstacles in examining behavioral interviews is the lack of a coherent research base. Many advances have been made in the behavioral literature regarding the use of multiple methods, sources, and settings. Indeed, one need only turn to the empirical literature to find numerous treatment studies that have used interviews along with other assessment methods for measuring behaviors and outcomes. At present, however, we are left to our own devices to bring the data together with regard to a "test review" approach to behavioral interviews. Although there is a large body of studies that can provide evidence for reliability and validity, we have made no attempt to engage in an exhaustive search of the research base. Rather, we have chosen to focus primarily on research that has been conducted using the behavioral consultation interview method. Our purposes for restricting our review is twofold: First, the semistructured, problem-solving interview method used in behavioral consultation is arguably the most widely used interview method in school settings. Second, the behavioral consultation research base includes studies that have examined verbal behaviors with methods such as the CAR. Because interviewing is a verbal enterprise, we believe an examination of this research base is necessary to advance our knowledge of behavioral problem-solving interviews.

Reliability of Behavioral Interviews

Within informant interviews, error is most likely to occur as interviewer drift, method error within the interview itself, and source error (e.g., retrospective information and perceptions of parents and teachers). Therefore, there are three major sources of error in practice and research for which we must account: (1) interviewer, (2) interview, and (3) interviewee.

Internal Consistency

Internal consistency refers to the ability of a measure to evidence consistent patterns of responses within a domain of interest. Methods for examining internal consistency typically use a correlational method (e.g., Cronbach's alpha, Kuder–Richardson 20) to examine the extent to which items are consistently measured, that is, are free from error. The concept of internal consistency, however, is not often applied to behavioral interviews. A generalized application of the logic of internal consistency to behavioral interviews is to assess whether the interview objectives are consistently used by interviewers. Kratochwill, Elliott, and Busse (1995) and Sheridan (1992) examined the integrity (i.e., consistent application of interview objectives) of behavioral interviews used in consultation with teacher interviewees. Consultants received training in behavioral consultation interviewing skills. Based on the standardized interview items (see Table 10.2), consultants in both studies adhered to an average 88% of the objectives, which indicates that the interview items were used consistently.

Another generalized application of internal consistency can be found in research that has used the CAR. Several researchers have found that verbalizations used in behavioral consultation interviews follow a similar trend, that is, evidence consistency (e.g., Bergan & Tombari, 1976; Busse, Kratochwill, & Elliott, 1999; Hughes & DeForest, 1993; Martens, Lewandowski, & Houk, 1989; McDougall, Reschly, & Corkery, 1988). For example, Martens, Lewandowski, and Houk (1989) and Busse, Kratochwill, and Elliott (1999) explored verbal behaviors of consultants during consultation problem-identification interviews with teachers and found 43% and 37%, respectively, of content statements occurred in the Behavior subcategory. Percentages reported for the subcategories of Behavior Setting also were similar. Results from Busse and colleagues, however, indicated greater frequency of Observation statements (12% vs. <3.5%). For teacher verbalizations, the results were nearly identical for the major subcategories although Observation statements again were more frequent in Busse and colleagues' study. (These differences may be an artifact of the length of the interviews used in the analyses. Specifically, Martens et al. used 15-minute interview segments, whereas Busse et al. coded entire case interviews.)

These results also were similar to those of Hughes and DeForest (1993), who presented percentages for consultant statements in the process category. These authors reported the percentages of consultant statements in the Positive Evaluation subcategory as 3%, Inference as 8%, Summarization as 14%, and Positive Validation as 36%, compared to 4%, 4%, 14%, and 36% in Busse and colleagues. The results from Martens and colleagues' study were similar, although Positive Validation statements in Martens and colleagues' work comprised over half (54%) of the consultants' total statements. Specification statements were greater for consultants in Busse and colleagues (43%) than for Martens and colleagues (29%) or Hughes and DeForest (37%). Finally, the percentages of consultants' control statements were comparable across the three studies. Taken together, the results from these three independent studies provide some evidence for the consistency of verbalizations that occur during problem-identification interviews. Unfortunately, most research with the CAR has focused on problem-identification to the exclusion of problem-analysis interviews.

These studies provided evidence that general behavioral interview objectives can be consistently used, however, researchers have not examined the internal consistency of behavioral interviews with regard to specific problems or cases. Traditional internal consistency estimation is premised on patterns of responses that are applicable for structured interview formats which, as noted earlier, is one of the advantages of structured interviews. The application of traditional methods for ascertaining internal consistency also can be readily applied to many behavior-specific and disorder-specific interviews, because the content remains consistent across cases. Problem-solving interviews, however, pose difficulty because the general objectives remain consistent, but the specific content changes with a given problem within an interview.

One method for applying the logic of internal consistency to problem-solving interviews is to assess whether the number and nature of problems in an interview are consistent at different points in the interview (Gresham & Davis, 1988). This method could involve response frequencies and/or ratings of the consistency of verbalizations on a specific problem or problems. One could gain specificity by dividing interviews into different problem foci (e.g., externalizing vs. internalizing behaviors) and examining the consistency with which interviews remain focused on those behaviors.

Interobserver Agreement

Interobserver or interrater agreement is a measure of the reliability or consistency between two or more observers. Kratochwill and coworkers (1995) calculated interobserver agreement data on the standardized interview objectives for 122 training and case interviews and found an agreement of 88% (range 67–100%). Sheridan (1992) reported nearly identical results across the three interview phases. Regarding the verbal content of behavioral interviews, several researchers have found raters can reliably code the broad categories of content, process, and control in analogue and actual case interviews. For example, Bergan and Tombari (1975) found that inter-observer agreements ranged from .87 to .92 for content across the three consultation interviews, .87 to .94 for the process category, and perfect agreement for the control category. Several researchers have reported similar findings using agreement percentages and/or kappa coefficients (e.g. Busse et al., 1999; Hughes & DeForest, 1993; Martens et al., 1989; McDougall, Reschly, & Corkery, 1988). Martens and colleagues (1989) also examined the interobserver agreement for the CAR subcategories (e.g., Behavior, Summarization) and found that, whereas the mean agreement was 96%, the Behavior Setting subcategory agreement evidenced a low range of 60%.

Although these data provide some evidence that the verbalizations categories can be consistently coded, the data are limited with regard to interviewer consistency and the level of examination. Specifically, there are no data that ascertain whether two interviewers would focus on the same behaviors in separate interviews, that is, if two interviewers independently engage in problem solving for the same case or client, do they focus on the same behaviors and engage in similar patterns of verbalizations? Further, there are limited data regarding the reliability of coding verbalizations. Most researchers have reported data on the broad domains of content, process, and control, rather than the specific subcategories subsumed within the content and process categories. Thus little is known about the interobserver agreement on the more important components of behavioral interviews, such as behavior and behavior setting. More data are needed regarding the reliability of these subcategories and, to ensure more reliable coding, minimum criteria need to be established for the coding process. For example, Busse and colleagues (1999) set a minimum criterion of 70% agreement for each of the broad categories which, albeit probably overly liberal, provided a basis for more reliable codings. Interviews with interobserver ratings or codings that did not meet the criterion were recoded until the criterion was met. A minimum criterion standard, perhaps set at a conservative level of 80% (e.g., Benes, Gutkin, & Kramer, 1995) could be applied to both broad categories and subcategories to strengthen future reliability studies.

Interobserver agreement at the interviewee level has received little empirical attention. Sheridan (1994, cited in Sheridan et al., 1996) provided some evidence for interobserver agreement in conjoint consultation interviews. Parents and teachers were found to engage in similar proportions of verbalizations in the background environment and behavior-setting categories. These results, however, only indicate that the frequency of statements was similar, not that the specific behavior related statements were consistent. Research clearly needs to be conducted on teacher–parent agreement, and on parent–parent agreement regarding the nature of target behaviors.

Test–Retest Reliability

Temporal stability can be an important component of an assessment tool. If behaviors are maintained and manifest across time, the method used to assess those behaviors should evidence high levels of test–retest reliability, particularly across relatively brief time periods such as two weeks or one month. Although there is evidence that across cases behavioral interviewers can consistently use the behavioral interview objectives and consistently engage in verbalizations as measured by the CAR, nothing is known about the temporal stability of the specific case content of behavioral interviews. One method for evaluating the temporal stability of behavioral interviews is to engage in separate interviews across time. This method would allow for determining whether the interview focus remained consistent. Obvious problems that are inherent in any retest study need to be considered, such as recency effects and potential changes in the person or environmental variables that may alter the target behavior and/or setting.

Validity of Behavioral Interviews

Validity is the extent to which an assessment procedure or test actually measures what it purports to measure. An interview, for example, may be highly reliable but fails to measure what it is intended to assess. Thus reliability is considered necessary but not sufficient for determining whether a test or measure should be used for a given purpose. Validation of an assessment measure involves a variety of conceptual domains that provide evidence for internal and external validity, many of which are applicable to behavioral interviews. We have adopted the approach that all validity evidence (indeed all reliability evidence) is subsumed under construct validation (e.g., Messick, 1995). The construct validity of behavioral interviews can be evaluated by examining how interviews are related to what the interview is designed to assess (Bergan & Kratochwill, 1990).

Content Validity

Content validity refers to the ability of an assessment procedure to represent a domain or universe of behavior. A general method for evaluating the content validity of a measure is through expert evaluations. Behavioral interviews have received prima facie content validation through general agreement in the literature on the important variables to include as objectives in a behavioral assessment. Thus the standard objectives in behavioral consultation interviews, for example, are assumed to possess valid content through the representation of domains deemed important in behavioral assessment, such as operationalization of target behavior and identification of behavior settings. Further evidence for the content validity of behavioral interviews is found through the use of the CAR, which includes defined subdomains seen as important in behavioral assessment (Gresham & Davis, 1988).

Whereas these aspects of content validation are important, there is a decided lack of specific research on the content validity of behavioral interviews. General agreement on major aspects of behavioral interviewing are necessary components, however, we are not aware of any validation studies that have used expert panels or quantitative methods to systematically assess the content of interview objectives or the content of the CAR categories and subcategories. Indeed, the CAR categories, although relatively well defined, were drawn from work on verbal behaviors in psychotherapy and extended to reflect a behavioral model (Bergan & Tombari, 1975). Several aspects of the coding format appear to be designed to measure dimensions that are theoretically important in interviewing (e.g., evaluation, individual characteristics), but need to be substantiated through content validation to establish their internal validity within a behavioral framework.

Criterion-Related Validity

Criterion-related validity is the extent to which a measurement device is related to a criterion or standard against which the measure can be judged. A diagnostic interview outcome, for example, should correlate with the appropriate psychiatric diagnosis. Two forms of criterion-related validity typically are used in validation studies. *Concurrent* validity, as the name implies, refers to the degree to which a measure is related to a criterion or standard that is obtained at the same point in time. *Predictive* validity is the extent to which the measure is related to a criterion that is temporally distant, that is, future oriented.

There are several criteria with which behavioral interviews should be related, such as behavioral observations, behavior rating scales, and measures of interview effectiveness (Gresham & Davis, 1988). Indirect evidence for concurrent validity of behavioral interviews can be found by examining studies that have incorporated criteria such as observations and rating scale data. For example, Sheridan and colleagues (1996) reported on case studies using conjoint behavioral consultation wherein concordance was found across interview data and various methods of assessment. For example, in the case of "Sherry" the conjoint problem identification interview revealed social initiation as the target behavior. Data also were obtained from several criteria: a self-report measure, parent and teacher social rating scales, a sociometric measure, observations by parent and teacher, and independent observations of Sherry and a comparison child. All data revealed that social initiation was correctly and adequately identified in the interview from both an idiographic and normative level.

Concurrent validity evidence also can be found by comparing verbalizations in behavioral interviews to the criterion of Bergan and Tombari's (1975; see Table 10.3) guidelines for effective occurrences of consultant verbalizations. Busse and colleagues (1999) examined 37 cases and found consultant verbalizations occurring during behavioral consultation interviews followed rather closely the major guidelines, and teacher verbalizations followed consultants' statement patterns. For problem identification interviews, consultants' statements accounted for 37% of the total (combined consultant and teacher) verbalizations. The largest amount of content verbalizations for consultants occurred in the Behavior subcategory (14%), followed by Behavior Setting (10%), and Observation (4%). The remainder of the subcategories accounted for 3% or less each of the total verbalizations. The amount of consultants' process verbalizations were 16% for Specification, 13% for Positive Validation, 5% for Summarization, with the remainder of subcategories each accounting for 3% or less of the total statements. For the control category, consultants' emitters constituted 27% of the total control verbalizations, and elicitors accounted for 10%. Teacher-consultees' statements accounted for the majority (63%) of the total verbalizations during the PII and, as expected, teachers' content verbalizations followed a pattern similar to that of the consultants: Behavior (25%), Behavior Setting (22%), and Observation (4%). Process verbalizations were predominately in the subcategory Specification (44%), followed by Positive Validation (10%), and Inference (4%). Teachers verbalized 62% of the emitters and 1% of elicitors. The researchers also found that consultant and teacher verbalizations in problem-analysis and treatment-evaluation interviews followed the expected patterns.

Another avenue for examining the concurrent validity of behavioral interviews involves their relation to interviewee outcomes as a criterion. In an early examination of teacher/consultee verbal behaviors, Tombari and Bergan (1978) found specific behavioral elicitors when compared to more general medical-model elicitors differentially impacted teacher behaviors. Using the CAR to measure teachers' content verbalizations, the researchers found each type of cue extracted verbal responses and problem definitions that were congruent with the elicitors. Further, behavioral cues were more likely to enhance teachers' expectations about ability to solve a problem in their classrooms.

In a related study, Anderson, Kratochwill, and Bergan (1986) analyzed verbal behaviors in a study which involved training teachers in behavioral consultation and behavior modification. Fifty-two teachers were assigned randomly to either an experimental training group or a nonspecific training control group. Participants in each condition were then assigned to one of two videotaped, analogue consultation conditions defined as general or specific in terms of consultant elicitors. Training teachers in behavioral consultation resulted in significant main effects for behavior specification responses during the problem-identification interview. Further, specific consultant elicitors resulted in greater numbers of verbalizations in behavior-setting specification. In problem analysis, a significant training effect was found for plan specification. No effects were found for problem evaluation. Although limited by the analogue nature of the study and the brief duration of the "interviews," the results provided evidence that specific consultant elicitors are more likely to be accompanied by specific teacher responses.

Evidence for the predictive validity of behavioral interviews was found in an early regression model application of the CAR. Bergan and Tombari (1976) measured the relations among consultant variables, the implementation of consultation, and consultation outcomes. Transcripts were coded for problem-identification and problem-analysis interviews conducted by 11 psychologists trained in behavioral consultation. An initial sample of 806 children in preschool through third-grade who were referred for services participated in the study. No information was provided regarding teacher demographics. The regression included the four measures of interviewing skill computed from the CAR: (1) content relevancy, (2) content focus, (3) verbal effectiveness, and (4) message control. Three other consultant variables included in the regression equation were two efficiency variables (i.e., time from referral to problem identification, case load) and flexibility (using a variety of interventions). It was hypothesized that these consultant predictor variables would be related positively to effective consultation.

Results were based on multiple regressions with dichotomous (i.e., coded 0 or 1) dependent variables of whether the problem identification interview occurred, whether there was plan implementation, and if the identified treatment goal was achieved. Results indicated problem identification occurred for 43% ($n = 347$) of the 806 cases, plan implementation for 31% ($n = 250$), and problem solution occurred for 30% ($n = 242$) of the cases. The seven variables accounted for 41% of the variance in problem identification. Of the four interviewing skills, only message control was reported as contributing significantly to the regression equation for problem identification, and none of the skills contributed significantly to plan implementation nor problem resolution. Time from referral to problem identification and flexibility contributed 5% and 13%, respectively, of the changes in the variance. For plan implementation, only the occurrence of the problem identification interview contributed significantly, accounting for 59% of the change in variance. Plan implementation contributed to 95% of the variance for problem resolution. Finally, the findings indicated that plan implementation occurred for 31% of the cases with all but 1% ($n = 8$) achieving problem solution as measured dichotomously by whether the goal identified in problem identification was achieved. Thus it appears that problem identification predicted whether treatment plans would be implemented and, once in place, whether treatments resulted in overwhelmingly positive outcomes.

The Bergan and Tombari (1976) study was an important stepping stone for research on verbal behaviors in behavioral consultation interviews and is one of the most frequently cited studies in the area. There are, however, several issues related to the variables included in the analyses that warrant consideration. First, it appears that the regressions were conducted on the entire sample of 806 children referred for services. It is puzzling to include in the analyses those cases ($n = 459$) for which consultation did not occur. A second issue involves the multiple regression for predicting the occurrence of problem identification. Consultant variables of verbal behaviors were included in the analysis as predictor variables of whether the problem identification interview occurred. The issue is that verbal behaviors cannot be coded on the CAR if no interview has taken place, therefore it appears the regression included variables which do not affect the dependent variable. It may be that these variables could be predictive of whether consultees engaged in subsequent consultations, although that was not the question addressed in the study.

The variables included in the regression for plan implementation also are puzzling. The results indicated that the occurrence of problem-identification interviews predicted whether a plan was implemented. This finding can be simply interpreted as indicating that once consultations are initiated there is a high probability that the consultation will continue. Thus consultant verbal behaviors would not be expected to be related to whether a plan is implemented, which was exactly what the results indicated. Consultant verbal behaviors may be related to whether teachers implement treatments, but intervening factors may occur that are more strongly related to plan implementation. It is important to note that for 97 cases plan implementation did not follow problem identification. The authors did not specify why these cases did not continue. It may be that early terminations occurred because children moved, problems were resolved without intervention, the school year was ending, or a variety of other reasons. Furthermore, the authors did not operationalize problem resolution beyond noting if the goal identified during problem identification was achieved.

Busse and colleagues (1999) also provided evidence for the predictive validity of behavioral interviews in an investigation of the relations among consultant and teacher verbalizations during behavioral interviews and behavioral consultation treatment outcomes. The independent variables were categories of verbal behaviors coded on the CAR. The dependent variables were teachers' perceptions of consultant effectiveness, and treatment outcome indices of convergent evidence scaling, and single-case effect sizes. As expected, analysis of variance results indicated consultants exerted control over the consultation process, that is, used elicitors to guide interviews. A series of multiple regressions was conducted to test a hypothesized model that consultant control, behavior specification, and plan specification, and teacher positive validation would account for significant variance in consultation outcomes. Results indicated that consultant control was not predictive of treatment outcomes. Teachers' positive validation statements were predictive of their perceptions of consultant effectiveness, but were not predictive of child outcomes. Interestingly, the results indicated that consultant behavior specification and plan specification verbalizations were *negatively* related to treatment indices, such that less frequent use of these types of statements resulted in more positive child outcomes. These results may indicate that the efficient use of behavior and plan specification statements were predictive of positive outcomes. (Alternatively, the negative relations may be indicative of problems that were less amenable to teacher-mediated interventions.) These results, however, must be interpreted cautiously because of the small number of cases ($n = 37$) and the nature of the CAR data (i.e., frequency counts). Furthermore, the strongest findings indicated the predicted model accounted for only 30% to 34% of the variance on outcomes, leaving the majority of variance unexplained.

Hughes and DeForest (1993) used the process and control categories in a modified version of the CAR to investigate consultant directiveness and support as predictors of consultation outcomes. The dependent variables were the Consultant Evaluation Form (CEF; Erchul, 1987), one item which measured teachers' perceptions of problem improvement, and a somewhat nebulous item on the impact on teachers doing "anything differently as a result of this consultation." The teachers expressed overall satisfaction with the consultants, as reflected on the CEF. Most (76%) of the teachers stated they did something differently, with 50% reporting the problem had improved. Significant correlations were evidenced between the CEF and positive validation elicitors ($r = -.62$), inference emitters ($r = .48$), and supportive verbalizations ($r = .47$), with near significance for total elicitors ($r = -.46$) and positive evaluation emitters ($r = .46$). No relations were found between problem improvement and the verbalization categories. The authors concluded that consultants who provide personal support and offer causal hypotheses during initial interviews may be perceived as more effective by teachers.

Other investigators also have used the CAR to examine the relation between consultant verbal behavior and teacher perceptions. Martens, Lewandowski, and Houk (1989) used the CAR to code 15-minute problem identification interviews conducted by two consultants with 20 teachers who rated subsequent perceptions of satisfaction on a measure similar to the CEF (Erchul, 1987). The results were based on percentages, correlations, sequential analysis, and multiple regression. Teachers' behavior inference emitters and consultant positive validation emitters were correlated significantly ($r = .53$ and .54) with the teachers' perceptions of satisfaction. Sequential analysis revealed one sequence that was related significantly ($r = .53$) to teachers' satisfaction: teacher behavior specification emitters followed by consultant positive validation emitters. These significant correlations and the significant sequence were regressed on teacher perceptions and accounted for 42% of the variance of the satisfaction ratings. As with the results from Hughes and DeForest (1993), the use of only initial problem-identification interviews may have constricted the usefulness of the scale used to measure perceptions of the consultation process. Furthermore, the use of only two consultants may have restricted variability in the interviews, thereby attenuating the generalizability of the results.

Taken together, these studies strengthen an earlier conclusion by Gresham and Davis (1988) that behavioral interviews conducted in consultation evidence expected patterns and relations with various criteria, particularly for various aspects of interviewing effectiveness and interviewee outcomes. The data are limited, however, regarding the relations among behavioral interviews and other measures of behavior. Although one may indirectly evaluate convergence among data obtained during interviews and other methods such as observations, self-monitoring, and rating scales, concerted efforts that examine these criteria are lacking. As with content validity, evidence for the criterion-related validity of behavioral interviews could be strengthened through studies that specifically address these important relations. For example, correlational methods could be used to examine the magnitude of relations among a target behavior and setting variables identified during problem identification interviews and other assessment methods. Problem-solving behavioral interviews also could be evaluated with regard to their concurrent and predictive relations to diagnostic or psychoeducational categories.

Convergent/Congruent Validity

Further validity evidence is found when a measure is positively related to another measure of the same (convergent) or similar (congruent) construct of interest. For example, one expects that two measures of depression are related and a measure of depression and anxiety are related. Sheridan (1994, cited in Sheridan et al., 1996) provided some evidence for the convergent validity of behavioral interviews in a comparison of the verbalizations of teachers and parents during conjoint and parallel (teacher-only) problem-identification interviews. The results, which were limited to selected variables, indicated the proportion of behavior setting statements were .25, .26, and .28, respectively, for consultants, teachers, and parents in conjoint interviews, and .32 and .35, respectively, for consultants and teachers in the teacher-only interviews. As expected, teachers made fewer overall statements during conjoint interviews, which indicates that parents and teachers shared in providing information. Interestingly, consultants made 56% of the statements during conjoint interviews, compared to 26% during teacher-only interviews, which indicates that consultants provided more direction during conjoint interviews.

Evidence of the congruent validity of behavioral interviews can be found in a series of studies (Erchul, 1987; Erchul & Chewning, 1990; Witt, Erchul, McKee, Pardue, & Wickstrom, 1991) that included verbal coding methods used in research on counseling interviewing. The dependent variables were consultant perceptions of teacher participation in baseline data collection and plan implementation, and consultee perceptions on the Consultant Evaluation Form (CEF). Verbal interactions were analyzed for 8 to 10 cases drawn and extended from Erchul (1987). Taken together, the results indicated consultant control was positively related to consultation outcomes, whereas teachers' attempts at control were negatively related to their participation and to their perceptions of the consultants.

Further evidence for the congruent validity of behavioral interviews is found in Martens, Erchul, and Witt (1992), who compared verbalizations from the CAR with the counseling coding systems discussed above. Data consisted of four problem-identification interviews drawn from Erchul (1987). The four coding schemes yielded consistent descriptions of the interpersonal processes that occurred during the consultation interviews. Specifically, consultants: (1) exerted control over the verbal relationship through elicitors or requests; (2) asked questions in a polite manner by using dominant-affiliative and submissive bids; (3) typically focused on the client (child); (4) initiated most topic changes; and (5) summarized and validated teacher verbalizations. Teacher verbalizations most often were characterized as topic-following and as providing information. Teachers seldom asked questions or made bids/requests, and seldom were successful at topic determination.

This vein of research on verbal interactions and subsequent relations to the process of consultation interviews and outcomes has been extended to include resistance. Wickstrom (1991) examined verbal interactions with a content coding system for measuring resistance and cooperation. Consultant verbal behaviors included categories labeled support, information seek, teach, disagree/confront, and a miscellaneous category. Teacher verbal behaviors were coded on indices labeled cooperate, answer, generate hypothesis, resist, question, and other. Dependent variables included teachers' perceptions of satisfaction with consultants and the consultation process, and perceptions of the effectiveness and success of interventions. Results indicated that teachers' statements occurred most frequently in the cooperate category, with consultants' verbalizations most frequent in support statements. Significant correlations were found between teachers' positive perceptions of the consultations and consultant support statements. Positive correlations also were found between verbal sequences coded support-cooperate and ratings of teacher satisfaction. Interestingly, information seeking by consultants was negatively correlated with each of the outcome indices. These findings, however, must be interpreted with caution because of the small sample size ($n = 9$).

There is a growing body of evidence to support the congruent validity of behavioral interviews, particularly regarding verbalization coding research. Less is known, however, about the convergent validity of behavioral interviews. The research base could be greatly strengthened by comparing behavioral interviewing methods to assess the level of convergence among interview objectives and identified problems. For example, further research on the comparison between conjoint and teacher/parent-only interviews can serve to strengthen the validity of both approaches. It also would be informative to compare the outcomes of interviews conducted within the indirect consultation method and a direct behavioral approach. Another validation method is to compare behavioral problem-solving interviews with other semi-structured interviews, such as behavior-specific formats.

Divergent Validity

Divergent or discriminant validity is evidenced when measures of unrelated or negatively related constructs are shown to indeed be unrelated. A measure of happiness, for example, should be negatively related to depression. One method for evaluating the divergent validity of behavioral interviews is to engage comparisons with other theoretically based interviewing methods. For example, micro-level differences between counseling and behavioral consultation interviews were examined by Henning-Stout and Conoley (1987). In this study verbal interactions were examined from counseling and consultation interviews with 30 graduate-student counselors and 30 graduate-student consultants matched on age, sex, and level of training. Verbal interactions were coded with a measure developed by Larabee (1980, cited in Henning-Stout & Conoley, 1987), called the Counselor Verbal Behavior Analysis system, which was designed to measure restrictiveness in the counseling process. Results indicated that behavioral interviews were characterized by more restrictive verbalizations (e.g., directions, suggestions) than counseling interviews. Less restrictive verbalizations (e.g., reflection, paraphrasing) were used with equal frequency by both groups. These authors concluded that, although further study is warranted, the results were indicative of divergence in verbal behaviors used in the two interview methods.

In a more recent study, Erchul, Covington, Hughes, and Meyers (1995) explored relational communication across different methods of consultation interviewing such as mental health consultation, behavioral consultation, and an "eclectic approach of these and other models of consultation" (p. 622). The consultants were composed of 26 graduate students who served an equal number of teachers. Using a request-centered system to code initial interviews, no significant correlations were found between consultant bids and CEF scores. Interestingly, when the data were analyzed for cases ($n = 14$) that were behavioral consultations, significant results were found. Dominant bids (i.e., commands or instructions) were negatively correlated ($r = -.67$) with the CEF, whereas dominant-affiliative bids (i.e., requests or validation elicitors) were positively correlated ($r = .52$) with the CEF. These results may indicate that the type of control exerted by consultants is important toward teachers' subsequent perceptions. The results also provide evidence for the divergence of behavioral and mental health interview approaches.

In an interesting study, Curtis and Watson (1980) examined outcomes of behavioral interviews conducted by four high-skilled and four low-skilled consultants. A problem-identification checklist was used to assess the consultants' problem-clarification skills, which included indices of factual versus inferential statements, and the occurrence of specifications of the target behavior, desired outcome, and observation methods. The results indicated divergence between the two groups, such that higher skilled consultants evidenced more effective interviewing skills as measured by the content relevancy and control indices of the CAR, and focused more on factual information. Further, interviews conducted by high-skilled consultants elicited better problem clarification skills from teachers.

Target behaviors and settings identified in behavioral interviews also should demonstrate divergence. For example, the case of "Sherry" presented by Sheridan and colleagues (1996) showed expected divergence between the target child's social withdrawal behaviors and those of a comparison child. Other methods that can provide expected divergence include comparing a child's behavioral strengths with identified problem behaviors. Few studies, however, include the assessment of alternative or incompatible behaviors; rather, most often the target behavior is measured alone. If a behavior such as aggression is validly assessed during behavioral interviews (and subsequently treated), an incompatible socially appropriate behavior can be concurrently assessed to measure the divergent validity of the assessment (and treatment).

Social Validity

Social validity of behavioral interviews can be garnered from judgments of the social importance of the goals, processes, and outcomes of interviews (e.g., Wolf, 1978). Several of the studies covered in this chapter have included consultant and treatment satisfaction and effectiveness ratings by teachers and, to a lesser degree, parents. Researchers who have used the Consultant Evaluation Form and similar measures typically report that consultants are viewed positively by teachers (e.g., Erchul, 1987; Kratochwill et al., 1995; Martens et al., 1989).

Research also has shown that interventions implemented after behavioral consultation interviews often are perceived as acceptable to teachers and parents (e.g., Kratochwill et al., 1995; Sheridan et al., 1996). Unfortunately, little is known about the social validity of behavioral interviews per se. There is some evidence to indicate that interviewers' supportive statements (Hughes & DeForest, 1993; Wickstrom, 1991), and affiliative control of the interviewing process (Erchul, 1987, Erchul et al., 1995) are related to teachers' satisfaction with the interviewer-consultant, and excessive use of behavior and plan statements are related to negative outcomes (Busse et al., 1999). These findings point to the importance of engaging in further research toward understanding variables related to interviewees' perceptions of the acceptability and significance of the content and process of behavioral interviews.

Treatment Validity

A final and important aspect for consideration rests within the concept of treatment validity. Treatment validity of an assessment measure is demonstrated when the measure enhances treatment outcome (Nelson & Hayes, 1979), wherein outcomes include appropriate problem identification, treatment selection, and beneficial treatment outcomes (Braden & Kratochwill, 1997). In many ways, treatment validity is related to social validity, in that a measure should be evaluated with regard to its social and clinical implications (Messick, 1995). Treatment validity is perhaps the most important aspect of an assessment measure and is of paramount importance for problem-solving interviews. With informant interviews, the concept of treatment validity extends to outcomes for each interview role, that is, interviewer, interviewee, and child/client.

Several of the studies presented in this chapter provide some evidence for the treatment validity of behavioral interviews. For interviewer outcomes, training in behavioral interviewing methods, not surprisingly, facilitates skills in behavior, observation, and plan specification (Kratochwill et al., 1995; Sheridan, 1992). At the interviewee level, positive outcomes have been reported for teachers' specification skills (e.g., Anderson et al., 1986; Curtis & Watson, 1980) and teachers' perceptions of their ability to solve problems (Tombari & Bergan, 1978). For the children whom the interviews serve, the literature is replete with indirect evidence for positive intervention outcomes derived from behavioral interviews. Several of the studies presented in this chapter resulted in positive treatment outcomes for children and provide somewhat more direct evidence of the treatment validity of behavioral interviews (Bergan & Tombari, 1976; Busse et al., 1999; Hughes & DeForest, 1993).

Although these studies support the treatment validity of behavioral interviews, the data are extremely limited. Indeed, the data are scant across all assessment methods with regard to treatment validity or utility of assessment (Braden & Kratochwill, 1997). Within the research base on behavioral consultation interviews, major deficits include inadequate outcome indices (e.g., dichotomous data and perceptions of treatment effectiveness), a paucity of treatment-integrity assessment (Gresham, 1989; Wickstrom, Jones, LaFleur, & Witt, 1998), and a lack of research on the relations between problem analysis and positive treatment outcomes. Therefore, although behavioral interviews are conducted to aid in functional assessments of behavior and to facilitate individualized intervention, the treatment validity of behavioral interviews remains questionable. The most reliable measure that demonstrates the highest levels of validity in all areas save treatment validity remains of little use. Moreover, it is not known whether other methods of interviewing or assessment may demonstrate greater treatment validity.

CONCLUSION

Informant interviews are a major component of assessments of children. Gathering information from multiple sources has the potential to increase our understanding of a child's difficulties and to facilitate possible interventions. There are obvious holes, some gaping, in our understanding of behavioral interviews with parents and teachers. It is clear that we know more than we did, yet, at the risk of triteness it is clear that more needs to be done, particularly regarding the treatment validity of behavioral interviews. Furthermore, our coverage of the literature reveals that the preponderance of research on behavioral interviews has been conducted with teacher informants. Parental figures assume an important role in the assessment process, yet little is known beyond the conceptual sphere about the specifics of behavioral interviews with parents. As research on behavioral interviews continues, parent variables need to be incorporated and vigorously studied.

In this chapter we presented an overview of informant interviewing formats and methods. Several advances in informant interviewing have been made since the publication of the previous edition of this volume. Foremost are the advances regarding the psychometric properties of informant interviews, particularly for diagnostic omnibus and behavior-specific interviews. Our understanding of behavioral problem-solving interviews also has shown significant advancements, especially within the context of criterion-related and congruent validity. Our level of understanding, however, leaves much to be desired. As we continue to adhere to informant interviews we must examine their validity and ask ourselves if we are using the most effective and efficient method for desired outcomes.

References

Achenbach, T., McConaughy, S., & Howell, C. (1987). Child/adolescent behavioral and emotional problems: Implications of cross informant correlations for situational specificity. *Psychological Bulletin, 101*, 213–232.

American Psychiatric Association. (1987). *Diagnostic and statistical manual of mental disorders* (3rd ed., rev.). Washington, DC: Author.

Anderson, T. K., Kratochwill, T. R., & Bergan, J. R. (1986). Training teachers in behavioral consultation and therapy: An analysis of verbal behaviors. *Journal of School Psychology, 24*, 229–241.

Apter, S. J. (1982). *Troubled children/troubled systems*. Elmsford, NY: Pergamon Press.

Benes, K. M., Gutkin, T. B., & Kramer, J. J. (1995). Lag sequential analysis: Taking consultation communication research methodology to the movies. *School Psychology Review, 24*, 694–708.

Bergan, J. R (1977). *Behavioral consultation*. Columbus, OH: Merrill.

Bergan, J. R., & Kratochwill, T. R. (1990). *Behavioral consultation and therapy*. New York: Plenum Press.

Bergan, J. R., & Tombari, M. L. (1975). The analysis of verbal interactions occurring during consultation. *Journal of School Psychology, 13*, 209–225.

Bergan, J. R., & Tombari, M. L. (1976). Consultant skill and efficiency and the implementation and outcomes of consultation. *Journal of School Psychology, 14*, 3–14.

Braden, J. P., & Kratochwill, T. R. (1997). Treatment utility of assessment: Myths and realities. *School Psychology Review, 26*, 475–485.

Breton, J. J., Bergeron, L., Valla, J.-P., Berthiaume, C. & St-Georges, M. (1998). Diagnostic interview schedule for children (DISC-2.25) in Quebec: Reliability findings in light of the MECA study. *Journal of the American Academy of Child and Adolescent Psychiatry, 37*, 1167–1174.

Bruininks, R. H., Woodcock, R. W., Weatherman, R. F., & Hill, B. K. (1996). *Scales of independent behavior-Revised*. Chicago, IL: Riverside Publishing.

Busse, R. T., & Beaver, B. R. (2000). Informant reports: Functional assessment interviewing with parents and teachers. In E. S. Shapiro & T. R. Kratochwill (Eds.), *Conducting school-based assessments of child and adolescent behavior*. New York: Guilford Press.

Busse, R. T., Kratochwill, T. R., & Elliott, S. N. (1999). Influences of verbal interactions during behavioral consultations on treatment outcomes. *Journal of School Psychology, 37,* 117–143.

Chambers, W., Puig-Antich, J., Hirsch, M., et al. (1985). The assessment of affective disorders in children and adolescents by semi-structured interview: Test–retest reliability of the Schedule for Affective Disorders and Schizophrenia for School-Age Children, Present Episode version. *Archives of General Psychiatry, 42,* 696–702.

Cone, J. D. (1977). The relevance of reliability and validity for behavioral assessment. *Behavior Therapy, 8,* 411–426.

Curtis, M. J., & Watson, K. L. (1980). Changes in consultee problem clarification skills following consultation. *Journal of School Psychology, 18,* 210–221.

Edelbrock, C. (1988). Informant reports. In E. S. Shapiro & T. R. Kratochwill (Eds.), *Behavioral assessment in schools: Conceptual foundations and practical applications* (pp. 351–383). New York: Guilford Press.

Edelbrock, C., & Costello, A. J. (1990). Structured interviews for children and adolescents. In G. Goldstein & M. Hersen (Eds.), *Handbook of psychological assessment,* second edition (pp. 308–323). New York: Pergamon Press.

Erchul, W. P. (1987). A relational communication analysis of control in school consultation. *Professional School Psychology, 2,* 113–124.

Erchul, W. P., & Chewning, T.G. (1990). Behavioral consultation from a request-centered relational communication perspective. *School Psychology Quarterly, 5,* 1–20.

Erchul, W. P., Covington, C. G., Hughes, J. N., & Meyers, J. (1995). Further explorations of request-centered relational communication within school consultation. *School Psychology Review, 24,* 621–632.

Frick, P. J., Silverthorn, P., & Evans, C. S. (1994). Assessment of childhood anxiety using structured interviews: Patterns of agreement among informants and association with material anxiety. *Psychological Assessment, 6,* 372–379.

Gresham, F. M. (1984). Behavioral interviews in school psychology: Issues in psychometric adequacy and research. *School Psychology Review, 13,* 17–25.

Gresham, F. M. (1989). Assessment of treatment integrity in school consultation and prereferral intervention. *School Psychology Review, 18,* 37–50.

Gresham, F. M., & Davis, C. J. (1988). Behavioral interviews with teachers and parents. In E. S. Shapiro & T. R. Kratochwill (Eds.), *Behavioral assessment in schools: Conceptual foundations and practical applications* (pp. 455–493). New York: Guilford Press.

Groth-Marnat, G. (1997). *Handbook of psychological assessment* (3rd ed.). New York: Wiley.

Gutkin, T. B., & Curtis, M. J. (1999). School-based consultation theory and practice: The art and science of indirect service delivery. In C. R. Reynolds & T. B. Gutkin (Eds.), *The handbook of school psychology* (3rd ed., pp. 598–637). New York: Wiley.

Harrison, P. L. (1984). The application of the Vineland Adaptive Behavior. Scales in educational settings. *Techniques, 1,* 101–112.

Haynes, S. N., & Uchigakiuchi, P. (1993). Incorporating personality trait measures in behavioral assessment. *Behavior Modification, 14,* 297–306.

Henning-Stout, M., & Conoley, J. C. (1987). Consultation and counseling as procedurally divergent: Analysis of verbal behavior. *Professional Psychology: Research and Practice, 18,* 124–127.

Hodges, K. (1993). Structured interviews for assessing children. *Journal of Child Psychology and Psychiatry, 34,* 49–68.

Hodges, K. (1997). *Child assessment schedule (CAS).* Ypsilanti, MI: Eastern Michigan University.

Hodges, K., Gordon, Y., & Lennon, M. (1990). Parent–child agreement on symptoms assessed via a clinical research interview for children: The Child Assessment Schedule (CAS). *Journal of Child Psychology and Psychiatry, 31,* 427–436.

Hodges, K., & Zeman, J. (1993). Interviewing. In T. H. Ollendick & M. Hersen (Eds.), *Handbook of child and adolescent assessment* (pp. 65–81). Boston: Allyn & Bacon.

Houk, J. L., & Lewandowski, L. J. (1996). Consultant verbal control and consultee perceptions. *Journal of Educational and Psychological Consultation, 7,* 107–118.

Hughes, J. N., & DeForest, P. A. (1993). Consultant directiveness and support as predictors of consultation outcomes. *Journal of School Psychology, 31,* 355–373.

Ivey, A. E. (1994). *Intentional interviewing and counseling: Facilitating client development in a multicultural society.* Pacific Grove, CA: Brooks/Cole.

Kamphaus, R. W., & Frick, P. J. (1996). *Clinical assessment of child and adolescent personality and behavior.* Boston: Allyn & Bacon.

Kanfer, F. H., & Grimm, L. G. (1977). Behavioral analysis: Selecting target behaviors in the interview. *Behavior Modification, 4,* 419–444.

Kaufman, J., Birmaher, B., Brent, D., Rao, U., Flynn, C., Moreci, P., Williamson, D., & Ryan, N. (1997). Schedule for affective disorders and schizophrenia for school-age children—present and lifetime version (K-SADS-PL): Initial reliability and validity data. *Journal of the American Academy of Child and Adolescent Psychiatry, 36,* 980–988.

Kratochwill, T. R., & Bergan, J. R. (1990). *Behavioral consultation in applied settings: An individual guide.* New York: Plenum Press.

Kratochwill, T. R., Elliott, S. N., & Busse, R. T. (1995). Behavioral consultation training: A five-year evaluation of consultant and client outcomes. *School Psychology Quarterly, 10,* 87–117.

Lentz, F. E., & Wehmann, B. A. (1995). Best practices in interviewing. In A. Thomas & J. Grimes (Eds.), *Best practices in school psychology* (3rd ed., pp. 637–649). Washington, DC: National Association of School Psychologists.

Linehan, M. M. (1980). Content validity: Its relevance to behavioral assessment. *Behavioral Assessment, 2,* 147–159.

Lord, C., Rutter, M., & Le Couteur, A. (1994). Autism Diagnostic Interview–Revised: A revised version of a diagnostic interview for caregivers of individuals with possible pervasive developmental disorders. *Journal of Autism and Developmental Disorders, 24,* 659–686.

Martens, B. K., Erchul, W. P., & Witt, J. C. (1992). Quantifying verbal interactions in school-based consultation: A comparison of four coding schemes. *School Psychology Review, 21,* 109–124.

Martens, B. K., Lewandowski, L. J., & Houk, J. L. (1989). Correlational analysis of verbal interactions during the consultative interview and consultees' subsequent perceptions. *Professional Psychology: Research and Practice, 20,* 334–339.

Mash, E. J., & Terdal, L. G., (1981). Behavioral assessment of childhood disturbance. In E. J. Mash & L. G. Terdal (Eds.), *Behavioral assessment of childhood disorders.* New York: Guilford Press.

McDougall, L. M., Reschly, D. J., & Corkery, J. M. (1988). Changes in referral interviews with teachers after behavioral consultation training. *Journal of School Psychology, 26,* 225–232.

Messick, S. (1995). Validity of psychological assessment. *American Psychologist, 50,* 741–749.

Nelson, R. O. (1983). Behavioral assessment: Past, present, and future. *Behavioral Assessment, 5,* 195–206.

Nelson, R. O., Hay, L. R., & Hay, W. M. (1977). Comments on Cone's "The relevance of reliability and validity for behavioral assessment." *Behavior Therapy, 8,* 427–420.

Nelson, R. O., & Hayes, S. C. (1979). Some current dimensions of behavioral assessment. *Behavioral Assessment, 1,* 1–16.

Piotrowski, C., & Keller, J. W. (1984). Psychodiagnostic testing in APA-approved clinical psychology programs. *Professional Psychology: Research and Practice, 15,* 450–456.

Raggio, D. J., & Massingale, T. W. (1990). Comparability of the Vineland Social Maturity Scale and the Vineland Adaptive Behavior Scale—Survey Form with infants evaluated for developmental delay. *Perceptual and Motor Skills, 71,* 415–418.

Raggio, D. J., & Massingale, T. W. (1993). Comparison of the Vineland Social Maturity Scale, The Vineland Adaptive Behavior Scales—Survey Form, and the Bayley Scales of Infant Development with infants evaluated for developmental delay. *Perceptual and Motor Skills, 77,* 931–937.

Reich, W. (1996). *Diagnostic Interview for Children and Adolescents—Revised (DICA-R) 8.0.* St. Louis: Washington University.

Reynolds, C. R., & Kamphaus, R. W. (1992). *Behavior assessment system for children.* Circle Pines, MN: American Guidance Service.

Ribera, J. C., Canino, G., Rubio-Stipec, M., Bravo, M., Bauermeister, J. J., Alegria, M., Woodbury, M., Heurtas, S., Guevara, L. M., Bird, H. R., Freeman, D., & Shrout, P. E. (1996). The Diagnostic Interview Schedule for Children (DISC-2.1) in Spanish: Reliability in a Hispanic population. *Journal of Child Psychology and Psychiatry, 37,* 195–204.

Sattler, J. M. (1998). *Clinical and forensic interviewing of children and families: Guidelines for the mental health, education, pediatric, and child maltreatment fields.* San Diego: Author.

Schwab-Stone, M. E., Shaffer, D., Dulcan, M. K., Hensen, P. S., Fisher, P. Bird, H. R., Goodman, S. H., Lahey, B. B., Lichtman, J. H., Canino, G., Rubio-Stipec, M., & Rae, D. S. (1996). Criterion validity of the NIMH Diagnostic Interview Schedule for Children Version 2.3 (DISC-2.3). *Journal of the American Academy of Child and Adolescent Psychiatry, 35,* 878–888.

Shaffer, D., Fisher, P., Dulcan, M. K., Davies, M., Piacentini, J., Schwab-Stone, J. E., Lahey, B. B., Bourdan, K., Jensen, P. S., Bird, H. R., Canino, G., & Regier, D. (1996). The NIMH Diagnostic Interview Schedule for Children Version 2.3 (DISC-2.3): Description, acceptability, prevalence rates, and performance in the MECA study. *Journal of the American Academy of Child and Adolescent Psychiatry, 35,* 865–877.

Shapiro, E. S. (1996). *Academic skills problems: Direct assessment and intervention* (2nd ed.). New York: Guilford Press.

Shapiro, E. S., & Kratochwill, T. R. (in press). *Conducting school-based assessments of child and adolescent behavior.* New York: Guilford Press.

Sheridan, S. M. (1992). Consultant and client outcomes of competency-based behavioral consultation training. *School Psychology Quarterly, 7,* 245–270.

Sheridan, S. M. (1997). Conceptual and empirical bases of conjoint behavioral consultation. *School Psychology Quarterly, 12,* 119–133.

Sheridan, S. M., & Kratochwill, T. R. (1992). Behavioral parent–teacher consultation: conceptual and research considerations. *Journal of School Psychology, 30,* 117–139.

Sheridan, S. M., Kratochwill, T. R., & Bergan, J. R. (1996). *Conjoint behavioral consultation: A procedural manual.* New York: Plenum Press.

Sheridan S. M., & Steck, M. C. (1995). Acceptability of conjoint behavioral consultation: A national survey of school psychologists. *School Psychology Review, 24,* 633–647.

Sparrow, S. S., Balla, D. A., & Cicchetti, D. V. (1984). *Vineland Adaptive Behavior Scales: Interview edition survey form manual.* Circle Pines, MN: American Guidance Service.

Sparrow, S. S., Balla, D. A., & Cicchetti, D. V. (1985). *Vineland Adaptive Behavior Scales: Classroom edition manual.* Circle Pines, MN: American Guidance Service.

Tombari, M. L., & Bergan, J. R. (1978). Consultant cues and teachers verbalizations, judgments, and expectancies concerning children's adjustment problems. *Journal of School Psychology, 16,* 212–219.

Wickstrom, K. F. (1991). *Consultant–consultee verbal interaction in school-based consultation: Cooperative and resistant behavior.* Paper presented at the annual convention of the National Association of School Psychologists, Dallas, TX, March.

Wickstrom, K. F., Jones, K. M., LaFleur, L. H., & Witt, J. C. (1998). An analysis of treatment integrity in school-based behavioral consultation. *School Psychology Quarterly, 13,* 141–154.

Witt, J. C., Erchul, W. P., McKee, W. T., Pardue, M. M., & Wickstrom, K. F. (1991). Conversational control in school-based consultation: The relationship between consultant and consultee topic determination and consultation outcome. *Journal of Educational and Psychological Consultation, 2,* 101–116.

Wolf, M. M. (1978). Social validity: The case for subjective measurement or how applied behavior analysis is finding its heart. *Journal of Applied Behavior Analysis, 11,* 203–214.

Yssledyke, J. E., & Christensen, S. L. (1993). *The Instructional Environment System–II.* Longmont, CO: Sopris West.

CHAPTER 11

Self-Reports

Theory and Research in Using
Rating Scale Measures

TANYA L. ECKERT
ERIN K. DUNN
KATIE M. GUINEY
ROBIN S. CODDING
Syracuse University

A number of self-report rating scales have been developed for assessing children's and adolescent's emotional and behavioral functioning. This chapter describes the use of child and adolescent self-report measures within the context of a multimethod behavioral assessment. Because this type of assessment methodology includes a wide range of considerations, our goal in this chapter is to outline the basic concepts and methods that characterize this approach to behavioral assessment. First, we define self-report measures and discuss the definitional and conceptual underpinnings of these measures. Second, we outline the benefits of using self-report measures and review the literature regarding practical considerations in the use of these measures. Third, we provide an overview of measures currently available for measuring two broad domains of behavior: externalizing and internalizing disorders. We conclude with a discussion of current limitations and future directions.

SELF-REPORT MEASURES

Definition and Background

Self-report ratings scales require the direct response of an individual to a set of structured written statements (Reynolds, 1993). Data obtained from self-report rating scales include quantitative and qualitative information regarding attitudes, beliefs, feelings, opinions, and physical states. What differentiates self-report measures from informal cognitive measures or projective assessment techniques is the standardization of response items and administration procedures. Data obtained from standardized, self-report measures can be readily quantified and compared with normative information. However, it is important to note that self-report rating measures are not considered objective reports of behavior (McConaughy & Ritter, 1995). Although self-report measures can be reliably and accurately administered, scored, and interpreted, the accuracy of data obtained from self-report measures may be biased, disputable, or unreliable (Martens, 1993). Therefore, only self-report measures with adequate psychometric properties should be utilized within the context of a multimethod behavioral assessment (Breen, Eckert, & DuPaul, 1996; Martens, 1993; McConaughy & Ritter, 1995).

The process of completing self-report measures has been conceptualized as a form of direct assessment (Witt, Cavell, Heffer, Carey, & Martens, 1988); however, data gathered from self-report measures are typically considered an indirect form of assessment (Cone, 1978). That is, data obtained from self-report measures represent an individual's perceptions of behavior that may have occurred during a different time or under different environmental conditions. These data serve as retrospective accounts of behavior relative to the assessment occasion (Kratochwill & Shapiro, 1988). In many cases, the extent to which data obtained from self-report measures can be objectively verified is limited because of the covert or unobservable nature of the reported information. For example, it is impossible to corroborate information pertaining to an individual's emotions that occurred during a previous activity. Therefore, self-report measures may provide valuable information that can be used to complement other sources of information, such as behavioral observations and intervention formulation (Elliott, Busse, & Gresham, 1993).

Two distinct categories of self-report measures are available: broadband behavior rating scales and narrowband behavior rating scales (Eckert & DuPaul, 1996). Broadband rating scales are defined as measures that assess behavioral assets and deficits across broad domains of behavior, such as internalizing and externalizing dimensions (Achenbach, McConaughy, & Howell, 1987). Both the Behavior Assessment System for Children (BASC; Reynolds & Kamphaus, 1992) and the Youth Self Report (Achenbach, 1991c) incorporate a broadband taxonomy. Use of a broadband rating scale allows information to be gathered regarding a child's perceived level of functioning in relation to broad categories of behavioral disturbances. Narrowband ratings scales are defined as measures that assess a specific area of behavior (e.g., depression, conduct disorder). Use of narrowband rating scales allows a comprehensive analysis of a child's perceived level of functioning in a specific dimension of behavior. Both the Children's Depression Inventory (Kovacs, 1992) and the Reynolds Child Depression Scale (Reynolds, 1989) are conceptualized as narrowband self-report measures of depression.

The use of broadband self-report measures in conjunction with narrowband self-report measures can provide important clinical information within the context of a multimethod behavioral assessment. That is, data gathered from broadband and narrowband self-report measures can be used for screening, classification, treatment planning, and progress monitoring (Breen, Eckert, & DuPaul, 1996). This type of assessment approach uses broadband self-report measures to screen and identify potential behavioral problems along the continuum of internalizing and externalizing disorders. Narrowband self-report measures are then employed to identify specific behavioral problems and obtain a more detailed examination of psychopathology.

Benefits of Using Self-Report Measures

In the assessment of childhood disorders, there are a number of advantages to using self-report measures within the context of a multimethod behavioral assessment (see Kratochwill, Sheridan, Carlson, & Lasecki, 1999; McConaughy & Ritter, 1995; Reynolds, 1993, for reviews). First, the technical adequacy of many commonly used self-report measures meets current standards for assessment instruments as described in the *Standards for Educational and Psychological Testing* (American Psychological Association, 1985). Most of the recently developed self-report measures address developmental issues, establish adequate psychometric standards, and demonstrate acceptable standardization samples. By addressing these methodological and psychometric issues, self-report measures can be incorporated in the school-based assessment of children's social and emotional functioning. Second, self-report measures allow for the collection of data on behaviors that may not be possible with other assessment techniques. That is, self-report measures provide unique information regarding the perceptions of children and adolescents. This information can be directly related to the child's or youth's behavior (e.g., "Do you attend school on a regular basis?"), cognitions (e.g., "Do you feel upset when you enter your school?"), and the environment (e.g., "Is your school a safe environment?"). This type of qualitative information may be particularly valuable in relation to aspects of child behavior that occur infrequently or covertly. Third, self-report measures permit the assessment of a broad and dissimilar range of behavioral domains. The diverse range of areas commonly contained on broadband self-report measures identifies dimensions of behavior, such as abuse or fears, which may not be typically addressed with other types of direct or indirect assessment methods. The identification of associated problem areas may direct additional assessment and treatment (Elliott, Busse, & Gresham, 1993). Fourth, self-report measures can be used as convergent sources of information within the context of a multimethod behavioral assessment (La Greca, 1990a). For example, data obtained from self-report measures can be compared with data from multiple informants to verify problem areas. Sixth, data obtained from self-report measures can be relevant to diagnostic and classification decisions. Because many self-report measures include normative data, significant deviations of self-reported behavior from the normative sample can be established. This, in turn, may explain the high prevalence of use among school-based practitioners (Stinnett, Havey, & Oehler-Stinnett, 1994). Seventh, there has been an increased emphasis in using data obtained from self-report measures in the treatment of childhood behavior problems. There have been a number of studies demonstrating that self-perceptions can mediate behavior and therefore should be used as targets for treatment (Mash & Terdal, 1997). In addition, self-report measures can be used to assess treatment effects and obtain data regarding the social validity of treatment and treatment effects. Finally, self-report measures are relatively inexpensive, easy to administer, readily quantifiable, and less obtrusive than other assessment techniques.

Considerations in the Use of Self-Report Measures

Although the use of self-report measures is considered an important component of behavioral assessment (Kratochwill, Sheridan, Carlson, & Lasecki, 1999; McConaughy & Ritter, 1995), there are a number of considerations that need to be recognized. First, a number of factors may influence respondents' reporting on self-report measures. These factors can include developmental issues, environmental influences, and demographic mediators (e.g., gender, ethnicity). Second, the correspondence between self-report measures and other measures, including direct observation and informant reports, can be equivocal. Third, a number of ethical issues need to be considered when using self-report measures.

Developmental Influences Relevant to Self-Report Measures

A number of developmental influences need to be considered when using self-report measures with children and adolescents. First, the child's language and reading skills need to be considered within the context of the assessment (Reynolds, 1993). Children who have limited reading abilities may require assistance completing self-report measures independently. Likewise, self-report measures with high readability indices may be inappropriate for young children. It has been recommended that self-report instruments be presented orally to young children (i.e., preschool) and elementary-aged children (Reynolds, 1993; Stone & LeManek, 1990). In a recent study, Walters and Merrell (1995) compared written versus oral administration of a self-report measure to 139 students in grades 3 through 6. Results of this study did not demonstrate significant differences in responses based on the two administration procedures, suggesting that oral administration of self-report measures may not affect younger children's responses.

A second influence that is important to consider when using self-report measures is the language abilities of the child or adolescent. From a developmental perspective, the language development of children and adolescents varies significantly. Research examining the linguistic competencies of preschool-aged children suggests that understanding covert behaviors or multiple perspectives may be extremely difficult (Bierman, 1983). Preschool-aged children are more likely to respond accurately to material that is presented in simple, concrete terms whereas elementary-aged children are more likely to understand complex constructs, such as concept of self or sadness, and be able to make inferences about these psychological constructs (Bierman, 1983; Stone & LeManek, 1990). In addition, elementary-aged children are more likely to provide accurate descriptive information pertaining to their thoughts and feelings than younger children. Research has demonstrated that children with higher cognitive abilities are more accurate in their ability to differentiate emotions and feelings then children with lower cognitive abilities (Carroll & Steward, 1984). It becomes necessary to assess the child's language and cognitive competencies. Elementary-aged children may also have difficulty understanding social roles and this may impact their ability to accurately respond. Furthermore, preschool and elementary-aged children may experience difficulty responding to self-report response formats. For example, Mischel, Zeiss, and Zeiss (1974) demonstrated that younger children were more likely to respond in the affirmative when presented with dichotomous (e.g., yes, no) response formats. Crandall, Katkovsky, and Crandall (1965) suggested that young children may experience difficulty remembering alternatives in polychotomous response formats and may respond affirmatively to the last alternative presented. While adolescents with normal language development have a greater understanding of complex or abstract concepts and social roles (Bierman, 1983), adolescents with delayed language development may experience difficulty understanding complex concepts and responding to complex response formats (i.e., 7-point Likert-type scale).

In addition to reading and language considerations, it is important for school-based practitioners to assess the psychosocial development of the child or adolescent before administering self-report measures. Young children may experience difficulty verbalizing feelings because of shyness or temperance (Sattler, 1992). Similarly, elementary-aged children and adolescents may be reluctant to share information about themselves because of issues of self-consciousness (Sattler, 1992). Finally, the content of some self-report measures may require children or adolescents to evidence a higher level of psychosocial maturity (Reynolds, 1993). For example, items from the Youth Self-Report (Achenbach, 1991c) require adolescents to respond to issues of sexual activity, drug usage, and larceny. Adolescents with limited exposure to these types of behaviors may experience discomfort completing self-report measures containing this type of content.

Environmental Influences Relevant to Self-Report Measures

A number of environmental factors may influence children and adolescent's responses on self-report measures. First, young children may be influenced by immediate events (Bierman, 1983). That is, young children may react negatively to working with a stranger. Similarly, children's behavior may be under the control of parents or environmental conditions (Mash & Terdal, 1997). This may result in children responding in ways that are not commensurate with their thoughts, feelings, or behavior. Second, the level of motivation exhibited by the child or adolescent should be assessed (La Greca, 1990b). Children or adolescents who are not motivated to complete self-report measures may provide information that is not representative. Third, a variety of social factors may influence children's responses on self-report measures. Children or adolescents may respond to demand characteristics of the examiner (La Greca, 1990b) and present a favorable evaluation to impress the examiner. Likewise, self-report data may be falsified to avoid treatment or harm to peers (Glennon & Weiss, 1978). In addition, children's responses may fluctuate as a result of environmental or social conditions. Tharinger and Stark (1990) demonstrated significant fluctuation in children's self-report data as a function of changes in environmental and social conditions. Therefore, school-based practitioners may need to assess environmental, social, or motivational factors that may influence responding on self-report measures.

Use of Self-Report Measures with Specific Populations

Although very few studies have examined the extent to which data obtained from self-report measures vary based on the type of population assessed, it has been suggested that gender, cultural, and developmental factors may influence responding (La Greca, 1990b; Mash & Terdal, 1997). In addition, the standardization sample of self-report measures should be closely examined to determine the applicability of using the measure with a specified population (La Greca, 1990b). If a self-report measure does not include a specific population in the standardization sample (i.e., ethnic group, special needs group), then it is inappropriate and invalid to use this measure with the population. Research investigating response differences based on specific populations has focused primarily on demographic factors such as gender. A number of epidemiological studies have demonstrated that prevalence rates and manifestations of behavior disorders will differ based on gender (Achenbach, 1993; Kavanagh & Hops, 1994; Zahn-Waxler, 1993; Zoccolillo, 1993). Furthermore, if a self-report measure has not been standardized with a specific population, then the content and format may not be appropriate for the population in question. For example, self-report measures that do not include children with developmental disabilities or learning disabilities in the standardization sample may experience difficulties responding to self-report measures.

Variance in Self-Report Measures of Internalizing and Externalizing Behaviors

An examination of the literature investigating the accuracy of children's and adolescent's self-report measures of internalizing and externalizing behaviors reveals some interesting findings. First, research suggests that children tend to underreport overt behaviors, such as hyperactivity, inattention, and oppositional behaviors (Christensen, Margolin, & Sullaway, 1992; Edelbrock, Costello, Dulcan, Conover, & Kalas, 1986; Landau, Milich, & Widiger, 1991; Loeber, Green, Lahey, & Stouthamer-Loeber, 1989; Reich & Earls, 1987). Second, children tend to be accurate reporters of covert behaviors, such as depression and anxiety (Klein, 1991; La Greca, 1990a; Loeber et al., 1989; Shain, Naylor, & Alessi, 1990). This finding corresponds with many theories of externalizing disorders that emphasize the role of cognitive processes in emotional and behavioral disorders (Beck, 1971; Reiss, 1987). Although some evidence exists suggesting that children may overreport internalizing symptoms (Angold et al., 1987; Earls, Smith, Reich, & Jung, 1988; Herjanic & Reich, 1982; Reich & Earls, 1987), it has been recommended that child-report data be collected for assessing internalizing symptoms (Kazdin, 1989) and parent- or teacher-report data be collected for assessing externalizing symptoms (Loeber et al., 1989).

Ethical Concerns

A number of ethical concerns need to be considered when using self-report measures with children and adolescents. First, the psychometric properties of any self-report scale need to be evaluated. Areas that should be examined include the reliability and validity of the measure, the adequacy of the standardization sample, the relevancy of the standardization sample to the respondent, and the timeliness of the measure (Breen, Eckert, & DuPaul, 1996). Second, the emotional effects of completing self-report measures on children and adolescents need to be considered. As mentioned previously, young children or children with limited psychosocial maturity may experience negative emotional or physiological responses. Although no empirical data have supported a link between respondents experiencing negative affectivity and completing self-report measures, the emotional impact should nevertheless be considered by school-based practitioners (Koocher, 1993). Third, at-risk children may be identified as a result of the assessment process. Therefore, it becomes crucial that school-based practitioners adopt strategies for assisting at-risk children and adolescents once they have been identified. Finally, issues of confidentiality need to be addressed with children and adolescents prior to the completion of self-report measures (La Greca, 1990b). From an ethical and legal standpoint, it is important that school-based practitioners make children and adolescents aware of the limits of confidentiality in association with self-report measures (Jacob-Timm & Hartshorne, 1994).

SELF-REPORT MEASURES FOR ASSESSING BROADBAND BEHAVIOR PROBLEMS

A number of broadband self-report measures have been developed to provide an empirical basis for identifying children and adolescent's behavioral problems. These measures allow children and adolescents to report the number and intensity of features across a number of syndromes (Achenbach & McConaughy, 1987). Data obtained from broadband self-report measures allow school-based practitioners to quantify the degree to which each syndrome is manifested.

Broadband Measures: Internalizing and Externalizing Disorders

The Youth Self-Report (YSR; Achenbach, 1991c) was designed to identify syndromes of internalizing and externalizing problem behaviors as well as assess adolescents' judgments of social and activity competencies. The YSR was developed as part of a class of empirically based assessment tools that include the Child Behavior Checklist for Ages 2–3 (CBCL/2-3; Achenbach, 1992), the Child Behavior Checklist for Ages 4–18 (CBCL/4-18; Achenbach, 1991a), and the Teacher Report Form (TRF; Achenbach, 1991b). These measures can be used as part of a multiaxail assessment to illustrate possible discrepancies between children's and adolescents' views of their functioning with assessment information obtained from parents and teachers (Achenbach & McConaughy, 1987; McConaughy, 1993). The YSR can be used in a variety of applications including mental health, school, forensic, and medical settings (Achenbach, 1991c).

The YSR was intended for persons aged 11–18 years who demonstrate a fifth-grade reading level. However, the YSR can be read orally to individuals with limited reading proficiency. There are two primary scales measured on the YSR, the total competence scale and the total problem behavior scale. The competence scale contains 17 items that require respondents to rate themselves compared to peers on various activities and social behaviors. Three scaled scores are obtained and include: Activities, Social, and Total Competency. The problem behavior scale includes a total of 119 items, sixteen of which are socially desirable items that are not included in the total problem behavior score. Responses for the problem behavior scale describe a behavior that has occurred within the last six months and are recorded on a 3-point Likert-type scale where 0 = not true, 1 = somewhat or sometimes true, and 2 = very true or often true. In addition, several items on the problem behavior scale provide space for the respondent to clarify the nature of the problem. The problem behavior scale assesses two broadband domains: Internalizing and Externalizing problem behaviors. From these broadband domains, eight cross-informant scales were produced with similar problem dimensions for both males, females, and across all ages. These dimensions include: Aggressive Behavior, Anxious/Depressed, Attention Problems, Delinquent Behavior, Social Problems, Somatic Complaints, Thought Problems, and Withdrawn. The Internalizing problem domain is composed of the Withdrawal, Somatic Complaints, and Anxious/Depressed scales, whereas the Externalizing problem domain includes the Delinquent and Aggressive Behavior scales.

The normative sample of the YSR included 1,315 youths selected from 48 states with respect to ethnicity, socioeconomic status, region, and locale of residence. The normative sample included youths between the ages of 11 and 18 who were not receiving mental health services or remediation within the previous year. To derive the clinical sample, youths referred for mental health services were identified in 26 different settings. The clinical sample included a total of 1,272 youths across a wide distribution of socioeconomic and demographic characteristics.

The reliability of the YSR has been examined over short-term and long-term intervals. Across a seven-day interval, the mean test–retest reliability coefficients on the competence scale was .68 for adolescents ages 11–14, and .82 for adolescents ages 15–18. On the total problem behavior scale, the reliability coefficients for was .70 for youths ages 11–14 and .91 for youths ages 15–18. In a sample of youths ages 11–14, the mean stability coefficient over a seven-month period for the competence scale was .50 and for the problem scales was .49. A longitudinal study examining the long-term stability of the YSR as well as the CBCL/4-18 and TRF demonstrated significant predictive correlations between self-, parent, and teacher ratings across a three-year period (McConaughy, Stanger, & Achenbach, 1992).

Evidence for content and criterion-related validity is presented in the manual (Achenbach, 1991c). Content validity was demonstrated by the discrimination between demographically matched referred and nonreferred youths on the YSR items. Criterion-related validity was supported by the ability of the YSR to discriminate between referred and nonreferred youths after demographic effects were controlled. Additionally, clinical cutpoints have discriminated significantly between demographically matched referred and nonreferred youths.

Another broadband measure of internalizing and externalizing disorders is the Behavior Assessment System for Children (BASC; Reynolds & Kamphaus, 1992). The BASC is a multimethod assessment approach designed to aid in the diagnosis, educational classification, and treatment of emotional and behavioral disorders in children. The Self-Report of Personality (SRP) is one component of this integrated system (other components are: Teacher Rating Scales (TRS), Parent Rating Scales (PRS), Structured Developmental History (SDH), and Student Observation System (SOS)), which assesses children's emotions and self-perceptions. The SRP is a comprehensive personality inventory composed of adaptive and clinical scales that review and quantify children's thoughts, feelings, and perceptions. The clinical scales measure maladjustment and the adaptive scales measure positive adjustment. The SRP consists of positively and negatively worded statements that the child responds to as True or False. These items comprise ten clinical and four adaptive scales of the SRP. The clinical scales include: Anxiety, Attitude to School, Attitude to Teacher, Atypicality, Depression, Locus of Control, Sense of Inadequacy, and Social Stress. The two additional clinical scales, Sensation Seeking and Somatization, are only available for the adolescent form of the SRP. The adaptive scales include: Interpersonal Relations, Relations with Parents, Self-Esteem, and Self-Reliance.

The SRP includes separate forms for children (8–11 years) and adolescents (12–18 years). The two forms are similar in their scales, structure, and items. Both forms of the SRP include validity indexes that assess the quality of child and adolescent responses. The F index is designed to detect respondents who are trying to "fake bad." The V index identifies students who may have provided unusual answers because of poor reading comprehension, failure to follow directions, or poor contact with reality. The adolescent form also has an L index for identifying students who are attempting to "fake good."

The SRP was standardized on 9,861 children from four regions of the United States and offers examiners a choice of four norming samples: (1) General, (2) Male, (3) Female, and (4) Clinical. The General norms are based on a national sample that are considered representative of the general population of children with respect to sex, race/ethnicity, and clinical or special education classification. Psychometric data for the SRP is contained in the manual (Reynolds & Kamphaus, 1992). The manual reports two types of reliability (i.e., internal consistency and test–retest) for the scales and composites. Internal consistencies of the various scales of the SRP are high, averaging .80 at both age levels (child and adolescent). Composite score reliabilities are also very high, ranging from .87 to .96. In addition, the SRP shows high test–retest reliability with the median value for the scales being .76 at each age level. Test–retest reliabilities for the composites range from .78 to .84. Furthermore, the temporal stability of the instrument was assessed across a seven-month period. The SRP demonstrates a fair degree of stability with a median scale correlation of .51.

The manual presents several types of evidence about the validity of the SRP. The content validity of the measure is supported by a study comparing the SRP scales with scales created by expert judges. A group of clinical psychologists divided items from the SRP into categories representing various forms of adolescent psychopathology. The scales created by the expert judges correlated highly with the SRP (adolescent form) scales. In addition, the construct validity of the SRP was established by correlating the measure with the following instruments: Minnesota Multiphasic Personality Inventory (MMPI; Hathaway & McKinley, 1970), the Youth Self-Report (YSR; Achenbach, 1991c), the Behavior Rating Profile (BRP; Brown & Hammill, 1983), and the Children's Personality Questionnaire (CPQ; Porter & Cattell, 1975). The first three instruments show a number of high correlations with SRP scales, offering support for the construct validity of the SRP. The CPQ, which, unlike the other instruments, focuses on normal-range personality, correlates at a lower level with the SRP.

Broadband Measures: Internalizing Disorders

The Internalizing Symptoms Scale for Children (ISSC; Merrell & Walters, 1996) is a broadband, self-report measure of internalizing disorders for children in grades 3 through 6. The ISSC contains 48 items that examine the presence of internalizing disorders including depression, anxiety, social withdrawal, and somatic complaints. Items are rated on a 4-point Likert-type scale that ranges from never true to often true. Items provide information pertaining to two subscales: (1) Negative Affect/General Distress; and (2) Positive Affect. Item content is varied, wherein a majority of the items are worded in a manner indicative of the presence of an internalizing disorder and the remaining items are worded in a manner indicative of the absence of an internalizing disorder. Sample items of negatively worded statements include: "I am shy," "I worry that I will hurt someone," and "Lots of things scare me." Sample items of positively worded items include "I feel important" and "I feel happy."

A large national standardization of the ISSC is ongoing, with the first standardization sample consisting of over 1,700 children in grades 3 through 6 (Merrell, Crowley, & Walters, 1997). Respondents were sampled from five states representing northeast, northwest, and midwest geographical regions. An equal number of males and females participated in the standardization sample. The ethnicity of the standardization sample included respondents of European-American ancestry (i.e., 79%) and respondents of ethnic minority groups (i.e., 21%).

Reliability and validity information are provided in the technical manual (Merrell & Walters, 1996), as well as in three studies examining the construct validity of the scale (Merrell & Dobmeyer, 1996; Merrell, Gill, McFarland, & McFarland, 1996; Sanders 1996) and one study examining the convergent validity of the scale

(Merrell, Anderson, & Michael, 1997). The internal consistency of the ISSC Total Score was .92. The test–retest reliability of the ISSC Total Score was .86 over a two-week interval, .76 at a four-week interval, and .74 at a twelve-week interval (Michael, 1997). The construct validity of the scale has been established by examining gender differences of self-reported internalizing symptoms (Merrell & Dobmeyer, 1996). Results of this study indicated that the ISSC was accurate in predicting the gender of respondents. In addition, the social and emotional difficulties among students identified as gifted and talented has been examined using the ISSC (Merrell, Gill, McFarland, & McFarland, 1996). Results of this comparative validity study indicated that gifted-and-talented students exhibited significantly lower levels of internalizing symptoms in comparison to nongifted peers. Furthermore, the convergent validity of the scale was demonstrated by correlating the ISSC with the Youth Self-Report (Achenbach, 1991c), Children's Depression Inventory (Kovacs, 1992), and Revised Children's Manifest Anxiety Scale (Reynolds & Richmond, 1985; Merrell, Anderson, & Michael, 1997). Strong to moderate correlation coefficients were found across all three measures, (range, .75 to .86). Furthermore, the factor structure of the scale has been examined using exploratory and confirmatory factor analytic approaches (Merrell, Crowley, & Walters, 1997). Results of this study suggested a two-factor model assessing Negative Affect/General Distress and Positive Affect.

SELF-REPORT MEASURES FOR SPECIFIC INTERNALIZING BEHAVIOR PROBLEMS

Anxiety and Related Disorders

The assessment of anxiety and related disorders relies heavily on self-report measures for a number of reasons. First, anxiety and related disorders represent a broad domain of child and adolescent problems that may occur as part of the normal developmental process (Morris & Kratochwill, 1991). To differentiate pathological anxiety and related disorders from normal symptoms experienced by children and adolescents, self-report measures may be the only viable mechanisms for quantification. Second, a number of longitudinal and cross-sectional comorbities are unique to children and adolescents (Stallings & Marsh, 1995). Third, environment-specific factors may influence the presentation of specific anxieties, such as school phobia, among this population.

Most of the self-report measures of anxiety assess relatively stable symptom clusters across multiple domains or specific dimensions of anxiety. Although in theory many of these measures can be classified across state-versus-trait or global-versus-situation-specific dimensions (Roberts, Vargo, & Ferguson, 1989), this dichotomy has not been well supported in the literature (Stallings & March, 1995). For the purposes of this review, we will review a measure that is considered to be multidomain measures of anxiety.

Multidimensional Anxiety Scale for Children

The Multidimensional Anxiety Scale for Children (MASC; March, 1997) is a multidimensional self-report measure of anxiety. The MASC contains 39 items and is composed of two major indexes (i.e., Anxiety Disorders Index, Inconsistency Index) and a scale measuring total anxiety (i.e., Total Anxiety Scale). In addition, major factors and associated subscales of the MASC include the Physical Symptoms Scale (subdivided into the Tense Symptoms and Somatic Symptoms subscales), the Harm Avoidance Scale (subdivided into the Perfectionism and Anxious Coping subscales), and the Social Anxiety Scale (subdivided into the Humiliation Fears and Performance Fears subscales). Furthermore, a separate form containing ten items, the MASC-10, can be used in the assessment of general anxiety symptoms. Items on the MASC are rated on a 4-point Likert-type scale that ranges from 0 (never true about me) to 3 (often true about me). All items are positively phrased to minimize variance in responding. Examples of items include "I feel tense or uptight," "I get shaky or jittery," and "I stay away from things that upset me." A readability index of the MASC indicates that comprehension of item content requires a fourth-grade reading level.

The MASC was standardized on a sample of 2,698 children and adolescents between the ages of 8 and 19 years. All students participating in the normative sample were enrolled in general education classes. An attempt was made to obtain a normative sample that included a broad range of demographic variables. However, in comparison to the most recent United States census data, the author reports that the normative sample was more likely to live in poverty and less likely to graduate from high school. Separate normative data are provided for gender and age.

The reliability of the MASC was examined in terms of internal consistency and test–retest reliability (March, 1997). The internal consistency of the MASC scales and subscales was examined by age and gender, with coefficients ranging from .46 to .89. The test–retest reliability of the MASC was examined with a small sample of children across a 3-month period (March, Parker, Sullivan, Stallings, & Conners, 1997). Test–retest reliability coefficients ranged from .70 to .93 across the MASC scales. The validity of the MASC was examined in terms of factorial validity, discriminant validity, and construct validity (March, 1997). The results of a four-factor confirmatory factor analysis suggested that the model had adequate fit in both clinical and nonclinical samples, however, specific indices were not presented in the manual. The discriminant validity of the MASC was examined with a moderate sample of children diagnosed with an anxiety disorder and a nonclinical sample of children. Results of this analysis suggested that the correct classification rate of the MASC was 87%. The content validity of the scale was examined by comparing ratings on the MASC with other self-report measures of anxiety and depression. Moderate to high correlations were found with the Revised Children's Manifest Anxiety Scale (RCMAS; Reynolds & Richmond, 1985); however, moderate to low correlations were found with the Children's Depression Inventory—Short (CDI-S; Kovacs, 1992).

Depression

The most commonly used measures of depression in children and adolescents are self-reports (Curry & Craighead, 1993). In part, this is attributable to a number of internal and environmental factors that may not be readily observable. In addition, depression in children and adolescents may be associated with few behavioral correlates because of the subjective nature of key symptoms of depression, such as feeling of sadness, worthlessness, and despair (Compass, 1997). Childhood and adolescent depression has been conceptualized as a cluster of symptoms, with little empirical support documenting which symptoms constitute a valid syndrome of depression (Reynolds, 1994). Therefore, depression in children and adolescents is currently viewed as a constellation of symptoms that may vary in terms of severity and syndromal forms. Although most of the self-report measures of depression include central symptoms of depression (Reynolds, 1994), there is evidence suggesting that these measures may not be able to distinguish depression from other general negative emotions (Saylor, Finch, Baskin, Furey, & Kelly, 1984; Wolfe, Finch, Saylor, Blount, Pallmeyer, & Carek, 1987).

The comorbidity of depression and other behavior disorders is relatively high. A number of studies have reported the comorbidity of depression with internalizing disorders such as anxiety (Alessi & Magen, 1988; Finch, Lipovsky, & Casat, 1989; Kovacs, 1990; Strauss, Last, Hersen, & Kazdin, 1988) and eating disorders (Alessi, Krahn, Brehm, & Wittekindt, 1989). In addition, a number of students have documented that depression coexists with externalizing disorders such as attention-deficit/hyperactivity disorder (ADHD) (Alessi & Magen, 1988; Anderson, Williams, McGee, & Silva, 1987; Jensen, Burke, & Garfinkel, 1988), conduct disorder (Alessi & Magen, 1988; Kovacs, Paulauskas, Gastonis, & Richards, 1988; Puig-Antich, 1982), and substance abuse (Akiskal, Downs, Jordan, Watson, Daugherty, & Pruitt, 1985; Kashini, Keller, Solmon, Reid, & Mazzola, 1985; Levy & Deykin, 1989). Furthermore, while the relationship between suicide and depression may be equivocal, there is some evidence suggesting that suicidal behavior may be associated with depression (Reynolds, 1994). Examining the presence of comorbidity in related behavioral disorders is important, given preliminary evidence suggesting that depressed children and adolescents with comorbid disorders increases the potential for long-term mental health problems (Kovacs, 1990).

Children's Depressive Inventory and
Children's Depressive Inventory—Short Form

Originally adapted from the Beck Depression Inventory (Beck, Ward, Mendelson, Mock, & Erbaugh, 1961), the Children's Depressive Inventory (CDI; Kovacs, 1981; 1992) and the more recently developed Children's Depression Inventory—Short Form (CDI-S; Kovacs, 1992) were designed to measure symptoms of depression in children and adolescents ranging in age from 7 to 17. The CDI, which is composed of 27 items, is purported to measure five factors including (1) Negative Mood,

(2) Interpersonal Problems, (3) Ineffectiveness, (4) Anhedonia, and (5) Negative Self-Esteem. In contrast, the CDI-S, which contains 10 items, does not contain factor subscales. Items on the CDI and the CDI-S are structured so that the child or adolescent is presented with three alternative statements. The respondent must choose the statement that characterizes his or her behavior or attitudes within the last two weeks. For example, the child or adolescent may be presented with statements such as, "I have plenty of friends," "I have some friends but I wish I had more," and "I do not have any friends." Responses to items are scored on a scale of 0 to 2, with higher scores indicating more depressive-like symptoms.

The CDI and the CDI-S were standardized on a sample of 1,266 boys and girls (Kovacs, 1992). Although the sample was composed of individuals from a variety of ethnicities and socioeconomic backgrounds, the majority (77%) were Caucasian and of middle socioeconomic status. In addition, no comparison was made between the sample and census data. As a result, the generalizability of the CDI and the CDI-S is questionable.

The majority of evidence pertaining to reliability and validity of the CDI and CDI-S are relevant only to the CDI (Kazdin, French, Unis, Esveldt-Dawson, & Sherick, 1983; Kovacs, 1981; Saylor, Finch, Baskin, Furey, & Kelly, 1984; Saylor, Finch, Spirito, & Bennett, 1984). Reliability data of the CDI tends to range between adequate and moderate. Internal consistency coefficients and item–total score correlations as measured by Cronbach's alpha have been above .80. However, test–retest reliability coefficients have been in the moderate range, between .38 and .87 (Saylor, Finch, Spirito, & Bennett, 1984).

The concurrent validity of the CDI has been adequately established in numerous studies (Green, 1980; Weissman, Orvaschel, & Padian, 1980). Students' scores on the CDI correlated significantly ($r = .49$) when compared to the Hopelessness Scale for Children (Kazdin, Rodgers, & Colbus, 1986). In addition, a study of 349 eighth-grade students, suggested a significant correlation ($r = .79$) between scores on the CDI and scores on the Reynolds Adolescent Depression Scale (RADS; Reynolds, 1987) (Kahn, Kehle, Jenson, & Clark, 1990). Discriminative validity of both the CDI and the CDI-S has ranged from acceptable to equivocal (Hodges, 1990; Smith, Mitchell, McCauley, & Calderon, 1990; Wendel, Nelson, Politano, Mayhall, & Finch, 1988). Using the CDI, Wendel and colleagues (1988) noted that while 84% of respondents were correctly classified in a combined sample of children under psychiatric inpatient care and a normal control group, 100% of those under psychiatric care were incorrectly classified as normal.

Construct validity has been examined in several studies investigating the factor structure of the CDI (Helsel & Matson, 1984; Saylor, Finch, Spirito, & Bennett, 1984; Weiss & Weisz, 1988; Weiss, Weisz, Politano, Carey, Nelson, & Finch, 1991). Although the CDI manual indicates a five-factor model, most studies have suggested that a one-factor structure, reflecting depression in general, is most parsimonious. Furthermore, the CDI is one of the few self-report measures with demonstrated sensitivity to treatment. For example, a study by Garvin, Leber, and Kalter (1991) indicated a reduction in scores on the CDI following implementation of an intervention.

Reynolds Child Depression Scale and
Reynolds Adolescent Depression Scale

The Reynolds Child Depression Scale (RCDS; Reynolds, 1989) and the Reynolds Adolescent Depression Scale (RADS; Reynolds, 1987) were designed to assess depressive symptomology as outlined in the DSM-III in children between the ages of 8 to 12 and 13 to 18, respectively. Each scale contains 30 items rated on a 4-point Likert-type scale. Raw scores on the RCDS range from 30 to 121 and on the RADS from 30 to 120, with higher scores indicating more severe depression. Scores can be converted to percentiles calculated from the total standardization sample, as well as subsamples. In addition, clinical cutoff scores are suggested to identify students for whom further evaluation is recommended. Although the initial cutoff score was established at 74 (Reynolds,1989), more recent studies have suggested a cutoff score of 77 (Reynolds & Mazza, 1998).

The standardization sample of the RCDS included over 1,600 students who were heterogeneous with respect to age, gender, ethnicity, and socioeconomic status. In contrast, the RADS was normed on a sample of 2,460 adolescents from one geographical region. While the sample was heterogeneous with regard to race, gender, grade and, to some degree, socioeconomic status, it is important to note that both standardization samples were compared with 1977 U.S. census data.

Reliability data pertaining to the RCDS is adequate. Reynolds and Graves (1989) examined the test–retest reliability of 220 students over a four-week period and found an average correlation of .85. Test–retest coefficients over 6-week, 12-week, and one-year intervals have ranged from .63 (one-year) to .80 (6-week) (Reynolds, 1987). Internal consistency reliability has been examined with both split-half procedures and Cronbach's alpha coefficients. Split-half reliability coefficients have ranged from .88 to .92, and coefficient alphas for subsamples and total samples have ranged from .87 to .90 (Reynolds, 1989). Similarly, several studies have examined the technical adequacy of the RADS (Dalley, Bolocofsky, Alcorn, & Baker, 1992; Reynolds, 1987; Reynolds & Miller, 1989; Schonert-Reichl, 1994). Generally, reliability coefficients have been high, ranging from .91 to .96.

The validity of the RCDS has been established through a variety of means. Concurrent validity studies have demonstrated significant correlations between the RCDS and other depression rating scales such as the Children's Depression Rating Scale — Revised (Poznanski, Freeman, & Mokros, 1985). Moreover, the RCDS has been shown to correlate significantly with measures of self-esteem as well as anxiety (Reynolds, Anderson, & Bartell, 1985). In addition, the degree to which individual items reflect DSM-III classification criteria were calculated. The results of item–total correlations suggested that 24 of the 30 items correlated significantly. The construct validity of the RCDS has been examined through factor-analytic procedures. The results of the factor analysis support the five-factor model presented by Reynolds (1989). Furthermore, studies examining the utility of the RCDS to measure treatment effects suggest the RCDS is sensitive to changes in depression (Stark, Reynolds, & Kaslow, 1987).

Similar to the RCDS, several types of validity have been examined with respect to the RADS (Blumberg & Izard, 1986; Carey, Finch, & Carey, 1991; Reynolds, 1987; Shain, Naylor, & Alessi, 1990). Concurrent validity studies have suggested the RADS correlates significantly with several measures of depression. For example, in a study of 349 eighth-grade students, Kahn, Kehle, Jenson, and Clark (1990) found a significant correlation between student's scores on the RADS and scores on the Children's Depression Inventory (CDI; Kovacs, 1992). Similarly, Shain, Naylor, and Alessi (1990) found significant correlations between the RADS and the CDI for a sample of 45 adolescent inpatients diagnosed with major depression ($r = .87$). In addition, correlations between the RADS and clinical interviews such as the Hamilton Depression Rating Scale (HDRS; Hamilton, 1960) have also been demonstrated to be significant. Specifically, Reynolds (1987) examined the relationship between scores on the RADS and scores on the HDRS for a sample of 111 older adolescents and reported a correlation of .83.

The construct validity of the RADS has been examined through item–total correlations and factor analysis. Item–total correlations were calculated based on a sample of 2,296 adolescents, and were generally high, with most between .50 and .60. Although the results of the factor analysis did suggest a five-factor model, the majority of items loaded on the first factor, generalized demoralization. The remaining four factors were identified as despondency and worry, somatic vegetative, anhedonia, and self-worth (Reynolds, 1987). Studies examining the treatment sensitivity of the RADS have suggested it can be used as an outcome measure for evaluating treatments for depression (Hains, 1992; Kahn, Kehle, Jenson, & Clark, 1990; Reynolds & Coats, 1986).

Although the RADS was originally designed for use with students in grades 9 through 12, recently researchers have suggested its use with younger adolescents (Reynolds & Mazza, 1997). Reynolds and Mazza examined the reliability and validity of the RADS with a sample of ethnically diverse students from an inner-city school in grades 6 through 8. The study examined the internal consistency and test–retest reliability as well as the criterion-related validity of the RADS. In addition, the clinical screening efficacy of the RADS was examined by looking at sensitivity, specificity, and hit rates. The results of this study suggest the reliability of the RADS to be adequate when used with younger adolescents. Specifically, the internal consistency coefficient for the total sample was .93. Similarly, the test–retest reliability coefficient was .87 over a variable retest interval of one to five weeks. The criterion-related validity of the RADS with the HDRS was .76, with slightly higher correlations for females than males (.79 versus .72, respectively). Using a cutoff score of 77, the sensitivity of the RADS was 89%, that is, 89% of individuals were correctly classified as being depressed. The specificity of the RADS was 90%, suggesting 90% of those individuals not identified with depression according to the HDRS were not identified by the RADS. Therefore, the hit rate of the RADS, or the number of valid positives and valid negatives was 90%. However, the relatively low base rate of depression should be considered when interpreting these results. Although Reynolds and Mazza support the use of the RADS for screening young adolescents, they sound a cautionary note that a trend in over-identification does exist.

Peer Relationship and Social Skill Deficits

Difficulties with peer relations and social skills plays an integral role in the diagnosis of internalizing and externalizing behavior problems (Bierman & Welsch, 1997; Boivin, Hymel, & Bukowski, 1995). To date, only moderate correlations have been found between self-reports and informant reports of social relations (Ledingham, Younger, Schwartzman, & Bergeron, 1982). However, informant reports of social behavior may not be sensitive to critical events of social impact or relational difficulties that occur in restrictive settings (Foster & Ritchey, 1985). The extent to which informant reports (i.e., teachers, parents) accurately measure social behaviors occurring in restrictive settings is also unclear (Ruffalo & Elliott, 1997). For example, in a recent study examining teachers' and parents' ratings of children's social skills, Ruffalo and Elliott found moderate correlations between parents' ratings of their child's social behaviors. However, relatively weak correlations between parents' and teachers' ratings of children's social skills were observed. In addition, peer reports of social behavior may be misleading when information is obtained from opposite-genders (Landau & Milich, 1990). Because of the multifaceted nature of peer relations and social behavior, it has been recommended that assessment practices incorporate data from multiple sources, including self-report measures (Demaray et al., 1995; Merrell, 1998).

Social Skills Rating System

The Social Skills Rating System (SSRS; Gresham & Elliott, 1990) includes a self-report measure of social behavior as part of a comprehensive, multirater assessment package. The student form of the SSRS (SSRS-S) ranges from 34 to 39 items that can be used with children aged 3 through 17. Three separate instruments and norms are available for three developmental levels, and include preschool (ages 3 to 5), elementary level (grades K to 6), and secondary level (grades 7 to 12). Although three domains of social behavior are assessed by the SSRS (i.e., (1) Social Skills; (2) Problem Behaviors; (3) Academic Competence), only the Social Skills domain is assessed with the SSRS-S. Within the Social Skills domain, information pertaining to the teacher and peer relations is obtained using two types of ratings: frequency ratings and social behavior importance ratings. The frequency ratings assess how often a social behavior occurs on a 3-point Likert-type scale (never, sometimes, or very often). The importance ratings assess how important a behavior is perceived for social development on a 3-point Likert-type scale (not important, important, critical) and is only completed by adolescents aged 12 to 17. Using these item response formats, four subscales of social behavior can be measured and include: (1) Cooperation; (2) Assertion; (3) Self-Control; and (4) Empathy. Examples of items constituting the Social Skills domain includes, "Uses time appropriately while waiting for help," "Appropriately questions rules that may be unfair," and "Responds appropriately to peer teasing."

The SSRS was standardized on a sample of 4,170 children from grades 3 to 10 as well as smaller samples of preschool children ($n = 200$) and students in grades 11 and 12 (*n* = 124). Of the total sample, 83% were general-education students and 17% were special-education students. Although attempts were made to approximate national demographic characteristics, the standardization sample contains an over-representation of Caucasian (73%) and African American (18%) children as well as an underrepresentation of Hispanic/Latino (6%) children. Normative data are available for age, grade level, gender, and type of disability.

Reliability and validity information of the SSRS are reported in the manual as well as two studies examining the factor structure (Clark, Gresham, & Elliott, 1985; Gresham, Elliott, & Black, 1987) and two studies examining the construct validity (Chewning, 1992; Stinnett, Oehler-Stinnett, & Stout, 1989). Internal consistency for the Social Skills domain of the SSRS-S was .83. The test–retest reliability coefficient was .68 across a four-week interval. Interrater agreement between parents and children resulted in a coefficient of .24. While this coefficient is relatively low, the SSRS-S interrater reliability coefficient is slightly higher than other cross-informant measures (e.g., Achenbach, McConaughy, & Howell, 1987). Evidence of the criterion-related and construct validity was established by obtaining high correlations between the SSRS and other social behavior rating scales such as the Social Behavior Assessment (Stephens, 1978), the Piers–Harris Self-Concept Scale (Piers, 1984) the Walker–McConnell Scale of Social Competence and School Adjustment (Walker & McConnell, 1988) and the CBCL/4–18 (Achenbach, 1991a). The construct validity of the SSRS was investigated by examining developmental changes, gender differences, and group separation of the normative sample and are reported in the manual.

Assessment of Interpersonal Relations

One of the few self-report measures of interpersonal relations is the Assessment of Interpersonal Relations (AIR; Bracken & Kelley, 1993). This scale was developed to assess children's and adolescent's interpersonal relations with peers, parents and teachers. The scale consists of five subscales (i.e., (1) Mother, (2) Father, (3) Male Peers, (4) Female Peers, (5) Teacher) that assess the quality of interpersonal relations. Respondents are required to indicate the extent to which they agree with items related to interpersonal relationships and interpersonal situations on a 4-point Likert-type scale, ranging from strongly agree (4) to strongly disagree (1). Fifteen relationship characteristics are measured by the AIR and include: (1) companionship, (2) emotional support, (3) guidance, (4) emotional comfort, (5) reliance, (6) trust, (7) understanding, (8) conflict, (9) identity, (10) respect, (11) empathy, (12) intimacy, (13) affect, (14) acceptance, and (15) shared values. Furthermore, a total scale score, the Total Relationship Index (TRI), can be computed by summing the total item responses across the five subscales.

The AIR was standardized on a sample of approximately 2,500 children and adolescents between the ages of 9 and 19 years. The authors note that attempts were made to approximate national demographic characteristics with regard to gender, ethnicity, and family characteristics (Bracken & Kelley, 1993). The standardization sample included children and adolescents from 17 school sites across the four geographic regions of the United States.

Reliability and validity of the AIR are reported in the manual (Bracken & Kelley, 1993). Internal consistency coefficients for the five subscales and the TRI ranged from .93 to .96. Across a two-week period, the test–retest reliability coefficients of the five subscales of the AIR and the TRI ranged from .94 to .98.

Evidence for the discriminative validity of the AIR was established by correlating the measure with the Multidimensional Self-Concept Scale (MCSC; Bracken, 1992). Moderate to high correlations were found for six of the subscales of the MCSC. In a separate study, the relationship characteristics of the AIR were found to significantly discriminate adolescent runaways from nonrunaways (Newman, 1996). Furthermore, the discriminant validity of the AIR was established by comparing clinical and nonclinical adolescents (Kelley, 1990). Results of this study suggested that in comparison to nonclinical adolescents, adolescents attending an inpatient psychiatric center reported significantly lower interpersonal relations on all five subscales of the AIR.

Self-Concept

Self-concept is viewed as a critical variable related to an individual's social-emotional adjustment (Crain & Bracken, 1994). Many researchers have conceptualized that self-concept may serve as a moderator variable in relation to psychological or educational outcomes (Marsh, Barnes, & Hocevar, 1985; Shavelson, Hubner, & Stanton, 1976). Research has suggested that self-concept and associated variables (i.e., self-esteem) may serve as a protective factor in the onset of depression (Moran & Eckenrode, 1992) and substance abuse (Callahan & Jackson, 1986; Dielman, Leech, Lorenger, & Horvath, 1984; Thompson, 1989). In addition, self-concept has been identified as a factor related to social relationship problems (Bierman & Welsch, 1997). Although very few empirical studies have examined this relationship, there is some evidence to suggest that popular and rejected children differ in ratings of self-concept (Jackson & Bracken, 1998).

While self-report instruments for assessing global self-concept have a long-standing history (Coopersmith, 1967; Harter, 1983; Piers & Harris, 1963), recent research has proposed theoretical models of self-concept that are multifaceted and hierarchical in nature (Byrne, 1988; Marsh, 1990; Wigfield & Karpathian, 1991). These models are based on factor-analytic studies of self-concept measures as well as structural models related to other variables, such as achievement (Strein, 1993). However, this work runs counter to generalized models of self-concept, wherein self-concept is defined as a global trait. To date, little research has supported a generalized, global model of self-concept (Strein, 1993; Wigfield & Karpathian, 1991). Furthermore, research has demonstrated that domain-specific self-concept treatments may result in greater changes in self-concept than global treatments (Craven, Marsh, & Delous, 1991).

Multidimensional Self-Concept Scale

Based on the notion that self-concept is organized, multifaceted, hierarchical, stable, developmental, evaluative, and differentiable, Bracken developed the Multidimensional Self-Concept Scale (MSCS; Bracken, 1992). The MSCS, which is composed of 150 items, was designed to measure self-concept in children between the ages of 9 and 19. The self-report scale assesses global self-concept as well as six subscales of self-concept, including: (1) Social, (2) Competence, (3) Affect, (4) Academic, (5) Family, and (6) Physical, which contribute to an overall construct of self-concept. These six factors were developed conceptually and were not based on factor-analytic procedures. However, Bracken (1992) suggests that each 25-item subscale can be administered and interpreted in isolation. Items on the MSCS are constructed as statements such as, "Sometimes I feel worthless." Students are asked to rate their agreement with these statements on a scale of 1 to 4, where 1 indicates strongly disagree and 4 indicates strongly agree. Several of the items are reverse-scored, and a higher score indicates a more positive self-concept.

The standardization sample of the MSCS included 2,501 students in grades five through twelve (Bracken, 1992). The sample is consistent, according to gender and ethnicity, with the U.S. Census Bureau estimates. Because raw scores did not differ significantly with respect to age, gender, and ethnicity, only general norms are provided. In addition, a recent study examined the extent to which the MSCS could be used with children in third and fourth grades (Wilson, 1998). The results of this study suggested that the MSCS could be used with younger children. However, only the norms for the Academic and Physical subscales are applicable with this younger group of children.

Several studies have examined the reliability and validity of the MSCS (Bracken, 1992; Bracken & Mills, 1994; Crain & Bracken, 1994; Delugach, Bracken, Bracken, & Schicke, 1992). Bracken (1992) examined the test–retest reliability of 37 eighth-grade students over a four-week interval and found correlation coefficients to range between .73 and .81. Internal consistency studies, as measured by Cronbach's coefficient alpha across gender and grade, have produced coefficients between .85 and .97 for the MSCS subscales and .97 to .99 for the total score (Bracken, 1992).

The discriminant validity of the MSCS was examined by comparing the subscales of the MSCS to the Assessment of Interpersonal Relations (AIR; Bracken & Kelley, 1993). Results of this study indicate that predictions about the relationship between the two scales, based on item content, were confirmed. Correlations between the MSCS and other measures of self-concept, such as the Piers–Harris Children's Self-Concept Scale (Piers, 1984) and the Coopersmith Self-Esteem Inventory (Coopersmith, 1959), have ranged between .69 and .83, suggesting the MSCS has adequate criterion-related validity. Although a factor analysis of the MSCS was not conducted during the development of the measure, studies examining the factor structure have confirmed the presence of a six-factor model (Bracken, Bunch, Keith, & Keith, 1992; Keith & Bracken, 1994). In addition, Tansy and Miller (1997) conducted a confirmatory factor analysis using both Caucasian and Latino American students and found the factor structure to be consistent with that suggested by Bracken (1992) for both groups of students. Furthermore, domain-specific subscales of the MSCS have been found to discriminate student social status (Jackson & Bracken, 1998).

Piers–Harris Children's Self-Concept Scale

The Piers–Harris Children's Self-Concept Scale (PHCSCS; Piers, 1984) was designed to assess students' self-esteem with respect to several factors. The 80-item scale, developed for use with students between the ages of 8 and 18, measures six factors of self-esteem including (1) Behavior, (2) Intellectual and School Status, (3) Physical Appearance and Attributes, (4) Anxiety, (5) Popularity, and (6) Happiness and Satisfaction. Items on the PHCSCS are presented as declarative statements to which the student must reply on a binary scale (i.e., "yes", "no"). For example, the student may be asked to reply to such statements as, "My friends like my ideas," or "I am unhappy." Responses are scored on a binary scale (0–1); however, several items are reverse-keyed. A higher score on the PHCSCS represents a more positive self-concept.

A total of 1,183 students in grades 4 through 12 were included in the standardization sample. All students came from a single district in Pennsylvania, and no gender information is provided. Cluster scales were standardized on a sample of 485 public-school students (248 girls, 237 boys) in grades 4 through 12. Although one investigation examined the validity of using the PHCSCS with a small sample of third grade students, the results indicated that over half of the items were misinterpreted by the students who were asked to verbally explain the items. Therefore, practitioners should exercise caution when administering the PHCSCS to younger students. Because of the limited information regarding the total and cluster standardization samples, as well as their failure to represent the population as a whole, Piers (1984) recommends generating local norms in order to ensure representativeness.

Reliability and validity data pertaining to the PHCSCS is adequate (Piers, 1984; Guiton & Zachary, 1984; Mannarino, 1978; Coopersmith, 1959; Marx & Winne, 1978). Test–retest coefficients of the total test score ranged between .42 and .96 (median = .73) with intervals between testing ranging from two weeks to one year (Piers, 1984). Although the internal consistency coefficients of the total score, as measured by Cronbach's coefficient alpha is high (i.e., .90), internal consistency coefficients for cluster scales are slightly lower, ranging from .73 to .81 (Piers, 1984).

The validity of the PHCSCS has been examined in a number of studies (Piers, 1984). Mannarino (1978) conducted a study in which the PHCSCS was shown to discriminate between students who were involved in "chum" relationships and students who were not. In addition, concurrent validity studies have found significant correlations between the PHCSCS and a number of self-concept measures (Piers, 1984). Correlations between the PHCSCS total score and other self-concept measures have ranged from .32 to .85 (Piers, 1984). Several studies have also examined the discriminative and concurrent validity of the cluster scores (Moller & Schnurr, 1995; Marx & Winne, 1978; Winne, Marx, & Taylor, 1977). For example, Moller and Schnurr (1995) demonstrated a relationship between the physical attractiveness and attributes (PAA) scale of the PHCSCS and the Harter Self-Perception Profile (Harter, 1985). However, studies examining the discriminative validity of the PHCSCS have found indeterminate results (Marx & Winne, 1978; Winne, Marx, & Taylor, 1977).

In addition to concurrent and discriminative validity, the construct validity of the PHCSCS has been examined in studies subjecting the measure to factor analysis (Piers, 1984). However, the results of such studies have been equivocal. Therefore, caution should be used when interpreting cluster scores. Treatment validity studies have demonstrated an increase in PHCSCS scores of students undergoing a number of types of treatment to increase (Piers, 1984). Specifically, the PHCSCS is sensitive to the effects of cognitive–behavioral training in self-control strategies (Kendall & Braswell, 1982). In contrast, scores on the PHCSCS do not appear to be sensitive to the effects of imipramine (Werry, Aman, & Diamond, 1980).

SELF-REPORT MEASURES FOR SPECIFIC EXTERNALIZING BEHAVIOR PROBLEMS

Attention and Concentration Problems

Relatively few self-report measures of attention and concentration problems have been developed for use with children and adolescents. This is largely because of the research demonstrating low correspondence between self-report data and externalizing behaviors (Landau, Milich, & Widiger, 1991). However, several recent advances in the field of attention and concentration problems suggest that it may be important to obtain self-report data. First, because of the high comorbidity between attention-deficit/hyperactivity disorder (ADHD) and internalizing disorders, such as depression and anxiety (Biederman & Steingard, 1989; Biederman, Newcorn, & Sprich, 1991; Milberger, Biederman, Faraone, Murphy, & Tsuang, 1995), it has been suggested that an assessment of behaviors related to ADHD should examine the presence of self-reported internalizing symptoms (DuPaul & Hoff, 1998) and may be pertinent to the diagnosis of comorbid disorders (Hinshaw, 1994). Second, there is some evidence suggesting that self-report measures of behaviors related to ADHD may be better predictors of observed behaviors than maternal reports (Loney, Volpe, & Ye, 1998; Volpe, Loney, & Salisbury, 1997). In addition, there are data suggesting that children who self-identify as exhibiting ADHD-related behaviors may experience higher levels of internalizing symptoms (i.e., depression, anxiety) than children who do not self-identify as exhibiting ADHD-related behaviors (Volpe, DuPaul, Loney, & Salisbury, in press).

Given these findings, it appears beneficial to assess attention and concentration problems in children and adolescents. Two self-report measures, the ADD-H Adolescent Self-Report Scale (Conners & Wells, 1985) and the Self-Evaluation Self-Report for Teenagers (Gittelman, 1985), were developed for the assessment of ADHD in adolescents. However, both of these measures have been criticized because of insufficient normative and psychometric data, reliance on outdated diagnostic procedures, and limited clinical utility (Adams, Kelley, & McCarthy, 1997; Barkley, 1997; Barkley, Fischer, Edelbrock, & Smallish, 1990).

Adolescent Behavior Checklist

The only standardized self-report measure based on recent diagnostic criteria for adolescents with ADHD is the Adolescent Behavior Checklist (ABC; Adams, Kelley, & McCarhty, 1997). This is a 44-item measure designed to assess the three core symptom areas of ADHD (i.e., inattention, impulsivity, hyperactivity) as well as associated problem areas (i.e., conduct problems, academic difficulties, social skill deficits). Items on the ABC are rated on a 4-point Likert-type scale from 1 (not at all) to 4 (very much). Examples of items include "I purposely break rules or disobey instructions," "I talk too much," and "I have problems waiting my turn in games of group situations."

The ABC was standardized on a sample of 909 adolescents between the ages of 11 and 17. While care was taken to obtain a sample that included a broad representation of key demographic variables, the majority of participants were recruited from a single geographic region. Normative data are broken down by gender and ethnicity. Principal components analysis of the ABC revealed six factors that accounted for 48% of the total variance of the scale. These factors include: (1) Conduct Problems; (2) Impulsivity/Hyperactivity; (3) Poor Work Habits; (4) Inattention; (5) Emotional Lability; and (6) Social Problems. The internal consistency of the entire measure was .94 and ranged from .60 to .85 for the individual factors. Test–retest reliability correlation coefficients across a two-week interval ranged from .62 to .81 for the individual factors and total scale score. Convergent and divergent validity were examined by correlating ABC total and factor scores with subscales of the Youth Self-Report (YSR; Achenbach, 1991c), the Child Behavior Checklist (CBCL; Achenbach, 1991a), and the Conners Parent Rating Scale–48 (CPRS-48; Conners, 1989). Individual factor and total scale scores of the ABC were found to correlate significantly with the YSR (range, .10 to .73) and the CBCL and CPRS (–.01 to .34). Furthermore, the discriminant validity was investigated with a small sample of students diagnosed with ADHD ($n = 15$). Individual factor and total scale scores of the ABC, except for Conduct Problems, were significantly higher for the clinical sample ($p < .05$).

Conduct Problems

There are few self-report measures of conduct problems available for use with children and adolescents. Of those developed, none has been widely used in the assessment of conduct problems. This may be caused by concerns regarding children's estimation accuracy and comprehension of conduct problems (McMahon & Estes, 1997). In addition, it has been argued that children and adolescents may underreport antisocial behaviors, such as substance abuse and assault, which may be punishable by law. Interestingly, the research examining the extent to which child- and adolescent-completed measures accurately identify conduct problems has not substantiated the aforementioned concerns. A number of studies have demonstrated that conduct problems may be more readily and accurately reported by children and adolescents than by caregivers or related reports (Elliott & Ageton, 1980; Herjanic & Reich, 1982; Williams & Gold, 1972).

Conduct disorder often occurs with other externalizing disorders such as oppositional defiant disorder and ADHD (Faraone, Biederman, Keenan, & Tsuang, 1991; Spitzer, Davies, & Barkley, 1990). In addition, children and adolescents with conduct disorder may also experience internalizing disorders, such as anxiety, depression, and low self-concept (Loeber & Keenan, 1994; Mitchell, McCauley, Burke, & Moss, 1988; Zoccolillo, 1992). In a review of studies examining the comorbidity of conduct disorder with other internalizing and externalizing disorders, McConaughy and Skiba (1993) demonstrated moderate to high correlations among the syndromes of aggressive behavior, delinquent behavior, anxious/depression, and attention problems as measures on the CBCL/4–18 (Achenbach, 1991a) and TRF (Achenbach, 1991b). Using self-report measures to assess conduct problems and associated features may provide a more complete examination of problem areas and identify comorbid conditions (Walker, 1997). Therefore, it appears that self-report measures of conduct problems can provide meaningful information that may not be obtained via direct observation or informant reports.

Self-Report Delinquency Scale

One of the more widely used self-report measures for conduct problems is the Self-Report Delinquency Scale (SRD; Elliott, Huizinga, & Ageton, 1985). This measure was developed for youths ages 11 to 19 and is intended to measure the frequency of conduct problems during the past year. The scale consists of 47 items that assess criminal offenses, delinquent behaviors, and drug use. The frequency of item occurrence is rated on a 6-point categorical scale, ranging from once a month to two to three times a day. In a addition to computing a Total Self-Report Delinquency score that reflects the severity of delinquent behavior, items can be compiled to form six summary subscales, which include (1) predatory crimes against persons, (2) predatory crimes against property, (3) illegal service crimes, (4) public disorder crimes, (5) status crimes, and (6) hard drug use. Sample items of the SRD include "How many times in the last year have you stolen something worth more than $50?," and "How many times in the last year have you made obscene telephone calls?"

The standardization sample consisted of 1,726 youths between the ages of 11 and 17 (Elliott & Ageton, 1980). Based upon a comparison with U.S. Census Bureau estimates, the standardization sample appears representative with respect to age, gender, and ethnicity. However, it is important to note that this comparison was based on 1977 U.S. Census Bureau estimates. Furthermore, the SRD was not standardized on youths older than age 17. Therefore, it does not appear that this scale should be used with this age group, despite the test developers' recommendations.

Test–retest reliability for the total scale and subscales are reported as greater than .60, with the exception of two subscales. Internal consistency of the total scale score of the SRD is reported as .91. Validity of the scale has been demonstrated in a longitudinal study comparing scores on the SRD with official arrest data (Elliott, Huizinga, & Ageton, 1985; Loeber, Stouthamer-Loeber, Van Kammen, & Farrington, 1989). In addition, the SRD has been used as an outcome measure in a number of intervention studies (Kazdin, Siegel, & Bass, 1992; Scherer, Brondino, Henggeler, Melton, & Hanley, 1994) and has been demonstrated to be sensitive to the effects of treatments (Kazdin, 1995).

Computer-Generated Assessment of Conduct Problems

One advancement in the development of self-report formats for assessing conduct problems is the use of microcomputers to provide video representations of various situations relevant to children and adolescents. This approach requires children to respond directly to computer-generated scenarios by touching the computer screen. Walker and colleagues (Irvin & Walker, 1994; Irvin et al., 1992; Walker, Irvin, Noell, & Singer, 1992) have begun to examine the utility of this response format to directly assess children's skills in three domains relevant to conduct problems. These domains include (1) joining ongoing play groups; (2) coping with teasing; and (3) complying with adult commands and directives. Preliminary research indicates that this format can be used successfully to obtain self-report information that differentiates children and youth with conduct problems from normal children and youth in a clinic facility (Irvin & Walker, 1994). However, classroom-based applications of this assessment format have yet to be examined.

SELF-REPORT MEASURES: LIMITATIONS AND FUTURE RESEARCH DIRECTIONS

It is important that school-based practitioners consider the limitations associated with the use of self-report rating scales for assessing children's and adolescent's emotional and behavioral functioning. Self-report rating scales are considered one source of information that is gathered as part of multimethod behavioral assessment. Data obtained from self-report rating scales should be used in conjunction with other direct and indirect measures as part of a problem-solving approach to assessment. Although important clinical information can be gathered using self-report rating scales (i.e., screening, classification, treatment planning, progress monitoring), a number of factors can influence the accuracy of these measures. Therefore, it is important to examine the accuracy of self-report data within the context of the child, the environment, and assessment process.

While there are a number of limitations associated with the use of self-report rating scales, it appears that there are a number of areas for future investigation. First, it appears crucial to continue examining the relationship between self-report measures and other direct and indirect forms of behavioral assessment. A continued investigation of patterns of respondent variance, factors related to respondent variance, and identification of behavior disorders that do not display respondent variance appears worthy of future empirical studies. Second, continued investigation of issues related to the use of self-report rating scales with young children appears warranted. Areas that should be considered in future research studies include examining administration factors that may improve the reliability and validity of respondent data, as well as variations in response formats. Perhaps variations in administration procedures or response formats may improve the accuracy of data obtained from self-reports. Conversely, it may be important to examine administration procedures or response formats that invalidate or jeopardize the accuracy of data obtained from self-report measures. The use of computer-generated self-report measures appears to be an important medium for investigation. Finally, continued research is needed in the development and validation of self-report measures for children and adolescents. Additional self-report measures need to be developed to reflect changes in theoretical models of behavior as well as provide a comprehensive assessment of behavior. Given the comorbidity of various disorders, it may be important for this factor to be considered in the development of future self-report measures. Future self-report measures may benefit from combining broad- and narrowband assessment approaches across comorbid conditions or diagnostic criteria.

References

Achenbach, T. M. (1991a). *Manual for the Child Behavior Checklist/4–18*. Burlington: University of Vermont, Department of Psychiatry.

Achenbach, T. M. (1991b). *Manual for the Teacher's Report Form and 1991 Profile*. Burlington: University of Vermont, Department of Psychiatry.

Achenbach, T. M. (1991c). *Manual for the Youth Self-Report and 1991 Profile*. Burlington: University of Vermont, Department of Psychiatry.

Achenbach, T. M. (1992). *Manual for the Child Behavior Checklist/2–3 and 1992 Profile*. Burlington: University of Vermont, Department of Psychiatry.

Achenbach, T. M. (1993). *Empirically based taxonomy: How to use syndromes and profile types derived from the CBCL/4–18, TRF, and YSR*. Burlington: University of Vermont, Department of Psychiatry.

Achenbach, T. M., & McConaughy, S. H. (1987). *Empirically based assessment of child and adolescent psychopathology: Practical applications*. Newbury Park, CA: Sage.

Achenbach, T. M., McConaughy, S. T., & Howell, C. T. (1987). Child/adolescent behavioral and emotional problems: Implications of cross-informant correlations for situational specificity. *Psychological Bulletin, 101*, 213–232.

Adams, C. D., Kelley, M. L., & McCarthy, M. (1997). The Adolescent Behavior Checklist: Development and initial psychometric properties of a self-report measure for adolescents with ADHD. *Journal of Clinical Child Psychology, 26*, 77–86.

Akiskal, H. S., Downs, J., Jordan, P., Watson, S., Daugherty, D., & Pruitt, D. B. (1985). Affective disorders in referred children and younger siblings of manic-depressives: Mode of onset and prospective course. *Archives of General Psychiatry, 42*, 996–1003.

Alessi, N. E., Krahn, D., Brehm, D., & Wittekindt, J. (1989). Prepubertal anorexia nervosa and major depressive disorder. *Journal of the American Academy of Child and Adolescent Psychiatry, 28*, 380–384.

Alessi, N. E., & Magen, J. (1988). Comorbidity of other psychiatric disturbances in depressed psychiatrically hospitalized children. *American Journal of Psychiatry, 145,* 1582–1584

American Psychological Association (1985). *Standards for educational and psychological testing.* Washington, DC: Author.

Anderson, J. C., Williams, S., McGee, R., & Silva, P. A. (1987). DSM-III disorders in preadolescent children: Prevalence in a large sample from the general population. *Archives of General Psychiatry, 44,* 69–76.

Angold, A., Weissman, M. M., John, K., Merikangas, K. R., Prusoff, B. A., Wicramarantne, P., Gammon, G. D., & Warner, V. (1987). Parent and child reports of depressive symptoms in children at low and high risk of depression. *Journal of Child Psychology and Psychiatry and Allied Disciplines, 28,* 901–915.

Barkley, R. A. (1997). Attention-deficit/hyperactivity disorder. In E. J. Mash & L. G. Terdal (Eds.), *Assessment of childhood disorders* (pp. 71–129). New York: Guilford Press.

Barkley, R. A., Fischer, M., Edelbrock, C., & Smallish, L. (1990). The adolescent outcome of hyperactive children diagnosed by research criteria: I. An 8-year prospective follow-up study. *Journal of the American Academy of Child and Adolescent Psychiatry, 29,* 546–557.

Beck, A. T. (1971). Cognition, affect, and psychopathology. *Archives of General Psychiatry, 24,* 495–500.

Beck, A. T., Ward, C. H., Mendelson, M., Mock, J. E., & Erbaugh, J. K. (1961). An inventory for measuring depression. *Archives of General Psychiatry, 4,* 561–571.

Biederman, J., Newcorn, J., & Sprich, S. (1991). Comorbidity of attention deficit hyperactivity disorder with conduct, depressive, anxiety, and other disorder. *American Journal of Psychiatry, 148,* 564–577.

Biederman, J. & Steingard, R. (1989). Attention-deficit hyperactivity disorder in adolescents. *Psychiatric Annals, 19,* 587–596.

Bierman, K. L. (1983). Cognitive development and clinical interviews with children. In B. B. Lahey & A. E. Kazdin (Eds.), *Advances in clinical child psychology* (pp. 217–250). New York: Plenum Press.

Bierman, K. L., & Welsch, J. A. (1997). Social relationship deficits. In E. J. Mash & L. G. Terdal (Eds.), *Assessment of childhood disorders* (pp. 328–368). New York: Guilford Press.

Blumberg, S. H., & Izard, C. E. (1986). Discriminating patterns of emotions in 10– and 11–year-old children's anxiety and depression. *Journal of Personality and Social Psychology, 51,* 852–857.

Boivin, M., Hymel, S., & Bukowski, W. M. (1995). The roles of social withdrawal, peer rejection, and victimization by peers in predicting loneliness and depressed mood in childhood. *Development and Psychopathology, 7,* 765–785.

Bracken, B. A. (1992). *Multidimensional Self-Concept Scale: Examiner's manual.* Austin, TX: Pro-Ed.

Bracken, B. A., Bunch, S., Keith, T. Z., & Keith, P. B. (1992). *Multidimensional self-concept: A five instrument factor analysis.* Paper presented at the annual convention of the American Psychological Association, Washington, DC, August.

Bracken, B. A., & Kelley, P. (1993). *Assessment of interpersonal relations.* Austin, TX: Pro-Ed.

Bracken, B. A., & Mills, B. C. (1994). School counselors' assessment of self concept: A comprehensive review of ten instruments. *School Counselor, 42,* 14–31.

Breen, M., Eckert, T. L., & DuPaul, G. J. (1996). Interpreting child behavior questionnaires. In M. Breen & C. Fiedler (Eds.), *Behavioral approach to the assessment of emotionally disturbed youth: A handbook for school-based practitioners* (pp. 225–241). Austin, TX: Pro-Ed.

Brown, L. L., & Hammill, D. D. (1983). *Behavior Rating Profile.* Austin, TX: Pro-Ed.

Byrne, B. M. (1988). Measuring adolescent self-concept: Factorial validity and equivalency of the SDQ III across gender. *Multivariate Behavioral Research, 23,* 361–375.

Callahan, V., & Jackson, D. (1986). Children of alcoholic fathers and recovered alcoholic fathers: Personal and family functioning. *Journal of Studies on Alcohol, 27,* 180–182.

Carey, T.C., Finch, A.J., & Carey, M. P. (1991). Relation between differential emotions and depression in emotionally disturbed children and adolescents. *Journal of Consulting and Clinical Psychology, 59,* 594–597.

Carroll, J. J., & Steward, M. S. (1984). The role of cognitive development in children's understandings of their own feelings. *Child Development, 55,* 1486–1492.

Chewning, T. G. (1992). An investigation of the discriminant and concurrent validity of the Social Skills Rating System-Teacher form. *Dissertation Abstracts International, 53*, 1843A.

Christensen, A., Margolin, G., & Sullaway, M. (1992). Interparental agreement in children and adolescents. *Psychological Bulletin, 111*, 244–255.

Clark, R., Gresham, F. M., & Elliott, S. N. (1985). Development and validation of a social skills assessment measure: The TROSS-C. *Journal of Psychoeducational Assessment, 4*, 347–356.

Compass, B. E. (1997). Depression in children and adolescents. In E. J. Mash & L. G. Terdal (Eds.), *Assessment of childhood disorders* (pp. 197–229). New York: Guilford Press.

Cone, J. D. (1978). The behavioral assessment grid (BAG): A conceptual framework and a taxonomy. *Behavior Therapy, 9*, 882–888.

Connors, C. K. (1989). *Conners' Rating Scales Manual: Conners' Teacher Rating Scales, Conners' Parent Rating Scales*. North Tonawanda, NY: Multi-Health Systems.

Connors, C. K., & Wells, K. C. (1985). ADD-H Adolescent Self-Report Scale. *Psychopharmacologoy Bulletin, 21*, 921–922.

Coopersmith, S. (1959). A method for determining types of self-esteem. *Journal of Abnormal and Social Psychology, 59*, 87–94.

Coopersmith, S. (1967). *The antecedents of self-esteem*. San Francisco: W. H. Freeman.

Crain, R. M., & Bracken, B. A. (1994). Age, race, and gender differences in child and adolescent self-concept: Evidence from a behavioral-acquisition context-dependent model. *School Psychology Review, 23*, 496–511.

Crandall, V. C., Katkovsky, W., & Crandall, V. J. (1965). Children's beliefs in their own control of reinforcements in intellectual-academic achievement situations. *Child Development, 36*, 92–109.

Craven, R. G., Marsh, H. W., & Delous, R. L. (1991). Effects of internally focused feedback and attributional feedback on enhancement of academic self-concept. *Journal of Educational Psychology, 83*, 17–27.

Curry, J. F., & Craighead, W. E. (1993). Depression. In T. H. Ollendick & M. Hersen (Eds.), *Handbook of child and adolescent assessment* (pp. 251–268). Boston: Allyn & Bacon.

Dalley, M.B., Bolocofsky, D. N., Alcorn, M. B., & Baker, C. (1992). Depressive symptomatology, attributional style, dysfunctional attitude, and social competency in adolescents with and without learning disabilities. *School Psychology Review, 21*, 444–458.

Delugach, R. R., Bracken, B. A., Bracken, M. J., & Schicke, M. C. (1992). Self concept: Multidimensional construct exploration. *Psychology in the Schools, 29*, 213–223.

Demaray, M. K., Ruffalo, S. L., Carlson, J., Busse, R. T., Olson, A. E., McManus, S. M., & Levanthal, A. (1995). Social skills assessment: A comparative evaluation of six published rating scales. *School Psychology Review, 24*, 648–671.

Dielman, T. E., Leech, S. L., Lorenger, A. T., & Horvath, W. J. (1984). Health locus of control and self-esteem as related to adolescent health behavior and intentions. *Adolescence, 19*, 935–950.

DuPaul, G. J., & Hoff, K. E. (1998). Attention/concentration problems. In T. S. Watson & F. M. Gresham (Eds.), *Handbook of child behavior therapy* (pp. 99–126). New York: Plenum Press.

Earls, F., Smith, E., Reich, W., & Jung, K. G. (1988). Investigating psychopathological consequences of a disaster in children: A pilot study incorporating a structured diagnostic interview. *Journal of the American Academy of Child and Adolescent Psychiatry, 27*, 90–95.

Eckert, T. L., & DuPaul, G. J. (1996). Youth completed and narrowband child behavior questionnaires. In M. Breen & C. Fiedler (Eds.), *Behavioral approach to the assessment of emotionally disturbed youth: A handbook for school-based practitioners* (pp. 289–357). Austin, TX: Pro-Ed.

Edelbrock, C. S., Costello, A. J., Dulcan, M, K., Conover, & Kalas, R. (1986). Parent–child agreement on child psychiatric symptoms assessed via structured interview. *Journal of Child Psychology and Psychiatry, 27*, 181–190.

Elliott, D. S., & Ageton, S. S. (1980). Reconciling race and class differences in self-reported and official estimates of delinquency. *American Sociological Review, 45*, 95–110.

Elliott, S. N., Busse, R. T., & Gresham, F. M. (1993). Behavior rating scales: Issues of use and interpretation. *School Psychology Review, 22*, 313–321.

Elliott, D. S., Huizinga, D., & Ageton, S. S. (1985). *Explaining delinquency and drug use*. Beverly Hills, CA: Sage.

Faraone, S. V., Biederman, J., Keenan, K., & Tsuang, M. T. (1991). Separation of the DSM-III attention deficit disorder and conduct disorder: Evidence from a family genetic study of American
child psychiatric patients. *Psychological Medicine, 21,* 109–121.

Finch, A. J., Lipovsky, J. A., & Casat, C. D. (1989). Anxiety and depression in children and adolescents: Negative affectivity or separate constructs? In P. C. Kendall & D. Watson (Eds.), *Anxiety
and depression: Distinctive and overlapping features* (pp. 171–202). San Diego: Academic Press.

Foster, S. L., & Ritchey, W. L. (1985). Behavioral correlates of sociometric status of fourth, fifth, and
sixth grade children in two classroom situations. *Behavioral Assessment, 7,* 79–93.

Garvin, V., Leber, D., & Kalter, N. (1991). Children of divorce: Predictors of change following preventive intervention. *American Journal of Orthopsychiatry, 61,* 438–447.

Gittelman, R. (1985). Self-evaluation (teenager's) self-report. *Psychopharmacology Bulletin, 21,* 925–
926.

Glennon, B., & Weiss, J. R. (1978). An observational approach to the assessment of anxiety in young
children. *Journal of Consulting and Clinical Psychology, 46,* 1246–1257.

Green, B. J. (1980). Depression in early adolescence: An exploratory investigation of its frequency,
intensity, and correlates. *Dissertation Abstracts International, 41,* 3890B.

Gresham, F. M., & Elliott, S. N. (1990). *The social skills rating system.* Circle Pines, MN: American
Guidance Service.

Gresham, F. M., Elliott, S. N., & Black, F. (1987). Teacher-rated social skills of mainstreamed mildly
handicapped and nonhandicapped children. *School Psychology Review, 16,* 78–88.

Guiton, G., & Zachary, R. A. (August 1984). *Criterion validity of the Piers–Harris Children's Self-
Concept Scale.* Paper presented at the annual meeting of the American Psychological Association, Toronto, Canada.

Hains, A. A. (1992). Comparison of cognitive–behavioral stress management techniques with adolescent boys. *Journal of Counseling and Development, 70,* 600–605.

Hamilton, M. (1960). A rating scale for depression. *Journal of Neurology, Neurosurgery, and Psychiatry, 23,* 56–62.

Harter, S. (1983). The Perceived Competence Scale for Children. *Child Development, 53,* 87–97.

Harter, S. (1985). *Manual for the Self-Perception Profile for Children.* University of Denver, Denver,
CO.

Hathaway, S. R., & McKinley, J. C. (1970). *Minnesota Multiphasic Personality Inventory.* Minneapolis:
University of Minnesota Press.

Helsel, W. J., & Matson, J. L. (1984). The assessment of depression in children: The internal structure
of the Child Depression Inventory. *Behaviour Research and Therapy, 22,* 289–298.

Herjanic, B., & Reich, W. (1982). Development of a structured psychiatric interview for children:
Agreement between child and parent on individual symptoms. *Journal of Abnormal Child Psychology, 10,* 307–324.

Hinshaw, S. P. (1994). *Attention deficits and hyperactivity in children.* Thousand Oaks, CA: Sage.

Hodges, K. (1990). Depression and anxiety in children: A comparison of self-report questionnaires to
clinical interview. *Psychological Assessment, 2,* 378–381.

Irvin, L. K., & Walker, H. M. (1994). Assessing children's social skills using video-based microcomputer technology. *Exceptional Children, 61,* 182–196.

Irvin, L. K., Walker, H. M., Noell, J., Singer, G. H. S., Irvine, A. B., Marquez, K., & Britz, B. (1992).
Measuring children's social skills using microcomputer-based videodisc assessment. *Behavior
Modification, 16,* 475–503.

Jackson, L. D., & Bracken, B. A. (1998). Relationship between students' social status and global domain-
specific self-concepts. *Journal of School Psychology, 36,* 233–246.

Jacob-Timm, S., & Hartshorne, T. S. (1994). *Ethics and law for school psychologists.* New York: Wiley.

Jensen, J. B., Burke, N., & Garfinkel, B. D. (1988). Depression and symptoms of attention deficit disorder with hyperactivity. *Journal of the American Academy of Child and Adolescent Psychiatry,
27,* 742–747.

Kahn, J. S., Kehle, T. J., Jenson, W. R., & Clark, E. (1990). Comparison of cognitive–behavioral, relaxation, and self-monitoring interventions for depression among middle-school students. *School
Psychology Review, 19,* 196–211.

Kashini, J. H., Keller, M. B., Solmon, N., Reid, J. C., & Mazzola, D. (1985). Double depression in adolescent substance users. *Journal of Affective Disorders, 8*, 153–157.

Kavanagh, K., & Hops, H. (1994). Good girls? Bad boys? Gender and development as contexts for diagnosis and treatment. *Advances in Clinical Child Psychology, 16*, 45–79.

Kazdin, A. E. (1989). Identifying depression in children: A comparison of alternative selection criteria. *Journal of Abnormal Child Psychology, 17*, 437–454.

Kazdin, A. E. (1995). Child, parent, and family dysfunction as predictors of outcome in cognitive–behavioral treatment of antisocial children. *Journal of Child and Family Studies, 1*, 3–20.

Kazdin, A. E., French, N. H., Unis, A. S., Esveldt-Dawson, K., & Sherick, R. B. (1983). Hopelessness, depression, and suicidal intent among psychiatrically disturbed inpatient children. *Journal of Consulting and Clinical Psychology, 51*, 504–510.

Kazdin, A. E., Rodgers, A., & Colbus, D. (1986). The Hopelessness Scale for Children: Psychometric characteristics and concurrent validity. *Journal of Consulting and Clinical Psychology, 54*, 241–245.

Kazdin, A. E., Siegel, T. C., & Bass, D. (1992). Cognitive problem-solving skills training and parent management training in the treatment of antisocial behavior in children. *Journal of Consulting and Clinical Psychology, 60*, 733–747.

Keith, L. K., & Bracken, B. A. (1994). *Factor analytic study of a multidimensional model of self-concept.* Paper presented at the annual convention of the National Association of School Psychologists, Seattle, WA, April.

Kelley, P. A. (1990). *Relationship between self-esteem, family environment, and interpersonal relations in a clinical and nonclinical sample of male and female adolescents.* Unpublished doctoral dissertation, Memphis State University, Memphis, TN.

Kendall, P. C., & Braswell, L. (1982). Cognitive behavioral self-control therapy for children: A components analysis. *Journal of Consulting and Clinical Psychology, 50*, 672–689.

Klein, R. G. (1991). Parent–child agreement in clinical assessment of anxiety and other psychopathology: A review. *Journal of Anxiety Disorders, 5*, 187–198.

Koocher, G. P. (1993). Ethical issues in the psychological assessment of children. In T. H. Ollendick & M. Hersen (Eds.), *Handbook of child and adolescent assessment* (pp. 51–64). Boston: Allyn & Bacon.

Kovacs, M. (1981). Rating scales to assess depression in school-aged children. *Acta Paedopsychiatria, 46*, 305–315.

Kovacs, M. (1990). Comorbid anxiety disorders in childhood-onset depressions. In J. D. Maser & C. R. Cloninger (Eds.), *Comorbidity of mood and anxiety disorders* (pp. 271–281). Washington, DC: American Psychiatric Press.

Kovacs, M. (1992). *Children's Depression Inventory.* Los Angeles: Multi-Health Systems.

Kovacs, M., Paulauskas, S. L., Gastonis, C., & Richards, C. (1988). Depressive disorders in childhood: III. A longitudinal study of comorbidity with and risk for conduct disorders. *Journal of Affective Disorders, 15*, 205–217.

Kratochwill, T. R., & Shapiro, E. S. (1988). Introduction: Conceptual foundations of behavioral assessment. In E. S. Shapiro & T. R. Kratochwill (Eds.), *Behavioral assessment in schools* (pp. 384–454). New York: Guilford Press.

Kratochwill, T. R., Sheridan, S. M., Carlson, J., & Lasecki, K. L. (1999). Advances in behavioral assessment. In C. R. Reynolds & T. B. Gutkin (Eds.), *Handbook of school psychology* (pp. 350–382). New York: Wiley.

La Greca, A. M. (1990a). *Through the eyes of the child: Obtaining self-reports from children and adolescents.* Needham Heights, MA: Allyn & Bacon.

La Greca, A. M. (1990b). Issues and perspectives on the child assessment process. In A. M. La Greca (Ed.), *Through the eyes of the child: Obtaining self-reports from children and adolescents* (pp. 3–17). Needham Heights, MA: Allyn & Bacon.

La Greca, A. M., & Stone, W. L. (1993). *Social Anxiety Scale for Children–Revised.* Factor structure and concurrent validity. *Journal of Clinical Child Psychology, 22*, 17–27.

Landau, S., & Milich, R. (1990). Assessment of children's social status and peer relations. In A. M. La Greca (Ed.), *Through the eyes of the child* (pp. 259–291). Boston: Allyn & Bacon.

Landau, S., Milich, R., & Widiger, T. A. (1991). Conditional probabilities of child interview symptoms in the diagnosis of attention deficit disorder. *Journal of Child Psychology and Psychiatry, 32,* 501–513.

Ledingham, J. E., Younger, A. S., Schwartzman, A. E., & Bergeron, G. (1982). Agreement among teachers, peers, and self-ratings of children's aggression, withdrawal, and likability. *Journal of Abnormal Child Psychology, 10,* 363–372.

Levy, J. C., & Deykin, E. Y. (1989). Suicidality, depression, and substance abuse in adolescence. *American Journal of Psychiatry, 146,* 1462–1467.

Loeber, R., Green, S. M., Lahey, B. B., & Stouthamer-Loeber, M. (1989). Optimal informants on childhood disruptive behaviors. *Development and Psychopathology, 1,* 317–337.

Loeber, R., & Keenan, K. (1994). Interaction between conduct disorder and its comorbid conditions: Effects of age and gender. *Clinical Psychology Review, 14,* 497–523.

Loeber, R., Stouthamer-Loeber, M., Van Kammen, W. B., & Farrington, D. P. (1989). Development of a new measure of self-reported antisocial behavior for young children: Prevalence and reliability. In M. W. Klein (Ed.), *Cross national research and self-reported crime and delinquency* (pp. 203–225). Dordrecht, The Netherlands: Kluwer-Nijhoff.

Loney, J., Volpe, R. J., & Ye, X. (1998). *Don't throw out the baby: The role of a child DSM interview in the assessment of inattention and hyperactivity.* Unpublished manuscript.

Mannarino, A. P. (1978). Friendship patterns and self-concept development in preadolescent males. *Journal of Genetic Psychology, 133,* 105–110.

March, J. S. (1997). *Multidimensional anxiety scale for children: Technical manual.* New York: Multi-Health Systems.

March, J. S., Parker, J. D. A., Sullivan, K., Stallings, P., & Conners, C. K. (1997). The Multidimensional Anxiety Scale for Children: Factor structure, reliability, and validity. *Journal of American Academy of Child and Adolescent Psychiatry, 36,* 554–565.

Marsh, H. W. (1990). The structure of academic self-concept: The Marsh/Shavelson model. *Journal of Educational Psychology, 82,* 623–636.

Marsh, H. W., Barnes, J., & Hocevar, D. (1985). Self–other agreement on multidimensional self-concept ratings: Factor analysis and multitrait–multimethod analysis. *Journal of Personality and Social Psychology, 49,* 1360–1377.

Martens, B. K. (1993). Social labeling, precision of measurement, and problem solving: Key issues in the assessment of children's emotional problems. *School Psychology Review, 2,* 308–312.

Marx, R. W., & Winne, P. H. (1978). Friendship patterns and self-concept development in preadolescent males. *Journal of Genetic Psychology, 133,* 105–110.

Mash, E. J., & Terdal, L. G. (1997). Assessment of child and family disturbance: A behavioral-systems approach. In E. J. Mash & L. G. Terdal (Eds.), *Assessment of childhood disorders* (pp. 3–70). New York: Guilford Press.

McConaughy, S. H. (1993). Advances in empirically based assessment of children's behavioral and emotional problems. *School Psychology Review, 22,* 285–307.

McConaughy, S. H., & Ritter, D. R. (1995). Multidimensional assessment of emotional or behavioral disorders. In A. Thomas & J. Grimes (Eds.), *Best practices in school psychology–III* (pp. 865–878). Washington, DC: National Association of School Psychologists.

McConaughy, S. H., & Skiba, R. J. (1993). Comorbidity of externalizing and internalizing problems. *School Psychology Review, 22,* 421–436.

McConaughy, S. H., Stanger, C., & Achenbach, T. M. (1992). Three-year course of behavioral/emotional problems in a national sample of 4- to 16-year-olds: I. Agreement among informants. *Journal of the American Academy of Child and Adolescent Psychiatry, 31,* 932–940.

McMahon, R. J., & Estes, A. M. (1997). Conduct problems. In E. J. Mash & L. G. Terdal (Eds.), *Assessment of childhood disorders* (pp. 71–129). New York: Guilford Press.

Merrell, K. W. (1998). Assessing social skills and peer relations. In H. B. Vance (Ed.), *Psychological assessment of children* (pp. 246–273). New York: Wiley.

Merrell, K. W., Anderson, K. E., & Michael, K. D. (1997). Convergent validity of the internalizing symptoms scale for children with three self-report measures of internalizing problems. *Journal of Psychoeducational Assessment, 15,* 56–66.

Merrell, K. W., Crowley, S. L., & Walters, A. S. (1997). Development and factor structure of a self-report measure for assessing internalizing symptoms of elementary-age children. *Psychology in the Schools, 34,* 197–210.

Merrell, K. W. & Dobmeyer, A. C. (1996). An evaluation of gender differences in self-reported internalizing symptoms of elementary-age children. *Journal of Psychoeducational Assessment, 14,* 196–197.

Merrell, K. W., Gill, S. G., McFarland, H., & McFarland, T. (1996). Internalizing symptoms of gifted and non-gifted elementary-age students: A comparative validity study using the Internalizing Symptoms Scale for Children. *Psychology in the Schools, 33,* 185–191.

Merrell, K. W., & Walters, A. S. (1996). *The Internalizing Symptoms Scale for Children: User's guide and technical manual.* Logan, UT: Utah State University, Department of Psychology.

Michael, K. D. (1997). An investigation of the temporal stability of self-reported internalizing symptoms of elementary-aged children. *Journal of Psychoeducational Assessment, 14,* 196–207.

Milberger, S., Biederman, J. Faroane, S., Murphy, J., & Tsuang, M. (1995). Attention deficit hyperactivity disorder: Issues of overlapping symptoms. *American Journal of Consulting and Clinical Psychology, 59,* 491–498.

Mischel, W., Zeiss, R., & Zeiss, A. (1974). Internal-external control and persistence: Validation and implications of the Stanford preschool internal-external scale. *Journal of Personality and Social Psychology, 29,* 265–278.

Mitchell, J., McCauley, E., Burke, P. M., & Moss, S. J., (1988). Phenomenology of depression in children and adolescents. *Journal of the American Academy of Child and Adolescent Psychiatry, 27,* 12–20.

Moller, L. C., & Schnurr, R. G. (1995). A comparison of self-esteem measures of attractiveness in a psychiatric population of adolescents: The Piers–Harris and the Harter scales. *Journal of Social Behavior & Personality, 10,* 445–454.

Moran, P. B., & Eckenrode, J. (1992). Protective personality characteristics among adolescent victims of maltreatment. *Child Abuse and Neglect, 16,* 743–754.

Morris, R. J., & Kratochwill, T. R. (1991). Childhood fears and phobias. In T. R. Kratochwill & R. J. Morris (Eds.), *The practice of child therapy* (2nd ed., pp. 76–114). New York: Pergamon Press.

Newman, V. L. (1996). An investigation of interpersonal relations among runaway and nonrunaway adolescents. *Dissertation Abstracts International, 57* (09A), 3829.

Piers, E. V. (1984). *Revised manual for the Piers–Harris Children's Self-Concept Scale.* Los Angeles: Western Psychological Services.

Piers, E. V., & Harris, D. B. (1963). *The Piers–Harris Self-Concept Scale.* Unpublished manuscript, Pennsylvania State University.

Porter, R. B., & Cattell, R. B. (1975). *Children's Personality Questionnaire.* Champaign, IL: Institute for Personality and Ability Testing.

Poznanski, E. O., Freeman, L. N., & Mokros, H. B. (1985). Children's Depression Rating Scale–Revised. *Psychopharmacology Bulletin, 21,* 979–989.

Puig-Antich, J. (1982). Major depression and conduct disorder in prepuberty. *Journal of the American Academy of Child Psychiatry, 21,* 118–121.

Reich, W., & Earls, F. (1987). Rules for making psychiatric diagnoses in children on the basis of multiple sources of information: Preliminary strategies. *Journal of Abnormal Child Psychology, 15,* 601–616.

Reiss, S. (1987). Theoretical perspectives on the fear of anxiety. *Clinical Psychology Review, 7,* 585–596.

Reynolds, C. R., & Kamphaus, R. W. (1992). *Behavior Assessment System for Children.* Circle Pines, MN: American Guidance Service.

Reynolds, W. M. (1987). *Professional manual for the Reynolds Adolescent Depression Scale.* Los Angeles: Western Psychological Services.

Reynolds, W. M. (1989). *Professional manual for the Reynolds Child Depression Scale.* Odessa, FL: Psychological Assessment Resources.

Reynolds, W. M. (1993). Self-report methodology. In T. H. Ollendick & M. Hersen (Eds.), *Handbook of child and adolescent assessment* (pp. 98–123). Boston: Allyn & Bacon.

Reynolds, W. M. (1994). Assessment of depression in children and adolescents by self-report question-naires. In W. M. Reynolds & H. F. Johnston (Eds.), *Handbook of depression in children and adolescents* (pp. 209–234). New York: Plenum Press.

Reynolds, W. M., Anderson, G., & Bartell, N. (1985). Measuring depression in children: A multi-method assessment investigation. *Journal of Abnormal Child Psychology, 13,* 513–526.

Reynolds, W. M., & Coats, K. I. (1986). A comparison of cognitive–behavior therapy and relaxation training for the treatment of depression in adolescents. *Journal of Consulting and Clinical Psychology, 54,* 653–660.

Reynolds, W. M., & Graves, A. (1989). Reliability of children's reports of depressive symptomatology. *Journal of Abnormal Child Psychology, 16,* 647–656.

Reynolds, W. M., & Mazza, J. J. (1998). Reliability and validity of the Reynolds Adolescent Depression Scale with young adolescents. *Journal of School Psychology, 36,* 295–312.

Reynolds, W. M., & Miller, K. L. (1989). Assessment of adolescents' learned helplessness in achievement situations. *Journal of Personality Assessment, 53,* 211–228.

Reynolds, W. M., & Richmond, B. O. (1985). *Revised Children's Manifest Anxiety Scale manual.* Los Angeles: Western Psychological Services.

Roberts, N., Vargo, B., & Ferguson, H. B. (1989). Measurement of anxiety and depression in children and adolescents. *Psychiatric Clinics of North America, 12,* 837–859.

Ruffalo, S. L., & Elliott, S. N. (1997). Teachers' and parents' ratings of children's social skills: A closer look at cross-informant agreements through an item analysis protocol. *School Psychology Review, 26,* 489–501.

Sanders, D. E. (1996). *Internalizing Symptoms Scale for Children: A validity study with urban, African-American, seriously emotionally disturbed and regular education students.* Unpublished doctoral dissertation, James Madison University, Harrisonburg, VA.

Sattler, J. M. (1992). *Assessment of children.* San Diego: Jerome M. Sattler.

Saylor, C. F., Finch, A. J., Baskin, C. H., Furey, W., & Kelly, M. M. (1984). Construct validity for measures of childhood depression: Application of multitrait–multimethod method. *Journal of Consulting and Clinical Psychology, 52,* 977–985.

Saylor, C. F., Finch, A. J., Spirito, A., & Bennett, B. (1984). The Children's Depression Inventory: A systematic evaluation of psychometric properties. *Journal of Consulting and Clinical Psychology, 52,* 955–967.

Scherer, D. G., Brondino, M. J., Henggeler, S. W., Melton, G. B., & Hanley, J. H. (1994). Multi-systemic family preservation therapy: Preliminary findings from a study of rural and minority serious adolescent offenders. *Journal of Emotional and Behavioral Disorders, 2,* 198–206.

Schonert-Reichl, K. A. (1994). Gender differences in depressive symptomatology and egocentrism in adolescence. *Journal of Early Adolescence,14,* 49–64.

Shain, B. N., Naylor, M., & Alessi, N. (1990). Comparison of self-rated and clinician-rated measures of depression in adolescents. *American Journal of Psychiatry, 147,* 793–795.

Shavelson, R. J., Hubner, J. J., & Stanton, G. C. (1976). Self-concept: Validation of construct interpretations. *Review of Educational Research, 46,* 407–411.

Smith, M. S., Mitchell, J., McCauley, E. A., & Calderon, R. (1990). Screening for anxiety and depression in an adolescent clinic. *Pediatrics, 85,* 262–266.

Spitzer, R. L., Davies, M., & Barkley, R. A. (1990). The DSM-III-R field trial of disruptive behavior disorders. *Journal of the American Academy of Child and Adolescent Psychiatry, 29,* 690–697.

Stallings, P., & March, J. S. (1995). Assessment. In J. S. March (Ed.), *Anxiety disorders in children and adolescents* (pp. 125–147). New York: Guilford Press.

Stark, K. D., Reynolds, W. M., & Kaslow, N. J. (1987). A comparison of the relative efficacy of self-control therapy and behavioral problem-solving therapy for depression in children. *Journal of Abnormal Child Psychology, 15,* 91–113.

Stephens, T. (1978). *Social skills in the classroom.* Columbus, OH: Cedars Press.

Stinnett, T. A., Havey, J. M., & Oehler-Stinnett, J. (1994). Current test usage by practicing school psychologists: A national survey. *Journal of Psychoeducational Assessment, 12,* 331–350.

Stinnett, T. A., Oehler-Stinnett, J., & Stout, L. J. (1989). Ability of the Social Skills Rating System–

Teacher version to discriminate behavior disordered, emotionally disturbed, and nonhandicapped students. *School Psychology Review, 18,* 526–535.

Stone, W. L., & LeManek, K. L. (1990). Developmental issues in children's self-reports. In A. M. La Greca (Ed.), *Through the eyes of the child: Obtaining self-reports from children and adolescents* (pp. 18–55). Needham Heights, MA: Allyn & Bacon.

Strauss, C. C., Last, C. G., Hersen, M., & Kazdin, A. E. (1988). Association between anxiety and depression in children and adolescents with anxiety disorders. *Journal of Abnormal Child Psychology, 16,* 57–68.

Strein, W. (1993). Advances in research on academic self-concept: Implications for school psychology. *School Psychology Review, 22,* 273–284.

Tansy, M., & Miller, J. A. (1997). The invariance of the self-concept construct across white and Hispanic student populations. *Journal of Psychoeducational Assessment, 15,* 4–14.

Tharinger, D. J., & Stark, K. (1990). A qualitative approach to evaluating the Draw-a-Person and Kinetic Family Drawing: A study of mood and anxiety-disordered children. *Psychological Assessment, 2,* 365–375.

Thompson, K. M. (1989). Effects of early alcohol use on adolescents' relations with peers and self-esteem: Patterns over time. *Adolescence, 24,* 837–849.

Volpe, R. J., DuPaul, G. J., Loney, J., & Salisbury, H. (in press). Alternative selection criteria for identifying children with attention deficit/hyperactivity disorder: Observed behavior and self-reported internalizing symptoms. *Journal of Emotional and Behavioral Disorders.*

Volpe, R. J., Loney, J., & Salisbury, H. (1997). *Self-reported behavioral and emotional symptoms as predictors of observed behavior in young referred boys.* Paper presented at the 8th Annual Scientific Meeting of the International Society for Research in Child and Adolescent Psychopathology, Paris.

Walker, H. M. (1997). *The acting out child: Coping with classroom disruption.* Longmont, CO: Sopris West.

Walker, H. M., Irvin, L. K., Noell, J., & Singer, G. H. S. (1992). A construct score approach to the assessment of social competence: Rationale, technological considerations, and anticipated outcomes. *Behavior Modification, 16,* 448–474.

Walker, H. M., & McConnell, S. R. (1988). *The manual for the Walker–McConnell Scale of Social Competence and School Adjustment.* Austin, TX: Pro-Ed.

Walters, A. S., & Merrell, K. W. (1995). Written versus oral administration of a social-emotional self-report test for children: Does method of execution make a difference? *Psychology in the Schools, 32,* 186–189.

Weiss, B., & Weisz, J. R. (1988). Factor structure of self-reported depression: Clinic-referred children versus adolescents. *Journal of Abnormal Psychology, 97,* 492–495.

Weiss, B., Weisz, J. R., Politano, M., Carey, M., Nelson, W. M., & Finch, A. J. (1991). Developmental differences in the factor structure of the Children's Depression Inventory. *Child Psychiatry and Human Development, 19,* 98–108.

Weissman, M. M., Orvaschel, H., & Padian, N. (1980). Children's symptom and social functioning self-report scales: Comparison of mothers' and children's reports. *Journal of Nervous and Mental Disease, 168,* 736–740.

Wendel, N. H., Nelson, W. M., Politano, P. M., Mayhall, C. A., & Finch, A. J. (1988). Differentiating inpatient clinically diagnosed and normal children using the Children's Depression Inventory. *Child Psychiatry and Human Development, 19,* 98–108.

Werry, J. S., Aman, M. G., & Diamond, E. (1980). Imipramine and methylphenidate in hyperactive children. *Journal of Child Psychology and Psychiatry and Allied Disciplines, 21,* 27–35.

Wigfield, A., & Karpathian, M. (1991). Who am I and what can I do: Children's self-concepts and motivation. *Educational Psychologist, 26,* 233–261.

Williams, J. R., & Gold, M. (1972). From delinquent behavior to official delinquency. *Social Problems, 20,* 209–229.

Wilson, P. L. (1998). Multidimensional self concept scale: An examination of grade, race, and gender differences in third through sixth grade students' self-concepts. *Psychology in the Schools, 35,* 317–326.

Winne, P. H., Marx, R. W., & Taylor, T. D. (1977). A multitrait–multimethod study of three self-concept inventories. *Child Development, 48*, 893–901.

Witt, J. C., Cavell, T. A., Heffer, R. W., Carey, M. P., & Martens, B. K. (1988). Child self-report: Interviewing techniques and rating scales. In E. S. Shapiro & T. R. Kratochwill (Eds.), *Behavioral assessment in schools* (pp. 384–454). New York: Guilford Press.

Wolfe, V. V., Finch, A. J., Saylor, C. F., Blount, R. L., Pallmeyer, T. P., & Carek, D. J. (1987). Negative affectivity in children: A multitrait-multimethod investigation. *Journal of Consulting and Clinical Psychology, 55*, 245–250.

Zahn-Waxler, C. (1993). Warriors and worriers: Gender and psychopathology. *Development and Psychopathology, 5*, 79–89.

Zoccolillo, M. (1992). Gender and the development of conduct disorder. *Development and Psychopathology, 5*, 65–78.

CHAPTER 12

Self-Reports

Theory and Practice in Interviewing Children

STEPHANIE H. McCONAUGHY

University of Vermont

Interviewing has long held a prominent position in mental health work with adults and children. Interviews are widely used by psychologists, psychiatrists, social workers, and other mental health workers for clinical assessment and psychotherapy. Clinical assessment interviews are designed to obtain data on an individual's behavioral, emotional, and social functioning in order to diagnose problems and develop treatment plans. Psychotherapeutic interviews, in contrast, are designed to alleviate stress and foster behavioral and emotional change (Sattler, 1998). In modern versions of behavioral assessment, interviews have also become key techniques for obtaining information from parents and teachers, as well as children (Hughes & Baker, 1990). This chapter will focus on interviewing children as a method of clinical assessment. (For brevity, the term "children" will be used to include adolescents.) While focusing on interviews, however, it is important to emphasize that no one method of assessment, including clinical interviewing, should be considered the "gold standard" for assessment. Because agreement among different data sources is low to moderate at best (Achenbach, McConaughy, & Howell, 1987), it is important to integrate child interview data with information from other sources, including parents and teachers, and to observe children's behavior in settings outside of the interview situation.

Within the context of multimethod assessment, interviewing children can have the following unique advantages:

1. While interviewing, clinicians can directly observe children's behavior, affect, and interaction styles;
2. Through questioning, clinicians can assess children's own perspectives of their problems and competencies;
3. Using behaviorally oriented questions and probes, clinicians can assess children's understanding of antecedents and consequences of specific problems;
4. Through observations and questioning, clinicians can assess directly whether children are amenable to different types of interventions;
5. Following interviewing, clinicians can compare their observations and children's self-reported problems to data obtained from other sources.

The format for conducting child interviews can vary from informal unstructured to semistructured and highly structured approaches. Unstructured formats are useful for establishing initial rapport and developing therapeutic alliances with children. However, unstructured interviews have limited value for clinical assessment because they have shown low levels of reliability for diagnosis and it is difficult to quantify their results (Young, O'Brien, Gutterman, & Cohen, 1987). Semistructured and highly structured interviews are more amenable to psychometric tests of reliability and validity because they are designed to produce quantitative data in the form of categorical diagnoses and/or continuous scores for rating observed problems and children's self-reports.

To familiarize school practitioners with research on child interviews, the next sections review the current status of several structured and semistructured diagnostic interviews for assessing child psychopathology. Five interviews designed to generate psychiatric diagnoses are discussed in detail, along with critiques of their psychometric properties and utility for child assessment. Later sections describe a semistructured clinical interview designed as a component of a multimethod empirically based assessment system. A final section covers applications of behavioral interviewing with children. Because the purpose of this chapter is to review research on child clinical interviews, readers are referred to other sources for practical guidelines for interviewing children (Hughes & Baker, 1990; McConaughy, 1996, 2000; McConaughy & Achenbach, 1994; Sattler, 1998).

STRUCTURED DIAGNOSTIC INTERVIEWS

Since the 1960s, several structured diagnostic interviews have been developed for use in epidemiological research and psychiatric practice (for additional reviews, see Hodges, 1993; Merrell, 1998; Sattler, 1998). Highly structured diagnostic interviews share several common features. First, they require strict adherence to standardized procedures for asking questions, recording responses, and sequencing items. They usually employ standard sets of questions and response categories, using a hierarchical system with skip procedures and probes. Within different content categories, questions are arranged so that the choice of the next question depends on the respondent's answer to the preceding question.

Second, most structured diagnostic interviews are designed to generate DSM diagnoses (*Diagnostic and Statistical Manual of Mental Disorders*; American Psychiatric Association, DSM-III, 1980; DSM-III-R, 1987; DSM-IV, 1994). Although originally designed for earlier versions of the DSM, most of the structured interviews have been revised to address the current DSM-IV nomenclature. The number of diagnoses vary across interviews, but most include common diagnoses attributed to children, such as attention-deficit/hyperactivity disorder (ADHD), conduct disorder, oppositional defiant disorder, affective disorders, and anxiety disorders. Some interviews also contain additional items for screening psychotic symptoms, substance abuse, and less common diagnoses. Diagnoses are scored dichotomously as present versus absent according to whether criteria have been met. Scores for individual symptoms may be scored as present versus absent or on multistep scales and are then aggregated according to computer algorithms or clinical judgments to obtain a yes/no decision for each diagnosis.

The structured diagnostic interviews differ in the length of time required for administration and in the experience required of the interviewer. Most require at least 45 to 60 minutes, but some can take as long as 4 hours or more, depending on the number of symptoms and complexity of problems reported by the respondent.

Diagnostic Interview for Children and Adolescents (DICA)

The DICA (Herjanic & Reich, 1982; DICA-R: Reich & Welner, 1992; DICA-IV: Reich et al., 1999) is an example of a highly structured diagnostic interview. The original DICA was developed as a child-oriented version of the Diagnostic Interview Schedule (DIS; Robins, Helzer, Ratcliff, & Seyfried, 1982) used in adult epidemiological research and clinical practice. The current version, the DICA-IV (Reich et al., 1997; Reich, 2000), has been revised for DSM-IV diagnoses and includes a self-report instrument for interviewing children aged 6 to 12 and 13 to 17, plus another version for interviewing parents. The two versions have similar questions with changes in wording appropriate to the particular respondent. The DICA-IV begins with a brief demographic section covering the child's age, level of education, favorite activities, and relationships with family, peers, and teachers. The major portion of the DICA-IV covers 28 diagnostic categories with over 1,600 possible questions. Questions are hierarchically organized into modules for each category, so that the user can choose whether to administer modules for any combination or all categories.

The DICA-IV can be administered via computer, either by having the interviewer ask questions and enter responses for the respondent or by having a child or parent enter responses on-line. The computer scoring program offers three report options: (1) a summary of responses that paraphrases each question and response; (2) a concise report that lists whether or not criteria have been met for possible diagnoses; and (3) a diagnostic report that lists criteria met, responses related to the criteria, plus positive responses to critical items for high-risk features (e.g., suicidal ideation, violent tendencies, drug abuse). There is also a paper-and-pencil version similar to the computer version, but it does not automatically branch questions or yield diagnostic reports. The DICA-IV requires 5 to 20 minutes for each module, with a maximum time of 2 to 9 hours if all modules are administered. However, the typical assessment time is 60 to 90 minutes, depending on the number of symptoms reported by the respondent. The DICA-IV can be administered by lay interviewers after training, but for clinical assessment it is preferable to have it administered by experienced clinicians.

Diagnostic Interview Schedule for Children (DISC)

The DISC (Costello, Edelbrock, Dulcan, Kalas, & Klaric, 1984; DISC-R; Shaffer et al., 1993; DISC-2.3; Shaffer, 1992; NIMH DISC-IV; Shaffer, Fisher, Lucas,

Dulcan, & Schwab-Stone, 2000) is another highly structured diagnostic interview that was developed primarily for epidemiologic research on the prevalence of psychiatric disorders in American children. The DISC has undergone many revisions, but is currently designed to generate DSM-IV diagnoses. Most of the published research on reliability and validity of the DISC has involved earlier versions generating DSM-III and DSM-III-R diagnoses.

The current NIMH DISC-IV (Shaffer et al., 2000) has separate formats for interviewing children aged 9 to 17 and interviewing parents. Over 1,500 questions are arranged in hierarchical order with skip procedures around criteria for different DSM diagnoses. The DISC can also provide ICD-10 diagnoses (*International Classification of Diseases–Tenth Edition*; World Health Association, 1992). Individual items or symptoms may be scored as present or absent or on multistep scales (e.g., no, sometimes/somewhat, yes, or don't know). As with the DICA, symptom reports are aggregated according to scoring rules to generate present versus absent decisions for each diagnosis. Administration of the child version of the DISC may take as little as 54 minutes, but can take as long as 4 hours or more if the respondent reports multiple symptoms (Shaffer et al., 2000). The DISC was designed to be administered by trained lay interviewers, but can also be used by clinicians who wish to obtain systematic symptom reports for psychiatric diagnoses.

Interviewer-Based versus Respondent-Based Interviews

Both the DICA and the DISC can be considered "respondent-based" interviews in contrast to "interviewer-based" approaches (Harrington et al., 1988). The respondent-based approach limits the range of responses to similar sets of questions for all respondents, and respondents' answers to the questions comprise the essential data obtained from the interview. As Costello, Burns, Angold, and Leaf (1993) explain, the aim of respondent-based interviews is "to structure the behavior of the interviewers in such a way that the 'stimulus' presented to each respondent is as similar as possible" (p. 1110). By thus standardizing the interaction between the interviewer and respondent, respondent-based interviews seek to reduce variability across interviews. In this respect, according to Costello and colleagues (1993), the DICA and DISC are similar to long questionnaires administered verbally.

"Interviewer-based" approaches, by contrast, allow more flexibility in questioning techniques and require clinical judgments for determining the presence of symptoms and diagnoses. In interviewer-based interviews, the interviewer decides whether a specific symptom is present based on the respondent's answers to questions. Symptom definitions are provided along with detailed questions to guide interviewer judgments and reduce variability between interviewers. Interviewer-based interviews are usually administered by experienced clinicians and employ semistructured formats, as discussed next.

SEMISTRUCTURED DIAGNOSTIC INTERVIEWS

Semistructured interviews are less rigid than structured interviews, employing open-ended questions that can be followed by probes when appropriate. The interviewer is free to alter questions and to vary the sequence of topics to follow the child's natural flow of conversation. Some semistructured interviews also include nonverbal activities, such as drawing and play materials, to provide more options for interacting and establishing rapport with the child.

Like the structured diagnostic interviews, most semistructured diagnostic interviews yield DSM diagnoses, and some generate ICD diagnoses. In addition to categorical diagnoses, some semistructured diagnostic interviews also yield scores for content areas, mental status, affect, observed behavior, and global ratings of psychopathology or total pathology scores. Scoring systems for semistructured diagnostic interviews generally include present versus absent ratings and/or multistep scales for rating the severity of problems.

Child Assessment Schedule (CAS)

The CAS (Hodges, McKnew, Cytryn, Stern, & Kline, 1982; Hodges, Cools, & McKnew, 1989; Hodges, Gordon, & Lennon, 1990) is intended to combine the standardized procedures of structured diagnostic interviews with the flexibility of semistructured interviews. Separate versions are used for interviewing children and parents. The CAS consists of 320 items organized into three broad sections. In the first section, the interviewer asks the child open ended questions concerning school, friends, activities, hobbies, family, and groupings of psychiatric symptoms. Questions are organized according to 11 content areas so that the interviewer can vary the sequence of topics to match the child's conversation. In the second section, the interviewer asks specific questions about the onset and duration of symptoms that were reported present in the first section. In the third section, after the interview is completed, the interviewer rates the child on 53 items covering behavior, affect, interpersonal interactions, and estimated cognitive ability, based on observations during the interview. Each CAS item is scored as "yes," "no," "ambiguous," or "unscorable." Response items are phrased such that a "yes" always indicates the presence of a symptom. The CAS can be scored by hand or computer to obtain a total pathology score, as well as scores for the content areas, symptom scales, and DSM diagnoses.

Child and Adolescent Psychiatric Assessment (CAPA)

The CAPA (Angold, Cox, Prendergast, Rutter, & Simonoff, 1987; Angold & Costello, 2000) is a semistructured interview for children aged 8 to 18. There are separate versions for interviewing children and their parents. The general format is semistructured, consisting of open-ended questions that introduce a particular topic area, followed by more specific probes tapping details of each topic for later scoring by the interviewer. The interview is divided into three broad sections: (1) introduction, (2) symptom review, and (3) incapacity ratings. The introduction, which is intended to establish rapport, includes general questions regarding home and family life, school, peer groups, and spare-time activities. The symptom review involves detailed questions about specific symptoms or problems that comprise 17 domains corresponding to psychiatric diagnoses. The CAPA protocol lists a definition of each symptom or problem along with open-ended questions, 1,401 emphasized probes, and 2,571 discretionary probes regarding the symptoms.

The CAPA interviewer must cover all symptoms, but can address sets of symptoms in a modular fashion (e.g., anxiety disorders, oppositional and conduct disorders, school-related problems, etc.). The interviewer starts with areas thought to be problematic for a particular child, as inferred from the child's responses in the introductory section. Following the symptom review, the interviewer questions the child about the effects of each reported symptom on 19 areas of "incapacity," or psychosocial impairment, such as relationships with parents, relationships with peers, homework, spare time activities, and the like. The interviewer must establish whether an "incapacity" is secondary to particular symptoms reported earlier (e.g., the child's reported loss of friends is because of a fear of leaving the home), rather than to some other factor separate from the symptom (e.g., the child's reported loss of friends is because of a move to a new community).

The CAPA interviewer also scores the reported symptoms for duration, frequency, time of onset, and intensity, according to a glossary of definitions for each symptom. Most CAPA items are rated on the basis of the three months preceding the interview, except for certain infrequent problems, such as setting fires or suicidal behavior. In addition to the symptom and incapacity ratings, the interviewer scores 67 observational items covering activity level, mood state, quality of social interaction during the interview, and psychotic behavior. The average time for administering the child version of the CAPA is approximately 60 minutes, with a range of 22 to 150 minutes reported for one study (Angold & Costello, 2000). An additional hour or more is also required for data coding, data entry, and supervisor review.

CAPA computer algorithms aggregate the interviewer's ratings to produce present or absent scores for some 40 DSM or ICD diagnoses and provide scores for the number of symptoms reported for each diagnosis and incapacity scores for each diagnosis. An optional section of the CAPA assesses critical life events impinging on the child's problems, and a companion interview has also been developed for assessing service utilization (Burns, Angold, Macgruder-Habib, Costello, & Patrick, 1992).

Schedule for Affective Disorders and Schizophrenia for School-Aged Children (K-SADS)

The K-SADS, or sometimes called the Kiddie-SADS (Ambrosini, 2000; Ambrosini, Metz, Prabucki, & Lee, 1989; Chambers et al., 1985; Puig-Antich & Chambers, 1978), is a semistructured interview developed as a downward extension of the Schedule for

Affective Disorders and Schizophrenia for adults (SADS; Endicott & Spitzer, 1978). The K-SADS is designed for children aged 6 to 18 with separate versions for interviewing children and their parents. Although its title suggests it is limited to affective and psychotic symptoms, the K-SADS assesses a broad range of symptoms to generate DSM diagnoses. The K-SADS has undergone many revisions. Three current versions are compatible with DSM-III-R and DSM-IV diagnoses. The K-SADS-P-IVR assesses present or current symptoms or episodes of psychopathology within the previous 12 months. The K-SADS-E (epidemiologic) assesses the most severe past episode and present episode of each diagnosis. The K-SADS-P/L assesses present and lifetime episodes for each diagnosis. In addition to diagnoses, the K-SADS-P-IVR includes ratings of depressive symptoms and clinical global impressions of overall psychopathology. The K-SADS contains over 800 questions, including open-ended and structured questions, with skip-out procedures, similar to the hierarchical organization of the DICA and DISC. Questions are organized around diagnostic categories and symptoms are scored on a 6-point scale. Diagnoses are generated by integrating parent and child data. (The issue of parent–child agreement will be addressed in a later section.) The K-SADS takes approximately 90 minutes for each parent and child for a total of 3 hours and requires a trained clinician.

RELIABILITY OF DIAGNOSTIC INTERVIEWS

Many studies have tested the reliability of the various structured and semistructured diagnostic interviews. To evaluate this research, the next sections describe reliability findings with respect to different diagnoses, reports of younger versus older children, child versus parent reports in clinical and community samples, parent–child agreement, and categorical diagnoses versus continuous symptom scores.

Reliability Differences among Diagnoses

Reliabilities have varied for different DSM diagnoses across the structured and semistructured diagnostic interviews. For example, the DICA-R demonstrated high agreement between clinician's judgments and interviewer's symptom scores for DSM diagnoses of conduct disorder, but low to moderate diagnostic agreement for other DSM diagnoses (Ezpeleta, de la Osa, Domenech, & Navarro, 1997). Different patterns of test–retest reliabilities have also occurred across diagnoses. These patterns are illustrated in Table 12.1, which lists test–retest kappa coefficients (a measure of agreement for categorical data) for DSM-III-R diagnoses generated from the child versions of four diagnostic interviews: (1) CAPA (Angold & Costello, 1995); (2) CAS (Hodges, 1993); (3) DICA-R (Boyle et al., 1993); and (4) DISC-2.1 (Jensen et al., 1995). For the DICA-R, Boyle and colleagues (1993) provided separate kappas for ages 6 to 11 and 12 to 16. Using Landis and Koch's (1977) criteria, kappas > .75 are considered excellent; kappa = .59–.75, good; kappa = .40–.58, fair; and kappa < .40, poor.

TABLE 12.1 Test–Retest Reliabilities (Kappa) for DSM-III-R Diagnoses from Child Versions of Four Diagnostic Interviews

Diagnosis	CAPA[a]	CAS[b]	DICA-R[c]	DISC 2.1[d]
Any anxiety disorder	.74/.56	.72	.04 (6–11) .56 (12–16)	.39
Any depressive disorder	.90/.75	.83	.21 (6–11) .38 (12–16)	.38
Attention-deficit/hyperactivity disorder	—	.43	.43 (6–11) .24 (12–16)	.59
Oppositional defiant disorder	—	—	.33 (6–11) .28 (12–16)	.46
Conduct disorder	.54	.71	.37 (6–11) .92 (12–16)	.86

[a]Angold & Costello (1995).
[b]Hodges et al. (1989).
[c]Boyle et al. (1993); age ranges in parentheses.
[d]Jensen et al. (1995) clinical sample.

As Table 12.1 shows, kappas for diagnoses of anxiety disorders (overanxious disorder/separation anxiety) were fair to good for the semistructured CAS and CAPA, but poor for the more highly structured DISC-2.1 and DICA-R for younger children. A similar pattern was found for depressive disorders (major depression/dysthymia), with the CAPA and CAS showing excellent test–retest reliabilities, but the DICA-R and DISC-2.1 showing poor reliabilities. Diagnoses of conduct disorder showed the opposite pattern, with the DICA for older children and DISC-2.1 showing excellent reliabilities, the CAS showing good reliability, but the CAPA showing only fair reliability. These findings suggest that the more flexible semistructured formats of the CAS and CAPA may be better for interviewing children about internalizing problems, such as anxiety and depression, whereas the flexibility of the format did not have as much effect on the reliability of diagnoses of externalizing conduct disorders, except for younger children. Diagnoses of attention-deficit/hyperactivity disorder and oppositional deficient disorder showed poor to good reliabilities across the different interviews, but particularly poor reliability for older children on the DICA-R.

Reliability for Younger versus Older Children

The DICA-R kappa coefficients listed in Table 12.1 for younger versus older children illustrate a general pattern found in several other studies: the reliability of highly structured diagnostic interviews decreases for younger children. Boyle and colleagues (1993) found particularly low reliabilities for internalizing disorders reported by 6–11-year olds, warranting cautions against relying on young children's reports for diagnosing these disorders. Reliabilities were higher for internalizing disorders reported by 12–16-year olds, except for separation anxiety disorder, but poor for oppositional defiant disorder and attention-deficit/hyperactivity disorder. For an early version of the DISC, Edelbrock, Costello, Dulcan, Kalas, and Conover (1985) also reported lower reliabilities for total symptom scores reported by younger versus older children. They obtained 9-day test–retest correlations of only .39 at ages 6 to 9 and .55 at ages 10 to 13, versus .81 at ages 14 to 18. In contrast, 9-day test–retest correlations for total symptom scores from parent versions of the DISC were .90 for the 6–9-year-olds and .78 for the 10–13-year-olds.

In a later study of a community sample of 109 6–11-year-old children interviewed with the DISC-R, children reported far fewer symptoms than their parents and were particularly unreliable in reporting time factors related to onset and duration of symptoms (Schwab-Stone, Fallon, Briggs, & Crowther, 1994). When duration was included among the criteria for diagnoses in this study, no reliabilities could be determined for child reports of overanxious disorder, oppositional defiant disorder or conduct disorder, and only poor to fair test–retest reliabilities were obtained for diagnoses of separation anxiety (kappa = .33) and attention-deficit/hyperactivity disorder (kappa = .41). In contrast, a study using the DISC-2.25 with a community sample of 145 adolescents aged 12–14 showed good test–retest reliability for separation anxiety (kappa = .59) and fair reliabilities for overanxious disorder (kappa = .53), depressive disorders (kappa = .55), and conduct disorder (kappa = .49) (Breton, Bergeron, Valla, Berthiume, & St-Georges, 1998). A study using the DISC-2.1 with a clinical sample of 299 12–17-year-old outpatients also showed fair test–retest reliabilities for any anxiety disorder (kappa = .44), any affective disorder (kappa = .53), any disruptive behavior disorder (kappa = .58), and any substance use disorder (kappa = .46) (Roberts, Solovitz, Chen, & Casat, 1996). In addition, 15–17-year-olds showed somewhat higher reliability for any diagnosis (kappa = .58) than did 12–14-year-olds (kappa = .44).

The higher reliabilities for older versus younger children on the DICA and DISC suggest that the rigid format of the highly structured diagnostic interviews may be incompatible with young children's communicative capacity and style of interaction. The length and detail of structured diagnostic interviews can pose formidable challenges to children's attention span and tolerance for verbal questioning. Interviewers may also find it hard to carry out complicated questioning and recording of responses with young children, while at the same time observing and maintaining rapport, particularly when interviewing children with challenging disruptive behavior.

Inappropriate formats are a particular problem for the respondent-based structured interviews. To standardize procedures across subjects, the respondent-based interviews use exactly the same questions with all children, regardless of age or cognitive level. As Costello and colleagues (1993) point out, this approach assumes that children, regardless of their developmental level, will "(1) understand the questions in the same way, (2) be equally capable of deciding whether they have experienced the phenomenon in question, and (3) be equally capable of deciding whether the level at which they experienced it falls into the range of deviance that interests the interviewer" (p. 1110).

Along with lower test–retest reliabilities for younger children, Edelbrock and colleagues (1985) reported that they seemed to employ a yea-saying set (i.e., responding "yes" to many symptoms) to initial DISC interviews and then switched to a nay-saying set (i.e., responding "no" to many of the same symptoms) in retest interviews. These researchers surmised that the change from yea-saying to nay-saying occurred because young children had learned that negative responses shortened the interview process. This produced large declines in child-reported symptom scores from Time 1 to Time 2. After closer examination of variables affecting the low reliabilities of 6–12-year-olds reports on the DISC, Fallon and Schwab-Stone (1994) came to the following conclusions: (1) test–retest reliability improves with age, but the reliability of 12-year-olds is still not equal to the reliability of adults' reports; (2) questions about observable behaviors elicited more reliable responses than questions about emotions or questions containing metaphors; and (3) questions requiring children to delineate time or to compare themselves to other children were particularly unreliable.

In the Fallon and Schwab-Stone (1994) study, the length or complexity of questions did not significantly affect reliability. However, when Breton, Bergeron, Valla, Lepine, Houde, and Gaudet (1995) directly tested 9–11-year olds' understanding of DISC questions, they found that children understood only 38 to 42% of questions as a whole and 26 to 30% of overall time concepts. In this study, shorter questions were significantly better understood than longer ones; questions with one time concept were grasped better than those with two or more time concepts; and durations of time (e.g., most of the day, two weeks) were better grasped than time periods (e.g., within the past 6 months) or frequencies (e.g., nearly every day, 1–6 days a week). Understanding of questions regarding diagnostic symptoms ranged from 16 to 56%, with the questions about simple phobias and conduct disorder understood best and questions about depressive symptoms understood least.

Because of the lower reliabilities obtained for young children, the current version of the DISC is recommended only for children aged 9–17 (Shaffer et al., 2000). Nonetheless, declines in DISC symptoms from Time 1 to Time 2 (*attenuation effects*) and lower test–retest reliabilities for younger than for older children have been found even for respondents above age 9. For example, test–retest kappas were significantly lower for 9–12-year-olds than for 13–18-year-olds for diagnoses of depression/dysthymia and conduct disorder, based on DISC-2.1 child interviews of community samples (Jensen et al., 1995). The tendency for subjects to report fewer symptoms at Time 2 than Time 1 did more to reduce test–retest reliability than did any other respondent characteristics, such as impulsive answers, being slow to warm up, or endorsement of many symptoms by "noncases" (Jensen et al., 1995). Similar attenuation effects have been found for the NIMH DISC-IV (Lucas et al., 1999), as well as other respondent-based interviews (Costello et al., 1993).

Child versus Parent Reports in Clinical and Community Samples

Reliability studies of diagnostic interviews have been conducted with both clinically referred and community samples of children and their parents or primary caregivers. In general, higher reliabilities have been found for clinically referred children than

TABLE 12.2 Test–Retest Reliabilities (Kappa) for Child, Parent, and Parent–Child Combined DSM-III-R Diagnoses from the Diagnostic Interview Schedule for Children (DISC-2.1 and 2.3)

Diagnosis	Clinical sample ($n = 97^a$)			Community sample ($n = 278^a/247^c$)		
	Child	Parent	Combined	Child	Parent	Combined
Any anxiety disorder	.39	.58	.50[b]	.30/.39	.40/.56	.32/.47
Any depressive disorder	.38	.69	.70[b]	.29/.35	.00/.50	.26/.45
Attention-deficit/ hyperactivity disorder	.59	.69	.68[b]	.43/.10	.57/.60	.62/.48
Oppositional defiant disorder	.46	.67	.61[b]	.23/.18	.65/.68	.51/.59
Conduct disorder	.86	.70	.71[b]	.60/.64	.66/.56	.64/.66

[a]Jensen et al. (1995).
[b]Clinical kappa > community kappa for Jensen et al. (1995) samples.
[c]Schwab-Stone et al. (1996).

children from community samples. These differences are illustrated in Table 12.2 for the DISC-2.1 from the first phase of the NIMH Methods for Epidemiology of Child and Adolescent Mental Disorders (MECA) study (Jensen et al., 1995). The MECA community sample included 278 youths aged 9 to 17 and their parent/primary caregiver drawn from probability samples in New York, Georgia, and Puerto Rico. The clinical sample included 97 9–17-year-olds and parents/caregivers recruited from clinical settings in the same three areas. Lay interviewers administered paper-and-pencil versions of the DISC-2.1 on two occasions to generate DSM-III-R diagnoses. Test–retest intervals ranged from 19 to 33 days across the three areas.

As Table 12.2 shows, when child and parent reports were combined to generate diagnoses (third and sixth columns), test–retest kappas were higher in the clinical versus the community samples for all diagnoses (Jensen et al., 1995). Within each sample, parents' reports of their children's symptoms showed significantly higher reliabilities than did children's reports for four out of five diagnostic categories. In the clinical sample, parent reports were more reliable for all diagnoses, except conduct disorder, where both parents and children showed good to excellent reliabilities. In the community sample, parent reports showed higher reliability for all diagnoses except depressive disorders, because too few parents reported depressive symptoms for their children.

Two later DISC studies conducted with community samples showed similar results for DSM-III-R diagnoses. One was a second phase MECA study of a community sample of 247 parent–youth pairs in New York, Georgia, Puerto Rico, and Connecticut (Schwab-Stone et al., 1996). This sample included 134 "screen-positive" youths with DSM-III-R diagnoses. Youths and parents were administered the DISC-2.3 via laptop computer over intervals of 1 to 15 days. Lay interviewers administered the DISC-2.3 at Time 1 whereas clinicians administered it at Time 2, but there were no significant interviewer effects on the reliabilities. The second community study used a French version of the DISC-2.25 with 2,400 Quebec youths aged 6 to 14 (Breton et al., 1998). Both of these studies produced fair to good test–retest reliabilities for the same five diagnostic categories listed in Table 12.2, based on parent reports. Kappa coefficients from the community sample in the second MECA study are listed after the slash in Table 12.2, showing fair to good reliabilities for all diagnoses, in contrast to poor reliability for depression/dysthymia in the first MECA community sample.

The data in Table 12.2 demonstrate how the highly structured format of the DISC consistently produced more reliable categorical diagnoses from parents' reports than from children's reports and more reliable reports from clinical versus community samples. Fair to good reliabilities in the second MECA community sample suggest that the DISC is appropriate for obtaining prevalence rates of DSM disorders, as long as parent reports are included to obtain diagnoses. The DISC-2.3 produced prevalence rates of 10.2% for any DSM-III-R based on parent reports alone and 20.9% based on combined parent and child reports (Schwab-Stone et al., 1996). These prevalence rates were defined by DSM diagnostic criteria, plus at least mild social and/or academic impairment indicated on the Children's Global Assessment Scale. When impairment criteria were not included to define "caseness," prevalence rates increased to 30.3% based on parent reports and 50.6% based on combined parent and child reports.

Shaffer et al. (2000) reported test–retest reliabilities for the NIMH DISC-IV derived from clinical samples of 84 parents and 82 youths aged 9 to 17 interviewed over an average of 6.6 days. For the parent version of the DISC-IV, reliabilities were good to excellent for diagnoses of attention-deficit/hyperactivity disorder (kappa = .79), major depression (kappa = .66), and two specific anxiety disorders, but only fair for oppositional defiant disorder (kappa = .54) and conduct disorder (kappa = .43). For the child version of the DISC-IV, reliabilities were fair to good for all diagnoses except major depression, for which reliability was excellent (kappa = .92).

Parent–Child Agreement in Diagnostic Interviews

Categorical diagnoses generated from a single source, such as a child interview, are often difficult to integrate with discrepant data obtained from other sources. Diagnoses based on separate interviews of children and their parents have generally shown only low to moderate agreement (for reviews, see Hodges, 1993; Young et al., 1987). Parent–child agreement has typically been moderate to high for externalizing symptoms, moderate for depressive symptoms, and low for anxiety symptoms (Edelbrock, Costello, Dulcan, Conover, & Kalas, 1986; Hodges, 1993; Hodges, Gordon, & Lennon, 1990). Such findings have raised questions about the validity of child diagnoses obtained from diagnostic interviews. However, such low to moderate parent–child agreement is consistent with the modest cross-informant agreement found in ratings of behavioral and emotional problems (Achenbach et al., 1987). Low parent–child agreement does not necessarily mean that one informant is right and the other wrong, but that both perspectives must be considered in assessing children's functioning.

Low agreement has also been found between DISC diagnoses and clinicians' diagnoses of the same subjects (Costello et al., 1984; Shaffer et al., 1988). A later study showed better agreement between clinician's diagnoses derived from a clinical style interview and DISC diagnoses based on parent reports, especially for attention-deficit/hyperactivity disorder and oppositional defiant disorder (Schwab-Stone et al., 1996). Agreement between clinician's and DISC diagnoses was lower for parent reports of conduct disorder, and fair to good for diagnoses of depressive and anxiety disorders. Agreement was poor between clinician's diagnoses and DISC diagnoses based on children's reports, except for fair agreement for conduct disorder (Schwab-Stone, et al., 1996).

Most experts now agree that data are needed from both children and parents, but no procedures have yet been agreed upon for deciding on categorical diagnoses derived from interviews of different informants (Hodges, 1993). Complex "optimal informant" procedures have been proposed for combining information across multiple sources and diagnoses (Loeber, Green, Lahey, & Stouthamer-Loeber, 1989). However, such procedures appear to have no more psychometric advantages than does a simple combination rule that acknowledges a diagnosis if symptoms are reported by either a child or parent (the "or" rule; Bird, Gould, & Staghezza, 1992; Hodges, 1993; Piacentini, Cohen, & Cohen, 1992). Using the "or" rule to combine child and parent data from the DISC-2.1 produced test–retest kappas ranging from .50 to .71 for the five diagnoses listed in Table 12.2 for the clinical sample (Jensen et al., 1995). Combined parent and child data from the DISC-IV clinical sample produced test–retest kappas ranging from .48 to .86 for eight diagnostic cateogries (Shaffer et al., 2000). In the community samples shown in Table 12.2, comparable test–retest reliabilities (kappas = .51 to .66) were also obtained with combined parent and child data for attention-deficit/hyperactivity disorder, oppositional defiant disorder, and conduct disorder. However, reliabilities remained lower for anxiety and depressive disorders (kappas = .26 to .47; Jensen et al., 1995; Schwab-Stone et al., 1996).

A problem related to modest parent–child agreement is the heavy reliance on the interview as the primary source of data on children's functioning. Although most experts now acknowledge the need for multiple data sources, "best estimate diagnoses" are still based primarily on interview data (Costello, 1989; Costello et al., 1993). However, interviews are vulnerable to errors even when questions and response formats are highly structured. For example, Young and colleagues (1987) listed several sources of potential error and misinformation affecting interviews, including the structure of the interview questions, characteristics of the respondent, and characteristics of the interviewer. Misinformation is further exacerbated when interviews are used to assess problems that might be better assessed in other ways. An example is asking children whether they are restless, fidgety, or have attention problems, rather than asking parents about these symptoms or assessing these behaviors through direct observations or standardized rating scales from parents and teachers.

Categorical Diagnoses versus Continuous Symptom Scores

The dependence on categorical DSM diagnoses as the primary product is a major limitation of the structured and semistructured diagnostic interviews for several reasons. First, the close tie to the DSM makes such interview formats vulnerable to the frequent revisions of the DSM. Each time the diagnostic nomenclature is revised, lay and clinical interviewers require new training in differential diagnosis and administration of the interviews (Costello et al., 1993; Young et al., 1987). As indicated earlier, the CAS, DICA, and DISC all now have versions for DSM-IV, but the research on these formats is limited.

Second, dichotomous categorization of symptoms and diagnoses can lose important information regarding the severity of problems. Although symptoms may be scored initially on more differentiated scales, the diagnostic algorithms for the structured and semistructured diagnostic interviews require categorization of each symptom as present or absent and each child as a "case" or "noncase" for a diagnosis, based on fixed cutpoints for diagnostic criteria. The sensitivity (percent of correctly identified cases) and specificity (percent of correctly identified noncases) for each diagnosis thus depend on the cutpoint used to identify cases (Rey, Morris-Yates, & Stanislaw, 1992). However, using an early parent version of the DISC, Edelbrock and Costello (1988) found that children who just met the minimum diagnostic criteria required for making a DSM-III diagnosis obtained significantly lower problem scores on the Child Behavior Checklist (CBCL; Achenbach & Edelbrock, 1983) than did children who exceeded the minimum criteria required for a diagnosis. The differences in CBCL scores demonstrated that important quantitative differences in the severity of problems were not reflected in the dichotomous categorizations for the DSM diagnoses.

Third, reliabilities have been consistently lower for categorical diagnoses than for continuous symptom scores. This has been demonstrated in several DISC studies that have compared reliabilities for categorical DSM diagnoses versus quantitative, continuous scores for symptom scales, and criteria counts for each diagnosis (Schwab-Stone et al., 1994: Schwab-Stone et al., 1996; Shaffer, Fisher, Dulcan, Davies, Piacentini, et al., 1996). Symptom scales were constructed by counting all symptoms reported present for each diagnosis, while criterion scales included positive symptoms plus positive criteria for frequency, duration, and severity of symptoms. These studies all showed higher test–retest reliabilities for the quantitative symptom and/or criterion scales than for the categorical classifications for most diagnoses. Quantitative scales from parent interviews continued to be more reliable than scales from child interviews, but the reliability differences between parents and children were less pronounced for the continuous scores than for the categorical diagnoses. Rubio-Stipec, Shrout, Canino, Bird, et al. (1996) also found good to excellent test–retest reliabilities for four factor-analytically derived symptom scales from the DISC 2.3: .80 to .86 for parent reports; .65 to .83 for child reports (ages 9–17); and .72 to .84 for combined parent and child reports. The higher reliabilities for the DISC symptom scales were comparable to reliabilities ranging from .57 to .88 for quantitative symptom scores derived from CAS interviews of 6–12-year old children (Hodges, Cools, & McKnew, 1989). These findings all demonstrate that continuous, quantitative scores produce more reliable information than do categorical diagnoses derived from interviews with parents as well as children.

Fourth, categorization according to DSM diagnoses can mask the variety of problems found in many children. This occurs because a particular diagnosis provides information only about the symptoms associated with that diagnosis. It does not include information about other problems that may exist but are not associated with that diagnosis and do not qualify for an additional diagnosis. For example, Edelbrock and Costello (1988) found that DSM diagnoses of depression and dysthymia, based on DISC parent interviews, correlated significantly with both Internalizing and Externalizing scores on the CBCL. The categorical diagnoses of depression and dysthymia, however, did not reflect the Externalizing problems also exhibited by the children.

Finally, categorical DSM diagnoses tell us little about children's thoughts or feelings about their problems, their understanding of the causes of their problems, the contexts in which problems occur, or problems that are omitted from the DSM criteria, all of which are important for assessment and treatment. With these issues in mind, the next sections describe a semistructured interview designed to produce continuous, quantitative scores for children's problems in contrast to the categorical DSM diagnoses.

SEMISTRUCTURED CLINICAL INTERVIEW
FOR CHILDREN AND ADOLESCENTS (SCICA)

The SCICA (McConaughy & Achenbach, 1994) is a standardized semistructured clinical interview for use with children aged 6 to 18. Like the CAS and CAPA, the SCICA incorporates the flexibility of a semistructured protocol, but has structured rating scales for scoring problems observed or reported during the interview. The SCICA differs from the structured and semistructured diagnostic interviews discussed previously in its empirically based, quantitative approach to assessing children's problems (Achenbach & McConaughy, 1997). The empirically based approach does not assume that children's (or parents') yes or no reports of problems dictate the presence or absence of symptoms or disorders. Instead of providing categorical classifications of problems, children's self-reports and interviewers' observations during the SCICA are quantified on rating scales, and scored on a profile of broad scales and "syndromes" developed through statistical analyses. By quantifying and grouping individual problems, measurement variations can be used to judge the severity of problems and multiple items can be used to sample each problem domain. (The DISC factor-analytic symptom scales [Rubio-Stipec et al., 1996] represented similar attempts to quantify problems reported in parent and child diagnostic interviews.) In addition, an individual child's scores on various problem items and SCICA scales are compared to reference samples of peers to provide a standard against which to judge deviance in problems.

The SCICA was designed as one component of a *multiaxial* approach to assessment (Achenbach & McConaughy, 1997) that assumes data will also be obtained from other key sources, including parent reports, teacher reports, standardized self-reports, direct observations, cognitive and achievement tests, and medical and physical exams, as appropriate. To facilitate multiaxial assessment, the SCICA was specifically designed to mesh with data obtained from parent ratings on the Child Behavior Checklist (CBCL; Achenbach, 1991a), teacher ratings on the Teacher's Report Form (TRF; Achenbach, 1991b), direct observations on the Direct Observation Form (DOF; see Achenbach, 1991a; McConaughy, Achenbach, & Gent, 1988) and self ratings on the Youth Self-Report (YSR; Achenbach, 1991c). The CBCL, TRF, and YSR are described by Merrell (Chapter 9, this volume) and Eckert (Chapter 11, this volume), along with other standardized rating scales.

SCICA Protocol Form

The SCICA Protocol Form outlines topics, questions, and tasks to be covered in nine broad areas: (1) activities, school, job; (2) friends; (3) family relations; (4) fantasies; (5) self-perception, feelings; (6) parent/teacher-reported problems; (7) achievement tests (optional); (8) for ages 6–12: Screen for fine and gross motor abnormalities; and (9) For ages 13–18: Somatic complaints, alcohol, drugs, trouble with the law. The protocol includes instructions and samples of open-ended questions for administering the interview and provides space for recording notes on observed behavior and children's self-reports. Table 12.3 lists issues covered in the nine topic areas. For the first five areas, the interviewer can alter the sequence of questions to follow the child's natural flow of conversation.

For children aged 6–12, the interviewer requests a Kinetic Family Drawing (KFD; "draw a picture of your family doing something together") and can administer optional standardized achievement tests, a writing sample, and gross motor screening to assess the child's functioning on more structured tasks. Play materials are also made available for use with young children who are reluctant to talk or participate in other tasks. For ages 13–18, more structured questions are included to assess somatic complaints, alcohol and drug use, and trouble with the law. The first six sections of the SCICA can usually be completed in 45 to 60 minutes, while the last three sections typically require an additional 10 to 15 minutes.

SCICA Observation and Self-Report Forms

After the SCICA is completed, the interviewer scores the child on the Observation and Self-Report Forms, using a 4-point rating scale: 0 *if there was no occurrence; 1 if there was a very slight or ambiguous occurrence; 2 if there was a definite occurrence with mild to moderate intensity and less than 3 minutes' duration; 3 if there was a definite occurrence with severe intensity or 3 or more minutes' duration.* The Observation Form contains 120 problem items, while the Self-Report Form has 114 items for ages 6–18 and 11 additional items for ages 13–18, plus open-ended items for adding other problems reported by the child or observed during the interview. Items were derived from the CBCL and TRF, reviews of the literature, and clinical observations by the developers.

TABLE 12.3 Topic Areas for the Semistructured Clinical Interview for Children and Adolescents (SCICA)

1. *Activities, school, job*

   Favorite activities, sports, organizations
   Attitudes toward school subjects and teachers
   Homework and study strategies
   Job (ages 13–18)

2. *Friends*

   Number and gender of friends
   Kids liked and disliked
   Problems in peer relations
   Problem solving strategies
   Dating and social life (ages 13–18)

3. *Family relations*

   People in family
   Rules, rewards, and punishments at home
   Relationships with parents and siblings
   Kinetic Family Drawing (ages 6–12)

4. *Fantasies*

   Three wishes
   Future goals
   Desired changes in self

5. *Self-perception, feelings*

   Feelings (happy, sad, mad, scared)
   Worries
   Strange experiences/suicidal tendencies

6. *Parent/teacher-reported problems*

   Six problems selected from the CBCL and/or TRF

7. *Achievement tests* (*optional*)

   Mathematics
   Reading recognition

8. *For ages 6–12: Screen for fine and gross motor abnormalities* (*optional*)

   Writing sample
   Gross motor screening

9. *For ages 13–18: Somatic complaints, alcohol, drugs, trouble with the law*

Note. Adapted from McConaughy & Achenbach (1994). Copyright 1994 by S. H. McConaughy and T. M. Achenbach. Adapted by permission.

SCICA Profile for Ages 6–12

To develop the SCICA Profile for Ages 6–12, McConaughy and Achenbach (1994) videotaped interviews for 168 clinically referred children. Each subject was scored on the SCICA Observation and Self-Report Forms by the interviewer and an independent rater of the videotapes. Principal components (PC)/varimax analyses applied to the averaged ratings of the interviewer and observer produced eight empirically based syndrome scales for the SCICA Profile: five scales from the observation items (Anxious, Attention Problems, Resistant, Strange, and Withdrawn), and three scales from the self-report items (Aggressive Behavior, Anxious/Depressed, and Family Problems). (Items scored for < 5% of the sample were excluded from the PC analyses.) Second-order principal factor analyses produced an Internalizing grouping comprising the Anxious and Anxious/Depressed syndromes and an Externalizing grouping comprising the Aggressive Behavior, Attention Problems, Resistant, and Strange syndromes. A clinically referred sample of 237 children was then used to derive normalized T-scores for the eight syndrome scales, Internalizing, Externalizing, Total Observations, and Total Self-Reports. McConaughy and Achenbach (1994) also provided means and standard deviations for comparisons to demographically matched samples of 53 clinically referred and 53 nonreferred children. Research is currently under way to develop a SCICA profile for adolescents.

Using a Dutch translation, Kasius (1997) administered the SCICA to 262 clinically referred and 148 nonreferred children aged 6 to 17. To construct syndromes for the Dutch SCICA Profile, Kasius applied PC/varimax analyses to SCICA ratings for a combined sample of 128 Dutch children aged 6–12 and McConaughy and Achenbach's sample of 168 American children. The Dutch PC analyses produced five syndromes scored from observation items (Attention Problems, Immature, Resistant, Strange, and Withdrawn) and four syndromes from self-report items (Aggressive Behavior, Anxious, Family Problems, Lonely). The names of the Dutch syndromes reflected four observation syndromes and two self-report syndromes that were similar to those derived from the American sample alone.

Reliability of the SCICA

McConaughy and Achenbach (1994) reported findings on the reliability of the original SCICA scales, while Kasius (1997) reported reliabilities for the Dutch SCICA scales. Reliabilities for both the American and Dutch samples are listed in Table 12.4 for similar SCICA scales. For each sample, interrater reliabilities (Pearson r) were obtained between raw scores from the interviewer and a videotape observer for each of the SCICA scales. For the broad scales, interrater reliabilities were fair to good for Total Observations ($r = .52$ and .61), fair to excellent for Total Self-Reports ($r = .58$ and .79) across the two samples, and consistently good for Internalizing ($r = .64$ and .66) and Externalizing ($r = .72$ and .74). For the syndromes, interrater reliabilities ranged from .45 for the Anxious syndrome to .85 for the Withdrawn syndrome with 11 of 17 correlations $\geq .69$. Mean scores for interviewers were significantly higher than means for videotape observers, suggesting that direct interviewing leads to more awareness of problems than does viewing videotapes.

Test–retest reliabilities were obtained by McConaughy and Achenbach (1994) for a sample of 20 American children aged 6–12 and by Kasius (1997) for a sample of 35 Dutch children aged 6–16. In both samples, children were seen in counterbalanced order by two different interviewers over a mean interval of 12 days. For the broad scales,

TABLE 12.4 Interrater and Test–Retest Reliabilities (Pearson *r*) for the Semistructured Clinical Interview for Children and Adolescents (SCICA)

	Interrater reliability		Test–retest reliability	
	American[a] (*n* = 168)	Dutch[b] (*n* = 24)	American[a] (*n* = 20)	Dutch[b] (*n* = 24)
Observation scales				
Anxious or	.45	.83	.75	.66
immature		.54		.71
Attention Problems	.57	.49	.71	.87
Resistant	.80	.64	.74	.80
Strange	.69	.77	.72	.86
Withdrawn	.76	.85	(.30)	.87
Self-report scales				
Anxious/Depressed or	.69		.54	
Lonely		.69		.74
Aggressive Behavior	.76	.82	.67	.81
Family Problems	.76	.65	.60	.75
Broad scales				
Internalizing	.64	.66	.69	.55
Externalizing	.72	.74	.84	.90
Total Observations	.52	.61	.89	.81
Total Self-Reports	.58	.79	.73	.84

[a]McConaughy & Achenbach (1994).
[b]Kasius (1997).

test–retest correlations were excellent for Total Observations (*r* = .89 and .81), good to excellent for Total Self-Reports (*r* = .73 and .84), fair to good for Internalizing (*r* = .55 and .69) and excellent for Externalizing (*r* = .84 and .90). For the syndromes, significant test-retest reliabilities ranged from .54 for Anxious/Depressed to .87 for Attention Problems and Withdrawn. A nonsignificant correlation for Withdrawn (*r* = .30) in the American sample suggested that children varied from one time to the next on this dimension, but this was not the case in the Dutch sample. No significant differences were found in either the American or Dutch samples in mean scores from Time 1 to Time 2 on any SCICA scale. Although these samples were relatively small, the lack of time effects showed that the SCICA did not manifest the attenuation effects that have been found for the DISC and other structured diagnostic interviews.

Relations Between the SCICA and DSM Diagnoses

Although the SCICA was not designed to generate specific DSM diagnoses, McConaughy and Achenbach (1994) assessed the reliability of DSM-III diagnoses based on information obtained from the SCICA, the CBCL, the TRF, and information in the child's clinical record. After rating a child on the SCICA Observation and Self-Report Forms, the interviewer and videotape observer independently assigned one or more DSM diagnoses for a sample of 106 referred children. Interrater reliabilities (kappas) were ≥ .70 for conduct disorders, oppositional disorders, anxiety disorders, and depressive disorders, and .51 for attention deficit disorders. These findings indicated that satisfactory agreement was obtained on major diagnoses when SCICA data were combined with information from other sources.

To directly assess relations between SCICA scales and DSM diagnoses, Kasius (1997) interviewed 175 parents and 44 children with the relevant versions of the DISC-2.3 to obtain DSM-III-R diagnoses. Comparisons of SCICA scales with DSM diagnoses from the child version of the DISC showed significant relations between Any Anxiety and Any Mood disorder and the SCICA Lonely syndrome, Internalizing, and Total Self-Reports, as well as significant relations between Any Disruptive disorder and SCICA Externalizing. SCICA Total Observations also showed significant relations with all DSM categories. When comparisons were made between SCICA scales and the parent version of the DISC, the SCICA Internalizing, Externalizing, Total Self-Reports, and all SCICA syndromes, except Immature, showed significant relations with the DSM categories. No significant relations were found between SCICA Total Observations and parent-reported DSM diagnoses. These findings indicated that the quantitative scales of the SCICA measured similar constructs to groupings of the categorical DSM diagnoses derived from the DISC, although there were not specific one-to-one relations with specific DSM diagnoses, as expected.

Validity of the SCICA

McConaughy and Achenbach (1994) tested the discriminative validity of the SCICA for differentiating demographically matched samples of referred versus nonreferred children ($n = 106$). Referred children scored significantly higher ($p < .05$) than nonreferred children on all SCICA scales, except Anxious, for which $p = .09$. McConaughy and Achenbach (1996) also found that children classified as having emotional or behavioral disorders (EBD) scored significantly higher ($p < .05$) than demographically matched nonreferred children on five SCICA syndromes (Anxious/ Depressed, Withdrawn, Attention Problems, Strange, Resistant), Externalizing, Total Observations, and Total Self-Reports. In the same study, combinations of SCICA, CBCL, and TRF scales produced exceptionally high classification rates for children with EBD versus nonreferred children, with misclassifications of only 3 to 4% in discriminant analyses.

Finally, significant moderate correlations have been found between comparable scales of the SCICA and CBCL, TRF, and YSR for the same subjects, as well as direct classroom observations of subjects scored on the DOF (Kasius, 1997; McConaughy & Achenbach, 1994). The moderate correlations indicated that data obtained from the SCICA were not redundant with data obtained from other sources. Such findings are consistent with meta-analyses on cross-informant agreement (Achenbach et al., 1987) and underscore the importance of conceptualizing child clinical interviews as components of multimethod assessment rather than as "gold standards" of single-source assessment. Although the SCICA does not have the extensive research base of the structured and semistructured diagnostic interviews, findings to date support its reliability and validity for multimethod assessment of children's problems. Let's now turn to behavioral interviews that might be used with children, as described in the following sections.

BEHAVIORAL INTERVIEWING

In contrast to the more comprehensive child clinical interviews that cover a wide range of problems, behavioral interviews are designed to pinpoint a limited number of specific problems that can be targeted for interventions. Behavioral interviews are widely used in school-based behavioral consultation (e.g., Gresham & Davis, 1988; Gutkin & Curtis, 1990; Sheridan & Kratochwill, 1992; Sheridan, Kratochwill, & Bergan, 1996; see McComas & Mace, Chapter 4, this volume, Busse, Chapter 10, this volume). As Sheridan and colleagues (1996) explain, "behavioral consultation involves indirect services to a client (e.g., child) who is served through a consultee (e.g., parent, teacher) by a consultant (e.g., a psychologist, special education teacher, social worker)." In most consultation models, a series of behavioral interviews are conducted between the consultant and consultee to identify specific problems in behavioral terms, analyze the circumstances surrounding the identified problems, and develop and evaluate interventions to address the problems. These generally occur in four discrete stages: (1) problem identification, (2) problem analysis, (3) treatment implementation, and (4) treatment evaluation (Bergan & Kratochwill, 1990). The first two stages of behavioral interviewing and consultation are intended to obtain a functional assessment of the problem behaviors.

Problem Identification

Problem identification involves selecting target behaviors and creating operational definitions of the behaviors. Global problems may be initially identified (e.g., inattention, aggression), but these must then be differentiated into specific behaviors that can become targets of interventions (e.g., off-task during independent work, hits other children). Once the problems have been identified, the interviewee is queried further about the intensity, frequency, and duration of each problem and the environmental circumstances surrounding the problem. If multiple specific problems are identified, they must be prioritized in terms of severity and/or need for intervention.

Sheridan and colleagues (1996) outline several considerations for selecting target behaviors. First priority is usually given to problems that are physically dangerous to the client or others or problems that are aversive to others because of their deviance or unpredictability. However, problems might also be targeted that promote long-term social good or problems that, if controlled, can have positive effects on other collateral behaviors. Sheridan and colleagues (1996) give an example of targeting tardiness to school for a child who is failing math because he often is late for class, doesn't have materials ready, and fails to turn in assignments. Behaviors can also be targeted that are likely to be maintained in the natural environment after interventions are terminated, such as appropriate social skills, promptness, work completion, and accuracy.

After target behaviors have been identified and prioritized, operational definitions must be developed that describe the behaviors in observable, concrete, specific, and measurable terms. Operational definitions are important to ensure that all persons involved in planned interventions clearly understand the problems to be addressed. It is also important to define the problems in terms of their behavioral manifestations or environmental events that can be altered, rather than in terms of internal conditions or environmental circumstances that are outside the realm of intervention. For example, Sheridan and colleagues (1996) suggested defining one boy's physical aggression as follows: "Kevin engages in negative physical contact (kicking, hitting, striking out) with peers 5 times per week," or "Kevin engages in negative physical contact (kicking, hitting, striking out) with peers when engaged in group activities on the playground." Such operational definitions are preferable to descriptions of the same problem in terms of an educational or diagnostic labels (e.g., behavior disorder) or family dysfunction, neither of which give much direction for what to do about the problem. Operational definitions are also essential for the data collection required in behavioral consultation models to validate descriptions of frequency, duration, and/or intensity of problems. Baseline data collection is usually accomplished by parents and/or teachers, but can also be done by consultants (Kratochwill, Bergan, Sheridan, & Elliott, 1998).

Problem Analysis

Problem analysis involves identifying antecedent, consequent, and sequential conditions that affect the target behaviors. Antecedents are events that precede the occurrence of a target behavior, while consequences are events that follow the behavior. Sequential conditions are common patterns across occasions, such as time of day or day of the week. For problem analysis, the interviewee is queried about situational and temporal variations in each target behavior, as well as specific environmental circumstances that maintain the behavior. Interviewees are also queried about specific consequences of the behavior (e.g., attention, reprimands, punishments, removal from an unpleasant situation or task). In addition, interviewees may be asked about their feelings and expectations regarding the behavior, and preferred behaviors to guide development of appropriate interventions. In Sheridan and colleagues' (1996) example, problem analysis might reveal that Kevin's physical aggression typically occurs after he fails to be selected for a team or after teasing by peers, and that after an act of aggression, Kevin is typically sent to the principal's office for punishment or is sent home. Sequential conditions for Kevin's physical aggression might involve days on which children are unsupervised at recess or times when children are not engaged in structured games at recess.

For some behaviors, Sheridan and colleagues (1996) add a skills analysis as well as a conditions analysis to determine the level of a child's social or academic skills related to the target behavior. This involves identifying the target skill that should be present, breaking the skill into its component parts, assessing the child's ability to perform the skill, and assessing the level of mastery required. Skills analysis should also address whether the child displays a skill deficit, which would require remediation, or a performance deficit, which would require operant techniques to reinforce using the skill.

Treatment Implementation and Evaluation

After problem analysis, behavioral consultation models usually proceed directly toward interventions to address identified problems. The third stage involves implementing an intervention plan and the fourth stage involves evaluating the effectiveness of the intervention. Both of these stages require additional interviewing and data collection to chart changes in targeted behaviors and to evaluate treatment integrity.

A sizable research literature has demonstrated the effectiveness of behavioral consultation with teachers and/or parents (for reviews, see Bergan & Kratochwill, 1990; Kratochwill et al., 1998; McComas & Mace, Chapter 4, this volume; Busse, Chapter 10, this volume). Effectiveness has been demonstrated for producing changes in clients' (children's) behavior as well as consultees' (teachers and parents) knowledge and use of behavioral strategies (e.g., Anderson, Kratochwill, & Bergan, 1986; Carrington Rotto, & Kratochwill, 1994; Galloway & Sheridan, 1990; Sheridan, Kratochwill, & Elliott, 1990).

Behavioral Interviews with Children

Because behavioral interviews are strongly associated with intervention planning, they have more often been used with parents and teachers, who are the mediators of the interventions, than with the children themselves. However, Merrell (1999) suggested that in many cases, the referred older child might also become a useful participant in behavioral interviews. When interviewing older children, Merrell recommended proceeding quickly from general questions for building rapport to specific questions regarding suspected problems. If the child is receptive to such direct questioning, the pattern of behavioral interviewing can follow the stages described for behavioral consultation with adults. Merrell also suggested combining problem identification and problem analysis into one interview with children if there are strong time pressures. However, combining the first two stages into one interview may forfeit the opportunity to collect baseline data, unless all parties involved agree to postpone interventions until after a period of data collection. For younger children (e.g., ages 6–9), behavioral interviewing is still likely to be more useful with adult informants than with the children themselves because of the level of logical reasoning and verbal sophistication required to obtain a functional assessment of problem behaviors.

In an attempt to use behavioral interviewing strategies directly with children, Kern and Dunlap developed the Student-Assisted Functional Assessment Interview (Kern & Dunlap, in press; Kern, Dunlap, Clarke, & Childs, 1994). In the first section of this interview, students respond to specific questions about features of the classroom environment and curriculum that may be contributing to problem behaviors. Several questions pertain to potential functions of the problem behaviors, such as attention (e.g., "Do you think people notice when you do a good job?"), escape (e.g., "In general, is your work too hard?"), or reinforcement (e.g., "Do you think you get the points or rewards you deserve when you do a good job?"). Other questions ask about features of the setting or time periods that may contribute to problems, such as whether there are distractions in the classroom or whether work periods are too long. Each question is answered "always," "sometimes," or "never." In two additional sections, children rank how much they like each academic subject on a 5-point scale and then answer open-ended questions about what they like and don't like about each subject.

Kern and Dunlap (in press) reported using the Student-Assisted Functional Assessment Interview with 15 students with emotional and behavioral disorders to develop hypotheses for functional behavioral assessment and intervention planning. They described one single-case study that showed improved on-task behavior after interventions that were developed from a functional assessment including the student interview. However, more research is needed with multiple cases to determine whether direct behavioral interviewing with children adds useful and valid information for functional assessment and intervention planning.

CONCLUSIONS

This chapter describes different methods for interviewing children to assess their emotional and behavioral problems. Direct interviewing has long been considered essential for clinical evaluation of children's problems. At the same time, child clinical interviews are likely to be most effective when used in the context of multimethod assessment rather than assuming that they alone represent the "gold standard" for clinical evaluation. Accordingly, practitioners are encouraged to seek data from multiple sources, including parents, teachers, and the children themselves, in order to obtain a comprehensive view of children's functioning. To provide a broad overview of interviewing techniques, this chapter describes several structured and semistructured diagnostic interviews, an empirically based semistructured clinical interview for children and adolescents, and behavioral interviewing techniques.

For many school-based assessments, the structured and semistructured diagnostic interviews may have limited utility, particularly when the purpose of assessment is to determine special education eligibility and to design school interventions (Gresham & Gansle, 1992; Martens, 1992; Sinclair & Forness, 1988). However, for broader purposes, the DSM diagnoses obtained from diagnostic interviews can be useful for descriptively classifying children's problems and communicating with mental health and medical professionals outside the school setting. With this in mind, the following conclusions can be drawn from this chapter's review of reliability studies of structured and semistructured diagnostic interviews: (1) Structured interviews with parents produce more reliable diagnoses than structured interviews with children; (2) Highly structured interviews are more reliable with older than younger children, particularly ages 12 or higher; (3) The reliabilities obtained from child interviews vary across different diagnostic categories, whereas reliabilities obtained from parent interviews remain consistently high across most diagnoses; (4) Combining information from parent and child interviews produces acceptable reliabilities for most diagnostic categories in clinical samples; and (5) Scores on continuous symptom and/or criterion scales produce higher reliabilities than categorical diagnoses and less pronounced differences between reliabilities for parents versus children.

Given the above findings, school-based practitioners might consider using a structured or semistructured diagnostic interview with parents to assess a child's DSM symptoms. However, even for parent interviews, the time requirements for most diagnostic interviews can be a limiting factor, although the new modular, computer-assisted format of the DICA-IV may render it a more viable option. Structured diagnostic interviews are not recommended as a primary assessment technique with children, especially children under age 12.

In contrast to the structured diagnostic interviews, the SCICA (McConaughy & Achenbach, 1994) provides a more flexible format for interviewing children and is more compatible with their interaction styles. The SCICA also provides a standardized profile for quantitatively scoring interviewers' observations of children's problems and children's self-reports during the interview. As part of a multiaxial empirically based assessment system, the SCICA was designed to dovetail with several other standardized rating scales: the CBCL (Achenbach, 1991a) for obtaining parent reports; TRF (Achenbach, 1991b) for teacher reports; YSR (Achenbach, 1991c) for youth self-reports; and DOF (Achenbach, 1986; McConaughy et al., 1988) for direct observations in school settings. Scores on the SCICA's broad scales and empirically derived syndromes can be compared to scores on similar scales of the CBCL, TRF, YSR, and DOF. Thus, unlike the structured diagnostic interviews, the SCICA yields continuous scores that can be easily integrated with other quantitative data in multimethod assessment. Research on the SCICA has been more limited than for the structured and semistructured diagnostic interviews, but the SCICA has demonstrated good to excellent reliabilities for most scales. The SCICA has also shown good validity for discriminating clinically referred from nonreferred children and discriminating children with emotional/behavioral disorders from nonreferred children.

A final section of this chapter reviewed behavioral interviewing techniques developed in the context of school-based behavioral consultation models. Although behavioral interviews have been used primarily with parents and/or teachers, Merrell (1999) suggested that similar strategies might be viable with older children. Because of their focus on problem identification and analysis, behavioral interviews are particularly well suited for functional assessment of children's problems (for reviews, see Lane, Umbreit, & Beebe-Frankenberger, 1999; McComas & Mace, Chapter 4, this volume). The 1997 amendments to the Individuals with Disabilities Education

Act (IDEA; P.L. 101-476, 1990; reauthorized P.L. 105-17, 1997) now require a functional behavioral assessment when certain discipline procedures and alternative educational placements are implemented for students with identified disabilities. This new requirement in the federal law is likely to increase the demand for functional assessments via behavioral interviewing techniques. Extensive research has demonstrated the effectiveness of behavioral interviewing with parents and teachers as an indirect method for assessing and treating children's problems. However, more research is needed to assess the viability of behavioral interviews as a method of direct assessment with children.

References

Achenbach, T. M. (1986). *The Direct Observation Form of the Child Behavior Checklist* (rev. ed.). Burlington: University of Vermont, Department of Psychiatry.

Achenbach, T. M. (1991a). *Manual for the Child Behavior Checklist/4–18 and 1991 Profile.* Burlington: University of Vermont, Department of Psychiatry.

Achenbach, T. M. (1991b). *Manual for the Teacher's Report Form and 1991 Profile.* Burlington: University of Vermont, Department of Psychiatry.

Achenbach, T. M. (1991c). *Manual for the Youth Self-Report Form and 1991 Profile.* Burlington: University of Vermont, Department of Psychiatry.

Achenbach, T. M., & Edelbrock, C. (1983). *Manual for the Child Behavior Checklist and Profile.* Burlington: University of Vermont, Department of Psychiatry.

Achenbach, T. M., & McConaughy, S. H. (1997). *Empirically based assessment of child and adolescent psychopathology: Practical applications.* Thousand Oaks, CA: Sage.

Achenbach, T. M., McConaughy, S. H., & Howell, C. T. (1987). Child/adolescent behavioral and emotional problems: Implications of cross-informant correlations for situational specificity. *Psychological Bulletin, 101,* 213–232.

Ambrosini, P. J. (2000). Historical development and present status of the schedule for affective disorders and schizophrenia for school-age children (K-SADS). *Journal of the American Academy of Child and Adolescent Psychiatry, 39,* 49–58.

Ambrosini, P. J., Metz, C., Prabucki, K., & Lee, J. (1989). Videotape reliability of the third revised edition of the K-SADS. *Journal of the American Academy of Child and Adolescent Psychiatry, 28,* 723–728.

American Psychiatric Association. (1980, 1987, 1994). *Diagnostic and statistical manual of mental disorders* (3rd ed., 3rd rev. ed., 4th ed.). Washington, DC: Author.

Anderson, T. K., Kratochwill, T. R., & Bergan, J. R. (1986). Training teachers in behavioral consultation and therapy: An analysis of verbal behaviors. *Journal of School Psychology, 24,* 229–241.

Angold, A., & Costello, E. J. (1995). A test–retest reliability study of child reported psychiatric symptoms and diagnoses using the Child and Adolescent Psychiatric Assessment (CAPA). *Psychological Medicine, 25,* 755–762.

Angold, A., & Costello, J. (2000). The Child and Adolescent Psychiatric Assessment (CAPA). *Journal of the American Academy of Child and Adolescent Psychiatry, 39,* 39–48.

Angold, A., Cox, A., Prendergast, M., Rutter, M., & Simonoff, E. (1987). *Child and Adolescent Psychiatric Assessment (CAPA).* Durham, NC: Duke University, Department of Psychiatry.

Bergan, J. R., & Kratochwill, T. R. (1990). *Behavioral consultation and therapy.* New York: Plenum Press.

Bird, H. R., Gould, M. S., & Staghezza, B. (1992). Aggregating data from multiple informants in child psychiatry epidemiological research. *Journal of the American Academy of Child and Adolescent Psychiatry, 31,* 78–85.

Boyle, M. H., Offord, D. R., Racine, Y., Sanford, M., Szatmari, P., Fleming, J. E., & Price-Munn, N. (1993). Evaluation of the diagnostic interview for children and adolescents for use in general population samples. *Journal of Abnormal Child Psychology, 21,* 663–681.

Breton, J. J., Bergeron, L., Valla, J. P., Berthiaume, C., & St-Georges, M. (1998). Diagnostic Interview Schedule for Children (DISC-2.25) in Quebec: Reliability findings in light of the MECA study. *Journal of the American Academy of Child and Adolescent Psychiatry, 37,* 1176–1174.

Breton, J. J., Bergeron, L., Valla, J. P., Lepine, S., Houde, L., & Gaudet, N. (1995). Do children aged 9 through 11 years understand the DISC Version 2.25 questions? *Journal of the American Academy of Child and Adolescent Psychiatry, 34,* 946–956.

Burns, B. J., Angold, A., Macgruder-Habib, K., Costello, E. J., & Patrick, M. K. S. (1992). *The Child and Adolescent Services Assessment (CASA).* Durham, NC: Duke University Department of Psychiatry.

Carrington Rotto, P., & Kratochwill, T. R. (1994). Behavioral consultation with parents: Using competency-based training to modify child noncompliance. *School Psychology Review, 23,* 669–693.

Chambers, W., Puig-Antich, J., Hirsch, M., Puez, P., Ambrosini, P., Tabrizi, M. Davies, M. (1985). The assessment of affective disorders in children and adolescents by semi-structured interview: Test–retest reliability of The Schedule for Affective Disorders and Schizophrenia for School-Aged Children, Present Episode Version. *Archives of General Psychiatry, 42,* 696–702.

Costello, E. J. (1989). Developments in child psychiatric epidemiology. *Journal of the American Academy of Child and Adolescent Psychiatry, 28,* 836–841.

Costello, E. J., Burns, B. J., Angold, A., & Leaf, P. J. (1993). How can epidemiology improve mental health services for children and adolescents? *Journal of the American Academy of Child and Adolescent Psychiatry, 32,* 1106–1113.

Costello, A. J., Edelbrock, C., Dulcan, M. K., Kalas, R., & Klaric, S. H. (1984). *Report on the Diagnostic Interview Schedule for Children (DISC).* Pittsburgh: University of Pittsburgh, Department of Psychiatry.

Edelbrock, C., & Costello, A. J. (1988). Convergence between statistically derived behavior problem syndromes and child psychiatric diagnoses. *Journal of Abnormal Child Psychology, 16,* 219–231.

Edelbrock, C., Costello, A. J., Dulcan, M. K., Conover, N. C., & Kalas, R. (1986). Parent–child agreement on child psychiatric symptoms assessed via structured interview. *Journal of Child Psychology and Psychiatry, 27,* 181–190.

Edelbrock, C., Costello, A. J., Dulcan, M. K., Kalas, R., & Conover, N. C. (1985). Age differences in the reliability of the psychiatric interview of the child. *Child Development, 56,* 265–275.

Endicott, J., & Spitzer, R. L. (1978). A diagnostic interview. The Schedule for Affective Disorders and Schizophrenia. *Archives of General Psychiatry, 35,* 837–844.

Ezpeleta, L., de le Osa, N., Domenech, J. M. & Navarro, J. B. (1997). Diagnostic agreement between clinicians and Diagnostic Interview for Children and Adolescents–DICA-R in an outpatient sample. *Journal of Child Psychology and Psychiatry and Allied Disciplines, 38,* 431–440.

Fallon, T., & Schwab-Stone, M. (1994). Determinants of reliability in psychiatric surveys of children aged 6–12. *Journal of Child Psychology and Psychiatry, 35,* 1391–1408.

Galloway, J., & Sheridan, S. M. (1990). Implementing scientific practices through case studies: Examples using home-school interventions and consultation. *Journal of School Psychology, 32,* 385–413.

Gresham, F. M., & Davis, C. J. (1988). Behavioral interviews with teachers and parents. In E. S. Shapiro & R. R. Kratochwill (Eds.), *Behavioral assessment in schools: Conceptual foundations and practical applications* (pp. 455–493). New York: Guilford Press.

Gresham, F. M., & Gansle, K. A. (1992). Misguided assumptions of the DSM-III-R: Implications for school psychological practice. *School Psychology Quarterly, 7,* 79–95.

Gutkin, T. B., & Curtis, M. J. (1990). School-based consultation: Theory, techniques, and research. In T. B. Gutkin & C. R. Reynolds (Eds.), *The handbook of school psychology* (pp. 577–611). New York: Wiley.

Harrington, R., Hill, J., Rutter, M., John, K., Fudge, H., Zoccollilo, M., & Weissman, M. M. (1988). The assessment of lifetime psychopathology: A comparison of two interviewing styles. *Psychological Medicine, 18,* 487–493.

Herjanic, B., & Reich, W. (1982). Development of a structured psychiatric interview for children: Agreement between child and parent on individual symptoms. *Journal of Abnormal Child Psychology, 10,* 307–324.

Hodges, K. (1993). Structured interviews for assessing children. *Journal of Child Psychology and Psychiatry, 34,* 49–68.

Hodges, K., Cools, J., & McKnew, D. (1989). Test–retest reliability of a clinical research interview for children: The Child Assessment Schedule. *Psychological Assessment, 1,* 317–322.

Hodges, K., Gordon, Y., & Lennon, M. (1990). Parent–child agreement on symptoms assessed via a clinical research interview for children: The Child Assessment Schedule (CAS). *Journal of Child Psychology and Psychiatry, 31,* 427–436.

Hodges, K., McKnew, D., Cytryn, L., Stern, L., & Kline, J. (1982). The Child Assessment Schedule (CAS) Diagnostic Interview: A report on reliability and validity. *Journal of the American Academy of Child Psychiatry, 21,* 468–473.

Hughes, J. N., & Baker, D. B. (1990). *The clinical child interview.* New York: Guilford Press.

Individuals with Disabilities Education Act (1990). Public Law 101-476. 20 U.S.C. §1401 et seq. (Reauthorized July, 1997). Public Law 105-17. 20 U.S.C. §1400 et seq.

Jensen, P., Roper, M., Fisher, P., & Piacentini, J., Canino, G., et al. (1995). Test–retest reliability of the Diagnostic Interview Schedule for Children (DISC 2.1): Parent, child, and combined algorithms. *Archives of General Psychiatry, 52,* 61–71.

Kasius, M. (1997). *Interviewing children: Development of the Dutch version of the Semistructured Clinical Interview for Children and Adolescents and testing of the psychometric properties.* Rotterdam, The Netherlands: Erasmus University.

Kern, L., & Dunlap, G. (in press). Assessment-based interventions for children with emotional and behavioral disorders. In A. C. Repp & R. H. Horner (Eds.), *Functional analysis of problem behavior: From effective assessment to effective support.* Monterrey, CA: Brooks/Cole.

Kern, L., Dunlap, G., Clarke, S., & Childs, K. E. (1994). Student-assisted functional assessment interview. *Diagnostique, 19,* 20–39.

Kratochwill, T. R., Bergan, J. R., Sheridan, S. M., & Elliott, S. N. (1998). Assumptions of behavioral consultation: After all is said and done more has been done than said. *School Psychology Quarterly, 13,* 63–80.

Kratochwill, T. R., & Sheridan, S. (1990). Advances in behavioral assessment. In T. B. Gutkin & C. R. Reynolds (Eds.), *The handbook of school psychology* (pp. 328–364). New York: Wiley.

Landis, J. R., & Koch, G. G. (1977). The measurement of observer agreement for categorical data. *Biometrics, 33,* 159–174.

Lane, K. L, Umbreit, J., & Beebe-Frankenberger, M. (1999). Functional assessment research on students with or at-risk for EBD: 1990 to the present. *Journal of Positive Behavioral Interventions, 1,* 101–111.

Loeber, R., Green, S. M., Lahey, B. B., & Stouthamer-Loeber, M. (1989). Optimal informants on child disruptive behaviors. *Development and Psychopathology, 1,* 317–337.

Lucas, C. P., Fisher, P., Piacentini, J., Zhang, H., Jensen, P., Shaffer, D., Dulcan, M., Schwab-Stone, M., Regier, D., & Canino, G. (1999). Features of interview questions associated with attenuation of symptom reports. *Journal of Abnormal Child Psychology, 27,* 429–437.

Martens, B. K. (1992). The difference between a good theory and a good treatment is a matter of degree. *School Psychology Quarterly, 7,* 104–107.

McConaughy, S. H. (1996). The interview process. In M. Breen & C. Fiedler (Eds.), *Behavioral approach to the assessment of emotionally/behaviorally disordered youth: A handbook for school-based practitioners* (pp. 181–223). Austin, TX: Pro-Ed.

McConaughy, S. H. (2000). Self-report: Child clinical interviews. In E. S. Shapiro & T. R. Kratochwill (Eds.), *Conducting school-based assessments of child and adolescent behavior.* New York: Guilford Press.

McConaughy, S. H., & Achenbach, T. M. (1994). *Manual for the Semistructured Clinical Interview for Children and Adolescents.* Burlington: University of Vermont, Department of Psychiatry.

McConaughy, S. H., & Achenbach, T. M. (1996). Contributions of a child interview to multimethod assessment of children with EBD and LD. *School Psychology Review, 25,* 24–39.

McConaughy, S. H., Achenbach, T. M., & Gent, C. L. (1988). Multiaxial empirically based assessment: Parent, teacher, observational, cognitive, and personality correlates of Child Behavior Profiles for 6–11-year-old boys. *Journal of Abnormal Child Psychology, 16*, 485–509.

Merrell, K. W. (1998). *Behavioral, social, and emotional assessment of children and adolescents*. Mahwah, NJ: Erlbaum.

Piacentini, J. C., Cohen, P., & Cohen, J. (1992). Combining discrepant diagnostic information from multiple sources. Are complex algorithms better than simple ones? *Journal of Abnormal Child Psychology, 20*, 51–63.

Puig-Antich, J., & Chambers, W. (1978). *The Schedule for Affective Disorders and Schizophrenia for School-aged Children (Kiddie-SADS)*. New York: New York State Psychiatric Institute.

Reich, W. (2000). Diagnostic Interview for Children and Adolescents. *Journal of the American Academy of Child and Adolescent Psychiatry, 39*, 59–66.

Reich, W., & Welner, Z. (1992). *DICA-R-C. DSM-III-R version. Revised version of DICA for children ages 6–12*. St. Louis, MO: Washington University, Department of Psychiatry.

Reich, W., Welner, Z., Herjanic, B., & MHS Staff. (1997). *Diagnostic Interview for Children and Adolescents-IV*. North Tonawanda, NY: Multi-Health Systems.

Rey, J. M., Morris-Yates, A., & Stanislaw, H. (1992). Measuring the accuracy of diagnostic tests using Receiver Operating Characteristics (ROC) analysis. *International Journal of Methods in Psychiatric Research, 2*, 39–50.

Roberts, R. E., Solovitz, B. L., Chen, Y. W., & Casat, C. (1996). Retest stability of DSM-III-R diagnoses among adolescents using the Diagnostic Interview Schedule for Children (DISC-2.1C). *Journal of Abnormal Child Psychology, 24*, 349–362.

Robins, L. N., Helzer, J. F., Ratcliff, K. S., & Seyfried, W. (1982). Validity of the Diagnostic Interview Schedule, Version II: DSM-III diagnoses. *Psychological Medicine, 12*, 855–870.

Rubio-Stipec, M., Shrout, P. E., Canino, G., Bird, H., Jensen, P., et al. (1996). Empirically defined symptom scales using the DISC 2.3. *Journal of Abnormal Child Psychology, 24*, 67–83.

Sattler, J. M. (1998). *Clinical and forensic interviewing of children and families*. San Diego: Author.

Schwab-Stone, M., Fallon, T., Briggs, M., & Crowther, B. (1994). Reliability of diagnostic reporting for children aged 6–11 years: A test–retest study of the Diagnostic Interview for Children — Revised. *American Journal of Psychiatry, 151*, 1048–1054.

Schwab-Stone, M., Shaffer, D., Dulcan, M. K., Jensen, P. S., Fisher, P., et al. (1996). Criterion validity of the NIMH Diagnostic Interview Schedule for Children Version 2.3 (DISC-2.3). *Journal of the American Academy of Child and Adolescent Psychiatry, 35*, 878–888.

Shaffer, D. (1992). *NIMH Diagnostic Interview Schedule for Children, Version 2.3*. New York: Columbia University, Division of Child Psychiatry.

Shaffer, D., Fisher, P., Dulcan, M., Davies, M., Piacentini, J., et al. (1996). The NIMH Diagnostic Interview Schedule for Children Version 2.3 (DISC-2.3): Description, acceptability, prevalence rates, and performance in the MECA study. *Journal of the American Academy of Child and Adolescent Psychiatry, 35*, 865–877.

Shaffer, D., Schwab-Stone, M., Fisher, P., et al. (1993). The Diagnostic Interview Schedule for Children — Revised Version (DISC-R) I: Preparation, field testing, interrater reliability, and acceptability. *Journal of the American Academy of Child and Adolescent Psychiatry, 32*, 643–650.

Shaffer, D., Fisher, P., Lucas, C. P., Dulcan, M., & Schwab-Stone, M. E. (2000). NIMH Diagnostic Interview Schedule for Children, Version IV (NIMH DISC-IV): Description, differences from previous versions and reliability of some common diagnoses. *Journal of the American Academy of Child and Adolescent Psychiatry, 39*, 28–38.

Shaffer, D., Schwab-Stone, M., Fisher, P., Davies, M., Piacentini, J., & Gioia, P. (1988). *A revised version of the Diagnostic Interview Schedule for Children*. New York: Columbia University, Division of Child Psychiatry.

Sheridan, S. M., & Kratochwill, T. R. (1992). Behavioral parent–teacher consultation: Conceptual and research considerations. *Journal of School Psychology, 30*, 117–139.

Sheridan, S. M., Kratochwill, T. R., & Bergan, J. R. (1996). *Conjoint behavioral consultation: A procedural manual*. New York: Plenum Press.

Sheridan, S. M., Kratochwill, T. R., & Elliott, S. N. (1990). Behavioral consultation with parents and teachers: Delivering treatment for socially withdrawn children at home and school. *School Psychology Review, 19,* 33–52.

Sinclair, E., & Forness, S. (1988). Special education classification and its relationship to DSM-III. In E. S. Shapiro & T. R. Kratochwill (Eds.), *Behavioral assessment in schools.* New York: Guilford Press.

Witt, J. C., Cavell, T. A., Carey, M. P., & Martens, B. (1988). Child self-report: Interviewing techniques and rating scales. In E. S. Shapiro & R. R. Kratochwill (Eds.), *Behavioral assessment in schools: Conceptual foundations and practical applications* (pp. 384–454). New York: Guilford Press.

World Health Organization. (1992). *Mental disorders: Glossary and guide to their classification in accordance with the Tenth Revision of the International Classification of Diseases* (10th ed.). Geneva: Author.

Young, J. G., O'Brien, J. D., Gutterman, E. M., & Cohen, P. (1987). Research on the clinical interview. *Journal of the American Academy of Child and Adolescent Psychiatry, 26,* 613–620.

PART III

Issues in Child and Adolescent Assessment

CHAPTER 13

Psychometric Qualities
of Professional Practice

DAVID W. BARNETT
FRANCIS E. LENTZ, JR.
University of Cincinnati

GREGG MACMANN
University of Kentucky

What information about the quality of assessment data would be most useful to professionals as they make decisions during problem solving? In this chapter we will examine the psychometric qualities of assessment that both guide and constrain the activities of professionals in their work with children, teachers, and parents. In order to accomplish our purpose, we will consider both the traditional and the behavioral assessment models. While we believe that the behavioral assessment approach has the strongest potential for helping professionals make decisions that resolve childhood problems, it is *how* measurement procedures are used that is critical, not which model best describes them. Typical psychometric constructs and evaluation methods can be important, but we will argue that, as they are currently used, they are insufficient as guides for practitioners.

Our major theme is that psychometric issues are best examined by focusing primarily on the effectiveness of context-specific decisions that are made during problem-solving processes, and with an ultimate regard to the *consequences* of these decisions. The appropriate unit for examining psychometric adequacy is a natural unit defined by a purposeful assessment process within the provision of psychological services. Within this theme, an evaluation of the ultimate technical adequacy of assessment data must also eventually involve an examination of the planning and other professional behaviors both prior to and during problem solving. These professional behaviors are related to decisions about which scales, instruments, or measurement procedures to use and how to draw inferences from the results. Our arguments are founded in behavioral assessment and applied behavior analysis (Baer, Wolf, & Risley, 1968; Baer, Wolf, & Risley, 1987; Wolf, 1978), psychometrics (Messick, 1995), decision theory (Tversky & Kahneman, 1984), research interpretation (Cohen, 1990), and criticisms of assessment practices that have never been resolved (Dawes, 1994; Meehl & Rosen, 1955; Mischel, 1968; Peterson, 1968).

Although psychometric variables such as reliability and validity have been traditionally seen as qualities of assessment instruments, we will strongly advocate that practitioners must consider the psychometric qualities of their *decisions* across the sequence of problem solving. The data on psychometric quality presented in test manuals do not sufficiently fit real-world decision contexts, nor do reliability and validity data collected during instrument development adequately generalize to questions of problem identification, classification, or problem solving. This criticism must be applied to so called traditional assessment, as well as to many of the methods that have been subsumed under the behavior assessment model. These gaps in the information related to psychometric quality are filled idiosyncratically by professional judgments (Barnett, 1988). However, professionals relying on traditional information about measurement quality without regard to research related to the problem situations and problem solving may have unwarranted confidence in their judgments. The *intent* of using psychometric data to improve decision making still must be met, but in ways that lead to confidence in the assessment-based understanding of both the problem context and likely consequences of subsequent decisions.

The meaning of traditional assessment data (i.e., test scores) has been dependent on differences among individuals or groups, and traditional psychometric analyses have been closely linked to studies of individual differences. Individual differences are not necessarily *meaningful* differences (e.g., Hart & Risley, 1995; Mischel, 1968); the meaning of individual differences is found within social contexts. We will outline our concerns that assessment decisions and their subsequent consequences have seldom been examined within psychometric research, much less been considered as prime criteria for choosing assessment procedures.

From a traditional viewpoint, evaluation studies of psychometric qualities have typically involved hypothesizing about the empirical and theoretical relationships among correlated variables, usually dichotomized into the constructs of reliability and validity. Examination of these constructs of psychometric quality is supposed to influence a number of professional activities such as selection of tests to use during assessment, score interpretation, including profile analysis (Kaufman, 1994), classification or diagnosis founded on the discrepancies among test or subtest scores (e.g., between high and low performances, patterns of performances, or differences between expected or desired performances), and intervention planning based on these results. Yet, when prevalent activities such as profile analysis or forms of child classification based on discrepancy analysis have been examined empirically, they have proven to be unsound or to lead to high rates of decision errors (Macmann & Barnett, 1985; Macmann & Barnett, 1994; Macmann & Barnett, 1997; Macmann & Barnett, 1999; Macmann, Barnett, Lombard, Belton-Kocher, & Sharpe, 1989) or, equally undesirable, to potentially meaningless decisions or the implementation of ineffective programs (Kavale & Forness, 1999).

Other coherent models of assessment, notably behavioral assessment and applied behavior analysis (considered conceptually as a form of behavioral assessment), yield alternative views of measurement qualities that provide clearer guidance for making decisions when working to resolve the problems of children and adolescents. The reason for this increased clarity in decision making stems from procedures that answer technical adequacy questions by directly collecting ongoing data on *both* problem variables and on the quality of those measures in the natural problem settings surrounding a referral. In other words, behaviors, other key variables (environmental events and interventions), and their technical adequacy can be all measured or sampled in phases of problem solving. Furthermore, the foundation research supporting behavior analysis and other types of behavioral assessment that has been conducted in problem settings can be more easily generalized to case-specific situations, as opposed to being generalized from group-specific information (e.g., from research on ADHD populations) and thus is more directly related to use in practice. These are the advantages; the complexities and challenges are reviewed in Nelson and Hayes (1986), as well as other sources (Johnston & Pennypacker, 1993).

This chapter is intended to help resolve questions concerning how to judge the appropriateness of assessment or measurement decisions and of the information used to make decisions. The fundamentals of psychometric quality should have to do with measuring (1) meaningful child-related variables, (2) within important natural contexts, and (3) for the purpose of guiding professional decisions. We warn that eclectic model mixes, such as adding traditional personality- or behavior-rating techniques to direct assessments of problem situations, are not panaceas. Such mixes may lead to a heightened sense of professional confidence while at the same time increasing rates of potential errors, obfuscating decision processes, and depleting time and resources. This chapter extends earlier work analyzing reliability and validity within decision contexts (Barnett & Macmann, 1992a; Barnett & Zucker, 1990; Macmann & Barnett, 1984; Macmann & Barnett, 1999; Macmann et al., 1996). We hope that this discussion will add impetus to the development of a common assessment lexicon that is based on the technical adequacy of actual problem solving within natural contexts.

HOW DOES PSYCHOMETRIC RESEARCH INFORM PROFESSIONAL BEHAVIOR?

Empirical answers to this question are difficult because there is very little actual information on the *behavior* of professionals related to assessment activities, including the selection of assessment procedures and the actual use of information (e.g., Wilson & Reschly, 1996). Assessment behaviors can be organized by several categories. First, there are those behaviors exhibited *prior* to problem presentation that result in establishment of relatively enduring personal instrument preferences or other highly probable but idiosyncratic chains of decision-making behavior. Second are the behaviors exhibited by professionals *during* problem solving, such as deciding on units of analysis: (1) child behaviors, child–peer, child–adult, or child–task behaviors, activities, and times; (2) planning behaviors, such as reviewing pertinent research or consulting with colleagues; and (3) organizing data or inferences to guide intervention development or other outcomes. Both of these categories of professional behavior are dynamic and, for a specific case, are under strong control of important events occurring before and during the case. Such important events could be related to nontechnical social interactions between those involved in assessment activities, or could occur within the assessment activities.

Likewise, it seems that the best psychometric data for guiding professional assessment decisions would have two characteristics. First, these data would provide direct information about how assessment data are likely to impact the quality of the decision in question. Second, the data would be derived from examination of the results of actual decisions that were informed by the assessment procedures being analyzed.

Although professionals should be guided by their understanding and knowledge of instrument quality and related criticisms, the lack of a commonly accepted model or set of criteria for using such information reinforces the need for an empirical database derived from observing what actually happens before and during problem solving. Furthermore, given the lack of universally accepted guiding principles, it would also seem important that professionals should communicate their values, preferences, and uncertainties to consumers. Unfortunately, the contact between a child and any specific instrument or procedure during problem solving may be actually a chance encounter based on idiosyncratic professional preferences (best practice would see this as highly negative). The outcomes associated with different instrument preferences are not likely to converge, and many differences in instrument use are probably not benign.

During the development of tests or other measurement tools such as standardized observational codes (Greenwood, Carta, Kamps, Terry, & Delquadri, 1994; Saudargas & Lentz, 1986), a wide array of information concerning psychometric quality is typically collected and reported in user manuals and, for many instruments, research continues after publication. When examining manuals for standardized scales used frequently by school psychologists, such as the Wechsler scales, or often recommended like the Child Behavior Checklist (Achenbach, 1991), most of these data would appear related to an *implicit* nomological network that is intended to demonstrate the meaning of measured constructs (validity, or internal structure, relationships with external measures, group differences), or to provide information about various measures of test error (reliability). However, in manuals for these instruments, there appear to be few if any data related to the reliability and validity of the outcomes of the proposed uses of test scores.

In user manuals for most assessment procedures, data are presented that have been collected on norm groups. Logical generalization is expected to be used by a practitioner to make the connection between the child who is referred and children who are represented in the manual's psychometric and statistical compilation. A "match" is typically "scored" if the characteristics of the child, information found in manuals or diagnostic guides, problem characteristics, and immediate assessment questions, overlap. As in the previous paragraphs, we have very little knowledge about the extent to which such a decision actually occurs. What may, in fact, occur is the nearly automatic selection of a test by a professional faced with some categorical question—special education classification, for example. Professional judgments based on test or instrument use are highly vulnerable to sources of influence such as pressures to diagnose and to predictable decision errors (termed *heuristics*) based on superficial similarity and resemblance ("the illusion of validity"), the ease to which a diagnosis comes to mind (i.e., the influence of attending a recent workshop on ADHD), and private anchors for inferences and adjustments in inferences in accord with preconceived ideas which may be out of practitioner awareness (Chapman & Chapman, 1969; Garb, 1998; Tversky & Kahneman, 1984).

Are the most serious problems pertaining to instrument use discussed in test manuals? Test or scale manuals generally lack clarity about how instruments are actually used in practice and how well they work given setting-specific base rate and selection ratio information for diagnostic disorders (Meehl & Rosen, 1955), and in the context of incremental validity (Sechrest, 1963). When profiles or patterns of subtests are to be used, how often is profile reliability and decision stability actually discussed? When manuals contain guides for using test data, how often is information regarding the effects and consequences of proposed uses actually provided? How are cost analyses of test or scale use portrayed (Sechrest, 1963)? We believe that the answer to these questions is essentially, "Never."

There are probably a number of ways in which published information regarding psychometric quality *could* actually affect the behavior of a professional. In this regard, the traditional process of making a decision to employ a measure or to use assessment results seems to be best described as weighing a wide array of evidence and somehow making the decision, most possibly without fully understanding the consequences of potential errors and subsequent actions. One way to conceptualize the possible impact of information about psychometric quality on professional decisions is based on whether data on the psychometric quality of a measure are collected directly during an individual case, or whether previous research data are used to guide either initial selection of measurement procedures or the subsequent development of inferences based on test data. Both of these methods are important to understand and they have their uses. There are at least three ways, all suggested within the literature on assessment, in which professional decisions can be affected by information about the psychometric quality of assessment data.

1. *Directly collecting data on the actual psychometric qualities of the measures that are used during problem solving.* Within many behavioral approaches to problem solving, the assessor may directly measure the quality of the actual data used during problem resolution. This is in contrast to using psychometric information collected in the past on groups of persons not directly involved in the current case (i.e., *reliability* and *validity* studies). For example, data may be collected by the professional decision maker (a) to estimate and even improve the accuracy of direct observation data (*interobserver agreement*); (b) to quantify problem presentations or to monitor progress; (c) to quantify and judge the significance of variables targeted for change and the quality of the goals of intervention (*social validity* or *acceptability*) to stakeholders; and (d) to determine the accuracy with which a treatment protocol is followed as a guide to making intervention changes (*treatment integrity*). All of these relate directly to the quality of the problem-solving process and, most importantly, they can set the occasion for subsequent professional behaviors aimed at improving the quality of data that will reciprocally affect professional decision making.

Although the exact topography of any of these measures of assessment quality will vary from case to case, intervention-planning models specifying procedures, decision points, collection of data on psychometric quality, and how to use data, have been developed and evaluated (Barnett et al., 1997; Barnett, Pepiton et al., 1999; O'Neill et al., 1997) using the judgment of beneficial outcomes to children as a criterion. While the various components of these assessment models have not been evaluated for all features of technical adequacy related to producing positive outcomes, examination of the published outcomes of such decision-based models can guide behavior during an actual case and allow a practitioner to better select procedures. The latter use is a direct analogue to the next category, which concerns information practitioners can use prior to selection of assessment procedures.

2. *Reviewing published data on the psychometric qualities of assessment procedures in order to select the most appropriate procedure for some purpose.* In an ideal world, a professional should use information about the nature of the referred problem and knowledge about assessment procedures to review possible methods (e.g., tests vs. observations) of collecting information to be used to make particular decisions. In the course of this implicit or explicit evaluation, data reflecting the required psychometric qualities of instruments should be examined. This information would be found in manuals, and by reading psychometric research published after the manuals are released. For example, if information concerning the "cognitive ability" of a child is presumed to be needed to make a classification decision during school-based multifactored evaluation, studies could be reviewed demonstrating that a test actually measured a desired construct, was useful in making a classification, that derived test scores lead to reliable decisions, and that consequences following classification are likely to be those that are desired. Based on available data and their perceived relevance to the individual case, a go/no-go decision (about using a particular instrument for example) would be made.

There are often such data about more direct and behavioral assessment methods such as observation codes (see, e.g., Greenwood et al., 1994; Saudargas & Lentz, 1986). Instrument or code-development data on the potential for observational accuracy/agreement, the importance of measured behaviors, and on standardized use are often reported in what are equivalent to user manuals for traditional tests. Less direct behavioral assessment procedures such as rating scales and checklists are accompanied by user manuals with a wide variety of technical data, including more traditional reliability estimates, intratest subscale relationships, norms, results of factor analysis, and correlations with other similar measures (Achenbach, 1991; Macmann & Barnett, 1999; Macmann, Barnett, & Lopez, 1993).

If the available data about use of particular assessment procedures by school psychologists are examined, it seems doubtful that selection being guided by evaluation of available psychometric data is often occurring (Wilson & Reschly, 1996). To further complicate this issue, there are several types of psychometric data, described earlier, that would typically *not* be available for consideration in selecting measurement procedures suitable for answering important assessment questions. This absence of pertinent information may not be noticed given the often overwhelming array of information provided in test manuals, and the equally large number of characteristics of the referral problem situation. From typical professional sources, it is not clear how practitioners do, or should, make logical generalizations and determine the suitability of a test score for making needed inferences. This process has been lumped into the concept of professional judgment (Barnett, 1988), and important ethical guides (American Psychological Association, 1992) make clear that an assessor must assume responsibility for assessment decisions. (This chapter is an elaboration of Standards 2.04[a] and [b] concerning assessment use.) It seems likely that completely explicit guides may be impossible (perhaps undesirable), and that some amount of subjective (meaning not understood) judgment will remain, but still judgments may be aided by appropriate data.

Other important types of data that *could* influence assessment choice would be those that reflect the actual outcomes of decisions, for example, the percent of false negatives or positives yielded by a screening project or the percent agreement about learning disability (LD) classification across two assessment occasions. To be useful, data should reflect empirical consequences of assessment decisions, for example, differences in the educational outcomes for children who were "false" negatives versus "true" positives after "risk" screening. The latter two types of information are very atypical for practitioners and, when it is presented, the use of the term *accuracy* is potentially highly misleading. *Agreement* is usually studied, not accuracy (which requires an incontrovertible criterion, not questionable diagnostic or risk status based on the results of similarly flawed diagnostic instruments to judge decisions as true or false).

Unfortunately, typical psychometric data are usually woefully inadequate for making clear analyses about the implications of a test-based decision and communicating these to consumers. Part of the reason for this conclusion is that data on psychometric quality are associated with single measures, while decisions are based on interactions of inferences developed from multiple data sources. A better type of psychometric information would be the actual data on the consequences of using particular test scores in ways that come as close as possible to how actual decisions may be made. In other words, what needs to be communicated as psychometric data would be a range of allowable inferences and error rates across different plausible instruments, raters, and occasions (Hall & Barnett, 1991; Ronka & Barnett, 1986). For example, Macmann and colleagues (1989) provide a set of data that allows one to estimate the actual probability that an LD classification decision (based on the discrepancy between a measure of cognitive ability and one of achievement) would be the same on a second testing occasion, or with a different pair of acceptable tests, or methods of discrepancy analysis.

Macmann and colleagues (1989) compared learning disability classification agreements based on the discrepancy between cognitive and achievement scores on a second occasion using the same instruments, or between results obtained across different pairs of commonly used instruments. Their data, and a review of other similar studies using different instruments and classifications, reveal three to five instances of disagreement (meets criteria one time but not the other) for every instance of agreement (meets or does not meet the same criteria across comparisons). The consequences of such uncertainty would seem staggering if selection decisions were being actually made by practitioners. Yet all of the instruments they examined would have been judged to have adequate to high reliability, and the studies *minimize* potential error sources.

The analyses of Macmann and others used some of the procedures long recognized within psychometric research but seldom documented in test manuals. These include analysis of incremental validity, analysis of false positives and negatives, use of base rates, and comparisons of decision outcomes across different cut scores, and examination of how well decisions generalize across methods. Manuals may report the size of differences between subtest scores necessary for statistical significance, for example, yet that also has little relationship to analysis of the nominal classifications that actually occur in practice. In the above example, the concept of error associated with actual practice is also not similar to the notion of standard error of test scores. The type of error probability analyzed by Macmann and colleagues (1989) is important for deciding to even use tests, much less which test to use. Note that neither the type of error discussed by Macmann and colleagues (1989), nor the analysis of validity and reliability data from more traditional methods, would necessarily inform us about the consequences of being labeled LD or not, just the stability of such decisions (which, not being up to professional standards, makes diagnostic applications questionable).

3. *Using information from previous research to predict a range of possible errors associated with any assessment inference.* Several inferences from test scores could be informed by data on psychometric quality. First, as Messick (1995) indicates, it is the inferences made from a measure that must be analyzed. In order to make an inference, the meaning of any construct being measured must be clearly understood and verified with data. Construct meaning is slippery at best. Certainly, professionals should review definitions and supporting evidence provided in test manuals in order to determine if tests measure the variable about which information is needed. Considering major cognitive tests such as the Wechsler scales or the Stanford–Binet IV (Thorndike, Hagen, & Sattler, 1986a, 1986b; Wechsler, 1991), examination of the stated theoretical definition of the intended constructs measured by the tests reveals widely different meanings.

If each test perfectly measured their constructs, would they be interchangeable in making inferences about child membership in a category such as learning disabilities? What contribution to the unsoundness of assessment decisions would accrue to selection of one instead of the other? When professionals review information about putative measures, how would this dilemma be resolved by review of available evidence? How does contextual use alter reliability and validity evidence? As an example of this last point, rarely discussed in practice, even varying the *sequences* of assessment events (what scales are given first, second, or third, etc.) may lead to a range of different outcomes (Mangold, 1982) that is akin to chaos theory. (Researchers counterbalance instrument administration order, but order is often uncontrolled in practice.) Based on data, conclusions about classification (or inferences) are not necessarily generalizable across tests or scales designed for similar or even the same purpose, or differences in actual use. These potential decision errors need to be communicated to consumers.

Irrespective of the meaning of a construct, direct interpretation of any specific score or score difference is not deemed appropriate; rather, some band of confidence needs to be established to ensure that potential error is factored into an inference (Anastasi & Urbina, 1997). There are a variety of ways to do this, all involving some form of standard error, estimated true scores, and confidence intervals (see Barnett & Macmann, 1992a). Error may be conceptualized as *standard* across the entire range of possible scores, *different* for different levels of scores or different cut scores (Thorndike, 1982), and even to some degree predetermined by item selection (Embretson, 1996). Irrespective of how it is calculated, error associated with a specific case must be inferred from error calculated from some research sample, and its relevance to the specific case assumed. Note that there are no previously collected data that directly bear on the actual measurement within the case, rather research data cue a decision around interpretation. In traditional measurement there are no *direct* measures of idiosyncratic errors in order to guide modification of assessment procedures once they have begun so that the data collected during a case can be made more useful.

There may be, of course, empirical evidence about differential error associated with particular problem situations, or even with particular characteristics of the child being assessed. For example, a meta-analysis of existing research (Fuchs & Fuchs, 1989) found that African American children perform less well than white children on tests administered by unfamiliar professionals. Other data would indicate that children with serious behavior problems may influence the behavior of adults in teaching situations in ways that may be similar to testing (e.g. Carr, Taylor, & Robinson, 1991) and may produce more erratic scores than other children. This information should be factored into inferences made by professionals, and into decisions about what to assess and how results should be interpreted. However, logical generalization from group data to the case at hand is still required, and existing data do not necessarily provide constructive guidance about what to do instead.

Data on the psychometric qualities of assessment procedures are certainly important. Psychometric data should guide professional practice far more than we suspect they actually do in practice. Yet we believe that the most important data to guide practice, information concerning the quality of our decisions, is virtually absent from traditional assessment models. A prime exception appears to occur within more behavioral approaches to treatment.

AN OVERVIEW OF PSYCHOMETRIC CONCEPTS

A Primer of Psychometric Models for Professionals: Reliability and Validity Revisited

Psychometric models exist to provide a logical framework from which to develop and make subsequent decisions about the appropriate uses of assessment procedures. Psychometric principles as used by professionals may also be conceptualized as a set of connected rules about the development and acceptable use of measurement procedures. Mirroring psychology in general, different measurement and supporting mathematical models have evolved. Given the radically divergent psychological views inherent in various models, an eclectic viewpoint could be considered untenable. However, we believe that there is a logical, consistent framework for the evaluation of measurement qualities that should guide professional practice that can encompass other existing models and that does not require an opportunistic eclecticism. Building on the research and arguments of many others, this framework must rest on strong empirical evidence of the net utility of assessment when potential consequences are weighed. Stated differently, confidence in assessment results and helpfulness in resolving problem situations are the mutually desirable and linked objectives of psychometric analyses of professional practice.

Detailed discussions of traditional notions of reliability and validity are widely available, and will not be rehashed here (Anastasi & Urbina, 1997; Nunnally & Bernstein, 1994). The most salient issue concerning traditional psychometrics for our discussion is that, in spite of a unifying criterion that measurement meets some purpose (Standard 2.02; American Psychological Association, 1992), utility is hardly ever actually addressed (Hayes, Nelson, & Jarrett, 1987). Rather, psychometric quality is usually treated as the separate facets of instrument reliability and validity. It is at least implicit that reliability and validity are connected qualities, but a framework for their integration into decision making is usually missing in practice. For example, manuals for major tests used in schools, such as the WISC-III, make virtually no effort to integrate evidence around any particular *use* of the respective instruments. This is an important point and will be elaborated below.

Reliability

The concept of reliability pertains to the consistency of a metric, and reliability estimation enables the quantification of a range of error associated with test use, both for judging the quality of potential assessment instruments and for identifying the uncertainties of using a test score to make inferences. Note that consistency actually applies to the inference(s) that are made from a metric, a very critical distinction for our arguments. There are a number of current models for the conceptualization and evaluation of reliability. The classical model developed by Spearman at the turn of the 20th century assumed that each score has two components: (1) a true score, which is estimated from an observed score, and (2) test error. Trait-like qualities (IQ, personality) as well as other characteristics (patterns of behavior, achievement) are typically assumed to be relatively stable qualities of individuals, and measurement error is assumed to be random. The reliability of a test score can be estimated through a single administration of a test using procedures such as Cronbach's alpha (Cronbach, 1951), by retesting the same individuals within a brief time interval (test–retest), by the proximate administration of different test forms (alternate forms), or through a study of the different factors influencing the variance of test scores (generalization study). With the exception of rarely used generalizability studies (Feldt & Brennan, 1989), different types of reliability estimation each account for different error sources that are actually *additive* with regard to individual inferences from test or scale use (Macmann & Barnett, 1997; Macmann & Barnett, 1999). To our knowledge, this has not been addressed in test manuals or in most guides to practice (although see, e.g., Anastasi & Urbina, 1997; Feldt & Brennan, 1989).

Other conceptual and methodological models for understanding reliability or reliability-like qualities have been derived from item–response theories or domain theory (Petersen, Kolen, & Hoover, 1989; Thorndike, 1982). These discussions are extremely complex, but irrespective of how reliability is conceptualized or measured, numerical estimates of instrument reliability and of the error associated with individual administrations are developed and are functionally similar for various scales. Practitioners are required as a professional standard to understand and use reliability evidence as criteria when they employ individual measures to make professional decisions. For example, when practitioners are comparing potential assessment instruments or methods to answer various questions, they are expected to consider reliability estimates. To help make a diagnosis, a practitioner could consider (1) estimates of diagnostic error associated with a single administration; (2) estimates of error, even hypothetical, if the test were administered again; or (3) administered by a different examiner—all would be used to predict the likelihood and soundness of a diagnosis. However, these relatively straightforward assertions about the use of reliability fail to account for *additive effects* of errors from different sources. There are, unfortunately, other special reliability problems related to many typical ways in which practitioners actually use test data.

Practitioners routinely go beyond drawing inferences from overall test scores to drawing inferences based on relationships among scores from batteries of tests, profiles across subtests from the same instruments, or discrepancies between subtests. In regard to the use of common cognitive tests or profiles from behavior ratings, this practice has been soundly criticized as providing little or error-prone information (Macmann & Barnett, 1997; Macmann & Barnett, 1999). However, the problems accrue from the interpretations of correlated measures, not the type of scale. When these types of multiscore analyses occur, then any such pattern is the source of an inference and needs to be subjected to psychometric analysis as a unit, not as separate scores.

Multiscore inference for individual children has numerous longstanding problems, including outcomes dependent on arbitrary instrument selection, conceptualization of these interpretive units, and the lack of attention to subsequent consequences for the child. (1) The chances of finding a problem or the probability of some statistical difference is partly a function of the number of scales and subscales in a battery of instruments. Practically speaking, finding a "problem" can become unconstrained given the possible number of unplanned comparisons of typical multiscale batteries that would defy the capabilities of research much less questions of individual practice ($n = 1$ with hundreds of possible comparisons; Cohen, 1990; Meehl, 1978). (2) Profiles derived from correlated scales are less reliable than the reported reliabilities of their parent scales or subscales (Macmann & Barnett, 1994). This outcome of profile reliability is true even with scales meeting ideal reliability standards if the correlations between instruments being compared are relatively high. As a simplified example, if a verbal scale (or externalizing scale, etc.) has an internal consistency reliability of .90, and a performance scale (or internalizing, etc.) also has a reliability of .90, and the correlation between scales is .60, the difference score reliability is .75, a result below accepted reliability standards for individual interpretation. Beyond the lower reliability, the difference score has unknown validity (it requires inventing a construct for interpreting the difference) (see Barnett & Macmann, 1992b, for elaborations). The test user would also need to consider other reliability facets, and even other scales that purport to measure the same construct in order to consider or communicate any level of decision confidence. Idiosyncratic or even standardized multiscale batteries, thought to be a panacea, create multiple problems for interpretation; the overall decision confidence is not reported in manuals, and they take the test user and consumer into uncharted territories that defy meaningful error calculation and human information processes capabilities.

In summary, beyond traditional estimates of reliability of scales, other psychometric qualities related to reliability are needed for scale use: additive effects of different error sources, as well as the reliability of profiles or other discrepancy-based interpretations. There are substantial errors associated with profile and discrepancy analysis that have received insufficient attention—topics to which we return.

Validity

Validity is a psychometric construct that usually focuses on what a test measures and on the generalizations that can be made from test results. Validity evidence is quantified and evaluated through conceptual, logical, statistical, or experimental procedures that are still evolving (Wainer & Braun, 1988). Reliability is a prerequisite (and limit) for any measure of validity, but different reliability estimates may be needed for different validity generalizations. As we have elaborated, decision reliability, which sets limits for validity estimates and ultimate usefulness, has been meager for many child-related referrals (Barnett & Macmann, 1992b).

A variety of methods have been employed to provide evidence for different types of validity, such as construct, content, criterion-related, and others. Instrument developers as well as post-publication researchers are supposed to provide evidence concerning the dimensions across which any index of validity can be generalized, such as age, gender, ethnicity, setting, or classification status (American Psychological Association, 1992). Instrument users are then expected to examine these dimensions of generalization as they relate to any specific questions they hope to answer through the use of test data. As discussed above, users are expected to make an *integrated* decision about the appropriateness of using any measure on a case-by-case basis. Unfortunately, this basic notion seems seldom to be employed within published test manuals. Rather, separate evidence for some of the many forms of validity is usually presented as evidence for the *validity of the test*, not inferences from test scores, and questions about integrating evidence across facets of validity (constrained by reliability evidence) for different uses is not made clear.

For an instrument user, the examination of the available validity evidence always yields a subjective judgment about the support for a particular measurement use. What pleases many developers or consumers in terms of validity evidence, such as correlations of a new test with an existing test, may be highly insufficient given alternative and more stringent analyses that take into account the extent of the relationships, allowable predictions and, again, how the test is actually used. Even if there are data that inferences from some score actually are useful for some purpose, there may be consequences of that use that are negative for a child. In our subsequent discussions we will emphasize a unified model of validity for understanding underlying constructs and the consequences of using measurement to make a decision (cf. Messick, 1995; Wolf, 1978).

Finally, comparison groups used in manuals from which facets of validity are estimated are built on prior information that may not be fully explained or revealed, but which may constrain generalizations about use. As an example, norm groups may be formed based on teachers' and parents' referrals, and the children may be given standardized scales to make diagnostic determinations. The parents and teachers then may be given the scale of interest (i.e., the one being developed) to again rate the children, but the group's diagnostic status is known to parents and teachers. Thus the system used for a scale's development and norm derivations may not generalize to first-time "diagnosis."

Test- and Scale-Based Measurement of Constructs versus Nominal Measurement of Constructs in Practice

Traditional measurement has usually been aimed at traits or constructs, which *should* derive their meaning from a well-defined nomological network supported by research data (Cronbach & Meehl, 1955). Traditionally, constructs are more or less abstract traits that are, in practice, represented by samples of items drawn from some domain(s) of items.

Two methods have been typically used to examine construct validity. Factor analysis represents a family of techniques used to simplify the complex correlation matrices in order to reveal the major dimensions that underlie a set of items. Factor-analytic studies of common instruments have yielded controversial results, especially when examined in the light of requirements for meaningful use (Macmann & Barnett, 1992; Macmann & Barnett, 1994; Macmann, Barnett, Burd, Jones, LeBuffe, O'Malley, Shade, & Wright, 1992; Macmann, Plasket, Barnett, & Siler, 1991). Second, multitrait–multimethod correlation matrices (MTMM) (Campbell & Fiske, 1959), can be used for partial validation of a construct whenever there is a clear nomological network and at least two related constructs are measured by two methods. An MTMM analysis examines convergent evidence whereby correlations intended to measure the same trait are expected to converge or be higher than those developed to measure different traits. MTMM analyses also enables a look at discriminant evidence, which is the predicted divergence of the traits. Dissimilar traits should have lower intercorrelations than those found for similar traits. MTMM is logical and powerful because it includes external estimates of constructs. Resulting analyses have generally provided weak to limited evidence for many child-related constructs (Barnett & Macmann, 1992a;

Fiske, 1982). However, either of these methods used to derive constructs misses the network of empirical relationships provided by the behavioral context. Constructs, in order to be meaningful within a consequence driven model of psychometrics, need to encompass the relationships among behaviors and situations, and need to include ongoing qualities of social validity appraisal (Schwartz & Baer, 1991).

Once meaning of a construct has been established (given the above, a very difficult proposition), other psychometric qualities should be evaluated in order to judge the appropriateness of using a measure for some purpose. Tests or scales provide one or more scores intended to represent the amount of some trait or construct possessed by an individual. A construct defines theoretical relationships "about the nature of human behavior" from the test developer's viewpoint (American Educational Research Association, American Psychological Association, & National Council on Measurement in Education, 1985, p. 9). Any attribute to be measured should be placed within a conceptual framework that provides the parameters for understanding the meaning of the construct, including the importance of measuring the construct within the purposes of assessment. The product of creating this framework is referred to as a nomological network (Cronbach & Meehl, 1955). The nomological network outlines the expected relationships among the target construct and measures of other constructs, observable behaviors or variables, and necessary qualities such as stability or other dimensions of generalizability.

Constructs conceptualized this way are used even within behavioral models, and the term ultimately refers to the meaningfulness of any target of measurement, whether it is social skills or intelligence. However, in actual school-based practice, many assessment activities are related to diagnosis, and assignment of a child to a particular diagnostic category is construct measurement of a different sort than test-derived construct validity associated with a test score. If a school psychologist gives several tests and/or uses other measures to determine whether a child has a specific learning disability, the professional has essentially measured the construct of learning disability at the nominal level. Traditional psychometrics do not account for this type of usage, and traditional ways of determining construct validity would seem insufficient.

The differences between traditional diagnostics and nomological context is critical. Diagnostic use is usually dichotomous, and nomological networks would need to be established in order to define the diagnosis. However, at this nominal level the construct is really represented by a network of relationships among measures of multiple constructs (intelligence, achievement, information processing, etc.). Psychometric qualities related to the nominal assessment of the presence of this diagnostic construct would seem highly related to the type of research done by Macmann and others (Macmann & Barnett, 1985; Macmann et al., 1989), because the level of measurement is a dichotomous one—a child is characterized as LD or not LD (or similar classifications or diagnoses). Simple examination of intercorrelations among measures may be necessary, but cannot take into account the reliability of that nominal measure. The prediction of correlational relationships remains important at the level of definition, yet completely insufficient in judging whether the construct can be measured at all at professional levels of confidence. In fact, the assessment of nominal agreement is perhaps the most practical meaningful measure of reliability, and reliability of this sort is closely tied to any concept of validity.

In summary, there are interrelated criticisms of reliability and validity as they are typically employed within traditional psychometric models.

1. *There is no direct or truly empirical link between an obtained score and any hypothetical true score*. In psychology, the true score is always inferred, and for many traits or constructs, critics have argued that the true score often seems to exist more vividly in the minds of instrument developers than in behavioral evidence. Further, many of the constructs that are actually assessed during most school-based assessment depend on intra- or interscore relationships or differences, and are not made from single observed scores. What would be a "true" score for such constructs? The meaning of high stakes difference scores is often invented or determined idiosyncratically through contemplation and without true experimentation (Kaufman, 1994).

2. *Reliability is not usefully separated from the idea of validity when examining appropriateness of test use, although it is conceptualized and nearly always employed separately in practice*. One reason is that the concept of reliability is directly related to construct meaning (validity), for example, the degree to which the measured concept should exhibit score stability, or reflect internal item homogeneity. Similarly, in the constructs measured by most traditional instruments, reliability and validity are treated as general, static qualities of the instrument, rather than as qualities of decision making across problem situations. Reliability is computed typically as part of test development, reported in test manuals, and is conceptually then the same across all instrument applications. While recognizing that some individual assessment situations have more "error" and that practitioners are expected to infer the existence of some special source of error for a particular case, it is the common range of errors across individuals that is supposed to be used to qualify any single measure. Most constructs in school-based practice are at the level of nominal diagnostic categories and reliability of such nominal categories would have to be examined by the probability of decision stability across occasions and different measures of "simpler" contributing concepts.

3. *In most cases, evidence for the validity of inferences from test scores depends on evidence about correlations among instruments, internal test structure including factor analysis of simple correlational matrixes across subtests, or differences among specific groups*. None of these data will directly inform practitioners about what happens during assessment and use of assessment data. This is complicated by the fact that tests are seldom used alone in school-based assessment. For example, if cut scores were used to make classification decisions (and, of course, they are), standard errors can be computed for the cut score and adjacent scores (Thorndike, 1982). However, that error will not allow a practitioner to fully understand the stability of any decision based on the cut score because that depends on many other variables such as base rates or relationships among all of the measures actually used to make decisions. When simple cut scores (e.g., some level of deviance from the mean) are intended to be used across instruments (activity level or IQ as examples), as is often the case in schools, the concept of decision stability is increasingly impacted in a negative man-

ner. In fact, the use of cut scores for decision making is not a psychometrically defensible professional procedure, and typical reliability estimates and resulting standard errors will not inform practitioners of the true nature of interpretive error, nor allow interpretive stability (Dwyer, 1996). When profiles or differences between two tests are used to make dichotomous decisions, for example, membership in a specific diagnostic category, then research indicates extreme variability of decisions and, in some high-incidence situations, disagreements may be more probable than agreements across occasions or instruments (Macmann et al., 1989).

4. *Assessment within school-based problem solving is fluid and occurs within changing contexts (Schön, 1983); problem solving involving actual problem behavior-in-context is the unit of analysis.* Decisions based on use of scores that result from examination of psychometric data are highly vulnerable to information arrays that include inconsequential and psychometrically weak data, and scores that are not context sensitive. There need to be acceptable guides, with accompanying psychometric qualities, that reflect the actual ongoing nature of assessment.

Behavioral Assessment as a Psychometric Model

Behavioral assessment (Nelson & Hayes, 1986) is a well-developed measurement model that stands in contrast to traditional models. Differences lie in a number of dimensions. First, behavioral assessment is oriented toward behaviors and their antecedent and consequences, as opposed to constructs that are solely internal to persons (e.g., Goldfried & Kent, 1972). Behaviors are assumed to be to some degree situationally specific instead of stable. Second, the purposes of assessment within this model have typically been intervention planning and evaluation—more specifically, identification of problem behaviors, selection of treatment targets, selection of interventions, and ongoing and summative evaluation of treatment outcomes. Third, the meaningfulness of measured variables characteristically requires low inference (e.g., the direct observation of a child's aggressive behavior vs. measurement of personality traits). Fourth, though experimental, appropriate classifications may be derived from the data that result from functional behavioral assessments and intervention plans (Barnett, Bell et al., 1999; Gresham, 1991).

For some behavioral assessors, there is overlap between traditional and behavioral assessment models, especially when paper-and-pencil measures such as behavior rating scales are involved. For measures such as the *Child Behavior Checklist* (CBCL; Achenbach, 1991) and the Behavioral Assessment System for Children (BASC; Reynolds & Kampaus, 1992), or other behavioral rating scales, traditional reliability and validity evidence has often been amassed in manuals and guidebooks, scores may be embedded within multicomponent assessment systems, and the different assumptions of traditional versus behavioral models in regard to such issues as situational specificity or constructs versus behaviors are so blurred as to be indistinguishable. For such behavior rating scales, psychometrics still appear to be evaluated as static qualities of instruments as in more traditional approaches, and will suffer from earlier criticisms.

On the other hand, assessment and intervention models such as applied behavior analysis provide distinctly different notions of psychometric qualities (Johnston & Pennypacker, 1993). Within applied behavior analysis, assessment is not separate from intervention; rather, both are fully integrated across problem-resolution activities; behaviors and the different situations in which they occur are the prime focus; and measurement quality is judged at the individual case level. In this regard, the accuracy of direct measures of behavior, as well the social significance of target behaviors and outcomes for a child, are expected to be assessed to some degree for individual cases as an *ongoing check* of the accuracy and utility of decisions made by consumers and change agents (Schwartz & Baer, 1991). This is a very important difference — intervention decisions, including judgment of errors associated with assessment, are idiosyncratic to a case and, more specifically, to the intervention or problem-solving phase (Macmann et al., 1996). Psychometrics applied to problem solving are less static qualities of instruments than they are *rules* that are intended to influence and guide ongoing decisions. In the model we will espouse, the rules of decision making, including use of information and sequence of decisions, should be the subject of psychometric analyses.

Within behavioral approaches, the ultimate criterion against which all activities (assessment and intervention) are judged is that efforts must produce socially significant outcomes for the target child and others who may be directly associated with a problem situation (Baer et al., 1968; Baer et al., 1987). Data-based decisions about measurement quality can be made for individual cases. For example, Ehrhardt, Barnett, Lentz, Stollar, and Reifin (1996) directly measured the satisfaction of parents and teachers throughout child-focused problem solving. Measurement was ongoing to ensure the implementation of collaborative interventions, the accuracy of data concerning changes in target behaviors, and the perceived significance of changes by parents or teachers for each case. These measures served as a quality control and were intended to affect the problem-solving behaviors of participants in interventions.

Practitioners following a behavioral assessment model will still need to evaluate potential assessment procedures, and for many direct measures this means evaluating the utility of a standardized *process* for creating case-specific measures as opposed to a standardized measure, for example, observational procedures (Saudargas & Lentz, 1986), or brief measures of the perceived significance of outcomes (Barnett et al., 1997; Ehrhardt et al., 1996). The actual topography of a measure would be idiosyncratic to a case. There remain many unknown factors within behavioral approaches, including the fact that there may be few data on the agreement across persons at critical decision points (target behavior definitions and selection, intervention selection, etc.). Understanding of the critical case variables that actually come to control the behavior of professionals is likewise unclear (Lentz & Daly, 1996), although control is intended by progress monitoring, direct assessment of measurement qualities, and other data. There are, however, numerous models that have been evaluated that establish procedures for collection of data on (1) target variables, (2) the quality of such measures, and (3) assessor responses to information, for example, functional behavioral assessment (Barnett et al., 1997; Barnett, Pepiton, et al., 1999; O'Neill et al., 1997). However, component understanding, even within these proven models, still requires research.

Unifying Nature of Constructs and Validity: Consequences and Values

Messick (1995) has articulated a model concerning the evaluation of the usefulness of assessment data that can help provide a unifying, *logical* (as opposed to methodological) structure across the various psychometric models. Essentially, from Messick, validity studies examine not only whether we *can* measure some variable, but also whether we *should* do so for some particular purpose. First, validity is a unitary concept that is studied within a specific decision context. The validity of an assessment procedure is ultimately judged by whether it accomplishes some clear purpose, *and* whether *consequences* for those assessed are positive. There are not types of validity; rather, there are definable characteristics of validity. He argues that there is a sequence of decisions that need be made about whether any metric should be used to help make a specified decision, a sequence that begins with demonstration that a construct to be assessed is meaningful. The characteristic of a meaningful, interpretable *construct* organizes and subsumes the various types of validities that have been discussed in the literature (predictive, construct, content, etc.). Messick argues that we must understand the meaning of variables and their metrics in order to use them appropriately within assessment.

Once construct meaning is demonstrated within Messick's model, evidence supporting specific use for measuring the construct is needed. This is the point where traditional psychometrics have typically stopped. However, Messick strongly advocates that there are values and consequences associated with assessment that are the final arbiters of whether assessment data *should* be used to make some decision. Thus a construct that may be measured with meaningfulness, and useful for some purpose, may not have ultimate validity if consequences of use are detrimental. Judgment of consequences would also take into account any negative values attached to the actual decision, which is of special importance considering the negative connotation many educational or diagnostic categories carry. The prototypical example is that of IQ testing and special education classification.

Judgments about the consequences and values attached to any measurement quantity are, by nature, subjective and value laden. These latter notions clearly fit such models as applied behavior analysis because it has as a standard the criterion of socially significant outcomes (Baer et al., 1968, 1987; Wolf, 1978), and would value directly measuring whether procedures and measures are, in fact, socially valid for individual cases.

While there has been much debate on methods of validating the meaningfulness of constructs, we are unaware of challenges to the merit of consequential criteria for validity (except that it has been avoided by test developers). It is one of the more appealing ways for understanding the ethics of test use and the robustness of validity questions. *Consequences* as the major criteria for judging ultimate validity incorporates considerations of the "appropriateness of interpretations and actions" of test scores or other assessment results and adds the appraisal of value implications of potential score use (Messick, 1995, p. 741). The idea of evaluating consequences includes those that may be intended or unintended. Messick (1995, p. 746) writes: "It is important to accrue evidence of . . . positive consequences as well as evidence that adverse consequences are minimal." The idea of consequences as a criteria for validity also may be linked to questions raised by behavioral ecology (Willems, 1974).

Is One Model Superior?

We believe that the behavioral assessment model offers the most potential in the resolution of childhood problems. However, particular methods or instruments that have been called behavioral assessment can still be used in ways that do not contribute to validity, as conceptualized above. Thus we will argue that it is not a question of which model is superior, but rather what *uses* of assessment data will contribute to validity that has positive consequences as a criterion. Within behavioral assessment models the notion of utility of treatment and importance of consequences have long been definitive, although not always characteristic of the use of behavioral assessment methods (see below) (Baer et al., 1968, 1987; Hayes et al., 1987). Any assessment procedure used during problem solving can incrementally increase positive consequences, although this is ultimately an empirical question within a values framework. Below we discuss a typical assessment process, diagnosis of ADHD, which usually involves use of behavioral assessment methods such as structured interviews, observations, and behavioral rating scales but whose decision error rates and overall validity as documented by consequences are unclear and have yet to be demonstrated. Practitioners will still need to understand the psychometric methods that we have called traditional and decide if these measures of psychometric quality are useful in validating various facets of some purposeful assessment. Irrespective of with which model of assessment any procedure is associated, practitioners are best informed about assessment if they consider validity as a unified construct, ultimately involving consideration of consequences of assessment.

Messick's Validity Construct and the Two Assessment Models

There is nothing about either model of the assessment models discussed that could not be subsumed under a unified concept of validity. We would propose, however, that there is only one clearly developed assessment/intervention model, applied behavior analysis (Baer et al., 1968, 1987), that actually has done so. Applied behavior analysis encompasses a view that what should be measured and what should be the target of subsequent intervention should involve the lowest degree of inference concerning targeted variables. Early comparisons of behavioral and traditional assessment noted that one of the distinguishing characteristics across these models was the level of inference involved in definitions of measurement targets (in essence, the constructs that are measured), with behavioral assessment conceptualized to require lower inference (Goldfried & Kent, 1972). Applied behavior analysis, to fully integrate assessment within an intervention approach, requires that assessment targets be observationally defined (this is a very low inference measurement construct); that the importance of what is measured should be directly assessed; that solving problems is considered the appropriate *unit* of analysis; and that the goal of assessment is to ultimately make socially significant differences for those assessed (Baer et al., 1968, 1987). These features fully overlap with the four aspects of Messick's notion of validity — (1) construct validity, (2) utility, (3) positive values, and (4) consequences for those assessed, although Messick is far from being a behaviorist (see, e.g., Messick, 1995, Messick, 1989).

As noted above, the validity of traditional assessment has very rarely been approached in a unified fashion. It seems appropriate to view much of the research that is contained in the manuals of typical child-related or school-based instruments (and even related published research) as involving the examination of the facet of construct validity. We say this because it relates primarily to establishing the meaning of some construct through examination of correlations with similar and dissimilar measures, internal structure analyses, and differences across groups. All of these types of data ultimately relate to the meaning of what is being assessed. Data on the utility of assessment to actually make decisions that also evaluate the associated values and consequences of assessment are seldom readily available to practitioners. We make the same conclusion about the available data on methods of behavioral assessment such as rating scales (see below), in regard to judging their ultimate validity against a consequential standard. In summary, when validity is viewed within the unified concept developed by Messick, procedures that are usually lumped together as behavioral assessment procedures because they target behavioral measurement are not, in fact, unified conceptually.

EXPANDED VIEW OF PSYCHOMETRIC QUALITIES ENCOMPASSING TRADITIONAL ASSESSMENT TASKS AND PROBLEM SOLVING

Appropriate Units of Psychometric Analysis for Practitioners

If single measures are seldom used alone to make decisions that can be validated as we describe above, then what are the appropriate units of validity analysis? In order to answer that question we first return to the previously discussed ways in which practitioners may be informed by data on psychometric quality. For the purpose of our discussion, we are focusing on (1) data previously collected on validity or potential error estimates that can guide assessment choices, and (2) data directly collected during assessment that can reciprocally influence professional behavior in order to improve positive outcomes (and thus improve validity from the perspective of a unified validity concept).

Validity Data Accessed by Practitioners as a Guide for Assessment Choices

Messick's model is an excellent validity framework for any model of assessment from the perspective of use to practitioners; however, it is still primarily articulated for inferences based on single test scores and single scores are seldom the basis for real-world decisions. For the purpose of helping practitioners to make assessment choices, we believe that the more useful unit for psychometric analysis for both the measurement models discussed above is defined by the overall *purpose* of an assessment activity, for example, problem solving, diagnosis, or screening. What is actually validated within this conceptualization is then an assessment process; and validity information for practitioners would be how well some "process" achieves positive outcomes for children. In essence, this validates *rules* that may be followed in successfully resolving a referred problem. The concept of purpose is critical and units for analysis need careful definition in this regard so that consequences of meeting some purpose can ultimately be part of validity evaluation.

Within any purpose-delineated analysis unit there will be multiple facets and inferences based on assessment data that can be meaningfully distinguished and perhaps analyzed separately. This is directly analogous to the facets of validity that Messick has defined. For example, in considering a problem-solving unit of analysis, the different facets for validity and practitioner inference that have been analyzed (and data published) include the following: (1) target behavior selection (inference about what needs to be changed); (2) hypotheses formation (inference about why a problem exists); (3) accuracy of direct data collected on target behaviors (inference about whether data should be used for decisions); (4) acceptability of interventions; (5) match between hypothesis and intervention; and (6) social significance of outcomes (inference that the changes from problem solving are important for a child). For a diagnostic unit of analysis, facets would include (1) the meaning and utility of the diagnostic construct, (2) accuracy and/or stability in making a diagnosis across different instruments, time, etc.; (3) values associated with assignment of a diagnostic label; and (4) the consequences of being diagnosed for the child. We do not believe that complete diagnostic systems exist that have positive data for all of these facets. Separate analysis of validity facets also would constitute an analysis of incremental validity in the sense that individual contribution of inferences toward positive outcomes for children may be determined.

Data Collected during an Assessment Process to Improve Inferences and Outcomes by Reducing Errors in Inference

Of the two measurement models we compare, only behavioral assessment seems to offer much in the regard of psychometric data oriented at quality control during assessment. For example, to use behavior analysis as a guide, a practitioner should and can routinely collect data on the psychometric quality of information used to make problem-solving decisions (Ehrhard et al., 1996; Lentz, Allen, & Ehrhardt,

1996). These include measuring observational accuracy or an analogue such as interobserver agreement (Cooper, Heron, & Heward, 1987), directly assessing social acceptability of interventions or significance of outcomes referred to as social validity (Wolf, 1978), and assessing the integrity of the treatment processes utilized in problem solving (Gresham, 1989). Such quality-control efforts are extremely important, we believe, to ensure that information used to make decisions is as free from errors as possible. Practitioners may consult the available empirical literature for guidance on how to do this, but the decision to *include* quality control within problem solving is idiosyncratic.

Summary

Irrespective of the separate, productive analysis of any of the facets discussed, judgment of validity always relates to the overall activities taken to resolve some presenting problem. Validity is a unitary concept and is ultimately judged by resulting consequences for children. Practitioners must understand the nature of their decisions and inferences, including the notion of the stability or replicability of decisions. The tangle of connections between facets of problem solving makes it nearly impossible to judge the *singular* effects of any facet on ultimate outcomes.

Of particular importance to this discussion is the idea that any information collected by an assessor should affect their subsequent problem-solving behaviors. Another way of saying this is that practitioners should be continually informed by the information they collect prior to and during an assessment process. In essence, the behavior of the assessor needs to come under control of assessment data and, if this is to occur most productively, then the events and sequence of assessment takes on additional importance. These ideas about control of assessor behavior provide a relatively new twist on the idea of incremental validity, which will be discussed in more detail, and has similarity to response guided experimentation (Edgington, 1996; Hayes, Barlow, & Nelson-Gray, 1999). Particular data may have valid uses only at certain points in a sequence, for example, data from a structured problem-identification interview. Use of information at another point in the sequence may actually have detrimental effects on the ultimate positive consequences for individuals. This means that incremental validity relates to use of information and is a property of inferences and not of any metric. A unit of psychometric analysis would be incomplete without the foundation of reciprocity between the assessor's behavior and data.

The study of consequential validity requires a decision context. Teaming among professionals, and between parents and professionals, provides the context for many educational decisions. In contrast, although mental health professionals outside of schools are often expected to diagnose, and although they rely heavily on observations of others, teaming may not be the expected relationship. These differences are not trivial, and expectations regarding the variables controlling assessor behavior in different decision contexts need to be further clarified. In schools, parents and professionals may participate by bringing information (or impressions) to guide discussions and activities toward predictions about problem situations (e.g., likely patterns of behavior with and without intervention), intervention selection, expected intervention outcomes, or the beliefs about the need for special educational services. There is both a "within the professional" process involving the construction of an assessment system for the individual case, and an interpersonal process among team members. Within both processes, different data sources and methods will not have equal influence on decisions, and planners may not be able to notice or reflect on what influences them. Some team members are more likely to be impressed, for example, with a parent's or teacher's natural observations; others would like to see these observations in the form of ratings; still others may prefer anchoring expectations about behavior to IQ scores. Interpretive confidence in the data across planners is unfortunately not always related to the quality of the data, nor to consideration of outcomes. Thus the actual concepts and methods that *may be applied* to examine decision making are outrageously complex and still evolving, even within a relatively consistent theoretical approach such as behavioral assessment.

To simplify some of these complexities, we will focus on the game plan of the professional. Energy and time given to assessment related activities are finite—therefore, a key question is how should effort be distributed? For the so-called behavioral assessor following professional guidelines (Mash & Terdal, 1997), there would be many choices in building an assessment system for the individual case. Interpretations within idiosyncratic, case-specific assessment relies on professional judgment (irrespective of which measurement model is used) about an array of information of often unknown quality, even when there is research on the psychometric qualities of some of the data that is contained in a manual or published in a journal.

If typical professional sources are used to guide typical school-based assessment, a huge quantity of data can be generated (scores, subscores, difference scores of perhaps several multidimensional scales, observations, academic products, interview results). This is commonly referred to as *multimethod assessment*, but it provides no guarantee for improving clarity—just the opposite may happen. The equivalence of the assessment events (which interview questions? with whom? which rating scale? compare which scores? observe what and when?) and the potential influence of event sequences (what comes first, second, etc.) cannot be presumed and differences may be unknown. As mentioned, the amount of information challenges human information processing. In the next section we will selectively review some of the current issues in assessment that relate to our conceptualization of psychometrics.

Constructs of Childhood, Psychometric Qualities, and Relationships to Practice

We move from the general to the specific in this section to help illustrate the issues of psychometric quality and the criterion of consequence, and to illustrate that it is not necessarily the measurement model associated with a particular procedure that is important, but how measurement is used within assessment procedures. To accomplish this, we will take a closer look at the diagnostic context, using empirical syndromal research related to ADHD as the example. Despite much debate, the assessment and definitions of constructs of childhood are ubiquitous and interest in them appears to be growing (Hibbs & Jenson, 1996). Some major texts in behavioral assessment clearly discuss many of the serious problems of construct-related assessments, yet ultimately still organize the text by them (e.g., Mash & Terdal, 1997). Ostensibly, psychometric constructs may be developed to guide the problem-solving process, but we see many problems with traditional diagnostics in this regard, and offer alternatives.

Of fundamental concern, advocates of classification (or related instrument use) have not studied the decision implications of their recommendations in light of an adequate range of psychometric issues pertaining to decision-making confidence and consequence of assessment. The construct-related measurement problems apply generally to correlated psychological and educational variables, but we offer one example here—that of ADHD diagnosis.

ADHD is a nominal diagnostic construct, or enterprise, whose assessment and consequences from assessment affect millions of children (Barkley, 1997). Barkley (1997), as well as many other authors, recommends the use of structured parental and/or teacher interviews, direct observations, and behavior rating scales, as well as other assessment techniques, to help establish and refine the diagnosis of ADHD. Most of these procedures would be considered as behavioral assessment methods, although it remains to be seen if diagnosis of ADHD as a unit of psychometric analysis has been validated with regard to outcomes. It is, however, as we have previously noted, a construct measured at the nominal level by multiple separate measures, and by different assessment processes. We emphasize the use of behavior rating scales within measurement of this diagnostic construct, although similar issues could be raised about other techniques. The issues we raise are as follows:

1. *A determination of the construct validity of ADHD in the sense of making an "accurate diagnosis" with confidence is not possible; there can only be studies of ADHD diagnostic agreement because there is not an incontrovertible criterion for ADHD.* Despite this fact, ADHD assessors compare their results to an ADHD unknown, considering conduct problems, academic problems, depression, and other potentially strong influences on behavior. The result is that individual error rates associated with ADHD and similar classifications may be functionally unknown, with intractable measurement problems (interpreting profiles of correlated variables, arbitrary cut score use) preventing perhaps even acceptable levels of agreement on diagnostic status much less accuracy. Researchers are most interested in "pure" ADHD cases. By doing so, proponents of this diagnosis set the stage for a nomological nightmare for practitioners in regard to constructs, measurements, and decision making: understanding the interrelationships of conduct disorders, academic difficulties, disturbed peer relationships, internalizing disorders, and so forth. However, these combinations of problems represent real-world concerns of parents and teachers—not often the search for pure syndromes (if they exist) or debates of primacy or comorbidity.

2. *Behavior rating scales are currently "in," and they are often used to anchor ADHD diagnosis within multimethod assessments, but because they behave theoretically as correlated variables, profile interpretations with them have all of the same problems as IQ or other profiles.* Although the estimates of scale reliabilities used for diagnosis may appear adequate, such estimates are only loosely related to resulting decision reliabilities. When studied, decision reliabilities have been found to be much lower than the scale reliabilities from which they are derived (Macmann & Barnett, 1999).

In assessing for the "presence" of the construct, the professional may select from many different broadband behavior rating scales (e.g., from Barkley, 1998; the CBCL, BASC, PIC), or more numerous narrowband scales measuring specific ADHD characteristics. Contact with any of these instruments is chance-related. There are no acceptable and practical ways to "combine" or compare various allowable or recommended data sources for individual diagnostic accuracy and utility. As mentioned, the additive effects of error as separate facets of reliability (internal consistency, retest, and in the case of behavior rating scales, interrater, and difference score reliability) with regard to diagnostic inferences generally has been unexamined.

3. *Choices in rating scales are likely to lead to different descriptions of the child with potentially different outcomes.* Even atypically high traditional validity coefficients, say, a correlation of .80 between two measures of construct-related behavior ostensibly measuring activity level, may not be a reason for diagnostic confidence of agreement across measures (64% of the variation in scores is shared and reliability is not taken into account with regard to the range of inferences that may be made) (see Macmann et al, 1989, for the decision-making implications of this type of validity coefficient). Under conditions that are rarely evaluated, even a relatively modest validity coefficient may imply information, but relatively high values also may suggest redundancy and ambiguity (Meehl & Rosen, 1955; Mischel, 1968; Sechrest, 1963) and may yield high diagnostic error rates. Data that would be more informative to practitioners would relate to the probability of certain conclusions under different assessment conditions. These data would best be developed in terms of agreement percentages given base rates and assessment criteria.

4. *Cross-informant ratings are frequently problematic because of predictable disagreements (comparisons between parents; comparisons between parent and teacher), and there is no set way to handle such discrepancies.* Moreover, they conflate raters and settings. Barkley (1997, p. 93) recommends that agreement across two raters is too stringent and that a disagreement may be dismissed. However, dismissal of one view involves a decision that needs appropriate validation also based on understanding consequences.

5. *Given the above concerns, and the lack of incontrovertible criteria for accurate ADHD diagnosis, the presence of this construct is decided probabilistically, but its utility may be even less certain.* Popular conceptualizations such as ADHD, and pressures for explanations strongly influence the game plan of the professional (Tversky & Kahneman, 1984). There is no question that psychologists play major roles in working with children referred for ADHD-related behaviors and that these behaviors represent very real concerns for all involved. However, questions that stem from the psychometry of practice within ADHD diagnosis include whether or not a decision about the presence or

absence of ADHD can be made reliably across different recommended methods, and the *decision implications* of construct meaning and consequences of outcomes.

Neither actual utility nor the range of consequences of ADHD diagnostic assessments have been addressed for any of the prominent published recommendations. For example, is the only outcome of ADHD diagnosis access to medication, or to a school-based 504 plan? A diagnosis is not needed to plan psychological treatment because such treatments need to be planned within a behavioral, problem-solving model. Furthermore, the types of psychological treatments shown effective with ADHD children may be effective with any child exhibiting similar problems. On the other hand, what would the consequences be if ADHD is deemed not present? Would medication improve symptoms of children who did not quite meet the criteria needed for a diagnosis of ADHD? ADHD diagnosis often leads to medication, but diagnosis is not clearly related to planning other interventions that may benefit children with similar behaviors who do not get the diagnostic label.

Assessment that leads to measurement of a diagnostic construct alone may not be completely validated within a framework of consequential validity, although it could, theoretically, add incremental validity to a valid process. However, moving from ADHD diagnosis to intervention is not consistent with a behavioral consultation problem-solving model prevalent in school psychology unless diagnosis provides data related to successful intervention. If assessment should be strongly linked to interventions (Lentz et al., 1996), the behavior ratings may be dropped from the proverbial assessment battery. In 30-plus years of development (Baer et al., 1968), behavioral assessment for intervention design has not *depended* on behavior ratings.

Summary

Diagnosis of one sort or the other remains a major activity for school psychologists. Questions of diagnostic practice are complex and, practically speaking, represent uncharted territory with regard to core questions of individual decision *outcomes*. Our key point is that constructs and associated recommendations for diagnosis based on use of procedures related to either traditional or behavioral assessment, and using various discrete facets of traditional reliability and validity as indices of psychometric quality, cannot provide meaningful guidance for practitioners. Only use validated by the criterion of positive outcomes should do that.

In contrast, assessment within problem solving starts with the development of a clear understanding of behavior in context early in the process, and it leads to appropriate questions of technical adequacy and direct assessment of measurement quality that is related to specific decisions and their consequences. If there are activities within a diagnostic sequence that add to this understanding, then they may be incrementally useful. In this regard, diagnostic sequences can be logically connected to problem solving, but with different driving purposes than "Is this child ADHD?" or designation of some other syndrome or diagnostic category. Diagnosis is an activity that would only be deemed useful if making a diagnosis clearly increased the probability of successful outcomes. Problem solving is based on a sequential and iterative process with questions like "What is the first most reasonable action?, The second most reasonable action?," and so on, with reasonableness judged by empirical data and social validity appraisal. Thus assessment information is used to help answer very specific questions related to the problem context and thus leads to more effective interventions—one of major differences between traditional assessment and behavioral assessment. Behavioral assessment methods may not be valid if they are not used in ways leading to positive outcomes. From Messick (1995), problem resolution provides the criterion for the validity of the process and problem resolution always resides in context.

Final Discussion of Incremental Validity

Although it is assessment processes that must ultimately be validated against consequences of use, and which provide a guidance structure for practitioners, there are certainly separate methods for assessing psychometric quality that are useful and important. We have referred to these types of psychometric methods as involving examination of incremental validity in the sense that evidence can be collected to demonstrate that a particular method adds some positive increment to positive outcomes. From a practitioner's perspective, incremental validity evidence provides some assurance that a particular assessment effort is useful within a process. In addition, some methods for demonstrating incremental validity are both exhibited in published research (guiding selection of assessment methods) and can be directly employed by a practitioner to reduce errors in decision making. These would include the following nonexhaustive examples: methods for assessing observational accuracy (Cooper et al., 1987); comparisons across methods of time sampling during observation (Saudargas & Lentz, 1986); demonstration or measurement of the social validity of outcomes or target measures (Schwartz & Baer, 1991; Wolf, 1978); direct assessment of treatment acceptability (Gresham, 1989); methods for generating hypotheses during problem analysis (Sasso et al., 1992; Taylor & Romanczyk, 1994); demonstration of important features or use of progress monitoring (Self, Benning, Marston, & Magnusson, 1991); and data on actual peer micronorms, or appropriate ways to collect such data to guide goal setting or target behavior selection (Bell & Barnett, 1999).

The idea of incremental validity can also be applied to the development of valid constructs that can be assessed during problem solving, although not perhaps in the traditional way. Examples of such constructs as assessment targets include: coercive cycles related to children's disruptive behavior as exemplified by Patterson and colleagues (Chamberlain & Patterson, 1995; Dishion, Patterson, & Kavanagh, 1992); ineffective discipline (Patterson & Bank, 1987); parent or teacher monitoring (Patterson & Bank, 1987; Sansbury & Wahler, 1992; Wahler & Sansbury, 1990); parental insularity (Wahler, 1980); keystone behaviors (Barnett, Bauer, Ehrhardt, & Lentz, 1996); and disability evaluation (Barnett, Bell et al., 1999). Although our examples are constructs related to the context of problem analysis or identification, diagnostic constructs as typically envisioned could be incrementally valid if they contribute increments to positive outcomes.

CONCLUSIONS

The responsibility for selection and use of assessment procedures in making decisions about the resolution of children's problems remains at the level of practitioner judgment. Published guides for the most commonly used assessment instruments do not provide sufficient information about valid use, if validity is seen as a unified construct that must be ultimately judged by the consequences of assessment decisions. Given that few of the reasons that initiate assessment activities can be satisfied with the use of single assessment measures, and the use of multiple measures without other criteria for adding or combining measures may actually make decision making less clear, the best type of psychometric evidence that may guide ethical practice is that which provides evidence that some assessment sequence or process, if followed appropriately, produces positive outcomes. We do not believe that assessment practices can be judged as ethical or not without an empirical base that supports the utility of a set of assessment procedures for some purpose, and that provides logic and evidence whose use will result in positive outcomes for children.

In this regard, even if school psychologists can collect assessment data that accurately reflect the presence of some diagnostic construct, whether they should do so is a very separate although related question. Traditional school-based diagnosis does not have a database supporting validity within the framework we have outlined. This does not, of course, mean that assessment packages involving diagnosis may not be positively supported at some point. Current assessment packages involving such procedures as functional assessment (Barnett et al., 1997; Barnett, Pepiton et al., 1999; O'Neill et al., 1997; Sasso et al., 1992; Taylor & Romanczyk, 1994), have databases that begin to support their consequential validity, although there are many technical adequacy facets that need additional research.

With a few exceptions, as reviewed above, practitioners are not yet able to depend on manuals to guide their assessment activities if they intend to follow the partially validated assessment/intervention models we have cited. This imposes an increased burden to remain current with a range of applicable research journals, and this is a behavior that may not be widely exhibited (Shapiro & Lentz, 1985). Also, we would advocate for publishers of user manuals accompanying traditional tests to accomplish several goals that may help clarify the concept of validity. First, they should provide clear nomological networks that organize their studies of construct validity. Second, if they have proposed uses, but no data directly validating (in terms of a facet of validity) that use, and no data on potential or actual consequences of that use, then a clear warning should appear about risks of using the measure for decisions in practice. Third, any validity data will almost always involve demonstrating that what is measured by a test provides some incremental validity within a multiple source assessment.

Finally, what all of us who conduct assessments in educational settings need are explicit sets of rules that we use to control (and communicate to others) our own assessment behaviors. This will invariably involve actively monitoring professional assessment behavior and routinely using direct measures of psychometric quality within problem solving.

References

Achenbach, T. M. (1991). *Manual for the Child Behavior Checklist/4–18 and 1991 profile*. Burlington: University of Vermont, Department of Psychiatry.

American Educational Research Association, American Psychological Association, & National Council on Measurement in Education (1985). *Standards for educational and psychological testing*. Washington, DC: Author.

American Psychological Association. (1992). *Ethical principles of psychologists and code of conduct*. Washington, DC: Author.

Anastasi, A., & Urbina, S. (1997). *Psychological testing* (7th ed.). Upper Saddle River, NJ: Prentice Hall.

Baer, D. M., Wolf, M. M., & Risley, T. R. (1968). Some current dimensions of applied behavior analysis. *Journal of Applied Behavior Analysis, 1*(1), 91–97.

Baer, D. M., Wolf, M. M., & Risley, T. R. (1987). Some still-current dimensions of applied behavior analysis. *Journal of Applied Behavior Analysis, 20*(4), 313–327.

Barkley, R. A. (1997). Attention-deficit/hyperactivity disorder. In E. J. Mash & L. G. Terdal (Eds.), *Assessment of childhood disorders* (3rd ed., pp. 71–129). New York: Guilford Press.

Barkley, R. A. (1998). *Attention-deficit hyperactivity disorder: A handbook for diagnosis and treatment* (2nd ed.). New York: Guilford Press.

Barnett, D. W. (1988). Professional judgment: A critical appraisal. *School Psychology Review, 17*(4), 658–672.

Barnett, D. W., Bauer, A. M., Ehrhardt, K. E., & Lentz, F. E. (1996). Keystone targets for change: Planning for widespread positive consequences. *School Psychology Quarterly, 11*(2), 95–117.

Barnett, D. W., Bell, S. H., Bauer, A., Lentz, F. E., Petrelli, S., Air, A., Hannum, L., Ehrhardt, K. E., Peters, C. A., Barnhouse, L., Reifin, L. H., & Stollar, S. (1997). The Early Childhood Intervention Project: Building capacity for service delivery. *School Psychology Quarterly, 12*(4), 293–315.

Barnett, D. W., Bell, S. H., Gilkey, C. M., Lentz, F. E., Graden, J. L., Stone, C. M., Smith, J. J., & Macmann, G. M. (1999). The promise of meaningful eligibility determination: Functional intervention-based multifactored preschool evaluation. *Journal of Special Education, 33*(2), 112–124.

Barnett, D. W., & Macmann, G. M. (1992a). Aptitude-achievement discrepancy scores: Accuracy in analysis misdirected. *School Psychology Review, 21*(3), 494–508.

Barnett, D. W., & Macmann, G. M. (1992b). Decision reliability and validity: Contributions and limitations of alternative assessment strategies. *Journal of Special Education, 25*(4), 431–452.

Barnett, D. W., Pepiton, A. E., Bell, S. H., Gilkey, C. M., Smith, J. J., Stone, C. M., Nelson, K. I., Maples, K. A., Helenbrook, K., & Hannum, L. E. (1999). Evaluating early intervention: Accountability methods for service delivery innovations. *Journal of Special Education, 33*(3), 177–188.

Barnett, D. W., & Zucker, K. B. (1990). *The personal and social assessment of children: Current status and professional practice issues*. Boston: Allyn & Bacon.

Bell, S. H., & Barnett, D. W. (1999). Peer micronorms in the assessment of young children: Methodological review and examples. *Topics in Early Childhood Special Education, 19*(2), 112–122.

Campbell, D. T., & Fiske, D. W. (1959). Convergent and discriminant validation by the multitrait-multimethod matrix. *Psychological Bulletin, 56*, 81–105.

Carr, E. G., Taylor, J. C., & Robinson, S. (1991). The effects of severe behavior problems in children on the teaching behavior of adults. *Journal of Applied Behavior Analysis, 24*(3), 523–535.

Chamberlain, P., & Patterson, G. R. (1995). Discipline and child compliance in parenting. In M. H. Bornstein (Ed.), *Handbook of parenting: Vol. 4. Applied and practical parenting* (pp. 205–225). Mahwah, NJ: Erlbaum.

Chapman, L. J., & Chapman, J. P. (1969). Illusory correlation as an obstacle to the use of valid psychodiagnostic signs. *Journal of Abnormal Psychology, 74,* 271–280.

Cohen, J. (1990). Things I have learned (so far). *American Psychologist, 45,* 1304–1312.

Cooper, J. O., Heron, T. E., & Heward, W. L. (1987). *Applied behavior analysis.* Columbus, OH: Merrill.

Cronbach, L. J. (1951). Coefficient alpha and the internal structure of tests. *Psychometrika, 16,* 297–334.

Cronbach, L. J., & Meehl, P. E. (1955). Construct validity in psychological tests. *Psychological Bulletin, 52,* 281–302.

Dawes, R. M. (1994). Psychological measurement. *Psychological Review, 101*(2), 278–281.

Dishion, T. J., Patterson, G. R., & Kavanagh, K. A. (1992). An experimental test of the coercion model: Linking theory, measurement, and intervention. In J. McCord & R. E. Tremblay (Eds.), *Preventing antisocial behavior: Interventions from birth through adolescence* (pp. 253–282). New York: Guilford Press.

Dwyer, C. (1996). Cut scores and testing: Statistics, judgment, truth, and error. *Psychological Assessment, 8*(4), 360–362.

Edgington, E. S. (1996). Randomized single-subject experimental designs. *Behaviour Research and Therapy, 34*(7), 567–574.

Ehrhard, K. E., Barnett, D. W., Lentz, F. E., Stollar, S. A., & Reifin, L. H. (1996). Innovative methodology in ecological consultation: Use of scripts to promote treatment acceptability and integrity. *School Psychology Quarterly, 11*(2), 149–168.

Embretson, S. E. (1996). The new rules of measurement. *Psychological Assessment, 8*(4), 341–349.

Feldt, L. S., & Brennan, R. L. (1989). Reliability. In R. L. Linn (Ed.), *Educational Measurement* (3rd ed., pp. 105–146). New York: Macmillan.

Fiske, D. W. (1982). Convergent-discriminant validation in measurements and research strategies. *New Directions for Methodology of Social and Behavioral Science, 12,* 77–92.

Fuchs, D., & Fuchs, L. S. (1989). Effects of examiner familiarity on black, Caucasian, and Hispanic children: A meta-analysis. *Exceptional Children, 55*(4), 303–308.

Garb, H. N. (1998). *Studying the clinician: Judgment research and psychological assessment.* Washington, DC: American Psychological Association.

Goldfried, M. R., & Kent, R. N. (1972). Traditional versus behavioral personality assessment: A comparison of methodological and theoretical assumptions. *Psychological Bulletin, 77,* 409–420.

Greenwood, C. R., Carta, J., Kamps, D., Terry, B., & Delquadri, J. (1994). Development and validation of standard classroom observation systems for school practitioners: Ecobehavioral Assessment Systems Software (EBASS). *Exceptional Children, 61*(2), 197–210.

Gresham, F. (1989). Assessment of treatment integrity in school consultation and preferral intervention. *School Psychology Review, 18,* 37–50.

Gresham, F. M. (1991). Whatever happened to functional analysis in behavioral consultation? *Journal of Educational and Psychological Consultation, 2*(4), 387–392.

Hall, J. D., & Barnett, D. W. (1991). Classification of risk status in preschool screening: A comparison of alternative measures. *Journal of Psychoeducational Assessment, 9,* 152–159.

Hart, B., & Risley, T. R. (1995). *Meaningful differences in the everyday experience of young American children.* Baltimore: Paul H. Brookes.

Hayes, S. C., Barlow, D. H., & Nelson-Gray, R. O. (1999). *The scientist practitioner: Research and accountability in the age of managed care* (2nd ed.). Boston: Allyn & Bacon.

Hayes, S. C., Nelson, R. O., & Jarrett, R. (1987). Treatment utility of assessment: A functional approach to evaluating the quality of assessment. *American Psychologist, 42,* 963–974.

Hibbs, E. D., & Jensen, P. S. (Eds.) (1996). *Psychosocial treatments for child and adolescent disorders: Empirically based strategies for clinical practice.* Washington, DC: American Psychological Association.

Johnston, J. M., & Pennypacker, H. S. (1993). *Strategies and tactics of behavioral research.* Hillsdale, NJ: Erlbaum.

Kaufman, A. S. (1994). *Intelligent testing with the WISC-III.* New York: Wiley.

Kavale, K. A., & Forness, S. R. (1999). Effectiveness of special education. In C. R. Reynolds & T. B. Gutkin (Eds.), *The handbook of school psychology* (3rd ed., pp. 984–1024). New York: Wiley.

Lentz, F., Allen, S., & Ehrhardt, K. (1996). The conceptual elements of strong interventions in school settings. *School Psychology Quarterly, 11*(2), 118–136.

Lentz, F. E., Jr., & Daly, E. J. I. (1996). Is the behavior of academic change agents controlled metaphysically? An analysis of the behavior of those who change behavior. *School Psychology Quarterly, 11*(4), 337–352.

Macmann, G. M., & Barnett, D. W. (1984). An analysis of the construct validity of two measures of adaptive behavior. *Journal of Psychoeducational Assessment, 2*(3), 239–247.

Macmann, G. M., & Barnett, D. W. (1985). Discrepancy score analysis: A computer simulation of classification stability. *Journal of Psychoeducational Assessment, 3*(4), 363–375.

Macmann, G. M., & Barnett, D. W. (1992). Redefining the WISC-R: Implications for professional practice and public policy. *Journal of Special Education, 26*(2), 139–161.

Macmann, G. M., & Barnett, D. W. (1994). Structural analysis of correlated factors: Lessons from the verbal-performance dichotomy of the Wechsler scales. *School Psychology Quarterly, 9*(3), 161–197.

Macmann, G. M., & Barnett, D. W. (1997). Myth of the master detective: Reliability of interpretations for Kaufman's "intelligent testing" approach to the WISC-III. *School Psychology Quarterly, 12*(3), 197–234.

Macmann, G. M., & Barnett, D. W. (1999). Diagnostic decision making in school psychology: Understanding and coping with uncertainty. In C. R. Reynolds & T. B. Gutkin (Eds.), *Handbook of school psychology* (3rd ed., pp. 519–548). New York: Wiley.

Macmann, G. M., Barnett, D. W., Allen, S. J., Bramlett, R. K., Hall, J. D., & Ehrhardt, K. E. (1996). Problem solving and intervention design: Guidelines for the evaluation of technical adequacy. *School Psychology Quarterly, 11*(2), 137–148.

Macmann, G. M., Barnett, D. W., Burd, S. A., Jones, T., LeBuffe, P. A., O'Malley, D., Shade, D., & Wright, A. (1992). Construct validity of the Child Behavior Checklist: Effects of item overlap on second-order factor structure. *Psychological Assessment, 4*(1), 113–116.

Macmann, G. M., Barnett, D. W., Lombard, T. J., Belton-Kocher, E., & Sharpe, M. N. (1989). On the actuarial classification of children: Fundamental studies of classification agreement. *Journal of Special Education, 23*(2), 127–149.

Macmann, G. M., Barnett, D. W., & Lopez, E. J. (1993). The Child Behavior Checklist/4–28 and related materials: Reliability and validity of syndromal assessment. *School Psychology Review, 22*(2), 322–333.

Macmann, G. M., Plasket, C. M., Barnett, D. W., & Siler, R. F. (1991). Factor structure of the WISC–R for children of superior intelligence. *Journal of School Psychology, 29*(1), 19–36.

Mangold, J. (1982). *A study of the primary process in children's kinetic family drawings as a function of predrawing activity.* Unpublished dissertation, Indiana State University, Terra Haute, IN.

Mash, E. J., & Terdal, L. G. (Eds.) (1997). *Assessment of childhood disorders* (3rd ed.). New York: Guilford Press.

Meehl, P. E. (1978). Theoretical risks and tabular asterisks: Sir Karl, Sir Ronald, and the slow progress of soft psychology. *Journal of Consulting and Clinical Psychology, 46*, 806–834.

Meehl, P. E., & Rosen, A. (1955). Antecedent probability and the efficiency of psychometric signs, patterns, or cutting scores. *Psychological Bulletin, 52*, 194–216.

Messick, S. (1989). Validity. In R. Linn (Ed.), *Educational measurement* (3rd ed., pp. 13–103). New York: Macmillan.

Messick, S. (1995). Validity of psychological assessment: Validation of inferences from persons' responses and performances as scientific inquiry into score meaning. *American Psychologist, 50*, 741–749.

Mischel, W. (1968). *Personality and assessment.* New York: Wiley.

Nelson, R. O., & Hayes, S. C. (Eds.). (1986). *Conceptual foundations of behavioral assessment.* New York: Guilford Press.

Nunnally, J. C., & Bernstein, I. H. (1994). *Psychometric theory* (3rd ed.). New York: McGraw-Hill.

O'Neill, R. E., Horner, R. H., Albin, R. W., Sprague, J. R., Storey, K., & Newton, J. S. (1997). *Functional assessment and program development for problem behavior: A practical handbook* (2nd ed.). Pacific Grove, CA: Brooks/Cole.

Patterson, G. R., & Bank, L. (1987). When is a nomological network a construct? In D. R. Peterson & D. B. Fishman (Eds.), *Assessment for decision* (pp. 249–279). New Brunswick, NJ: Rutgers University Press.

Petersen, N. S., Kolen, M. J., & Hoover, H. D. (1989). Scaling, norming, and equating. In R. L. Linn (Ed.), *Educational measurement* (3rd ed., pp. 221–262). New York: Macmillan.

Peterson, D. R. (1968). *The clinical study of social behavior*. New York: Appleton–Century–Crofts.

Reynolds, C. R., & Kampaus, R. W. (1992). *BASC: Behavior assessment system for children manual*. Circle Pines, MN: American Guidance Service.

Ronka, C. S., & Barnett, D. W. (1986). A comparison of adaptive behavior ratings: Revised Vineland and AAMD-ABS-SE. *Special Services in the Schools, 2,* 87–96.

Sansbury, L. L., & Wahler, R. G. (1992). Pathways to maladaptive parenting with mothers and their conduct disordered children. *Behavior Modification, 16*(4), 574–592.

Sasso, G., Reimers, T., Cooper, L., Wacker, D., Berg, W., Steege, M., Kelly, L., & Assaire, A. (1992). Use of descriptive and experimental analyses to identify the functional properties of aberrant behavior in school settings. *Journal of Applied Behavior Analysis, 25*(4), 809–821.

Saudargas, R. A., & Lentz, F. E. (1986). Estimating percent of time and rate via direct observation: A suggested observational procedure and format. *School Psychology Review, 15*(1), 36–48.

Schön, D. A. (1983). *The reflective practitioner: How professionals think in action*. New York: Basic Books.

Schwartz, I. S., & Baer, D. M. (1991). Social validity assessments: Is current practice state of the art? *Journal of Applied Behavior Analysis, 24*(2), 189–204.

Sechrest, L. (1963). Incremental validity: A recommendation. *Educational and Psychological Measurement, 23*(1), 153–158.

Self, H., Benning, A., Marston, D., & Magnusson, D. (1991). Cooperative teaching project: A model for students at risk. *Exceptional Children, 58*(1), 26–34.

Shapiro, E. S., & Lentz, F. E. (1985). A survey of school psychologists' use of behavior modification procedures. *Journal of School Psychology, 23*(4), 327–336.

Taylor, J., & Romanczyk, R. (1994). Generating hypotheses about the function of student problem behavior by observing teacher behavior. *Journal of Applied Behavior Analysis, 27*(2), 251–265.

Thorndike, R. L. (1982). *Applied psychometrics*. Boston: Houghton Mifflin.

Thorndike, R. L., Hagen, E. P., & Sattler, J. M. (1986a). *The Stanford–Binet Intelligence Scale: Fourth edition, Guide for administering and scoring*. Chicago: Riverside.

Thorndike, R. L., Hagen, E. P., & Sattler, J. M. (1986b). *The Stanford–Binet Intelligence Scale: Fourth edition, Technical manual*. Chicago: Riverside.

Tversky, A., & Kahneman, D. (1984). The framing of decisions and the psychology of choice. In G. Wright (Ed.), *Behavioral decision making* (pp. 25–41). New York: Plenum Press.

Wahler, R. G. (1980). The insular mother: Her problems in parent–child treatment. *Journal of Applied Behavior Analysis, 13*(2), 207–219.

Wahler, R. G., & Sansbury, L. E. (1990). The monitoring skills of troubled mothers: Their problems in defining child deviance. *Journal of Abnormal Child Psychology, 18*(5), 577–589.

Wainer, H., & Braun, H. I. (Eds.) (1988). *Test validity*. Hillsdale, NJ: Erlbaum.

Wechsler, D. (1991). *WISC-III Manual*. San Antonio, TX: Psychological Corporation.

Willems, E. P. (1974). Behavioral technology and behavioral ecology. *Journal of Applied Behavior Analysis, 7*(1), 151–165.

Wilson, M. S., & Reschly, D. J. (1996). Assessment in school psychology training and practice. *School Psychology Review, 25,* 9–23.

Wolf, M. M. (1978). Social validity: The case for subjective measurement or how applied behavior analysis is finding its heart. *Journal of Applied Behavior Analysis, 11,* 203–214.

CHAPTER 14

Legal and Ethical Issues in Child and Adolescent Assessment

JULIA E. McGIVERN
ANN M. MARQUART
University of Wisconsin–Madison

Describing the origins of children's psychological testing in schools in France, Koocher and Keith-Spiegel (1990) noted that "children were among the first beneficiaries of psychological testing and probably also among the first victims of its misuse" (p. 47). Over time, safeguards to protect children from the misuse of psychological tests have increased; today, federal and state laws, school district policies, and professional ethical standards strongly influence assessment practices in schools (e.g., Bersoff, 1995; Fischer & Sorenson, 1996; Jacob-Timm & Hartshorne, 1998). School practitioners are required to understand and abide by laws and ethics affecting their professions. The purpose of this chapter is to describe sources of law and ethics related to assessment in schools and to discuss assessment issues facing school practitioners that arise from legal mandates and ethical guidelines.

Salvia and Ysseldyke (1995) defined assessment as "the process of collecting data for the purpose of making decisions about students" (p. 5). Assessment is the broad process of identifying the concerns to be addressed, selecting measures/approaches to use, administering/applying the measures, and interpreting and communicating results. Assessment is frequently differentiated from "testing," which usually is seen as a component of assessment (e.g., Matarazzo, 1990). Matarazzo (1990) differentiated between assessment and testing based on the relationship between the examinee and examiner and the responsibility of the examiner. In testing, for example, when an examiner administers a group academic achievement test, the examiner may have little continuing relationship with the examinee and little responsibility for the selection of the test or its subsequent use. In contrast, in assessment there is a one-to-one relationship between the examiner and the examinee, and the examiner bears significant responsibility for selection, administration, interpretation, and application of the test and its results. Matarazzo (1990) further noted that although test administration can be objective, assessment involves a subjective component.

Abundant assessment information is gathered in schools today. In addition to classroom assessments, millions of students each year take standardized achievement measures administered by school districts or states (American Psychological Association [APA], 1985). Salvia and Ysseldyke (1995) identified four types of special education decisions made in schools based on assessment information: (1) pre-referral classroom decisions, which include classroom instructional decisions occurring prior to a student's referral for special education evaluation; (2) entitlement decisions, which are related to eligibility for special education services; (3) post-entitlement decisions, which involve instructional planning, setting, and progress evaluation for students who qualify for special education services; and (4) accountability/outcome decisions, which inform professionals and consumers about the effectiveness of school services. Assessment practices addressing these four types of decisions yield both process information, such as the activities and decisions occurring during assessment itself, and content information, the information collected during assessment (Witt, Elliott, Daly, Gresham, & Kramer, 1997). Legal and ethical guidelines govern both process and content practices within each type of decision described above. Examples of legal and ethical process and content questions raised in assessments are presented in Table 14.1.

TABLE 14.1   Examples of Legal and Ethical Questions to Be Asked in Four Types of Special Education Decisions

	Type of decision			
Type of question	Pre-referral decisions	Entitlement decisions	Post-entitlement decisions	Accountability decisions
Content questions	Which tools directly address issues of concern? Which measures provide direct link with intervention? Which measures allow progress monitoring?	Which measures best satisfy federal and state legal requirements for valid, unbiased assessment? Which measures provide relevant functional and developmental information?	Which assessment tools link directly with IEP goals? Which measures allow for progress monitoring? Which assessment tools address exit criteria?	Which tools allow progress toward IEP goals to be monitored? Does the content of state and/or district-wide assessments address the student's IEP goals?
Process questions	Should parental consent be obtained? How will interventions be monitored and evaluated? How long should prereferral process continue?	How will parental consent be obtained? How will assessment records be stored? Who has access to assessment results and records?	How frequently will parents be informed of student progress? Will the student be involved in programming decisions? If so, how?	Should accommodations be made in classroom and district/state assessments? How will results of assessments with accommodations be reported?

Although some assessment questions specifically relate to traditional psycho-educational practices (such as intelligence testing and use of other nationally normed tests), many questions relate directly to behavioral assessment. As noted by Kratoch-will, Sheridan, Carlson, and Lasecki (1999), many features of behavioral assessment and traditional psychoeducational assessment overlap; many so-called traditional measures are now used in behavioral assessment (Shapiro & Kratochwill, 1988). However, regardless of the assessment approach adopted, legal and ethical mandates govern the assessment practices of school professionals.

LAW AND PROFESSIONAL ETHICS

School personnel are guided in the conduct of assessments by several sources of law and ethics, including federal and state constitutions, federal and state case law and statutes, state credentialing standards, ethical principles and practice guidelines de-veloped and/or endorsed by professional organizations, and position statements pub-lished by professional organizations. In addition, specific published standards, such as the Standards for Educational and Psychological Testing (APA,1985), developed jointly by the American Educational Research Association, the American Psycho-logical Association, and the National Council on Measurement in Education, guide members of sponsoring organizations.

Definition of Professional Ethics

In the Principles for Professional Ethics, the National Association of School Psychologists (NASP) (1997) defined ethics as "the formal principles that eluci-date the proper conduct of a professional" (p. 1). Bersoff (1995) distinguished be-tween "descriptive ethicists," who gather data about the ethical beliefs of particu-lar groups, and "normative ethicists," who work to transform these beliefs and principles into concrete prescriptions designed to guide behavior. Professional codes of ethics are the expressions of normative ethics. Articulation of a profession's guid-ing principles and practices is a sign of the profession's maturity and is a service to the profession, its users, and the community (Bennett, Bryant, VandenBos, & Greenwood, 1995).

Professional ethical standards evolve over time; as Fischer and Sorenson (1996) stated: "ethics (like legal principles) are not unchangeable axioms but rather shared norms, beliefs, customs, and values that have stood the test of time—guiding prin-ciples to be renewed and reinvented, over time, as our best common understanding of right professional behavior evolves" (p. 3). However, as Bersoff and Keoppl (1993) noted, any professional code of ethics is "inevitably, anachronistic, conservative, protective of its members, the product of political compromise, restricted in its scope, and too often unable to provide clear-cut solutions to ambiguous professional predicaments" (p. 348). Therefore, the professional looking to an ethics code for guid-ance in a specific situation may be disappointed by the general and political nature of most ethical codes (see, e.g., Bersoff & Koeppl, 1993, for a discussion of the American Psychological Association's [1992] Ethical Principles of Psychologists and Code of Conduct).

Sources of Ethics

A number of professional organizations representing school-based professionals have developed ethical codes to guide the behavior of their members. Included among these are the American Counseling Association (ACA, 1995), the American Psychological Association (APA; Ethical Principles of Psychologists and Code of Conduct, 1992), the American School Counselor Association (ASCA; Ethical Standards for School Counselors, 1992), the National Association of School Psychologists (NASP; Principles for Professional Ethics, 1997), the National Association of Social Workers (NASW; Code of Ethics of the National Association of Social Workers, 1997), and the National Education Association (NEA; Code of Ethics of the Education Profession, 1975). Adherence to ethical standards is required for members of sponsoring organizations only; however, ethical standards may acquire the force of law if they are adopted by state licensing boards. For example, many states have adopted the American Psychological Association's Ethical Principles of Psychologists in laws and requirements regulating certification and licensure of psychologists (Bennett et al., 1995; Haas & Malouf, 1995). Generally, it is the responsibility of the individual professional to understand and comply with applicable ethical standards; ignorance of such guidelines is not an excuse for inappropriate practice (e.g., ACA, 1995; APA, 1992; NASP, 1997).

Some professional organizations (such as the American Psychological Association) maintain ethics committees that evaluate complaints against members and recommend sanctions. As an example, the sanctions available to the APA Ethics Committee include: cease-and-desist order, reprimand, censure, supervision requirement, rehabilitation requirement, probation, and recommendation that the individual be expelled or allowed to resign under stipulated conditions from the Association (APA Ethics Committee, 1998). Although loss of membership is the most serious sanction a professional organization can impose, these organizations can report ethical violations to other bodies such as state licensure boards and accrediting bodies, which can impose more serious sanctions.

Major Ethical Principles

Bersoff and Koeppl (1993) identified alternative ethical frameworks on which ethical codes can be built. One of these frameworks is Ross's (1930) notion of reliance on prima facie duties to which the ethical person is bound, including: nonmaleficence, fidelity, beneficence, justice, and autonomy. Bersoff and Koeppl identified nonmaleficence—"above all, do no harm" (p. 347)—as the "bedrock ethical duty required of psychologists and other professionals" (p. 347).

Haas and Malouf (1995) described three general characteristics of ethical acts. Ethical acts are (1) principled: the actor can justify the action as adhering to a generally accepted moral principle (such as honesty or respect for others); (2) reasoned: the actor is assumed to be capable of choice and responsible for basing actions on ethical principles; (3) universalizable: the actor must be able to recommend the same action to others in a similar situation.

The judgment of whether an act is ethical can be based on examination of the consequence of the act (teleological justification that more good than harm results from the act) or on examination of the actor's adherence to a moral characteristic (deontological justification that a moral principle was upheld) (Bersoff & Koeppl, 1993; Haas & Malouf, 1995). In schools and other settings, each type of justification has limitations. Teleological justification can be used to argue that the end justifies the means; deontological justification fails to provide the professional with a hierarchy of moral principles to consult when an act could support one principle (such as justice) and violate another (such as fidelity).

Ethical standards are written broadly to provide guidance to professionals in varied roles, settings, and situations. As explained in the introduction to the NASP Principles for Professional Ethics, "The practitioner must use judgment to infer the situation-specific rule from the general principle" (p. 1). Ethical principles developed by organizations that represent school professionals usually include both broad principles that could apply across disciplines (e.g., social work, psychology, school counseling, teaching), and specific principles unique to each profession. Whereas the ethical standards of organizations representing school-based professionals often share broad ethical themes, their assessment-specific guidelines vary by profession.

Sources of Law

"The law plays a part in everything that educators do. Some practices are required by law; some are prohibited, and the rest are permitted" (Imber & Van Geel, 1993, p. 14). Specific legal mandates derive from federal and state constitutions, statutes, regulations, and case (or common) law and local practices and policies.

Constitutional Law

The Constitution of the United States is the foundation for all U.S. law. The Constitution does not specifically address the provision of education services; however, the 10th and 14th Amendments to the Constitution have been interpreted by the courts as relevant to the provision of education. Through the 10th Amendment, which grants to states powers not delegated to the federal government, the Constitution gives to the States the authority to regulate and fund education. The 14th Amendment to the Constitution, which protects the rights of individual citizens, has been interpreted by the courts to apply to the provision of education by the states. Two provisions of the 14th Amendment have been judged particularly applicable. First, the equal-protection clause of the 14th Amendment prohibits states from denying any person equal protection of the law. Courts have interpreted "equal protection" to extend to provision of public school education. Several critical court decisions have relied on this 14th Amendment clause as a foundation for requiring equal educational opportunity for all students.

A second provision of the 14th Amendment, prohibiting states from depriving any person of "life, liberty, or property, without due process of law," has also been consistently applied to access to public schooling. Education has been decided by the courts to be a property right protected by the 14th Amendment (*Goss v. Lopez*, 1975). As such, states cannot deprive any person of the right to an education without due process. "Due process" has been interpreted by the courts to include "substantive" (relating to the content of the law) and "procedural" (relating to fairness procedures) due process (Jacob-Timm & Hartshorne, 1998, p. 27). Substantive due process prohibits states from depriving citizens of life, liberty, or property based on a law without a legitimate governmental interest. Procedural due process prohibits states from depriving citizens of life, liberty, or property without safeguards to protect them from unfair procedures.

In *Mills v. Board of Education* (1972) the court outlined due process procedures for labeling, placement, and exclusion of students with disabilities. The specific safeguards, which formed the basis for due process requirements in subsequent federal legislation, included the right to a hearing (with representation) and record, an impartial hearing officer, the right to appeal, the right to have access to records, and requirement of written notice at all stages of the process.

In addition to the federal Constitution, each of the 50 states has its own constitution. State constitutions may not deny persons rights guaranteed by the Constitution of the United States, but they may provide additional rights not specified in the federal Constitution. Although the federal Constitution does not address education rights specifically, each state includes an educational mandate in its constitution (Yell, 1998).

Statutory Law

Statutes are laws enacted by the U.S. Congress or by state legislatures. At the federal level, statutes must uphold rights guaranteed by the Constitution of the United States; at the state level, laws cannot abridge rights specified in the state or federal constitutions.

Federal statutes affecting education services have included program and civil rights legislation (Fiedler & Prasse, 1996). Program legislation (e.g., the Individuals with Disabilities Education Act, 1997) describes program components and provides funds to states for compliance with the law. Civil rights legislation requires compliance with the law, but does not provide specific funding. Some civil rights legislation (e.g., Section 504 of the Rehabilitation Act of 1973) applies only to agencies receiving federal funds; although the law does not provide additional funding contingent on compliance with the law, it does threaten withdrawal of any federally provided funds for noncompliance. Other civil rights legislation (e.g., the Americans with Disabilities Act of 1990), in some cases such as the workplace, applies more broadly, including to institutions not receiving federal funds (see following discussion of the Section 504 and ADA).

States also assume the responsibility for developing certification or licensure requirements for education professionals. In addition to requirements such as degree requirements, specific coursework to be completed, and hours of supervised experience, some states, in regulating professions such as psychologists, require adherence to specific ethical standards (e.g., the APA's Ethical Principles, 1992).

Regulatory Law

Federal and state regulations or rules are written to clarify the intent and application of laws enacted by Congress or state legislatures. Although regulations are developed by federal and state agencies (rather than by elected officials), once passed, regulations acquire the force of law. Federal statutes are published in the United States Code (USC); federal regulations can be found in the Code of Federal Regulations (C.F.R.). State education regulations are generally published by the state department of education or public instruction. Education professionals must be familiar with the specific education regulations of the state(s) in which they practice.

Case Law (or Common Law)

"Judge-made law is often called *case law* or *common law*, indicating that it has evolved from the common thought and experience of a people" (Fischer & Sorenson, 1996, p. 2). Case law derives from the federal court system, which is binding throughout its jurisdiction (which may include several states in the case of a district court, or the entire country, in the case of the Supreme Court), and from state court systems, binding within the state in which the decision was rendered.

The importance of case law rests on the tradition of precedents of published opinions. Courts today continue the tradition, rooted in English common law, of upholding prior legal decisions (Yell, 1998). In cases in which there are no statutory laws governing an issue, courts generally review decisions from prior similar cases in deciding current cases, thus creating a body of consistent case law on an issue. Many areas of education law, for example, regarding corporal punishment, derive from published case decisions rather than enacted statutes (Jacob-Timm & Hartshorne, 1998).

Ethical and Legal Conflicts

The potential for conflict between ethical principles and local, state, and federal law "is ever present" (Bennett et al., 1995; p. 22). When laws and ethical principles conflict, professionals are faced with a serious dilemma. As Pope and Bajt (1988) described, professionals may be forced to choose between absolute compliance with the law and selective noncompliance, and neither position may be acceptable. The APA Ethical Principles address this issue but do not provide clear guidance to members, stating, "If psychologists' ethical responsibilities conflict with law, psychologists make known their commitment to the Ethics Code and take steps to resolve the conflict in a responsible manner"(Ethical Standard 1.02). However, a clear definition of "responsible manner" is not provided. The APA Ethical Principles provide clearer guidance in Standard 8.01 to 8.07 regarding resolution of other ethical issues. For example, in Standard 8.02 psychologists are directed to consult other knowledgeable psychologists regarding ethical questions, and in Standards 8.04 and 8.05 psychologists are provided a process to follow in addressing potential ethical violations by other psychologists.

THE LAW AND STUDENTS WITH DISABILITIES

During the 1900s a number of significant legal events shaped the availability and delivery of education services to students with disabilities. Several federal laws were passed, including the Education of All Handicapped Children Act in 1975 (and subsequent reauthorization as the Individuals with Disabilities Education Act in 1990 and 1997), Section 504 of the Rehabilitation Act of 1973, and the Americans with Disabilities Act of 1990, all of which affect the provision of education to students with or suspected of having disabilities. In addition, a significant body of case law has addressed critical issues in education, including discrimination based on race and disability and access to and quality of educational services, and has shaped interpretation of federal and state statutes.

Individuals with Disabilities Education Act (IDEA)

PL 105-17, the Individuals with Disabilities Education Act Amendments of 1997, is the major federal law regulating education services to children with disabilities in the United States. The precursor to IDEA, the Education for All Handicapped Children Act (PL 94-142), passed in 1975, provided the first entitlement to public education with federal financial assistance for children with disabilities. IDEA provides funding to states to provide special education and related services to children with disabilities; in return, states must comply with IDEA regulations, which include developing a state plan for the provision of special education to all eligible children with disabilities. IDEA consists of four parts: Part A–General Provisions, Part B–Assistance for Education of All Children with Disabilities, Part C–Infants and Toddlers with Disabilities, and Part D–National Activities to Improve Education of Children with Disabilities. The major provisions of IDEA are described in Table 14.2.

As stated in Part A of the law, the purposes of IDEA include: ensuring that all children with disabilities have available to them a free appropriate public education that emphasizes special education and related services designed to meet their unique needs and prepare them for employment and independent living; to protect the right

TABLE 14.2   Major Provisions of the IDEA (1997)

Major provisions	Description
Zero reject	IDEA's purpose is to ensure that *all* children with disabilities receive a free appropriate public education.
Testing, classification, and placement	IDEA outlines the requirements of appropriate testing, classification, and placement practices for students with disabilities.
Appropriate education	IDEA defines specific standards by which an education can be evaluated (e.g., provided at public expense; meets state education agency standards) and requires that education be individualized to meet the student's needs.
Least-restrictive appropriate educational placement	IDEA directs SEAs and LEAs to assure that, to the maximum extent appropriate, students with disabilities are educated with students who do not have disabilities.
Procedural due process	IDEA requires that SEAs and LEAs adopt practices that safeguard a student's rights to protest the actions of the SEA or LEA.
Parent participation and shared decision making	IDEA identifies several ways in which parents of students with disabilities are to be included in educational evaluation, planning and decision making.

Note. Based on Turnbull & Turnbull (1998).

of children with disabilities and their parents; and to assess, and ensure the effectiveness of, efforts to educate children with disabilities (IDEA, 20 U.S.C.S. §1400[d], Lexis Law Pub., 1998).

IDEA outlines specific procedures governing special education services. Overall, IDEA provides a set of procedures for states and local educational agencies to follow in determining whether a student is eligible for special education services and in providing those services. Specific provisions address eligibility of students for special education, evaluation procedures, development of an individual education program (IEP) for the student, and due process protections for the student and parents.

IDEA identifies 10 disability categories—(1) mental retardation, (2) hearing impairments (including deafness), (3) speech or language impairments, (4) visual impairments (including blindness), (5) serious emotional disturbance, (6) orthopedic impairments, (7) autism, (8) traumatic brain injury, (9) other health impairments, and (10) specific learning disabilities—through which a student can become identified as a "child with a disability" (IDEA, 20 U.S.C.S. §1401[3][A], Lexis Law Pub., 1998) and be eligible for IDEA services, supports, and safeguards. States are allowed to develop their own definitions of these disability categories, which cannot be more restrictive than the federal definitions.

In addition to the 10 specific categories of disability identified in IDEA, the law allows children age 3 through 9 to be identified as a "child with a disability" if the student is experiencing delays (as defined by the state) in one or more of the following areas: physical development, cognitive development, communication development, social or emotional development, or adaptive development, and who needs special education and related services as a result (IDEA, 20 U.S.C.S. §1401[3][B], Lexis Law Pub., 1998). This provision allows children ages 3 through 9 to receive special education services without diagnosis of a specific disability category. IDEA Part C describes eligibility criteria and early intervention services for infants and toddlers age birth to three. Educators need to become familiar with their state's special education definitions and eligibility criteria to plan assessments that address eligibility criteria and meet specific assessment provisions of the law.

Influence of IDEA on Assessment Practices

Numerous provisions of IDEA directly influence assessment of students with or suspected of having disabilities. Most specifically, IDEA mandates assessment practices for use in the conduct of evaluations for special education. Specific evaluation procedures included in IDEA are outlined in Table 14.3.

Examination of the assessment practices required by IDEA reveals significant overlap between these legally mandated practices and assessment practices required by the ethical standards of many professional organizations. For example, both law and ethics require professionals to select assessment tools that are technically sound and valid for the purpose used, to select and administer tools so as not to be racially or culturally biased, and to use only tools they are trained to use (APA, 1992; NASP, 1997).

IDEA requirements, however, go beyond the specific assessment practices addressed in most ethical standards to include a focus on the multiple questions to be answered via assessments. According to IDEA, the school team (called the IEP team) is directed to review and/or produce certain types of data to answer specific questions, including:

- Whether a child has a disability;
- Present levels of performance and educational needs of the child;
- Whether the child needs special education and related services; and
- Whether additions or modification to the special education and related services are needed to enable the child to meet measurable annual goals set out in the IEP and to participate, as appropriate in the general curriculum (IDEA, 20 U.S.C.S. §1414[c], Lexis Law Pub., 1998).

In making these determinations the IEP team is directed to review existing information, including information provided by the child's parents, current classroom-based assessment and observations, teacher and related services providers observations and, if necessary, to generate additional data (IDEA, 20 U.S.C.S. §1414[c], Lexis Law Pub., 1998). IDEA also includes a focus on the link between assessment tools and information regarding the child's educational needs (see discussion of treatment utility of assessment). Some of the information required by the IEP team is often

TABLE 14.3   Specific Evaluation Procedures Required by IDEA (1997)

<u>Conduct of evaluations under IDEA</u>

In conducting the evaluation, the local educational agency shall

- Use a variety of assessment tools and strategies to gather relevant functional and developmental information, including information provided by the parent, that may assist in determining whether the child is a child with a disability and the content of the child's individualized education program.
- Not use any single procedure as the sole criterion for determining whether a child is a child with a disability or determining an appropriate educational program for the child.
- Use technically sound instruments that may assess the relative contribution of cognitive and behavioral factors, in addition to physical or developmental factors.

<u>Assessment requirements under IDEA</u>

Tests and other evaluation materials used to assess a child

- Are selected and administered so as not to be discriminatory on a racial or cultural basis.
- Are provided and administered in the child's native language or other mode of communication, unless it is clearly not feasible to do so.

Any standardized tests that are given to the child

- Have been validated for the specific purpose for which they are used.
- Are administered by trained and knowledgeable personnel.
- Are administered in accordance with any instructions provided by the producer of such tests.

The child is assessed in all areas of suspected disability.

Assessment tools and strategies that provide relevant information that directly assists persons in determining the educational needs of the child are provided.

A child shall not be determined to be a child with a disability if the determinant factor for such determination is lack of instruction in reading or math or limited English proficiency.

As part of an initial evaluation (if appropriate) and a part of any reevaluation under this section, the IEP Team and other qualified professionals, as appropriate, shall

- Review existing evaluation data on the child, including evaluations and information provided by the parents of the child, current classroom-based assessments and observations, and teacher and related services providers observation; and on the basis of that review, and input from the child's parents, identify what additional data, if any, are needed to determine whether the child is a child with a disability . . .

Note. See IDEA; 20 U.S.C.S. §1414(b) and (c) (Lexis Law Pub., 1998).

obtained via behavioral assessment methods, such as structured observations and interviews. Furthermore, the focus on the link between assessment data and the child's educational needs is consistent with the characteristics of behavioral assessment (Kratochwill et al., 1999).

Central to IDEA is the principle of multidisciplinary team involvement in evaluation and service planning. This principle has implications for school assessment practices. IDEA specifies the make-up of the IEP team to include parents of the child with a disability, at least one regular education teacher if the child participates or may participate in the general curriculum, at least one special education teacher or provider, an LEA (local education agency) representative, an individual who can interpret the educational implication of evaluation results, additional individuals as appropriate and, whenever appropriate, the child with a disability (IDEA, 20 U.S.C.S. §1414[d], Lexis Law Pub., 1998). School professionals must be familiar with the expertise their colleagues contribute to IEP teams and be trained in team skills to maximize the effectiveness of these teams (e.g., Reeder, Maccow, Shaw, Swerdlik, Horton, & Foster, 1997).

Behavioral Assessment and Intervention

Important for assessment practices is IDEA's focus on functional assessment and positive behavioral supports. Describing procedures required when implementing disciplinary measures and alternative educational placements for children with disabilities, the law states that "if the local educational agency did not conduct a functional behavioral assessment and implement a behavioral intervention plan for such child before the behavior that resulted in the suspension . . . , the agency shall convene an IEP meeting to develop an assessment plan to address that behavior" (IDEA, 20 U.S.C.S. §1415[k], Lexis Law Pub., 1998). IDEA thus requires that school professionals know how to conduct functional behavioral assessments with children with disabilities. Furthermore, describing development of the IEP, IDEA directs that the IEP team shall "in the case of a child whose behavior impedes his or her learning or that of others, consider, when appropriate, strategies, including positive behavioral interventions, strategies, and supports to address that behavior" (IDEA, 20 U.S.C.S. §1414[d][3][B], Lexis Law Pub., 1998). This provision requires professionals to be competent in evaluating behavioral problems and designing positive behavioral interventions effective with students with disabilities.

Reevaluations

The 1997 amendments to IDEA altered some requirements of reevaluations for special education services. Unlike earlier law that required only parental notice of an LEA's intent to reevaluate a child with a disability, IDEA (1997) requires that parental consent be obtained for reevaluations (unless the LEA can demonstrate that it has taken reasonable measures to obtain such consent and the child's parent has failed to respond) (IDEA, 20 U.S.C.S. §1414[c], Lexis Law Pub., 1998). In addition, IDEA 1997 allows the IEP team to determine, based on existing data, whether additional evaluation data are needed to determine whether a child continues to be a child with a disability; if the team determines that no additional data are needed, there they are not required to conduct an assessment unless requested to by the child's parents (IDEA, 20 U.S.C.S. §1414[c], Lexis Law Pub., 1998).

Section 504 of the Rehabilitation Act of 1973

In 1973 Congress passed and President Nixon signed a revision of the Rehabilitation Act extending protection from discrimination based on disability to individuals with disabilities. Later clarifications (such as the 1974 amendments to the law and, finally, the 1977 regulations) provided civil rights protections to persons with disabilities by extending to them the rights and protections specified in the Civil Rights Act of 1964. (See Yell, 1998, for a description of this lengthy and contentious process.) Section 504 prohibits discrimination against persons with disabilities in programs receiving federal funds. Table 14.4 summarizes the definitions included in Section 504 and its regulations.

Although Section 504 provides no new funding to programs complying with its antidiscrimination provisions, it does threaten revocation of federal funds from programs not in compliance with the law. In some cases Section 504 provides broader protection to persons with disabilities than IDEA. Under IDEA a person must meet the federal and state definitions of the handicapping condition and, because of that handicapping condition, need special education services as prerequisites to receiving those services. In contrast, a person gains the protection of Section 504 by meeting its definition of impairment and by being discriminated against on the basis of that disability. To use an example cited by Turnbull and Turnbull (1998), a student with HIV could meet the Section 504 definition of disability (either as someone having an impairment or someone regarded as having such an impairment) and access protection of the law if discriminated against; however, that student might not be eligible for services under IDEA if the HIV infection has not resulted in a need for special education services.

TABLE 14.4 Definitions of Key Terms Used in Section 504

Person with a disability is one who
- Has a physical or mental impairment which substantially limits one or more of the person's major life activities;
- Has a record of such an impairment; or
- Is regarded as having such an impairment [29 U.S.C.§706 (1996)]

Physical or mental impairment is
- Any physiological disorder or condition, cosmetic disfigurement, or anatomical loss affecting one or more of the following body systems: neurological; musculoskeletal; special sense organs; respiratory, including speech organs; cardiovascular; reproductive, digestive, genitourinary; hemic and lymphatic; skin; and endocrine; or
- Any mental or psychological disorder, such as mental retardation, organic brain syndrome, emotional or mental illness, and specific learning disabilities. (Regulations implementing § 504 [30 C.F.R., Part 104])

Major life activities mean
- Functions such as caring for oneself, performing manual tasks, walking, seeing, hearing, speaking, breathing, learning, and working. (Regulations implementing § 504 [30 C.F.R., Part 104])

Section 504 states that "no otherwise qualified individual with a disability" shall be discriminated against solely on the basis of disability. The definition of "otherwise qualified" was clarified in a U.S. Supreme Court case, *Southeastern Community College v. Davis* (1979). In this case the Supreme Court held that "otherwise qualified" meant qualified *in spite of* the impairment rather than qualified *except for* the impairment (Turnbull & Turnbull, 1998).

Americans with Disabilities Act of 1990

In 1990 Congress passed the Americans with Disabilities Act, broad antidiscrimination legislation intended to accomplish multiple goals, including:

1. To provide a clear and comprehensive national mandate for the elimination of discrimination against individuals with disabilities;
2. To provide clear, strong, consistent, enforceable standards addressing discrimination against individuals with disabilities;
3. To ensure that the federal government plays a central role in enforcing the standards established in the Act on behalf of individuals with disabilities; and
4. To invoke the sweep of Congressional authority, including the power to enforce the Fourteenth Amendment and to regulate commerce, in order to address the major areas of discrimination faced day-to-day by people with disabilities. (ADA, 42 U.S.C. § 12101)

The ADA is composed of five titles affecting (1) Employment, (2) Public Services, (3) Public Accommodations and Services Operated by Private Entities, (4) Telecommunications, and (5) Miscellaneous Provisions. The Section 504 definition of persons with disabilities also applies to the ADA. Although the ADA provides no additional student rights guarantees beyond those provided in IDEA and Section 504 (Yell, 1998), education is affected by this law, particularly by Title II (Public Services) and Title III (Public Accommodations Operated by a Private Entity). Public schools are considered public entities and so are subject to provisions of Title II. Title III specifically includes places of education among its 12 categories of public accommodations owned by private entities; private schools are covered by this subchapter of ADA. Both discrimination on the basis of disability and "practices and structures that effectively discriminate against persons with disabilities" (Yell, 1998; p. 137) are prohibited by the ADA.

Impact of Section 504 and ADA on Educational
Assessment Practices

School practitioners must understand the legal requirements and prohibitions of Section 504 of the 1973 Rehabilitation Act and the Americans with Disabilities Act (1990). Whereas IDEA is program entitlement legislation that provides funding to states for programs for students with disabilities, Section 504 and the ADA are anti-discrimination legislation that prohibit discrimination based on disability. Section 504 goes beyond the reaches of IDEA by extending protection from discrimination to all institutions receiving federal monies, including employment settings and institutions of higher education. The ADA further extends antidiscrimination protections to public entities, including private schools. As discussed earlier, some public school students may be identified as persons with disabilities under Section 504 who would not qualify under IDEA. School personnel must be familiar with the definitions of disability and impairment under 504 to provide appropriate services to these students.

ISSUES IN ASSESSMENT OF STUDENTS FROM MINORITY BACKGROUNDS

General Ethical Guidelines for Working with Students from Minority Backgrounds

As indicated in data collected from the 1990 U.S. Census, this country is becoming increasingly multilingual, multicultural, and multiracial (Sue, Arredondo, & Davis, 1995). Statistics suggest that less than 20 years from now racial and ethnic minorities will represent the majority of individuals living in the United States. More importantly, schools are being impacted by the rapid diversification of this country, and professionals working in schools need to be prepared to respond to changing student populations and the various types of learning needs that arise.

Ethical guidelines provided by professional organizations such as NASP and APA have established standards by which professionals should develop awareness, knowledge, and skills for conducting assessments with students from ethnic and cultural minority backgrounds. The NASP Principles, the APA Ethical Standards, the Standards for the Provision of School Psychological Services (NASP, 1997), and the Guidelines for Providers of Psychological Services to Ethnic, Linguistic, and Culturally Diverse Populations (APA, 1993) are all documents that provide ethical guidelines and standards regarding assessment practices with students from minority backgrounds. Common to all of these documents is the mandate for school professionals to exhibit respect for individual differences and diversity, including physical, mental, emotional, political, economic, social, cultural, ethnic, and racial characteristics, gender and sexual orientation, religion, age, national origin, and native language (NASP, 1997; APA, 1992). Respect for differences includes recognition that ethnicity and culture have an impact on individuals' behavior, and school professionals should be aware of this when working with ethnic/racial groups (APA, 1993).

Ethical Guidelines and Nonbiased Assessment

School professionals are expected to be knowledgeable about the validity, reliability, standardization, outcome studies, and proper application of the assessment tools they use with students (NASP, 1997; APA, 1992). They select assessment tools that have current standardization data, are appropriate and beneficial to students, and provide information that helps to maximize educational achievement and success in the general school environment. At the same time, the students' cultural, ethnic, and linguistic background should be addressed in all assessment decisions (NASP, 1997). School professionals are also aware of potential limitations of using particular assessment instruments with certain populations. When interpreting the results obtained from assessments, school-based professionals must consider characteristics of the test and of the particular individual being assessed that may influence their interpretation of the results. They clearly communicate the reservations they may have about the data and/or their interpretation of it (APA, 1992). Further, specific recommendations for considering cultural and linguistic factors when conducting assessments can be found in Cummins (1984), Lopez (1995; 1997), Thomas-Presswood, Sasso, and Gin (1997), Serna (1998), and Valles (1998).

Test Bias

Legal and ethical guidelines for school-based professionals emphasize use of assessment practices that are nonbiased, valid, and reliable for the individuals and concerns being addressed (NASP, 1997; IDEA, 1997). Therefore, it is important to be aware of potential bias in the content, administration, interpretation, and use of assessments. Test bias and how it should be defined is an issue that has caused considerable debate for many years. Reynolds and Kaiser (1990) asserted that validity is central to the issue of test bias; these authors describe bias as affecting content, construct, and criterion validity.

Bias in Content Validity

Reynolds and Kaiser (1990) defined content bias as follows:

> An item or subscale of a test is considered to be biased in content when it is demonstrated to be relatively more difficult for members of one group than another when the general ability level of the groups being compared is held constant and no reasonable theoretical rationale exists to explain group differences on the item (or subscale) in question. (p. 498)

Reynolds (1995) also distinguished between *cultural loading* and *cultural bias*, defining cultural loading as "the degree of cultural specificity present in the test or the individual items within it" (p. 550). He stated that all tests possess some degree of cultural specificity, and cultural loading should be viewed as a continuum ranging from general to specific cultural specificity. This position is consistent with the idea that the more culturally specific the content of an item, the higher the probability that the item will be biased when used with individuals from different cultures.

Similarly, an item that is broadly culturally loaded may not necessarily be biased. Reynolds (1995) pointed out that basically all tests will contain some degree of cultural loading and this relates to the difficulties inherent in creating "culture-free" tests. Reynolds asserted that a test developed within a particular culture can only predict behavior within that cultural context, and the generalizability of that test to other cultures must be examined empirically.

Both empirical and qualitative strategies have been used to determine whether test items are culturally biased. Empirical procedures for assessing item bias include approaches such as examining group × item interactions produced through analysis of variance or by assessing the difficulty of items within groups and comparing item difficulties across groups. If certain items stand out as being exceptionally difficult for a particular group, then those items are considered to be possibly biased and may be extracted from the measure. Interestingly, however, studies have shown that withdrawal of potentially biased items and rescoring of tests has little impact on mean differences in scores obtained by different groups on tests that have already been standardized (Reynolds, 1995; Sandoval & Mille, 1979). In addition, group × item interactions account for only a fraction of variance. However, statistical methods should be used to assess item bias when a test is in the process of being developed and standardized (Reynolds, 1991).

Reynolds (1995) also discussed the practice of providing "armchair" inspection of test items to determine the presence of bias. In this approach, professionals in the area of testing and often members of different minority groups are asked to review test items to determine whether the content of particular items is biased. This is essentially the process that Judge Grady used in the case of *P.A.S.E v. Hannon* (1980), in which he examined every individual item on an intelligence test to determine whether it was biased (Bersoff & Hofer, 1990). Studies that have examined the reliability and accuracy of this approach in identifying biased items have shown that neither testing experts nor minority judges are able to detect biased items with high levels of accuracy (Sandoval & Mille, 1979). However, many individuals in the field believe that this "face validity" approach has value in obtaining the public's perceptions of what content is fair or unfair on a test. As discussed by Sandoval and Mille (1979), gaining support from individuals from different minority groups and others who inspect tests for bias helps to communicate to the general public that tests are generally nonbiased and fair. Reynolds (1995) recommended that this "subjective-judgment approach" be used only to supplement, rather than replace, empirical psychometric analyses.

Bias in Construct Validity

A test demonstrates a lack of bias in construct validity by measuring the same hypothetical traits for different groups consistently. Therefore, a test is considered biased if it measures different traits across different ethnic groups or varies in the accuracy with which it measures the same trait for different groups (Millsap & Everson, 1993). Factor analysis is a technique frequently used to examine construct validity. It is a statistical analysis that determines which items or subtests of a test cluster together, or are highly correlated with one another, and which items/subtests are not. Reynolds and Kaiser (1990) described the results of several studies that utilized one common approach to interpreting factor analysis results. Most often, studies assess factoral similarities and use techniques such as calculating coefficients of congruence between factor loadings of corresponding factors between two groups. For example, Reschly (1978) compared the factor structures of the WISC-R for four ethnic groups, (1) Caucasian, (2) Mexican American, (3) African American, and (4) Native American, by examining the congruence of the Verbal and Performance factors for each group. He obtained congruence coefficients of .97 to .99 for all comparisons between groups, which suggests nearly equivalent factor structures across groups. A variety of other methodologies have been used to investigate construct validity (e.g., internal consistency reliability estimates across groups) and, as summarized by Reynolds (1995), "No consistent evidence of bias in construct validity has been found with any of the many tests investigated. This leads to the conclusion that psychological tests, especially aptitude tests, function in essentially the same manner, test materials are perceived and reacted to in a similar manner, and that tests measure the same construct with equivalent accuracy for blacks, whites, Mexican-Americans, and other American minorities of both sexes and at all levels of SES" (p. 563).

Bias in Criterion/Predictive Validity

Bias in predictive validity can occur as the result of bias not only in the test (predictor) but also in the criterion measure (Reynolds & Kaiser, 1990). According to Reynolds and Kaiser (1990), a definition of predictive validity that has received wide acceptance by researchers and many psychologists is Cleary and colleagues' (1975) definition: "A test is considered biased with respect to predictive validity when the inference drawn from the test scores is not made with the smallest feasible random error or if there is constant error in an inference or prediction as a function of membership in a particular group" (p. 511). To evaluate for test bias using this definition, the relationship between a predictor and a criterion is plotted to form a regression line. If fairness in predictive validity exists, then the regression lines formed for each group demonstrating the relationship between the predictor and criterion should be identical. If the slope or intercept of the regression lines differ significantly when two or more groups are compared, then bias in prediction exists. Reynolds (1991, 1995) reviewed several studies that utilized a variety of statistical strategies with many different types of standardized tests to assess and compare their predictive validity across ethnic groups. The summary of this sizable pool of empirical research suggests that tests generally demonstrate fairness in prediction across groups. He found that bias rarely occurs in the use of instruments with adequate reliability and internal validity. Studies that have shown tests to predict differentially across groups consistently overpredict the performance of students from low socioeconomic and ethnic minority backgrounds, which reveals that predictive validity is less likely the culprit in the overrepresentation of minority students in educable mentally retarded special education classes (Reynolds, 1995).

Regardless of how bias may exist within these types of validity, many have held the view that tests are biased if mean differences are obtained between ethnic groups on cognitive tests (Reynolds, 1995). In an extensive discussion of this issue, Reynolds points out that "the overlap among the distributions of intelligence test scores for the different races is much greater than the degree of differences between the various groups" (Reynolds, 1995, p. 546). There continues to be much debate over this issue, however, and the reader can refer to Reynolds (1995) and Reynolds, Lowe, and Saenz (1999) for further information regarding test bias and mean differences across ethnic groups. In addition to this issue, some have questioned the role cultural factors may play in the statistical procedures themselves that are used to examine the presence of bias in tests. For example, Helms (1992) hypothesized that cultural borrowing may take place between ethnic groups, which reduces the cultural independence of groups and thereby possibly restricts the range of responses of different groups to particular test items.

Assessment of Minority Children and the Law

IDEA (1997) outlines specific assessment practices to ensure that assessments are not biased (see Table 14.3). IDEA also addresses the issue of disproportionate representation of minority students in special education programs. The law directs each state to collect data on the number of students representing different racial backgrounds who have been identified as having disabilities, their specific types of disabilities, and the educational placement of these students. If a disproportionate number of minority students is found to be identified as having disabilities (or being placed in a specific disability category), then the state must review and, if appropriate, revise its "policies, practices, and procedures" regarding the identification and placement of students so that they are in compliance with all requirements of this law (IDEA, 20 U.S.C.S. §1418[c], Lexis Law Pub., 1998).

Bias in Test Use

An important factor to consider when using tests to assess various behavioral, academic, and emotional issues with children is how the information from tests is used in making decisions regarding children's education. Messick stated that the "key issues of test validity are the meaning, relevance, and utility of scores, the import or value implications of scores as a basis for action, and the functional worth of scores in terms of the social consequences for their use" (1989, p. 5). Just as there has been significant controversy about the internal validity (i.e., content, construct validity) of tests and their usefulness in predicting future behavior and outcomes, there has also been major legal and ethical debate about the use of tests in educational planning for children from different ethnic groups.

A major outcome of *Larry P. v. Riles* (1972, 1974, 1979, 1984) was the attention it drew to the stigmatization that can occur with educational classification or labeling. Intelligence tests were used as the primary basis for placing African American students in educable mentally retarded (EMR) classes (de la Cruz, 1996; Reschly, Kicklighter, & McKee, 1988). Judge Peckham's description of the EMR classes as "dead-end" and "inferior" conveyed the belief that the educational services these African American children were receiving as a result of the IQ scores they obtained were not equivalent to those of students in other educational programs. Therefore, the ban he placed on the use of IQ tests for EMR placement decisions impacts the policies and procedures regarding use of assessments (de la Cruz, 1996).

Issues Related to the Misclassification of Students

As noted by numerous authors (e.g., Artiles & Trent, 1994; MacMillan & Reschly, 1998), there are many factors to consider when examining the possible causes and outcomes of the misclassification and overrepresentation of minority students in special education programs. In particular, the overclassification of minority students with mild mental retardation (MMR) has long been debated as a possible outcome signifying bias in the use of test results with minority student populations. Artiles and Trent (1994) cautioned that an analysis of data regarding the overrepresentation of minority students in particular special education programs is not as straightforward as comparing ethnic group enrollment in general versus special education programs. They highlight at least four factors that should be considered when examining overrepresentation data, which include (1) the proportion of minority population in a given region, (2) the size of an educational program, (3) the type of special education program, and (4) the specific ethnic group. MacMillan and Reschly (1998) also identified three primary issues related to the overrepresentation of minority students in special education programs, including (1) inconsistent methods for calculating overrepresentation data, (2) consideration of other factors that may contribute to the overrepresentation of minority students in special education, and (3) the question of whether overrepresentation of minority students in special education results in differential outcomes for these students.

MacMillan and Reschly (1998) examined the issue of various methods being used to calculate ratios of minority students in special education programs. Central to this issue is the fact that overrepresentation data cannot be compared across schools and districts if different ratios are computed to produce these estimates. Therefore, it is also problematic to make any attributions about why the overrepresentation of minority students exists. MacMillan and Reschly point to two different types of ratios that can be calculated regarding the percentages of minority students in special education. The first of these is the "percent of category or program by group" (1998, p. 2), which refers to the percentage of children in a disability category who are members of a particular ethnic group. For example, using this ratio the numerator would reflect the number of Hispanic children classified as having a learning disability and the denominator would reflect the total number of children classified as having a learning disability (MacMillan & Reschly, 1998). MacMillan and Reschly state that this ratio was used in litigation such as *Larry P.* (1984) and Marshall (1984, 1985). MacMillan and Reschly use the case of *Larry P.* to illustrate: In 1971, African Americans constituted 10% of California student enrollment but 25% of total enrollment in MMR programs.

A second calculation for estimating overrepresentation results in a "percent of group in category" (MacMillan & Reschly, 1998, p. 2), which assesses the percentage of minority students enrolled in special education programs. The numerator for this calculation is the same as that used in the formula presented above (i.e., number of minority children classified in particular special education program) but the denominator is different. The denominator for this calculation is the total number of children from a particular minority background in the district, state, or national school population (MacMillan & Reschly, 1998). Using the example of *Larry P.* again, MacMillan and Reschly computed that only 1.1% of all African American students in California were placed in MMR programs.

As one can see by comparing the representation estimates produced using these two different calculations (i.e., 25% vs. 1.1%), one could get a very different impression of the extent to which minority students are represented in particular special education programs in various schools and districts. Each type of estimate may be useful depending on the question being investigated; however, when describing representation estimates it is critical to identify how the data were derived to understand how to interpret findings.

A second related issue that MacMillan and Reschly (1998) discussed is the need to specify more clearly individuals' ethnicities when classifying students into special education categories. They argue that current methods for documenting students' ethnic backgrounds force many parents to identify their children as being from only one racial and/or ethnic group, when many children have a multiracial background.

Issues in Assessment of Students with Limited English Proficiency

"Limited English proficient" (LEP) refers to individuals who were not born in the United States and whose native language is other than English, or to students who come from environments in which a language other than English is dominant (U.S. Department of Education, 1994). Legal and ethical directives governing assessment of students with limited English proficiency are clear. Federal regulations governing implementation of IDEA specify that "tests and other evaluation materials used to assess a child with or suspected of being a child with a disability are provided and administered in the child's native language or other mode of communication, unless it is clearly not feasible to do so" (34 C.F.R. §300.532, 1999). These regulations further stipulate that "materials and procedures used to assess a child with limited English proficiency are selected and administered to ensure that they measure the extent to which the child has a disability and needs special education, rather than measuring the child's English language skills" (IDEA, 34 C.F.R. §300.532, 1999).

Ethical standards for assessment of students with LEP are also clear in documents such as APA's (1993) *Guidelines for Providers of Psychological Services to Ethnic, Linguistic, and Culturally Diverse Populations* and (1985) *Standards for Educational and Psychological Testing*, and professional ethical standards (e.g., NASP, 1997). However, the scarcity of professionals trained to assess students with LEP (e.g., Lopez, 1995) raises serious ethical issues for educators today. Cummins' (1984) distinction between basic interpersonal communicative skills (which may require two to three years to acquire) and cognitive academic language proficiency skills (which may take five to seven years to acquire) suggests that students with LEP may require and/or benefit from assessment in their primary language for a significant length of time. Educators may be faced with ethical dilemmas in which the student's need for evaluation and services is in conflict with the professional's limited competence to assess the student and the limited availability of qualified examiners.

One avenue professionals have used to address the limited availability of bilingual examiners is to employ interpreters in the assessment process. However, Lopez (1995) described this practice as "risky, speculative, and plagued with conjecture. They should therefore, be the absolute last resort" (p. 1119). Lopez noted several specific barriers to effective assessment that may arise with the use of interpreters, including errors in translation, lack of understanding of the testing process, reduced establishment of rapport, and difficulty caused by dialectical differences within languages.

PRIVACY AND INFORMED CONSENT FOR ASSESSMENT

Privacy

Siegel (1979) defined privacy as "the freedom of individuals to choose for themselves the time and the circumstances under which and the extent to which their beliefs, behavior, and opinions are to be shared or witheld from others" (p. 251). In schools, students' and parents' privacy rights are protected by federal statutes, such as the Protection of Pupil Rights Amendment (PPRA) or "Hatch Amendment," originally enacted in 1978 and amended in 1994; the Family Educational Rights and Privacy Act of 1974; and IDEA 1997. The implications of these statutes regarding assessment in schools are discussed in the following sections.

Federal statutes and case law extend protection of privacy rights to certain assessment activities in schools, but not to others. As part of their educational mission, schools are allowed to assess student progress and to monitor program effectiveness. Also, courts have upheld the rights of schools to determine their effectiveness through student minimum-competency testing or exit examinations (e.g., *Brookhart v. Illinois State Board of Education*, 1982, 1983; *Debra P. v. Turlington*, 1984). However, when assessment occurs because a student is suspected of having an educational disability, parental consent (or consent from a legal guardian) for assessment is required by law (IDEA, 1997; discussion follows).

Students' privacy rights are also protected by ethical codes. For example, the APA's Ethical Principles (1992) direct psychologists to include in written and oral reports and consultations "only information germane to the purpose for which the communication is made" to minimize intrusions on privacy (Ethical Standard 5.03).

Informed Consent

Some educational professionals are required by law and by ethical codes to obtain "informed consent" of the client (or parent/legal guardian if the client is a minor) prior to provision of services. Informed consent is generally considered to include three components (Bersoff, 1983; Bersoff & Hofer, 1990). The first component is knowledge; the person seeking consent is required to provide enough information, in an understandable manner, for the individual providing consent to make an informed decision. The second component is voluntariness; the individual must provide consent without being coerced or unduly influenced. The third component is capacity; the individual providing consent must be legally competent to give consent. In school settings, children are generally seen as incapable of giving consent for assessment; informed consent is sought from the student's parent or legal guardian. In addition to knowledge, voluntariness, and capacity, the American Psychological Association's 1992 Ethical Principles of Psychologists include appropriate documentation of informed consent as a critical component (Ethical Standard 4.02). (For a detailed discussion of informed consent, see Bersoff & Hofer, 1990.)

Child Competence and Consent

"In the main, the law considers children generally incapable of knowing what is best for themselves" (Bersoff, 1983, p. 165). Adults are considered competent unless adjudicated incompetent. However, children are generally considered legally incompetent, regardless of their actual competence (Weithorn, 1983). "A minor child is presumed incompetent for most purposes without any concern for whether he or she has the capacity to make the requisite decision in a practical sense" (Koocher & Keith-Spiegel, 1990, p. 12). However, as noted recently (e.g., DeKraai, Sales, & Hall, 1998; Sales, Krauss, Sacken, & Overcast, 1999) empirical research suggests that children have more competence than has been recognized historically by the legal system. In addition, there is evidence that children who participate in treatment decisions may improve their attitudes toward and outcomes from treatment (e.g., Taylor, Adelman, & Kaser-Boyd, 1985). Consequently, legal exceptions to the presumption of child incompetence have emerged, including those for mature minors and emancipated minors, and in the case of specific treatments, such as drug rehabilitation and pregnancy counseling (DeKraai, Sales, & Hall, 1998). Because most legal and ethical discussions of child consent and competence address issues related to *treatment* rather than *assessment* per se (e.g., Taylor & Adelman, 1989; Taylor, Adelman, & Kaser-Boyd, 1985), the issue of students' legal right to provide consent for assessment remains in question. In the case of *Merriken v. Cressman* (1973) the court had the opportunity to address the question of whether denying children the opportunity to provide informed consent for invasion of privacy was constitutional; however, the court declined to address this question, choosing instead to focus on the lack of informed consent provided by parents for invasion of their privacy rights (Bersoff, 1983).

Child consent for assessment is not required by laws specifically mandating informed consent (e.g., IDEA, 1997). As Fleming and Fleming (1987) observed, "although many children have a relatively high amount of first-hand knowledge about the impact of various special educational options, their rights to participate in relevant decision-making are practically nonexistent" (p. 390). IDEA does require, however, that "whenever appropriate, the child with a disability" shall be included as a member of the IEP team (IDEA, 20 U.S.C.S. §1414[d][1][B], Lexis Law Pub., 1998). In addition, some ethical codes specifically address the importance of informing students of the parameters of services and gaining their voluntary participation. For example, the NASP Principles for Professional Ethics (1997) state "When another party initiates services, the school psychologist will make every effort to secure voluntary participation of the child/student" (Principle III.B.3). In addition, the NASP Principles require that "school psychologists explain important aspects of their professional relationships with students and clients in a clear understandable manner. The explanation includes the reason why services were requested, who will receive information about the services, and the possible outcomes" (Principle III. B2). Weithorn (1983) suggested that "professionals who work with children involve their clients, subjects, and patients in decisions regarding their own welfare to the maximum extent possible given the minor's own desire for involvement, the minor's capacity for meaningful participation, and the legal standards regarding consent requirements" (p. 257). These ethical directives can raise dilemmas for professionals. For example, behavioral assessment employing observation in the classroom may be most effective if unobtrusive to reduce the target student's reactivity (e.g., Kratochwill et al., 1999). Yet the observer may perceive an ethical need to inform the student of the on-going assessment.

Informed Consent and the Law

IDEA requires that "informed consent from the parent" be obtained prior to initial evaluation of a student suspected of having a disability (IDEA, 20 U.S.C.S. §1414[a][1][C], Lexis Law Pub., 1998). If a parent refuses consent for the evaluation, IDEA permits the local education agency to continue to pursue evaluation by utilizing mediation and due process procedures specified in the law (IDEA, 20 U.S.C.S. §1414[a][1][C], Lexis Law Pub., 1998).

Parental consent prior to *reevaluation* of a student determined to have a disability is also required by IDEA 1997 (IDEA, 20 U.S.C.S. §1414[c][3], Lexis Law Pub., 1998). (Prior to the 1997 amendments to IDEA, only parental *notice* of reevaluations was required.) In the case of reevaluations, informed parental consent is required except when the LEA "can demonstrate that it had taken reasonable measures to obtain such consent and the child's parent has failed to respond" (IDEA, 20 U.S.C.S. §1414[c][3], Lexis Law Pub., 1998).

Assessments administered to entire groups of students (such as standardized school-wide achievement measures) are not considered individualized assessments that must comply with IDEA provisions for nondiscriminatory assessment and parental consent if these assessment results are not used to evaluate or reevaluate a child for special education eligibility or services (*Rettig v. Kent City School District*, 1980; Turnbull & Turnbull, 1998). Yell (1998) noted that pre-referral assessments, typically based on assessments such as classroom tests, daily observations, and interviews, "are not subject to the strictures of the IDEA" (p. 226). However, some schools and districts choose to obtain parental consent prior to pre-referral assessment.

Informed Consent and Ethical Codes

Some professional ethical codes require practitioners to obtain parental informed consent prior to providing services. For example, the American Psychological Association's Ethical Principles of Psychologists (1992) require psychologists to obtain informed consent for therapy or "related procedures" (EP 4.02). The National Association of School Psychologists' Principles for Professional Ethics (1997) do not use the term "informed consent" or even "consent" in addressing the ethics of school service provision. (However, "informed consent" is discussed relative to record release; see following section.) This may be because there are circumstances in which assessment of a minor may be legal and required of a professional without parental consent (e.g., in a case in which parental consent for reevaluation was sought but the parent failed to respond [IDEA 1997]). However, the NASP Principles for Professional Ethics are clear in emphasizing the importance of providing information for parents (and students) about services in advance: "parents and students are to be fully informed about all relevant aspects of school psychological services in advance. The explanation should take into account language and cultural differences, cognitive capabilities, developmental level, and age so that the explanation may be understood by the student, parent, or guardian" (Principle III.A.4). Further, the NASP principles stress the importance of parental involvement at all levels of service provision. Principle III.C.2 states: "School psychologists recognize the importance of parental support and seek to obtain this by assuring that there is direct parent contact prior to seeing the student/client on an on-going basis." Principle III.C.3 continues this theme in saying, "School Psychologists encourage and promote parental participation in designing services provided to their children. When appropriate, this includes linking interventions between the school and the home, tailoring parental involvement to the skills of the family, and helping parents to gain the skills needed to help their children."

CONFIDENTIALITY AND EDUCATIONAL RECORDS

The confidentiality of student communications and records is protected by law and ethical codes. As Turnbull and Turnbull (1998) observed, "Clearly, access to records and confidentiality of records are two different, but related, ways to hold the schools accountable" (p. 231). Parents must have access to school records to be informed about school practices, and because of the large amount of student and family information that may appear in records, these records must be kept confidential to protect student and family privacy.

Confidentiality and Privileged Communication

Confidentiality is a concept rooted originally in professional ethics (Keith-Speigel & Koocher, 1985). Discussing confidentiality, Taylor and Adelman (1989) stated, "Confidentiality is an ethical concern. The fundamental intent is to protect a client's right to privacy by ensuring that matters disclosed to a professional will not be relayed to others without the informed consent of the client" (pp. 79–80). Ethical codes guiding school practitioners, such as those of the APA (1992), the NASP (1997), and the ASCA (1992), address the importance of respecting client confidentiality.

Privileged communication, in contrast to confidentiality, is "a legal term that describes the quality of certain specific types of relationships that prevent information, acquired in such relationships, from being disclosed in court or other legal proceedings" (Keith-Spiegel & Koocher, 1990, p. 58). Privilege belongs to the client; it cannot be invoked by the professional if the client wants confidential information released. As Haas and Malouf (1995) noted, privilege is a "legally guaranteed right of the consumer, whereas confidentiality is an ethical obligation of the service provider" (pp. 35–36).

Some states protect the confidentiality of information shared with specific school personnel and extend the right to privileged communication to school personnel, including counselors, social workers, and psychologists (Fischer & Sorenson, 1996). However, laws regarding confidentiality and privilege vary considerably across states; school professionals must become familiar with the laws of their states to determine whether they are granted privileged communication rights and whether their communications with students are considered confidential (e.g., Haas & Malouf, 1993; Jacob-Timm & Hartshorne, 1998).

The confidentiality of information shared by students, even when protected by law, is not absolute. Law and ethical codes consistently delineate several circumstances in which professionals generally are expected to release confidential information. These instances include:

1. *Cases of suspected child abuse or neglect.* Discussing confidentiality, Boomer, Hartshorne, and Robertshaw (1995) stated, "The law on confidentiality is clear only in very narrow, factual situations such as statutes that prescribe reporting of information on child abuse and neglect" (p. 20). All states require school officials to report suspected child abuse; professionals must be familiar with the laws of their states regarding mandated reporting (Haas & Malouf, 1995; Sales et al., 1999).

2. *Cases in which the student or another individual might be harmed.* Subsequent to the Tarasoff rulings (*Tarasoff v. Regents of University of California*, 1974/

1976), some states have established dangerous person reporting requirements or duty to protect requirements for mental health providers (DeKraai, Sales, & Hall, 1998). In the Tarasoff case the California Supreme Court ruled that a therapist has a duty to take reasonable action to protect a potential victim when the therapist knows—or should reasonably know—that a client poses a threat to a potential victim. (For further discussion of the implications of the Tarasoff decisions and duty to protect laws see DeKraai et al., 1998). In addition to their need to consider a duty to protect potential third-party victims, school personnel also must consider their overarching duty to safeguard the welfare of students within the school. At times this may require release of confidential information without student consent. For example, in a case in which a student committed suicide following disclosure of such intent to school personnel, the Maryland Supreme Court ruling affirmed the duty of school personnel to protect pupils from harm (*Eisel v. Board of Education*, 1991). Such rulings have been interpreted to suggest that school personnel must inform parents of the child's threat to commit suicide (see McCarthy & Sorenson, 1993, for further discussion). This reasoning is consistent with ethical principles that emphasize the responsibility of school professionals to protect the welfare of students (e.g., NASP's Principle III.A.1: "School psychologists are committed to the application of their professional expertise for the purpose of promoting improvements in the quality of life for students, their families, and the school community").

3. *Cases in which the practitioner is obligated to testify in a court of law.* Fischer and Sorenson (1996) identified circumstances in which a practitioner might be compelled to release confidential information. These include cases in which a defendant seeks access to confidential communications to present a complete defense and cases in which confidential communications may help the court determine what is in the best interests of a child.

4. *Cases of malpractice filed against the professional.* Professionals are allowed to reveal confidential information in self-defense (Koocher & Keith-Spiegel, 1990).

Ethical standards (e.g., APA, 1992; ASCA, 1992; NASP, 1997) enjoin professionals to define the limits of confidentiality "at the outset of the relationship and thereafter as new circumstances may warrant" (APA Ethical Standard 5.01). The need to release confidential information is often thought to arise in counseling relationships, but this need may also arise in the course of school assessment. For example, during the course of assessment, a school professional could observe injuries or behavior that would raise suspicion regarding child abuse. The APA Ethical Principles make specific reference to minor clients, requiring psychologists to define the limits of confidentiality and the foreseeable uses of information obtained throughout their services with persons "including to the extent feasible minors and their legal representatives" (APA Ethical Standard 5.01).

"In summary, it is simply not clear how much confidentiality a student may expect in dealings with school personnel. It depends on the nature of the communication, to whom the communication is directed, and the particular status of state law" (Sales et al., 1998, p. 1135).

EDUCATIONAL RECORD KEEPING

There are numerous laws and ethical guidelines regarding the acquisition, storage, and release of student records related to assessment. Three major pieces of legislation significantly shape school practices concerning assessment records: the Family Educational Rights and Privacy Act of 1974 (FERPA), the Grassley Amendment to the Goals 2000: Educate America Act (1994), and the Individuals with Disabilities Education Act (1997).

Family Educational Rights and Privacy Act of 1974 (FERPA)

In 1974 Congress enacted FERPA (also called the Buckley Amendment, because it was introduced by Senator James Buckley of New York), an amendment to legislation extending the Elementary and Secondary Education Act of 1965. The law was proposed as a response to complaints from parents about inaccuracy and inaccessibility of school records (Prasse, 1995). The purpose of FERPA is "to guarantee parental access to student records as well as to prohibit access to those records by persons without legitimate reasons to know their contents" (Yell, 1996; p. 44). FERPA and its federal regulations provide detailed, complex guidelines regarding the confidentiality of student records and the rights of students and parents regarding those records. The main provisions of FERPA are outlined in Table 14.5.

   FERPA contains two major provisions: First, it authorizes withdrawal of federal funding from an educational agency or institution that denies or prevents parents from exercising their right to inspect and review the educational records of their children. Second, FERPA authorizes withdrawal of federal funds from schools that permit the release of educational records of students without the written consent of their parents. FERPA's definition of "parent" includes a "natural parent, a guardian, or an individual acting as a parent in the absence of a parent or a guardian" (34 C.F.R. § 99.3). FERPA allows release of educational records without parental consent in specific circumstances, including to other school officials who have been determined to have a legitimate educational interest (FERPA; 20 U.S.C. § 1232). (See Table 14.5 for further exemptions.) The rights to review educational records and consent to their release generally transfer to the student at the age of 18 or upon attendance at a postsecondary institution, at which time the student becomes an "eligible student" under FERPA (34 C.F.R. § 99.3).

   The FERPA definition of educational records is broad, applying to all records, files, documents, and other materials that contain personally identifiable information about a student that are maintained by the educational agency or by a person acting for that agency. Boomer and colleagues (1995), discussing the definition of educational records in FERPA, noted, "essentially any information becomes an educational record when it is communicated to others for educational purposes" (p. 19). FERPA exempts from its definition records kept by a law enforcement unit of a school district created only for the purpose of law enforcement and job-related records of students employed by the school (34 C.F.R. § 99.3). Also exempted from the definition of educational records are those records that are in the "sole possession" of the maker

TABLE 14.5 Main Provisions of the Family Educational Rights and Privacy Act (FERPA, 1974)

<hr>

Educational records

Include: Records directly related to a student containing personally identifiable information and maintained by an educational agency. Includes information recorded in any way, including but not limited to handwriting, print, tape, film, microfilm, and microfische.

Exclude: Records of school personnel kept in the sole possession of the maker and not revealed to others except as a substitute; records of school-based law enforcement units maintained for law enforcement; records of employees (but records of students employed as a result of student status are not exempt); records of eligible students made by a physician, psychiatrist, psychologist, or related professional working in a treatment capacity (unless related to remedial educational activities or instruction).

Rights

Parents and eligible students have the right to:

See and inspect educational records. School personnel must explain and interpret records to parents if parents so request. Parents may obtain copies of records if not procuring copies effectively prevents parents from reviewing records.

Request that the school amend records the parent believes are inaccurate or misleading.

Responsibilities

School officials must:

Establish written policies regarding student records.

Inform parents of current students annually of their rights under FERPA.

Establish procedures for complaints and destruction of records.

Comply with parental requests to inspect educational records "in a reasonable time frame" (no longer than 45 days after request).

Obtain written parental consent to disclose personally identifiable information from the educational record of a student with the following exceptions:
  • School personnel with legitimate educational interests
  • Officials representing schools to which the student has applied
  • Persons responsible for determining eligibility for financial aid
  • Judicial orders for release
  • In emergency situations to protect the health and safety of the student.

Destroy records when no longer needed.

Directory information

School personnel may release "directory information" (to be determined by the school) if it has given public notice to parents of students and eligible students of the types of information designated as "directory information" and the period of time within which the parent or eligible student must notify in writing that they do not want such information released.

<hr>

and are not revealed to any other individual except as a substitute for the maker. The law does not grant eligible students the right to see records of a physician, psychologist, or other recognized professional used only in connection with their treatment.

Under FERPA, parents are entitled to inspect and review a child's educational records, challenge the accuracy of student records (including a right to a hearing if the school refuses to amend records; if as a result of the hearing the district decides the records are accurate, the parent or eligible student may place comments in the record), and obtain copies of educational records "where failure of the agency or institution to provide the copies would effectively prevent a parent or eligible student from exercising the right to inspect and review the education records" (34 C.F.R. § 99.11). School personnel must explain and interpret educational records to parents if parents so request.

There is a vast amount of information collected about students today and "the technological explosion of the 1980s and 1990s has dramatically changed the manner in which we collect, disseminate and store information. For this reason, FERPA is even more significant today than it was when first introduced on the floor of Congress in 1974" (Fry, 1997, p. 44). However, several questions raised by FERPA still have not been definitively answered. One important question related to assessment involves whether raw test data (specifically, test protocols and responses) are subject to parental inspection. In a 1987 Illinois appellate court decision (*John K. and Mary K. v. Board of Education for School District 65*) the court ruled that test protocols (in this case, verbatim responses to the Rorschach Inkblot test) fall under the FERPA definition of educational records and may be inspected by parents if so requested. "The court was not persuaded either by professional standards or by federal regulations that the psychologist cited in support of nondisclosure" (Prasse, 1995, p. 49). However, as Prasse (1995) and others have noted, parental access to test protocols does not necessarily mean obtaining copies of protocols, which are often copyrighted materials. School professionals attempting to comply with FERPA and with ethical guidelines regarding test security (e.g., APA's Ethical Standard 2.10) may experience conflict. Jacob-Timm and Hartshorne (1998) recommended that practitioners establish collaborative relationships with families early in their work together, explain parents' rights and issues of test security, and provide parents with sufficient information about assessment results to avoid ethical conflicts.

The effects of the FERPA provisions have been far reaching. Because of this and subsequent legislation (e.g., IDEA, 1997), teachers are prohibited from publically posting students' grades and even engaging in "lounge talk" about students in which students are personally identified and private information is divulged (Yell, 1996). (For further discussion of FERPA, see Fischer, Schimmel, & Kelly, 1995; Jacob-Timm & Hartshorne, 1998; Yell, 1998.)

IDEA

IDEA (1997) affirms for students with disabilities the same rights guaranteed by FERPA (1974); the provisions of both laws apply to students with disabilities. Beyond the protections provided by FERPA, IDEA provides additional protections to students with disabilities by requiring educational agencies to permit a representative of parents to inspect the student's education record, to appoint a qualified person at each school to protect the confidentiality of all personally identifiable educational records, to inform parents when information is no longer needed to provide education services, and to destroy records at the request of parents (NFES, 1997; Yell, 1998).

Goals 2000: Educate America Act (1994)

In March, 1994, Congress passed the Goals 2000: Educate America Act. This act includes the Grassley Amendment, which replaced and modified the Hatch Amendment (or Protection of Pupil Rights Amendment, 1978). This statute prohibits schools receiving U.S. Department of Education funding from requiring students to submit to surveys, analysis or evaluation revealing:

1. Political affiliations;
2. Mental and psychological problems potentially embarrassing to the student or family;
3. Sex behavior and attitudes;
4. Illegal, antisocial, self-incriminating, and demeaning behavior;
5. Critical appraisals of other individuals with whom the students have close family relationships;
6. Legally recognized privileged or analogous relationships, such as those of physicians, lawyers, or ministers; or
7. Income, except for information required to determine eligibility for financial assistance. (20 U. S.C. § 1232 h)

The Amendment mandates that written consent of parents or eligible students must be obtained prior to requiring students to reveal such information; it also provides parents, guardians, or eligible students the right to inspect certain materials used in schools. All instructional materials, including teachers' manuals, films, tapes, or other materials used in connection with any survey, analysis, or evaluation must be made available for inspection by parents, guardians, or eligible students. The 1994 revision expanded coverage to include all survey, analysis, or evaluation projects; prior to 1994 only research programs targeting development of new teaching methods were addressed (Yeager, 1994).

Ethical Considerations in Record Keeping

Ethical standards of school practitioners also mandate protection of educational records. Educational records are addressed in ethical provisions regarding confidential communications and in specific references to record keeping. For example, specifically addressing record keeping the NASP Principles state, "School psychologists comply with all laws, regulations, and policies pertaining to the adequate storage and disposal of records to maintain appropriate confidentiality of information" (Principle IV.E.5).

Maintaining the confidentiality of electronically stored and transmitted records is critical. In recognition of the frequency of electronic storage and transmission of records and the inherent threats to confidentiality therein, the NASP Principles state, "To ensure confidentiality, student/client records are not transmitted electronically without a guarantee of privacy. (For example, a receiving FAX machine must be in a secure location and operated by employees cleared to work with confidential files; e-mail messages must be encrypted or else stripped of all information that identifies the student/client)" (Principle IV.C.8).

Subpoenas and Court Orders to Provide Information

Education practitioners, particularly school psychologists, may face an ethical dilemma in situations in which they receive a subpoena to produce a student's education records without the parent's consent or they are asked to provide raw psychological data, including test responses, test scores, test protocols, or test manuals to non-experts. As Tranel (1994) noted, "At the center of the problem is the fact that there is a direct conflict between law and ethics where it comes to the release of raw psychological data. The law says one thing ('Provide the data'); the ethics code says the opposite ('Do not provide the data')" (p. 34). The APA's (1992) Ethical Standard 2.02(b) states, "Psychologists refrain from misuse of assessment techniques, intervention results and interpretations and take reasonable steps to prevent others from misusing the information these techniques provide. This includes refraining from releasing raw test results or raw data to persons, other than to patients or clients as appropriate, who are not qualified to use such information." Release of raw or standardized scores and test responses to nonexperts could lead to misuse of information; release of test protocols or test manuals could violate copyright laws and test security, which psychologists are ethically bound to uphold (e.g., APA's Ethical Standard 2.10).

Because of the numerous queries received by the APA about this issue, the Committee on Legal Issues of the APA (1996) summarized the issues involved and outlined potential courses of action for professionals. The Committee defined relevant terms, including *subpoenas* (legal commands to appear to provide testimony), *subpoenas duces tecum* (legal commands to appear and bring along specific documents) and *court orders* (to provide testimony or produce documents). The Committee noted that "a subpoena requesting testimony or documents, even if not signed by a judge, requires a timely response, but it may be modified or quashed (i.e., made void or invalid). However, once a court order for testimony or documents is issued and any attempt (made in a timely manner) to have the court vacate or modify its order has been unsuccessful, a psychologist may be held in contempt of court if he or she fails to comply" (p. 245).

Tranel (1994) and the APA Committee on Legal Issues (1996) suggested similar strategies for reacting to subpoenas and court orders which place the professional in an ethical dilemma, including:

1. Determine whether the request for information carries the force of law. For example, determine whether the court issuing the subpoena has jurisdiction over the practitioner.
2. Contact the client. Discuss the implications of the demand with the client.
3. Negotiate with the requester. If the client has not agreed to release of the information, contact the legal counsel for the requesting party and discuss concerns regarding release.
4. Seek guidance from the court. Explain the ethical dilemma.
5. Consult the client's attorney. File a motion to quash the subpoena.
6. Consult your own or the school district's legal counsel.

TECHNICAL ADEQUACY OF ASSESSMENTS

Ethical principles and legal guidelines specifically address the need for professionals conducting assessments in schools to be aware of and understand the technical properties of assessment tools. For example, the APA's Ethical Principles (1992) state that "Psychologists who develop, administer, score, interpret, or use psychological assessment techniques, interviews, tests, or instruments do so in a manner and for purposes that are appropriate in light of the research on or evidence of the usefulness and proper application of the techniques" (Ethical Standard 2.02 [a]). These Principles state further that "Psychologists who perform interventions or administer, score, interpret, or use assessment techniques are familiar with the reliability, validation, and related standardization or outcome studies of, and proper applications and uses of, the techniques they use" (Ethical Standard 2.04[a]). These and similar ethical guidelines direct professionals to understand concepts such as reliability, validity, and standardization, concepts that in some cases (and particularly in the case of validity) are evolving in meaning and application (e.g., Anastasi, 1988; Geisinger, 1992; Messick, 1995).

Reliability

Reliability can be considered " the degree to which test scores are free from errors of measurement" (APA,1985, p. 19). Measures of reliability allow us to estimate what proportion of the total variance in two sets of test scores is attributable to measurement error versus true variance in the target characteristic or behavior (Anastasi, 1988). All tests scores contain some measurement error; however, what is considered error variance in scores versus what is considered true variance can differ across assessments. For example, if we are measuring behavior we expect to be consistent across settings, such as hearing, variance in performance across settings would be considered error variance. But if we are measuring behavior we expect might be influenced by settings, such as attention to task, variance in performance would be considered true variance related to the purpose of measurement.

Multiple forms of reliability have been identified to provide evidence of test consistency, including test–retest, alternate form, split-half, internal consistency, and interrater reliabilities (e.g., Anastasi, 1988; Cone, 1981). Educational professionals must understand what type(s) of reliability are critical for the particular assessment they are using; in addition, they must be able to interpret reliability data provided by test publishers and/or gather relevant reliability data themselves (such as interrater reliability of classroom observations).

Validity

The Standards for Educational and Psychological Testing (APA, 1985) describe validity as "the most important consideration in test evaluation. The concept refers to the appropriateness, meaningfulness, and usefulness of the specific inferences made from test scores" (p. 9). Defining validity, Messick (1995) noted:

> Validity is not a property of the test or assessment as such, but rather of the meaning of the test scores. In particular, what needs to be valid is the meaning or interpretation of the score, as well as any implication for action that this meaning entails (Cronbach, 1971) . . . The principles of validity apply not just to interpretive and action inferences derived from test scores as ordinarily conceived, but also to inferences based on any means of observing or documenting consistent behaviors or attributes. Thus, the term *score* is used generically in its broadest sense to mean any coding or summarization of observed consistencies or performance regularities on a test, questionnaire, observation procedure, or other assessment devices such as work samples, portfolios, and realistic problem simulations. (p. 741)

Test validity has been identified in statutory and case law as a fundamental component of appropriate assessment (e.g., IDEA, 1997; *Larry P. v. Riles*, 1972, 1979, 1984, 1986; *P.A.S.E. v. Joseph P. Hannon*, 1980). The concept of validity has traditionally been divided into three categories: (1) content-related, (2) criterion-related, and (3) construct-related validity (e.g., APA, 1985). Examining the uses of validity evidence, Foster and Cone (1995) summarized six validity judgments that can be made regarding tests: (1) face validity—whether the test looks appropriate for a particular use; (2) content validity—whether the test is made up of stimuli calling for construct-relevant responses; (3) criterion-related validity—whether responses to the test stimuli relate to other types of responses, either concurrently available or to be available sometime in the future; (4) construct validity—whether relationships entered into by scores on the test are consistent with theory; (5) treatment validity (Hayes, Nelson, & Jarrett, 1987)—whether predictions based on test scores add incremental value in decision-making in intervention planning; and (6) consequential validity (Messick, 1994)—whether the measure fulfills its intended purposes and is consistent with other social values. According to Foster and Cone, assessment of validity should vary across measures and should depend on what is being measured (construct, behavior, or response class) and why (purpose of assessment). These authors distinguished between *representational* validity—evidence that the measure assesses what it claims to measure, and *elaborative* validity—"the theoretical or applied utility of the measure . . . whether it can be used to understand, predict control or monitor changes in other phenomena" (p. 250). As they noted, "no single, easily specified litmus test of validity exists. Thus, assessors should articulate what they wish to assess and for what purposes, and then evaluate their instruments in light of those requirements" (p. 258).

Messick (1995) described a unified concept of validity in which six aspects of validity—(1) content,(2) substantive, (3) structural, (4) generalizability, (5) external, and (6) consequential—are subsumed within a comprehensive theory of construct validity. In this framework, two major threats to construct validity include construct underrepresentation (in which the assessment is too narrow and does not include critical aspects of the construct being measured) and construct-irrelevant variance (in which the assessment is too broad and results include excess reliable variance attributable to other constructs or sources).

In Messick's framework of construct validity, test interpretation and use are evaluated on both an evidential basis (including both general evidence supportive of score meaning and specific evidence for the relevance of scores applied to a specific purpose and setting) and consequential basis (including both the value implications of a test and the social consequences of test use). Messick (1988, 1995) defined the consequential aspect of validity as both the value implications of score meaning and the social consequences (intended and unintended) of test use. According to Messick, "validity judgments *are* value judgments" (1995, p. 748).

Discussing the social consequences of test use, Messick (1995) noted:

> What matters is not only whether the social consequences of test interpretation and use are positive or negative, but how the consequences came about and what determined them. In particular, it is not that adverse social consequences of test use render the use invalid but, rather, that adverse social consequences should not be attributable to any source of test invalidity. . . . (p. 748)

Educators and lawmakers alike recognize the potential life-long impact of educational placement and programming for children. Recent laws (e.g., IDEA, 1997), professional ethical principles, and professional standards (e.g., APA, 1985) direct practitioners conducting assessments and using assessment data to evaluate validity of assessment tools broadly—not only whether a tool appears to measure the construct in question or whether it does so as well as other measures—but also the potential use of interpretations based on assessment data. This focus on the consequential validity of assessments has raised the standards by which education professionals evaluate their tools. Summarizing the evolution of the concept of test validation, Geisinger (1992) stated, "The notion of validation has changed from test validity— with emphasis on the test itself—to the validation of a test for a specific use with a specific population in a given setting, and finally to providing evidence to support particular inferences based on test scores" (p. 217).

Treatment Utility of Assessment

Revisions to IDEA in 1997 have increased the emphasis in the law on the link between assessment and intervention. The focus of IDEA is no longer accessibility of appropriate educational services, but the quality of educational interventions (Turnbull & Turnbull, 1998). The purposes of the law are clearly stated, including "to ensure that all children with disabilities have available to them a free appropriate public education that emphasizes special education and related services designed to meet their unique needs and prepare them for employment and independent living" and "to assess, *and ensure the effectiveness of*, efforts to educate children with disabilities" (IDEA, 20 U.S.C.S. §1400[d], Lexis Law Pub., 1998, emphasis added).

The concept of treatment utility of assessment was originally defined by Hayes, Nelson, and Jarrett (1987) as "the degree to which assessment is shown to contribute to beneficial treatment outcome. An assessment device, distinction, or strategy has this kind of utility if it can be shown that treatment outcome is positively influenced by this device, distinction, or strategy" (pp. 963–964). Several provisions within IDEA direct that assessment tools and data be linked and that assessments demonstrate treatment utility. First, and most clearly, describing the conduct of evaluations, IDEA directs LEAs to ensure that "assessment tools and strategies that provide relevant information that directly assists persons in determining the educational needs of the child are provided" (IDEA, 20 U.S.C.S. § 1414[b][3], Lexis Law Pub., 1998).

Second, describing additional requirements of evaluations and reevaluations, IDEA directs the IEP team to identify the information needed to answer multiple questions, including:

- Whether the child has a category of disability;
- Present levels of performance and the educational needs of the child;
- Whether the child needs (or continues to need) special education and related services;
- Whether any additions or modifications to the special education and related services are needed to enable the child to meet the measurable annual goals established in the IEP and to participate in the general curriculum. (IDEA, 20 U.S.C.S. § 1414[c][1][B], Lexis Law Pub., 1998)

The last provision directly links assessment data to annual goals established for the child in the IEP. These mandates influence the type of assessment information that will be collected in schools; assessment data need to be useful for multiple purposes (identification, intervention planning, and progress monitoring), and educational practitioners need to evaluate the appropriateness of measures to accomplish diverse goals. IDEA (and some ethical principles) specifies that no one assessment tool be used for special education classification decisions (see Table 14.3).

Numerous authors have argued that tools often used in special education decision making (in particular, intelligence tests) have limited treatment utility (e.g., Gresham & Witt, 1997; MacMillan, Gresham, Siperstein, & Bocian, 1996; Reschly, 1996; Reschly and Ysseldyke, 1995). These authors argue for selecting assessment tools that will contribute valuable information to intervention planning and monitoring. Elliott and Fuchs (1997) asserted that measures with high treatment validity or utility should be used not only in intervention planning, but also in eligibility determination. These authors outlined three technical requirements an assessment tool must demonstrate to contribute sound data to special education eligibility decision making: (1) it must be capable of modeling learning; (2) it must be capable of informing instructional planning; and (3) it must be capable of documenting treatment effects.

ASSESSMENT ACCOMMODATIONS

In special and general education there is a trend toward greater accountability for services delivered (e.g., Graden, Casey & Bonstrom, 1985; Thurlow, Ysseldyke, & Silverstein, 1995). Like many other organizations today, schools are being asked to provide evidence of effectiveness. No longer is *access* to public education the primary concern; evidence of accountability now requires *outcome data* that document student gains (e.g., Illback, Zins & Maher, 1999; Salvia & Ysseldyke, 1995; Turnbull & Turnbull, 1998). These data may be acquired through classroom assessments; increasingly they are gathered through school- and districtwide assessments.

Most states and many school districts administer assessments designed to provide information about the achievement of students. According to Thurlow, Seyfarth, Scott, and Ysseldyke (1997), in 1996 48 states either had statewide testing programs in place or were developing them. However, states, districts within states, and even schools within districts vary in the degree to which students with handicapping conditions identified in IDEA are included in these assessments. As Thurlow, Elliott, and Ysseldyke (1998) observed, "It is important also to realize that education has been woefully negligent in promoting accountability for *all* students" (p. 12). Thurlow and colleagues (1998) estimated that in those states with regular accountability systems, most include less than half of their students with disabilities in state assessments.

IDEA 1997 now requires that "Children with disabilities are included in general State and district-wide assessment programs, with appropriate accommodations, where necessary" (IDEA, 20 U.S.C.S. §1412[a][17], Lexis Law Pub., 1998). In addition, the law mandates that each state (1) develop guidelines for the participation of children with disabilities in alternate assessments for those children who cannot participate in regular assessment programs; (2) conduct such alternate assessments beginning no later than July 1, 2000; (3) report the number of children with disabilities participating in regular and alternate assessments; (4) report the results of assessments of students with disabilities if so doing is statistically sound and would not result in disclosure of results identifiable to individuals (IDEA, 20 U.S.C.S. §1412[a][17], Lexis Law Pub., 1998). Finally, IDEA also requires that if the IEP Team determines that a student with a disability will not participate in a state or district-wide assessment, the IEP Team will include in the IEP a statement of why the assessment is not appropriate for the student and how the child will be assessed (IDEA, 20 U.S.C.S. §1414[d][1][A], Lexis Law Pub., 1998).

Thurlow and colleagues (1998) identified five reasons (in addition to legal directives) to include students with disabilities in state and district-wide assessment: (1) Inclusion of students with disabilities provides us with a more accurate picture of the outcomes of education; (2) For students with disabilities to benefit from school reform efforts we need to accrue outcome data regarding their performance; (3) We need information from comparable populations across states to make fair and accurate comparisons; (4) Exclusion of students with disabilities from such assessments can produce unintended consequences; and (5) Inclusion of students with disabilities in assessments promotes high expectations for all students.

A key concept in the requirements of IDEA regarding student participation in state or district-wide assessments is the requirement that such participation occur with appropriate accommodations where necessary. It is important to note that not all students with disabilities will need accommodations to participate, and not all students will be able to participate, even with accommodations. But the law directs states and districts to provide appropriate accommodations where necessary. Thurlow and colleagues (1998) defined accommodations as "changes in testing materials or procedures that enable the student with disabilities to participate in an assessment in a way that allows abilities to be assessed rather than disabilities" (pp. 27–28). Accommodations may include adaptations in setting, timing, scheduling, presentation, student response or other factors (Thurlow et al., 1998). Thurlow and colleagues (1997) reported that testing accommodations have become very common, with nearly every state having a policy offering some accommodations. These authors further reported that the most commonly offered accommodations include Braille or large-print editions of tests, the use of a proctor or scribe, extended time, and allowing for individual or small group administration of assessments. Controversial accommodations (i.e., those offered by some states and prohibited by others) include reading a test aloud and use of calculators.

Uncertainty regarding the application of testing accommodations stems from the lack of specific legal guidelines about which students need accommodations and which accommodations are acceptable (e.g., Phillips, 1994; Thurlow et al.,1998). Primary among concerns regarding testing accommodations is the question of whether scores from measures taken with and without accommodations are comparable (e.g., Phillips, 1994). As Phillips (1994) noted, "When judging the appropriateness of a particular accommodation, measurement specialists should consider its effect on the validity of the inference to be made from the test score" (p. 97). The validity of a test given with accommodation is dependent on the objective of the assessment; can the same inferences about the construct in question be drawn from performance by groups of students using the accommodation and groups not using the accommodation? In specific, skills intended to be measured on the assessment must continue to be measured when an accommodation is introduced, and access skills unrelated to the skill being measured (such as reading skill on a math computation test) must be neutralized (Thurlow, Ysseldyke, & Silverstein, 1995; Tindal, Heath, Hollenbeck, Almond, & Harniss, 1998).

Several state and federal court decisions have addressed the complex issues regarding "reasonable accommodations" required by Section 504, ADA, and IDEA.

For example, in *Brookhart v. Illinois State Board of Education* (1982; 1983) the court interpreted the Section 504 requirement for reasonable accommodations for a disabled person who is otherwise qualified to require physical accommodations but not accommodations that "substantially modified" the test.

The Standards for Educational and Psychological Testing (APA, 1985) specifically address assessment of individuals with disabilities. In Chapter 14, titled "Testing People Who Have Handicapping Conditions" the Standards state that "Although the development of tests and testing procedures for such people is encouraged by the *Standards*, it should be noted that all relevant individual standards given elsewhere in this document are fully applicable to the testing applications considered in this chapter" (p. 77). Additional standards for testing individuals with disabilities are articulated in this document, including Standard 14.1:

> People who modify tests for handicapped people should have available to them psychometric expertise for so doing. In addition, they should have available to them knowledge of the effects of various handicapping conditions on test performance, acquired either from their own training or experience or from close consultation with handicapped individuals or those thoroughly familiar with such individuals. (p. 79)

Little empirical research has been conducted to examine the effects of specific accommodations or test modifications. As Tindal and colleagues (1998) noted, "we are making important decisions using tests which require complex clusters of skills to complete, and for which accommodations frequently are allowed, all done in the absence of data" (p. 440). Well-designed research will help validate specific accommodations by demonstrating that the accommodations benefit the specific subgroup of interest but do not benefit students without disabilities (Phillips, 1994; Tindal et al., 1998).

Thurlow and colleagues (1998) have identified criteria for local decision makers to use to guide decisions about accommodations for individual students participating in state and district-wide assessments. These criteria are presented in Table 14.6.

ROLE OF TECHNOLOGY IN ASSESSMENT

"Schools across the nation have married the computer for better or worse, with wedding expenses in the $30 billion range" (Tennyson & Morrison, 1999, p. 885). Assessment-related tasks are included among the rapidly increasing applications of computers in schools. Jacob and Brantley (1987a), for example, found that 72% of school psychologists surveyed used computers in assessment work.

Maddux and Johnson (1998) identified six assessment-related tasks that may be carried out partially or completely by computers, including:

1. Administration of standardized tests;
2. Scoring of test items;
3. Arithmetic manipulation or transformation of test or subtest scores;

TABLE 14.6   Criteria for Good Accommodations Decisions

1. Decisions are made by people who know the student, including the student's strengths and weaknesses.
2. Decision makers consider the student's learning characteristics and the accommodations currently used during classroom instruction and classroom testing.
3. The student's category of disability or program setting does not influence the decision.
4. The goal is to identify accommodations that the student is using in the classroom during instruction and in classroom testing situations; new accommodations should not be introduced for the district or statewide assessment.
5. The decision regarding accommodations is made systematically, using a form that lists questions to answer or variables to consider in making the accommodation decision. On this form, the decision about recommended accommodations and the reasons for the decision are documented.
6. Parents (or students at an appropriate age) are involved in the decision by either participating in the decision-making process or at least being given the analysis of the need for accommodations and by signing the form that indicates accommodations that are to be used.
7. The decision is documented on the student's IEP.

Note. Based on Thurlow, Elliott, & Ysseldyke (1998).

4. Interpretation of test results;
5. Production of test or assessment reports; and
6. Storage of test scores or other assessment data.

However, many ethical concerns have been raised about the use of computers in assessment (e.g., Bersoff & Hofer, 1991; Jacob & Brantley, 1987a, 1987b; Maddux & Johnson, 1998; Matarazzo, 1986; Sattler, 1988). As Haas and Malouf (1995) noted:

Testing programs are no better than the humans behind them, although they give the impression of being comparable to objective physical laboratory measurements in their precision and apparent completeness. Using such reports without awareness of the fact can lead to difficulty as easily as misuse of the test itself. (p. 164)

Guidance regarding use of computers in assessment is provided by a number of sources, including the ethical principles of some professional organizations. For example, the APA (1992), NASP (1997), and the ASCA (1992) address the use of computerized assessment, scoring, and interpretation in schools. In addition, the Standards for Educational and Psychological Testing (APA, 1985) provide practice standards regarding computer use in assessment. As noted in the Standards Introduction, "Although in some instances specific standards have been stated for tests administered by computer, all the standards apply with equal force to such tests. In many instances, the switch from paper and pencil to computer assessment will require additional evidence that relevant standards have been met in the new testing mode" (p. 4).

Maddux and Johnson (1998) identified arithmetic manipulation or transformation of scores as the most appropriate of all possible uses for computers in assessment.

This application matches well the strengths of computers to manipulate numbers with speed and accuracy. However, practitioners who choose to use such computer applications retain responsibility for the accuracy of the software programs used.

A growing area of computer use in assessment lies in employing computers to administer tests (Braden, 1997). Advantages of computerized test administration can include time saved, guaranteed standardized administration, increased flexibility in assessment settings and times, and more active participation on the part of the test-taker (e.g., Kratochwill, Doll, & Dickson, 1985; Maddux & Johnson, 1998; Matarazzo, 1986; Sattler, 1988; Witt, Elliott, Gresham, & Kramer, 1988). However, in computer-administered assessment, as in any testing situation, the clinician retains the responsibility for ensuring that the testing conditions are appropriate (APA, 1985). "For example, such matters as whether a client who needs glasses or a hearing aid has them available during testing can affect the validity of test results" (p. 45).

Maddux and Johnson (1998) described two types of computerized assessment that may be used in schools: (1) computer-based tests, in which a computer is used to administer a conventional test, which was often developed originally as a paper-and-pencil test, and (2) computer-adaptive tests in which a measure has been developed specifically for computerized administration (items presented to the test-taker are dependent on the test-taker's performance on previous items). Several critical concerns have been raised regarding computer-based test administration (e.g. Jacob & Brantley, 1987b; Maddux & Johnson, 1998). Primary among these concerns is the potential lack of equivalence between computerized administration of a measure and the original paper-and-pencil measure. As Maddux and Johnson (1998) asserted, *"As a general rule, the computer version of a test cannot be assumed to be equivalent to the original, paper-and-pencil version . . .* This is unfortunate, indeed, since lack of equivalence means that the computer version of the test must be restandardized and renormed, a costly and time-consuming process" (p. 94).

Additional sources of error may be introduced in computerized assessment. Some test publishers have produced computer-administered versions of paper-and-pencil tests that have not been normed using computerized administration. It is imperative that test-users carefully evaluate computer-administered tests to determine their validity (e.g., NASP Ethical Principle IV.B.2 states: "School psychologists are knowledgeable about the validity and reliability of their instruments and techniques, choosing those that have up-to-date standardization data and are applicable and appropriate for the benefit of the student/client"; and NASP Ethical Principle IV.C.6 states: "School psychologists maintain full responsibility for any technological services used. All ethical and legal principles regarding confidentiality, privacy, and responsibility for decisions apply to the school psychologists and cannot be transferred to equipment, soft-ware companies or data processing departments").

Computers have also been employed in recent years to carry out direct assessment of specific skills. They have been particularly useful in behavioral assessment, because of its focus on observation and direct assessment of behavior (e.g., Kratochwill et al., 1999). For example, computers have a history of use in psychophysiological assessment (Kratochwill et al., 1985). Computer administration of assessment tools can facilitate standardized administration of measures, and rapid coding, analysis, and graphing of data, often critical in behavioral assessment. Computerized assessment can include administration of standardized measures, analogue assessment of a skill or content area (e.g., Gettinger, 1988), in which authentic classroom materials are presented to the student, and laboratory-based measures assessing specific skills hypothesized to relate to performance in natural settings (e.g., Gordon & Barkley, 1998). For example, one area of increasing computer use is in the assessment of attention deficits. Measures such as variations of the continuous performance task (CPT) are frequently administered to evaluate vigilance, impulsivity, and inhibition of response. Although multiple variations of CPTs are available, in the most common format the student is required to respond (e.g., either press a button or release a button) when a target stimulus or set of stimuli are presented. Use of such measures has been controversial, however. Studies evaluating the discriminative validity of CPT measures have demonstrated mixed results. For example, the Gordon Diagnostic System has been found to have a false-positive rate of 2–17%, but an alarming high false-negative rate of 15–52% in discriminating children with ADHD from normally developing children (Gordon & Barkley, 1998). Some authors question the ecological validity of CPT assessments conducted in laboratory settings (e.g., DuPaul & Stoner, 1994; Landau & Burcham, 1995). Landau and Burcham (1995) noted, "Under the best of circumstances (i.e., adequate normative data and sufficient reliability and validity), knowing the child's performance on one or more of these lab techniques contributes little to an understanding of how the child functions in the classroom. In addition, these procedures are incapable of revealing controlling variables that could be targeted for intervention" (p. 825).

The availability and widespread use of such evaluation tools raise ethical issues for professionals. It is incumbent on the professional to evaluate the purpose of the assessment (e.g., Is this a screening in which a high rate of false negatives may be of greater concern in an assessment tool than a high rate of false positives?), the reliability of the assessment procedure, the validity of the assessment for the purpose intended, and the treatment utility of the tool.

An area of long-standing and continuing concern in the use of computers in assessment is computerized test interpretation and report writing (e.g., Bersoff & Hofer, 1991; Haas & Malouf, 1995; Maddux & Johnson, 1998; Matarazzo, 1986). Ethical mandates require that school practitioners take responsibility for assuring that assessment results are analyzed and interpreted within the context of specific assessment circumstances (e.g., Was the student healthy? Engaged in the task? Familiar with the keyboard?) and that interpretations and conclusions are communicated accurately. For example, APA's Ethical Standard 2.08 (c) states: "Psychologists retain appropriate responsibility for the appropriate application, interpretation, and use of assessment instruments, whether they score and interpret such tests themselves or use automated or other services." NASP's Ethical Principle IV.C.5 states: "School Psychologists do not promote or encourage inappropriate use of computer generated test analyses or reports. For example, a school psychologist would not offer an unedited computer report as one's own writing, nor use a computer scoring system for tests in which one has no training. They select scoring and interpretation services on the basis of accuracy and professional alignment with the underlying decision rules." As discussed earlier in reference to FERPA (1974), confidentiality of educational records is required by law and ethical standards. Computerized records are no exception.

In a 1997 statement addressing delivery of psychological services by telephone, teleconference, and the Internet, the APA Ethics Committee noted such services constitute a "rapidly evolving area" (APA, 1998; p. 979) which is not specifically addressed in the 1992 Ethics Code. The Ethics Committee recommended that psychologists adhere to Ethical Standard 1.04 (c), Boundaries of Competence, which states: "In those emerging areas in which generally recognized standards for preparatory training do not yet exist, psychologists nevertheless take reasonable steps to ensure the competence of their work and to protect patients, clients, students, research participants, and others from harm."

CONCLUSIONS

School professionals who are assessing students must be aware of the legal and ethical mandates governing their practices. It is particularly critical that professional safeguard the welfare of child clients who are likely unable to protect themselves (Koocher & Keith-Spiegel, 1990). As Witt, Elliott, Daly, Gresham, and Kramer (1998) noted, "the overriding purpose of all assessments is to gather information to facilitate effective decision making" (p. 17). Legal and ethical mandates influence the assessment tools chosen, the inferences drawn from them, the use made of these inferences, and the professional's behavior during the entire process. Regardless of the type of assessment tool employed and the type of decision being made (Salvia & Ysseldyke, 1995), school professionals must perform within legal and ethical boundaries.

References

American Counseling Association. (1995). *American Counseling Association code of ethics and standards of practice*. Alexandria, VA: Author.

American Psychological Association. (1985). *Standards for educational and psychological testing*. Washington, DC: Author.

American Psychological Association. (1992). Ethical principles of psychologists and code of conduct. *American Psychologist, 47*, 1597–1611.

American Psychological Association. (1993). *Guidelines for providers of psychological services to ethnic, linguistic, and culturally diverse populations*. Washington, DC: Author.

American Psychological Association Committee on Legal Issues. (1996). Strategies for private practitioners coping with subpeonas or compelled testimony for client records or test data. *Professional Psychology: Research and Practice, 27*(3), 245–251.

American Psychological Association Ethics Committee. (1998). Report of the Ethics Committee, 1997. *American Psychologist, 53*(8), 969–980.

American School Counselor Association. (1992). *Ethical standards for school counselors*. Alexandria, VA: Author.

Americans with Disabilities Act of 1990, 42 U.S.C., § 12101 *et seq.*

Anastasi, A. (1988). *Psychological testing* (6th ed.). New York: Macmillan.

Artiles, A. J., & Trent, S. C. (1994). Overrepresentation of minority students in special education: A continuing debate. *Journal of Special Education, 27*(4), pp. 410–437.

Bennett, B. E ., Bryant, B. D., VandenBos, G. R. & Greenwood, A. (1995). *Professional liability and risk management.* Washington, DC: American Psychological Association.

Bersoff, D. N. (1983). Children as participants in psychoeducational assessment . In G. B. Melton, G. P. Koocher, & M. J. Saks (Eds.), *Children's competence to consent* (pp. 149–177). New York: Plenum Press.

Bersoff, D. N. (1995). *Ethical conflicts in psychology.* Washington, DC: American Psychological Association.

Bersoff, D. N., & Hofer, P. J. (1990). The legal regulation of school psychology. In C. R. Reyolds & T. B. Gutkin (Eds.), *The handbook of school psychology* (2nd ed.), (pp. 937–961). New York: Wiley.

Bersoff, D. N., & Hofer, P. J. (1991). Legal issues in computerized psychological testing. In T. B. Gutkin & S. L. Wise (Eds.), *The computer and the decision-making process* (pp. 225–243). Hillsdale, NJ: Erlbaum.

Bersoff, D. N., & Koeppl, P. M. (1993). The relation between ethical codes and moral principles. *Ethics and Behavior,* 3(3 & 4), 345–357.

Boomer, L. W., Hartshorne, T. S., & Robertshaw, C. S. (1995). Confidentiality and student records: A hypothetical case. *Preventing School Failure,* 39(2), 15–21.

Braden, J. P. (1997). The practical impact of intellectual assessment issues. *School Psychology Review,* 26(2), 242–248.

Brookhart v. Illinois State Board of Education, 534F Supp. 725 (CD Ill) 1982. 697F 2d 179 (CA7) 1983.

Cleary, T. A., Humphreys, L. G., Kendrick, S. A., & Wesman, A. (1975). Educational uses of tests with disadvantaged students. *American Psychologist,* 30, 15–41.

Cone, J. D. (1981). Psychometric considerations. In M. Hersen & A. S. Bellack (Eds.), *Behavioral assessment: A practical handbook* (2nd ed., pp. 38–68). New York: Pergamon Press.

Cronbach, L. J. (1988). Five perspectives on the validity argument. In R. Wainer & H. I. Braun (Eds.), *Test validity* (pp. 3–17). Hillsdale, N.J.: Erlbaum.

Cummins, J. (1984). *Bilingualism and special education.* Clevedon, England: Multilingual Matters.

Debra P. v. Turlington, 730 F.2d 1405 (11th Cir. 1984).

DeKraii, M. B., Sales, B. D., & Hall, S. R. (1998). Informed consent, confidentiality, and duty to report laws in the conduct of child therapy. In R. J. Morris & T. R. Kratochwill (Eds.), *The practice of child therapy.* Boston: Allyn & Bacon.

de la Cruz, R. E. (1996). Assessment-bias issues in special education: A review of the literature. (ERIC Document Reproduction Service No. ED 390 246).

Diana v. State Board of Education, Civ. Act. No C-70–37 (N.D. Cal., 1970).

DuPaul, G. J., & Stoner, G. (1994). *ADHD in the schools: Assessment and intervention strategies.* New York: Guilford Press.

Education for All Handicapped Children Act (1975), 20 U.S.C., Chapter 33.

Eisel v. Board of Education of Montgomery County, 597 A.2d 447 (Md. 1991).

Elliott, S. N., & Fuchs, L. S. (1997). The utility of curriculum-based measurement and performance assessment as alternatives to traditional intelligence and achievement tests. *School Psychology Review,* 26(2), 224–233.

Family Educational Rights and Privacy Act of 1974. 20 U.S.C. § 1232g.

Fiedler, C. R., & Prasse, D. P. (1996). Legal and ethical issues in the educational assessment and programming for youth with emotional or behavioral disorders. In M. J. Breen & C. R. Fiedler (Eds.), *Behavioral approach to assessment of youth with emotional/behavioral disorders: A handbook for school-based practitioners* (pp. 23–79). Austin, TX: Pro-Ed.

Fischer, L., Schimmel, D., & Kelly, C. (1995). *Teachers and the law.* White Plains, NY: Longman.

Fischer, L., & Sorenson, G. P. (1996). *School law for counselors, psychologists and social workers* (3rd ed.) White Plains, NY: Longman.

Fleming, E. R., & Fleming, D. C. (1987). Involvement of minors in special educational decision-making. *Journal of Law and Education,* 16(4), 389–402.

Foster, S. L., & Cone, J. D. (1995). Validity issues in clinical assessment. *Psychological Assessment,* 7(3), 248–260.

Fry, B. G. (1997). The Family Educational Rights and Privacy Act of 1974. In M. T. Ruzicka & B. L. Weckmueller (Eds.), *Student records management: A handbook* (pp. 43–57). Westport, CN: Greenwood Press.

Geisinger, K. F. (1992). The metamorphosis of test validation. *Educational Psychologist, 27* (2), 197–222.

Gettinger, M. (1988). Analogue assessment: Evaluating academic abilities. In E. S. Shapiro & T. R. Kratochwill (Eds.), *Behavioral assessment in schools: Conceptual foundations and practical applications* (pp. 247–290). New York: Guilford Press.

Gordon, M., & Barkley, R. A. (1998). Tests and observational measures. In R. A. Barkley (Ed.), *Attention-deficit hyperactivity disorder: A handbook for diagnosis and treatment* (pp. 294–311). New York: Guilford Press.

Goss v. Lopez, 419 U.S. 565 (1975).

Graden, J. L., Casey, A., & Bonstrom, O. (1985). Implementing a prereferral intervention system: Part II. The data. *Exceptional Children, 51*(6), 487–496.

Gresham, F. M., & Witt, J. C. (1997). Utility of intelligence tests for treatment planning, classification, and placement decisions: Recent empirical findings and future directions. *School Psychology Quarterly, 12*(3), 249–267.

Guadelupe Organization, Inc. v. Tempe Elementary School District No. 3, No. 71–435 (D. Ariz., 1972) (Consent Decree).

Haas, L. J., & Malouf, J. L. (1995). *Keeping up the good work: A practitioner's guide to mental health ethics* (2nd ed.). Sarasota, FL: Professional Resource Press.

Hayes, S. C., Nelson, R. O., & Jarrett, R. B. (1987). The treatment utility of assessment. *American Psychologist, 42*(11), 963–974.

Helms, J. (1992). Why is there no study of cultural equivalence in standardized cognitive ability testing? *American Psychologist, 47*(9), 1083–1101.

Hobson v. Hansen, 269 F. Supp. 401 (D.D.C., 1967), *aff'd sub nom, Smuck v. Hobson*, 408 F.2d 175 (1969).

Illback, R. J., Zins, J. E., & Maher, C. A. (1999). Program planning and evaluation: Principles, procedures, and planned change. In C. R. Reynolds & T. B. Gutkin (Eds.), *The handbook of school psychology* (3rd ed., pp. 907–932). New York: Wiley.

Imber, M. & Van Geel, T. (1993). *Education law.* New York: McGraw-Hill.

Individuals with Disabilities Education Act (1990, 1997), 20 U.S.C. Chapter 33, § 1400 *et seq.*

Jacob, S., & Brantley, J. C. (1987a). Ethical-legal problems with computer use and suggestions for best practices: A national survey. *School Psychology Review, 16*(1), 69–77.

Jacob, S., & Brantley, J. C. (1987b). Ethical and legal considerations for microcomputer use in special education. In D. L. Johnson, C. D. Maddux, & A. C. Candler (Eds.), *Computers in the special education classroom* (pp.185–194). New York: Haworth Press.

Jacob-Timm, S., & Hartshorne, T. S. (1998). *Ethics and law for school psychologists* (3rd ed). New York: Wiley.

John K. & Mary K. v. Board of Education for School District 65, Cook County, 504 N.E. 2d 797 (Ill. App.1 Dist. 1987).

Keith-Spiegel, P., & Koocher, G. P. (1985). *Ethics in psychology: Professional standards and cases.* Hillsdale, NJ: Erlbaum.

Koocher, G. P., & Keith-Spiegel, P. C. (1990). *Children, ethics and the law: Professional issues and cases.* Lincoln: University of Nebraska Press.

Kratochwill, T. R., Doll, E. J., & Dickson, W. P. (1985). Microcomputers in behavioral assessment: Recent advances and remaining issues. *Computers in Human Behavior, 1*, 277–291.

Kratochwill, T. R., Sheridan, S. M., Carlson, J., & Lasecki, K. K. (1999). Advances in behavioral assessment. In C. R. Reynolds & T. B. Gutkin (Eds.), *The handbook of school psychology* (3rd ed., pp. 350–382). New York: Wiley.

Landau, S., & Burcham, B. G. (1995). Best practices in the assessment of children with attention disorders. In A. Thomas & J. Grimes (Eds.), *Best practices in school psychology* (3rd ed., pp. 817–829). Washington, DC: National Association of School Psychologists.

Larry P. v. Riles, 343 F. Supp. 1306, (N.D. Cal. 1972), *aff'd*, 502 F.2d 963 (9th Cir. 1974), further proceedings, 495 F. Supp. 926 (N.D. Cal. 1979), *aff'd*, 502 F. 2d 693 (9th Cir. 1984).

Lopez, E. C. (1995). Best practices in working with bilingual children. In A. Thomas & J. Grimes (Eds.), *Best practices in school psychology* (3rd ed., pp. 1111–1121). Washington, DC: National Association of School Psychologists.

Lopez, E. C. (1997). The cognitive assessment of limited English proficient and bilingual children. In D. P. Flanagan, J. L. Genshaft, & P. L Harrison (Eds.), *Contemporary intellectual assessment: Theories, tests, and issues* (pp. 503–516). New York: Guilford Press.

MacMillan, D. L., & Reschly, D. J. (1998). Overrepresentation of minority students: The case for greater specificity or reconsideration of the variables examined. *Journal of Special Education, 32,* 15–24.

Maddux, C. D., & Johnson, L. (1998). Computer-assisted assessment. In H. B. Vance (Ed.), *Psychological assessment of children: Best practices for school and clinical settings* (2nd ed., pp. 87–106). New York: Wiley.

Marshall v. Georgia, No. CV482-233 (S.D. Ga., 1984), *aff'd sub. Nom. Georgia State Conferences of Branches of NAACP v. Georgia*, 775 F.2d 1403 (11th Cir. 1985).

Matarazzo, J. D. (1986). Computerized clinical psychological test interpretations: Unvalidated plus all mean and no sigma. *American Psychologist, 41,* 14–24.

Matarazzo, J. D. (1990). Psychological assessment versus psychological testing: Validation from Binet to the school, clinic, and courtroom. *American Psychologist, 45*(9), 999–1017.

McCarthy, M. M., & Sorenson, G. P. (1993). School counselors and consultants: Legal duties and liabilities. *Journal of Counseling and Development, 72,* 159–167.

MacMillan, D. L., Gresham, F. M., Siperstein, G., & Bocian, K. (1996). The labyrinth of I.D.E.A.: School decisions on referred students with subaverage intelligence. *American Journal on Mental Retardation, 101,* 161–174.

Melton, G. B. (1983). Children's competence to consent: A problem in law and social science. In G. B. Melton, G. P. Koocher, & M. J. Saks (Eds.), *Children's competence to consent.* (pp. 1–18). New York: Plenum Press.

Merriken v. Cressman, 364 F. Supp. 913 (1973).

Messick, S. (1988). The once and future issues of validity: Assessing the meaning and consequences of measurement. In R. Wainer & H. I. Braun (Eds.), *Test validity* (pp. 33–45). Hillsdale, NJ: Erlbaum.

Messick, S. (1989). Meaning and values in test validation: The science and ethics of assessment. *Educational Researcher, 18*(2), 5 –11.

Messick, S. (1994). Foundations of validity: Meaning and consequences in psychological assessment. *European Journal of Psychological Assessment, 10,* 1–9.

Messick, S. (1995). Validity of psychological assessment: Validation of inferences from persons' responses and performances as scientific inquiry into score meaning. *American Psychologist, 50*(9), 741–749.

Mills v. Board of Education of District of Columbia, 348 F. supp. 866 (1972); contempt proceedings, EHLR 551:643 (D.D.C. 1980).

Millsap, R. E., & Everson, H. T. (1993). Methodology review: Statistical approaches for assessing measurement bias. *Applied Psychological Measurement, 17*(4), 297–334.

National Association of School Psychologists. (1997). *Professional conduct manual* (3rd ed.). Silver Spring, MD: Author.

National Association of Social Workers. (1997). *National Association of Social Workers Code of Ethics.* Washington, D.C.: Author.

National Education Association. (1975). *Code of ethics of the education profession.* Washington, DC: Author.

National Forum on Education Statistics. (1997). *Protecting the privacy of student records: Guidelines for education agencies.* Washington, DC: Author.

P.A.S.E. (Parents in Action on Special Education) v. Hannon, 506 F.Supp. 831 (N.D. Ill. 1980).

Phillips, S. E. (1994). High-stakes testing accommodations: Validity versus disabled rights. *Applied Measurement in Education, 7*(2), 93–120.

Pope, K. S., & Bajt, T. R. (1988). When laws and values conflict: A dilemma for psychologists. *American Psychologist, 43,* 828–829.

Prasse, D. P. (1995). Best practices in school psychology and the law. In A. Thomas & J. Grimes (Eds.), *Best practices in school psychology* (3rd ed., pp. 41–50).Washington, DC: National Association of School Psychologists.

Protection of Pupil Rights Amendment (1978). Amendment to ESEA; amended in 1994).

Reeder, G. D., Maccow, G. C., Shaw, S. R., Swerdlik, M. E., Horton, C. B. & Foster, P. (1997). School psychologists and full-service schools: Partnerships with medical, mental health, and social services. *School Psychology Review, 26*(4), 603–621.

Reschly, D. J. (1978). Concepts of bias in assessment and WISC-R research with minorities. In H. Vance & F. Wallbrown (Eds.), *WISC-R: Research and interpretation.* Washington, DC: National Association of School Psychologists.

Reschly, D. J. (1997). Diagnostic and treatment utility of intelligence tests. In D. P. Flanagan, J. L. Genshaft, & P. L. Harrison (Eds.), *Contemporary intellectual assessment: Theories, tests, and issues.* New York: Guilford Press.

Reschly, D. J., & Bersoff, D. N. (1999). Law and school psychology. In C. R. Reynolds & T. B. Gutkin (Eds.), *Handbook of school psychology* (3rd ed., pp. 1077–1112). New York: Wiley.

Reschly, D. J., Kicklighter, R., & McKee, P. (1988). Recent placement litigation, Part I, II, and III. *School Psychology Review, 17,* 9–50.

Reschly, D. J., & Ysseldyke, J. E. (1995). School psychology paradigm shift. In A. Thomas & J. Grimes (Eds.), *Best practices in school psychology* (3rd ed., pp. 17–32).Washington, DC: National Association of School Psychologists.

Rettig v. Kent City School District, 788 F. 2d 328 (6th Cir. 1980).

Reynolds, C. (1991). Methods for studying bias in psychological and educational tests. *Diagnostique, 17,* 21–39.

Reynolds, C. (1995). Test bias and the assessment of intelligence and personality. In D. H. Saklofske & M. Zeidner (Eds.), *International handbook of personality and intelligence* (pp. 545–573). New York: Plenum Press.

Reynolds, C., & Kaiser, S. (1990). Test bias in psychological assessment. In C. R. Reynolds & T. B. Gutkin (Eds.), *The handbook of school psychology* (2nd ed., pp. 487–525). New York: Wiley.

Reynolds, C. R., Lowe, P. A., & Saenz, A. L. (1999). The problem of bias in psychological assessment. In C. R. Reynolds & T. B. Gutkin (Eds.), *The handbook of school psychology* (3rd ed., pp. 549–595). New York: Wiley.

Ross, W. D. (1930). *The right and the good.* Oxford, England: Clarendon.

Sales, B. D., Krauss, D. A., Sacken, D. M., & Overcast, T. D. (1999). The legal rights of students. In C. R. Reynolds, & T. B. Gutkin (Eds.), *The handbook of school psychology* (3rd ed., pp. 1113–1145). New York: Wiley.

Salvia, J., & Ysseldyke, J. E. (1995). *Assessment* (6th ed.) Boston: Houghton Mifflin.

Sandoval, J., & Mille, M. (1979). Accuracy judgments of WISC-R item difficulty for minority groups. Paper presented at the annual meeting of the American Psychological Association, New York.

Sattler, J. M. (1988). *Assessment of children* (3rd ed.). San Diego: Jerome M. Sattler.

Serna, L. A. (1998). Intervention versus affirmation: Proposed solutions to the problem of disproportionate minority representation in special education. *Journal of Special Education, 32,* 48–51.

Shapiro, E. S., & Kratochwill, T. R. (Eds.). (1988). *Behavioral assessment in schools: Conceptual foundations and practical applications.* New York: Guilford Press.

Siegel, M. (1979). Privacy, ethics, and confidentiality. *Professional Psychology, 10,* 249–258.

Southeastern Community College v. Davis, 442 U.S. 397 (1979).

Sue, D. W., Arredondo, P., & McDavis, R. J. (1995). Multicultural counseling competencies and standards: A call to the profession. In J. G. Ponterotto, J. M. Casas, L. A. Suzuki, & C. M. Alexander (Eds.), *Handbook of multicultural counseling* (pp. 624–644). Thousand Oaks, CA: Sage.

Tarasoff v. Regents of University of California, 118 Cal.Rptr. 129, 529 P.2d 553 (Cal. 1974). *Tarasoff v. Regents of University of California,* 131 Cal Rptr. 14, 551 P.2d 334 (Cal. 1976).

Taylor, L., & Adelman, H. S. (1989). Reframing the confidentiality dilemma to work in children's best interests. *Professional Psychology: Research and Practice, 20*(2), 79–83.

Taylor, L., Adelman, H. S., & Kaser-Boyd, N. (1985). Minors' attitudes and competence toward participation in psychoeducational decisions. *Professional Psychology: Research and Practice, 16*(2), 226–235.

Tennyson, R. D., & Morrison, D. (1999). Computers in education and school psychology: The existing and emerging technology knowledge base supporting interventions with children. In C. R. Reynolds & T. B. Gutkin (Eds.), *The Handbook of school psychology* (3rd ed., pp. 885–906). New York: Wiley.

Thomas-Presswood, T. N., Sasso, J., & Gin, G. (1997). Cultural issues in the intellectual assessment of children from diverse cultural backgrounds. *Journal of Social Distress and the Homeless, 6*(2), 113–127.

Thurlow, M. L., Elliott, J. L., & Ysseldyke, J. E. (1998). *Testing students with disabilities: Practical strategies for complying with district and state requirements.* Thousand Oaks, CA: Corwin Press.

Thurlow, M. L., Seyfarth, A. L., Scott, D. L., & Ysseldyke, J. E. (1997). State assessment policies on participation and accommodations for students with disabilities: 1997 Update. National Center on Educational Outcomes.

Thurlow, M. L., Ysseldyke, J. E., & Silverstein, B. (1995). Testing accommodations for students with disabilities. *Remedial and Special Education, 16*(5), 260–270.

Tindal, G., Heath, B., Hollenbeck, K., Almond, P., & Harniss, M. (1998). Accommodating students with disabilities on large-scale tests: An experimental study. *Exceptional Children, 64*(4), 439–450.

Tranel, D. (1994). The release of psychological data to nonexperts: Ethical and legal considerations. *Professional Psychology: Research and Practice, 25*(1), 33–38.

Turnbull, H. R., & Turnbull, A. P. (1998). *Free appropriate public education: The law and children with disabilities* (5th ed.). Denver: Love.

U.S. Department of Education. (1994). *Summary of the bilingual education state educational agency program survey of states' limited English proficient persons and available educational services (1992–1993): Final report.* Arlington, VA: Development Associates.

Valles, E. C. (1998). The disproportionate representation of minority students in special education: Responding to the problem. *Journal of Special Education, 32,* 52–54.

Weithorn, L. A. (1983). Involving children in decisions affecting their own welfare: Guidelines for professionals. In G. B. Melton, G. P. Koocher, & M. J. Saks (Eds.), *Children's competence to consent* (pp. 235–260). New York: Plenum Press.

Witt, J. C., Elliott, S. N., Daly, E. J., Gresham, F. M., & Kramer, J. J. (1998). *Assessment of at-risk and special needs children* (2nd ed.). Boston: McGraw-Hill.

Witt, J. C., Elliott, S. N., Gresham, F. M., & Kramer, J. J. (1988). *Assessment of special children: Tests and the problem-solving process.* Glenview, IL: Scott Foresman.

Yeager, J. D. (1994). *Confidentiality of student records: A guide for school districts establishing policies and procedures with special emphasis on alcohol and other drug use.* Portland, OR: Northwest Regional Education Laboratory.

Yell, M. L. (1996). Education and the law: Managing student records. *Preventing School Failure, 41*(1), 44–46.

Yell, M. L. (1998). *The law and special education.* Upper Saddle River, NJ: Prentice-Hall.

CHAPTER 15

Assessment of Ethnic and Linguistic Minority Children

STEPHEN M. QUINTANA
ELISA M. CASTILLO
MANUEL X. ZAMARRIPA
University of Wisconsin–Madison

Ethnic and linguistic minority children constitute the most rapidly growing segment of the youth population in the United States. In fact, ethnic minority youth now constitute 35% of the U.S. public school population and more than 50% of the student population in many large urban school districts and several large states (e.g., Texas). Currently, approximately 16% of students are African American, 12% are Hispanic, 3% are Asian or Pacific Islander, and 1% are American Indian or Alaskan Native. About 14% of students in grades K through 12 speak languages other than English at home and we estimate another 8% or more may speak a nonmainstream dialect (e.g., Black English).

Relatively little information is available to aid psychologists and educators in their assessment of problems, needs, and strengths of these young people. The lack of appropriate instrumentation and practices in the assessment of children and adolescents from ethnic and linguistic minority (ELM) backgrounds has been considered a pervasive problem in education and psychology (Padilla & Medina, 1996). This problem stems from many sources, including historical bias in the development of psychological assessment procedures that have been applied to ELM children, disproportionate representation of ELM populations as research participants and as researchers, and the ecological or contextual issues that may contribute to mistrust of the psychological profession on the part of some ELM communities (see Table 15.1). Finally, assessment of ELM children may be significantly more complicated than it is for monolingual English-speaking, white children. For example, understanding the process by which bilingual children process educational material in their nondominant language requires awareness of bilingual issues in addition to the educational issues associated with monolingual children. On the other hand, there are some encouraging trends in the current technology related to psychological services (e.g., dynamic and authentic assessment procedures), which we believe have the potential to improve the appropriateness of psychological assessment procedures for ELM children.

TABLE 15.1   Barriers in the Psychological Profession to Assessment of ELM Children

Ethnocentric bias
   Deficit model applied to ELM children
   Paucity of information about:
      Normal development of ELM children
      Strengths and resilience of ELM children
      Psychological impact of racism and bias on ELM children

Representation problems
   ELM children historically underrepresented in development of assessment procedures
   Research tends to be cross-cultural rather than culturally specific or culturally
      pluralistic in origin

Sources of cultural mistrust
   History of ELM communities reaction to standardized assessments
   Psychologists lacking sensitivity and competence to work with ELM children
   Interethnic conflict

Complexity of assessment with ELM children
   Culture considered in primarily ad hoc fashion
   Understanding psychological functioning is more complex in multicultural context
      than in monocultural context

HISTORICAL BIAS

The history of psychology and the application of psychological science reflects a pervasive ethnocentric bias in the practice and science of psychology (Hall, 1997). Ethnocentrism has been defined as, to paraphrase Helms (1992, p. 1093), *the use of particular cultural groups' behavioral and psychological functioning (e.g., behavior, values) as the standard or norm against which to judge other cultural groups' psychological functioning.* In this context, psychological functioning that departs from the standard or norm is usually considered a deficiency. Historically, ELM children have been interpreted as pathological or, more commonly, deficient. A review of literature published in developmental journals indicates that only a small proportion of research (approximately 20%) includes samples diversified across race or ethnicity (McPhee, Kreutzer, & Fritz, 1994). However, of those studies including ethnically and racially diverse samples, most focused on deviancy rather than normal developmental processes. This pattern is all too typical for psychological research: When studying normal process researchers look to white, usually middle-class populations; when defining deviancy, researchers turn to ELM populations. Generally, there have been four broad models which have been used to conceptualize the perceived deficiency of ethnic minority children: (1) genetic deficiency, (2) cultural deficit, (3) social disorganization, and (4) social pathology. The perceived genetic deficiency of some ethnic and minority children was particularly popular in the Eugenics movement, but apparently continues to be accepted by some (e.g., Herrnstein & Murray, 1996). Frequently, the implicit implication drawn from this model is that there should be genetic, educational, social, and occupation segregation (see Herrnstein & Murray, 1996). The cultural deficit model attributes problems of ethnic minority children to their culture with the implicit implication that ELM children should assimilate to white cultural norms (see García Coll et al., 1996). In the social disorganization and social pathology models, problems are attributed to either the perceived disintegration of values or to the effects of a social pathology (e.g., drugs, violence, poverty) in ethnic minority communities, resulting in the apparent loss or absence of adaptive culture. The implicit implication of these two models is that ELM children should assimilate to dominant cultural norms to replace the perceived loss of adaptive culture (Rollack & Terrell, 1996). Two important considerations are missing in these four traditional models: (1) the strengths, resources, and resilience of ethnic minority cultures and communities, and (2) the role of outside forces (e.g., racism, discrimination, and bias) in the creation and maintenance of many problems that face ELM children (García Coll et al., 1996).

PROBLEMS WITH REPRESENTATION

As mentioned, a disproportionately small amount of psychological research has investigated children of ELM backgrounds when the focus of the study is on normal educational or developmental processes (Graham, 1994; McPhee et al., 1994). Of this research, most could be classified as cross-cultural in nature rather than either culturally pluralistic or culturally specific. By cross-cultural we mean that research was developed for one population and applied to another population. Conversely, culturally specific or culturally pluralistic approaches often attempt to represent and examine processes using procedures indigenous to the culture of interest rather than ones that have been transported or translated from another culture. A metaphor may be instructional to illustrate the differences between cross-cultural and the other two kinds of approaches: When traveling to a foreign language country, a visitor may attempt to translate signs and communications into his or her own language (cross-cultural approach) or may attempt to become fluent in the other language and understand the communication in its original language (pluralistic or culturally specific approach). The obvious problem with relying on translations is that much may be lost in the translation and, analogously, the problem with cross-cultural research is that features specific to one culture may not be applicable or generalizable to another.

CULTURAL MISTRUST

For a variety of reasons, many in ELM communities may view psychologists and psychological assessments suspiciously (Baker & O'Neil, 1996). In part, this suspiciousness has been generalized from distrust of the meaningfulness of results from psychological instruments. A variety of legal challenges have been initiated that have attacked the manner in which psychological assessments, particularly standardized intellectual and achievement tests, have been developed, administered, and used for ELM children (see Lopez, 1997; Valencia & Aburto, 1991). Cultural mistrust appears to exist for psychological instruments when employed in "high stakes" testing (Valencia & Guadarrama, 1996). High stakes refers to those situations in which decisions about critical educational placement (e.g., special education), and/or admissions (entrance exams) are based, in part or whole, on results from tests (Valencia & Aburto, 1991).

Another reason for cultural mistrust or suspicions is that psychologists may not be demonstrating appropriate levels of sensitivity or competency when working in cross-cultural or cross-linguistic contexts. Indeed, special task forces of the American Psychological Association and individual surveys of training programs repeatedly find that the training programs in psychological professions are ill-equipped to provide effective and relevant services for ELM children (e.g., Quintana & Bernal, 1995; Ramirez, Wassef, Paniagua, & Linskey, 1996). Ineffective professional services undermine essential trust between the psychological/educational professions and ELM communities (Hall, 1997).

A third reason for mistrust is based on historical and structural factors of interethnic conflict. Sociologists have described structural features within the society of, for example, the United States, in which some ethnic minority communities perceive barriers to their access of resources (e.g., jobs, educational opportunities, etc.) within the society (Ogbu, 1994). Moreover, these communities may suspect that professionals (e.g., educators and psychologists) perpetuate the inequities. Consequently, the decisions, services, and recommendations of these professions may be perceived as antithetical to the success of ELM children. Many times these services reflect lower expectations, less motivation, and less understanding relative to white, English-speaking children.

AREAS OF COMPLEXITY

Because most of the psychological technology was developed primarily for white, middle-class children, the adaptation of these instruments for ELM children requires that the role of culture and cultural context be considered. Unfortunately, the consideration of cultural or linguistic factors in the development of psychological assessment and theory usually occurs in an ad hoc fashion rather than as an essential component in the original formulation of the theory or assessment technology.

The introduction of cultural differences greatly complicates the adaptation of the assessment technology. Consider the need to assess the cognitive functioning of a Spanish-speaking Latino child. An administrator may be able to access a Spanish version of the WISC-III, but there may be dialect differences between the child's Spanish, the administrator's Spanish, and that of the translated version of the test. Moreover, the application of appropriate norms is further complicated given that the Spanish norms may have been developed in a context different from that of the child (e.g., standardization sample may have been from a different country) and that perhaps the child has been in English immersion classes for the last several years, but not long enough to become fluent in English at a level in order to process advanced academic materials but too long to process academic material proficiently in Spanish (e.g., Ortiz, 1997). Moreover, there may be different cultural definitions of intelligence between the authors of the instrument and that of the child's culture (e.g., relative weighting of cognitive and social components of intelligence). These comprise but a small subset of the ways in which cultural and linguistic differences serve to further complicate the application of psychological instruments.

BEHAVIORAL ASSESSMENT: IS IT NONBIASED?

Many of the problems described above are particularly characteristic of assessments that use norm-referenced procedures or assessments that require a high level of inference (e.g., projective assessments). Conversely, behavioral assessments avoid some of the problems endemic to these approaches when applied to culturally and linguistically diverse populations. Indeed, several have suggested that behavioral assessment may allow for a nonbiased or nondiscriminatory assessment. Of course, like all procedures, there are no guarantees that behavioral assessment will not be used in a discriminatory or biased fashion. Nonetheless there are several reasons why behavioral assessment has been found, in some ways, to be culturally appropriate for ethnic and linguistic minority (ELM) children. Behavioral assessment traditionally gathers information on the role environment plays in the child's identified problem and integrates information about the child's strengths. These are two areas that are often lacking in traditional assessments of ELM children. Also, behavioral assessment has been described as an effective strategy in the assessment and treatment of culturally diverse populations because of certain inherit characteristics that tend to be culturally congruent with such populations. For example, behavioral strategies tend to be concrete, action oriented, focused on the immediate and on learning (Paniagua, 1994). Although some features of behavioral assessment may increase the likelihood that they may be implemented in a nondiscriminatory fashion, we believe the goal of being nonbiased or nondiscriminatory is overly limited. Consequently, we review resources that attempt to increase the culturally appropriate nature of assessment that may be even more ambitious than simply reducing potential bias in the assessment.

In this chapter, we discuss four considerations in the assessment of ELM children we have identified as critical: (1) cultural and linguistic competencies of examiners, (2) cultural and linguistic characteristics of the child, (3) cultural or linguistic characteristics of the assessment instruments and procedures, and (4) cultural and linguistic characteristics of the context of assessment. In each of these sections we briefly summarize some of the important kinds of information, but cannot, of course, provide a comprehensive review of the material. Consequently, readers will need to consult other sources, depending on the nature of the specific assessment issue.

CULTURAL AND LINGUISTIC COMPETENCIES OF EXAMINERS

The cultural competency of the examiner is of great importance and may be more critical than the cultural relevance of the assessment instrument (Sue, 1998; Lopez,

1997; Arredondo et al., 1996; Sue, Arredondo, & McDavis, 1992). Psychologists and other examiners who are not culturally competent in working with ELM populations are unaware of the impact of their own personal and cultural characteristics on the (1) assessment process, (2) interpretations of assessment data, as well as (3) implications inferred from the assessment results. Additionally, examiners who are unaware of the impact of their cultural background may be unaware of the children's culturally based reactions to the assessment. Indeed, Ponterotto and Alexander (1996) suggest they would prefer a culturally biased instrument in the hands of a culturally competent clinician, than a culturally fair instrument in the hands of an examiner who lacks cultural competencies.

Arredondo and colleagues (1996) have identified for the counseling profession three categories of cultural competence ((1) knowledge, (2) beliefs/attitudes, and (3) skills) across three areas ((1) counselor's cultural background, (2) client's cultural background, and (3) cultural nature of psychological interventions). We extend this definition of cultural competency to be applicable for the conduct of psychological assessments.

Examiner's Self-Awareness of Cultural Background

Examiners who are culturally competent have knowledge about how their own cultural socialization influences personal and professional judgments. Many aspects of the examiner's professional behavior are greatly affected by cultural socialization. Some of these may be values about how professional relationships are structured (e.g., level of formality), the verbal characteristics used by the examiner (e.g., adherence to standard English), and implicit norms applied to judge children's behavior, to name only but a few examples.

Examiners need to be knowledgeable about how stereotyping and discrimination may cloud their professional judgments. We believe that it is nearly impossible to escape the cultural socialization that leads to stereotyping of ELM groups (see Quintana, 1998). Indeed, members of ELM groups are not immune from adopting stereotypes of even their own group (see Cross, 1995; Hall, 1997). Consequently, it is ethically incumbent on all examiners to be aware of stereotyping and take appropriate steps to neutralize the deleterious effect of these stereotypes on their work. One of the ways to reduce stereotyping is for examiners to have enough personal as well as professional contact with other cultural groups to replace misconceptions with more accurate and in-depth personal understanding of the nuances of different cultural groups.

Culturally competent examiners also need to be able to recognize the limits of their cultural competency. In this regard, examiners may need to find culturally appropriate resources when a case requires skills (e.g., linguistic) that they do not possess. Additionally, examiners may need to redress deficits in their cultural competence with additional professional development training. In short, the psychoanalytic mantra of "Know thyself" is an important facet of culturally competent assessment.

Examiner's Awareness of Child's Cultural Background

The second area of cultural competence requires that examiners have awareness of the child's cultural worldview and background. Importantly, culturally competent examiners are aware of potential sources of differences in cultural values, perceptions, and understandings between the examiner and child. The ability to detect these differences requires that examiners have specific knowledge about the cultural traditions, history, and values of the child's ethnic or linguistic group. Unfortunately, examiners' knowledge about other ethnic and linguistic groups is often sufficient only to generate stereotypes about the group. Consequently, it is critical that examiners be aware of their attitudes about the child's cultural background. We have found that many examiners hope to disguise their cultural stereotypes, but we have found that children are especially attuned to the cultural attitudes of others. For example, in interviews with elementary school children, Quintana (1994) found that children were skilled in identifying educators (e.g., teachers) who were culturally biased.

A particularly challenging area of cultural competency is being able to differentiate cultural differences from actual behavioral problems. A child's behavior may be identified as problematic only because the behavior reflects a cultural norm that is different from that of the examiner. For example, Hall (1997) suggested that Latino children's deference to authority may be improperly interpreted as passivity or resistance. In other situations, real problems in children's behavior may be ignored because it is assumed, incorrectly, that it reflects norms of the child's cultural group. Hall (1997) reported a case in which an African American boy's acting-out behavior was inappropriately attributed to perceived cultural norms of African Americans. Across these situations, examiners will need to be knowledgeable of behavioral norms within the child's cultural group. This kind of knowledge requires familiarity with general characteristics of various ethnic and linguistic groups as well as knowledge about cultural variations that occur within each ethnic or linguistic group (Lopez, 1997).

It is also critical that examiners become aware of the impact of sociocultural influences on the children, the children's families and, more broadly, on the cultural group of the children. A child's behavior may reflect a variety of coping strategies (e.g., coping with racism) in response to sociocultural history of his or her cultural group (García Coll et al., 1996). These coping strategies may be important sources of resiliency and, at other times, limit the development of other adaptive coping strategies. Finally, a culturally competent examiner should have the cultural skills necessary to conduct the assessment across several cultural contexts. In some situations, bilingual skills may be required and for other situations more subtle cultural skills may be necessary. For example, examiners may need to be skilled in sending and responding to a variety of verbal and nonverbal messages in order to respond in a culturally appropriate fashion to an ELM child.

An integration of (1) awareness of their own cultural background with (2) awareness of the child's cultural background allows the examiner to shift cultural perspectives between the examiner's culture and that of the child. In Piagetian theory, the ability to assume another's perspective allows for the reduction of developmental egocentricism. We believe the ability to assume another's cultural perspective would result in a reduction in ethnocentrism. In the context of assessment this cultural shift in perspective, allowing the examiner to apply the cultural worldview of the child's culture, reduces the potential for ethnocentric bias undermining the integrity of the assessment process.

Examiner's Awareness of Cultural Aspects of Assessment Procedures

The third major area of cultural competency is the examiner's awareness of the cultural implications of psychological assessments and the examiner's ability to implement culturally appropriate assessment procedures. This kind of competency would require that the examiner be aware of the underlying assumptions of the assessment procedures. Many assumptions underlying assessment procedures are culturally determined (e.g., preference for subdued behavior, abstract thought, etc.). That is, an assessment procedure may have been implicitly developed for one particular cultural population, although this may not have been an explicit intention. In addition, there may be important cultural features of a referral that may not be addressed by traditional assessment procedures. For example, a child may have been referred for assessment because of some behavioral problems and it may be that the behavioral problems originated in response to cultural mistrust or some cultural discrimination within the setting. If the original developers had not considered the potential for cross-cultural conflict as being a possible source of the child's problem, the assessment may not provide guidelines that would allow for this kind of contextual information to be gathered.

Perhaps more important, there may be critical modifications for tailoring assessments for a cross-cultural context. For example, additional time or procedures may be required to develop the necessary rapport in a cross-cultural context that may not be required in a monocultural context. Somewhat relatedly, there may be necessary adjustments in order to ensure cultural equivalence when generalizing cross-culturally. For example, in order to ensure cultural appropriateness of the procedures, the examiner may need to translate some of the concepts into the child's native language in order for the assessment results to be accurate. Additionally, there may be some procedures indigenous to the child's culture that could be implemented that may provide the most relevant information about the psychological functioning of the child. For example, in extended kinship contexts, the examiner may need to include more than the "nuclear family" in the procedures and include, for example, *padrinos* (godparents), religious leaders, or other influential persons in the child's socialization.

Examiner Competencies for Working with Linguistic Minority Children

In order to conduct valid assessments with bilingual children, Lopez (1997) recommends that the examiner have substantial proficiency in each of the child's languages, be knowledgeable about practices of nonbiased assessment, and have intimate experience with the child's linguistic group. Although these guidelines may seem ambitious, these guidelines have been implicitly followed for the assessment of nonminority language children.

In practice, the examiner of language minority children may not possess all of the requisite skills. To compensate, examiners have relied on interpreters to have the necessary language skills and familiarity with the cultural features of the linguistic group (Lopez, 1997). However, preliminary research suggests there are several problems with the use of interpreters in psychological assessments. Frequently, interpreters may lack critical information about principles of nonbiased assessment or may not have the professional knowledge necessary to make appropriate translations. Lopez (1992; cited in Lopez, 1997) found that interpreters made substantial changes in the meaning of test and interview items. In most situations, it is unlikely that the examiner would be aware of these translation problems. Hence, examiners would be unable to detect the erroneous and potentially misleading information. Lopez and Rooney (1997) found that schools rely on informal and unsystematic procedures for involving interpreters in assessment situations.

Even when the examiner may be bilingual, linguistic differences between the test and the child is not solved by the examiner translating the standardized test instrument (Braken & Barona, 1991). Test directions are often too technical for most "on the spot" translations, translated items rarely reflect equivalent meanings, and underlying constructs may not be equivalent across linguistic groups. Lopez (1997) suggested that the use of interpreters be "the absolute last resort." The long-range solution frequently recommended for appropriate assessment of language minority children is the training of bilingual examiners and development of instruments either indigenous to the child's linguistic group or thoroughly standardized on a wide variety of ELM populations (Lopez, 1997). Until there are more trained bilingual examiners, examiners need to be very strategic in the collection of information about the child, rely on multiple sources, make observations in different contexts, scrutinize the appropriateness of norms and standardized procedures, and work with multidisciplinary assessment and treatment teams which include bilingual, language, and cultural experts (Lopez, 1997; Ortiz, 1997).

To reiterate, cultural competencies of examiners requires that they become aware of how their own cultural and linguistic background affects their professional behavior, attitudes, judgments, and values. Cultural competence also requires that examiners become intimately aware of the way in which culture and language influences children's behaviors, attitudes, values, and experiences. Finally, examiners should be aware of the way in which culture and language influences the assessment procedures they use. In the next section we turn our attention to cultural and linguistic characteristics of children and in the subsequent section we discuss the cultural characteristics of the assessment procedures as further elaboration of the necessary features of cultural competency in assessment.

CULTURAL AND LINGUISTIC CHARACTERISTICS
OF THE CHILD

One of the most important features of cultural competency in the assessment process is for examiners to be able to integrate their awareness of the cultural characteristics of the child into the assessment process. Gibbs and Huang (1998) indicate four specific ways in which the child's culture can influence the assessment process: (1) Culture influences the child's belief systems about behaviors and characteristics associated with adjustment, (2) culture influences how disorders (e.g., fear, depression, guilt, anger) are expressed and manifested, (3) culture influences help-seeking behaviors, and (4) culture influences treatment acceptability and responsivity to treatment. Clearly, the child's culture has a significant impact on the assessment process.

There are many cultural characteristics associated with ELM children. We present several frameworks for conceptualizing characteristics that may have important implications to working with cultural and linguistic minority children. Specifically, in this section we address primary cultural characteristics (Ogbu, 1994), which are those characteristics in a culture group (e.g., Mexican Americans) that are manifest prior to contact with another cultural group (e.g., whites in the United States) and acculturation processes (Berry, 1993) that often mediate the manifestation of culture in children's behavior.

Primary Cultural Characteristics

Primary cultural characteristics are distinguished from secondary cultural characteristics in that the former occur prior to contact between the cultural groups whereas secondary cultural characteristics occur because of, or in response to the cultural contact between the cultural groups. Secondary cultural characteristics are discussed in a later section of this chapter. Examples of primary cultural characteristics of Mexican Americans would be Spanish and cultural values that can be traced to Mexico. In contrast, secondary cultural characteristics cannot be traced to cultural origins and arise out of the contact with another cultural group (Ogbu, 1994). For example, the mixture of Spanish and English, giving rise to "Spanglish," used by some Mexican Americans resulted from contact with English-speaking populations in the United States and could be considered a secondary cultural characteristic. Obviously, primary cultural characteristics will be most pronounced with those populations having strongest connections to their culture of origin (e.g., recent immigrants) and will be less characteristic of those populations having distant connections with their culture of origin. We would like to emphasize that *the origin of many, if not all, of these cultural characteristics can be traced to adaptation to environmental conditions.* Consequently, we view cultural differences as primarily different solutions to life's challenges.

One particularly important framework for understanding primary cultural characteristics is based on the extensive cross-cultural work of Triandis and colleagues (e.g., Triandis, Bontempo, Villareal, Asai, & Lucca, 1988). They have identified the individualism/collectivism continuum as a critical dimension with which to characterize cultural differences across many cultural groups around the world. Although most of the dominant cultures within the United States, as well as Northern and Western Europe are based on individualistic cultural orientations, most (estimated to be approximately 70%) of the world's population is considered collectivistic in orientation (Greenfield, 1994). Many of the ELM children in the United States may be more collectivistic in orientation than their nonminority peers. We present a summary of differences between individualistic and collectivistic orientations in Table 15.2, which is based on research described by Triandis and colleagues (1988). Although this summary represents general trends, it is important to note that most cultures represent integration of individualistic and collectivistic characteristics and that, within any culture, individuals may vary widely across this individualistic/collectivistic continuum. Cross-cultural research suggests that there are, nonetheless, general trends that make this framework useful in broadly conceptualizing general differences between cultures.

TABLE 15.2 Comparison of Individualistic and Collectivist Cultural Orientations

Dimensions	Individualistic orientation	Collectivistic orientation
Main emphasis	In-groups are chosen to be compatible with individual's interest	Individuals are encouraged to be compatible in-group
Values	Hedonism Achievement Self-direction Social power Stimulation	Group harmony Conformity Security Tradition
Common problems	Loneliness and alienation High rates of criminality and divorce	Restrictive conformity Economic problems may result from resistance to innovations
Antecedents	Affluence Geographic and social mobility Many immigrants Economic structure based on innovation	Security of resource Large families Economic structure based on cooperation (e.g., agriculture)
Socialization goals	Independence and autonomy Creativity Expression of individuality	Obedience to in-group Duty and sacrifice for the group Cooperation Interdependence
Relationship patterns	Many short-term relationships and acquaintances	Relatively few relationships which are stable but often not chosen by individual

Note. Compiled from Triandis et al. (1988).

Although ELM cultural groups within the United States vary in adherence to collectivistic goals, most are more collectivistic, in a general manner, than white children in the United States. For example, some Asian (e.g., Japanese, Chinese, Korean) cultures, in particular, tend to emphasize group harmony, personal modesty, obedience to authority, and filial piety. Children who are descendants of Latin Americans tend to value respect, preserving dignity, and cooperation (Triandis et al., 1988). Research has found, for example, that Latino children in the United States were willing to share lunch money even with peers that they did not like (Rotheram-Borus & Phinney, 1990). Some African-descent children may be socialized toward individual expressiveness (e.g., demonstrate individual talents), but be collectivistic in many other characteristics (Boykin, 1986). Some American Indian tribes (e.g., Navajos) tended to emphasize holistic cognitive processing (Tharp, 1994). Clearly, there are many more cultural differences between and within ethnic and linguistic cultural groups in the United States than we can describe here, but interested readers may wish to find other sources detailing these cultural differences (e.g., Greenfield & Cocking, 1994).

Acculturation

Research on ELM groups indicates that there are important sources of variation within each ethnic and linguistic group on the presence of primary cultural characteristics. Indeed, the framework on acculturation has been instrumental in identifying key forms of variation on cultural characteristics that have important implications for psychological assessment (Velasquez, 1998). Acculturation refers to the process of adjustment and adaptation that occurs when two cultural groups have contact. This contact often arises out of immigration, migration, or other sociological trends. Although traditionally we usually think of minority cultural or immigrant groups adjusting or adapting to the dominant cultural groups, Berry (1993) emphasizes that acculturation processes affect both minority and dominant groups.

The strongest markers of the degree of acculturation to dominant cultural norms are the child's language ability and usage, the length of stay in the dominant culture of the child or the child's family, and the extent of exposure to members of the dominant culture. Children whose first language is that of the dominant culture tend to be more acculturated than are children whose first language is not. Similarly, those children who are fluent in the language of the minority culture tend to be less acculturated than are children who are not fluent. The generational status of the child or the child's family is often associated with the level of acculturation to dominant culture, with those recent immigrants being less acculturated than are second- or third-generation families. Finally, the degree of the child's extended and intimate exposure to members of the dominant culture tend to be associated with acculturation status. Those children who live in integrated neighborhoods tend to be more acculturated than are those who live in segregated ethnic enclaves. For any individual child, these sociological markers of acculturation need to be supplemented with a more individualized exploration of the child's behavioral, social, attitudinal, and ideological dimensions of acculturation.

Several theorists have articulated psychological implications of Berry's (1993) essentially sociological framework. Importantly, LaFromboise, Coleman, and Gerton (1993) have suggested that attention be given to a particular dimension of acculturation: the process of second-culture acquisition. By this term, LaFromboise and colleagues refer to the process by which a second culture is learned and adopted. LaFromboise and colleagues and Coleman (1995) identified several strategies for coping with cultural diversity, which range from cultural segregation to assimilation to bicultural integration. Examiners could use this framework to understand the way in which an ELM child or family is coping with cultural diversity. Those that cope by separating or segregating themselves from other cultural groups may do so in response to racism and discrimination (Quintana, Vera, & Cooper, 1999). For these children, it seems important for the examiner to consider the role of racism, the child's perception of it, and the child's response to it in the assessment process. For other ELM children, there may be an attempt to assimilate into the dominant culture by adopting the characteristics of the dominant group while abandoning or losing the cultural characteristics of their own group. Between these two extreme orientations to coping with diversity there are a range of strategies for integrating the two cultures. Some may choose to interact only with the dominant culture for expedient purposes (access available resources in dominant culture). Others may choose to try to fuse the two cultures by including components of each culture in their social relationships and activities.

A particularly important means of coping with the cultural diversity for children of immigrant parents is the alternation strategy. Children of immigrant parents are often exposed to two very different cultures: (1) dominant school culture and (2) their parent's culture. For these children, it seems difficult, if not impossible, to try to fuse the two cultures in a meaningful fashion and they find themselves alternating between the two cultures. The alternation strategy involves, for example, the child conforming to the school culture when at school and following their parent's cultural patterns while at home. Although this strategy may be particularly viable for children of immigrants, other cultural groups may also benefit from using this strategy. In a recent study, Quintana and colleagues (1999) found that African American children following the alternation strategy evidenced positive signs of adjustment in their cultural coping.

There are important implications of the cultural characteristics and acculturation status of children for the assessment process. These cultural characteristics influence children's interpersonal behavior with instructors, examiners, and with peers (Rotheram-Borus & Phinney, 1990). These characteristics also influence parental beliefs, values, and expectations about their children's education. For example, Okagaki and Sternberg (1993) found that immigrant (Cambodian, Mexican, Filipino, and Vietnamese) parents valued children's conforming to external standards more than they valued autonomous behavior. Okagaki and Sternberg also found that noncognitive (e.g., deference to teachers) variables were as or more important to immigrant parents' conception of intelligence as were cognitive factors for their young children. Hence, cultural characteristics influence parental expectations of their children and the educational system. It is critical for examiners to evaluate the individual child's adherence to, and departure from, the cultural characteristics of their ELM community.

Linguistic Considerations of Children

Linguistic ability varies considerably for all children in the United States who are raised in homes in which standard English may not have been the dominant language. Children from limited English proficiency (LEP) homes may not develop fluency in English prior to their entry into elementary schools. Fortunately, there has been important research into second-language acquisition that has identified several trends in the development of verbal and academic skills. Unfortunately, there has been relatively little research into the implications of second-language acquisition specific for assessment purposes.

Research into second-language acquisition has made an important distinction between development of second language (e.g., English) and the development of verbal reasoning and understanding of academic concepts. This distinction is, of course, unnecessary when developing curricula for children whose native language is the dominant language. However, for bilingual children the development of advanced verbal and academic concepts may be in either their first or second language. In the United States, educators attempting to promote the English language skills of children have often recommended to parents of LEP children—who often themselves have only limited proficiency in English—that they speak more English to their children (Ortiz, 1997). This recommendation can have an ironic effect. To explain, LEP parents may be unable to provide the critical language stimulation for advanced verbal concepts in English that they could provide in their native language. In these cases, children may be robbed of an important source of language stimulation which potentially stunts their language development. Hence, parents should be advised to speak more, not less, of the child's native language in order to provide complex and stimulating language models for their children and thereby stimulate children's cognitive and intellectual development (Ortiz, 1997). The development of children's verbal skills in their native language promotes, not hinders, their academic achievement in English (Cummins, 1984).

Similarly, research investigating bilingual education suggests those children with late entry into English classrooms, compared to children who had early entry into English immersion classrooms, had high scores on achievement skills (e.g., reading, math), even though these skills were assessed in English (see Padilla et al., 1991). This pattern of findings contradicts prevalent views that early immersion in educational environments in which English is dominant promotes academic skills. Conversely, research suggests that proficiency in children's native language is a critical basis for learning English proficiency (Cummins, 1984). Several principles of second-language acquisition adapted from Lopez (1997) and Ortiz (1997) are worth noting (see Table 15.3).

Ortiz (1997) and Stockman (1986) invite us to generalize the principles of second-language acquisition to those situations in which children are exposed to Black

TABLE 15.3 Important Principles of Working with Linguistic Minority Children

1. Learning a second language is facilitated by exposure to natural, contextualized communication.
2. The quality of language exposure is as or more important than the quantity of exposure.
3. Maintenance of native language can facilitate, rather than retard, development of a second language.
4. Learning a second language can lead to the temporary regression of language skills in the first language.
5. Bilingual children may process information easier in a second language, even if this isn't their dominant language.

Note. Compiled from Lopez (1997) and Ortiz (1997).

English rather than standard English as the main basis for oral and written communication prior to beginning formal schooling. Clearly, it is critical for those conducting assessments and making recommendations for language minority children to become familiar with research on second-language acquisition.

Several practical guidelines have been recommended for psychologists in conducting assessments for bilingual and limited English proficiency children. First, it is critical that the child's language dominance be determined as well as the child's level of English proficiency. It is critical not to assume that the child's native language will be his or her dominant language. For example, as children are exposed to a second language, linguistic skills in their first language may regress (see Lopez, 1997). Consequently, the level of proficiency in each of the child's languages needs to be assessed prior to formal assessment. The assessment of language proficiency should be conducted in different contexts as language usage may vary depending on context (with family at home, with peers in recreation, in formal classrooms, etc.). In addition to estimating the general level of proficiency in each language, children can be assessed for the dynamic integration of linguistic skills. For example, children may prefer their first language for social contexts, but rely on their second language skills for academic tasks, especially if they learned these academic skills in their second language. Results obtained from assessments conducted in one language may not be replicated when the child is assessed in another language. For example, examiners have noted that bilingual children performed higher in a nondominant language than they did when assessed in their apparent dominant language. Research into the psychological assessment in which bilingual clients were interviewed in English and in their native language suggest that the ratings of level of pathology varied across the two languages (see Padilla et al., 1991). Similarly, Malgady (1998) found significant differences among ratings of pathology across English, Spanish, and bilingual interviews for the same clients. Hence, the current state of science does not allow examiners to assess bilingual children with the same level of consistency or reliability that there is for monolingual children.

CULTURAL NATURE OF ASSESSMENT PROCEDURES

Assessment instruments and procedures develop and are embedded within particular cultural contexts. The assessment technology necessarily reflects that cultural context. Although the cultural embededness of assessment technology is not problematic per se, the cultural embeddedness becomes potentially problematic when the assessment technology is applied to another cultural context. Consequently, we review some of the cultural characteristics of traditional assessment methodologies and review several recent innovations in assessment procedures that have important implications for ELM children.

Normative-Based Assessment

Several kinds of traditional assessment formats have been found to be problematic when applied to ELM populations. Standardized testing procedures exemplify the attempt to identify norms and to evaluate individuals based on their departure from the norms. These norms are often based on a predominately white population and the use of the tests often implicitly assume that adjustment (e.g., academic achievement) requires the same kind of characteristics in ELM populations as is required in nonminority populations.

Several strategies have been employed to redress the problems with norm-referenced or standardized testing for ELM populations. The movement to increase the demographic representativeness of the standardization population is laudable, but does not ensure the cultural appropriateness of the assessment. Specifically, greater representativeness in the standardization sample increases the precision with which the norm represents the larger society or population, but does not increase the utility of the test when applied to subpopulations. An example could illustrate: Although the inclusion of a group of children who do not speak English could be included in a standardization sample (proportionate to their representation in the population) of an English version standardized achievement test, their inclusion does not ensure that the results would be valid for them.

Other strategies to redress cultural problems with standardized assessments have been to strip cultural features from the test items. Specifically, test developers have attempted to modify items to be less culturally biased. Although important, these modifications rarely address the underlying cultural assumptions of the assessment instrument. Usually these assumptions involve what behavior or characteristics are considered normal or appropriate. These assumptions fail to take into account great variability in children and fail to consider that the goal of conforming to the generalized norm may not be possible or even desirable for some ELM children. A second strategy, to strip the cultural bias from assessment instruments has been to use instruments, such as nonverbal assessments, that are void of apparent cultural or linguistic bias. These include projective assessments as well as nonverbal assessments of intelligence. On the surface, these assessments appear to be nondiscriminatory. However, analysis of test bias often suggests that many of these so-called nondiscriminatory or nonverbal tests are actually more biased than are traditional assessment procedures (see, e.g., Suzuki &Valencia, 1997). Hence, stripping culture from the test items does little to address the embeddedness of culture within the assessment device.

Many of these concerns about the cultural appropriateness related to traditional assessment procedures are not specific to standardized assessments. Although standardized assessments rely on explicit norms or normative groups, implicit norms are often a component of nonstandardized assessment procedures. In behavioral assessment, implicit norms may involve, for example, rater's expectations about children's behavior (i.e., what kind of behavior is judged acceptable or appropriate). Teachers and psychologists may have acquired expectations about appropriate student behavior and these expectations may dictate referral for assessment or intervention. These expectations and implicit norms are often socially constructed and reflect the cultural values and experiences of the educators. When implicit norms developed in one cultural context are applied to other cultural contexts problems can arise. Baker and O'Neil (1996) provide a good illustration. They suggest that raters' valuing of "subdued and controlled" behavior may inappropriately affect their ratings of African American children. Although avoiding the problems associated with explicit norms, behavioral assessment procedures may still rely on implicit norms that have been culturally or socially constructed.

Innovative Assessment Procedures

There are two strategies attempting to increase the cultural appropriateness of psychological assessments for ELM populations: (1) recent innovative assessment strategies and (2) culturally centered assessments. The first strategy to address appropriate assessment across cultural groups is based on several trends in educational practices toward dynamic, individualized, and authentic assessment. Each of these practices redress problems with standardized assessment in one of several ways. The first kind of innovation involves the interaction of diagnosis, assessment, and intervention. Traditionally, there was an apparent assumption that accurate diagnosis held the key to effective intervention. The role of the assessment, therefore, was to yield an accurate diagnosis. Extending this assumption of the role of diagnosis to ELM populations would be that similar assessment procedures would yield accurate diagnosis across ELM and non-ELM populations and that similar diagnoses would implicate similar interventions across populations.

Conversely, dynamic assessment (Lidz, 1997) avoids this assumption about the universality of treatment response. Specifically, dynamic assessment modifies the traditional assessment–intervention strategy with a more interactive relationship between assessment and intervention. The dynamic assessment embeds the intervention within the assessment process in order to link more explicitly assessment with intervention implications. Indeed, the usual process of dynamic assessment is *pretest–intervention–posttest* or *intervention–posttest* (Lidz, 1997), where intervention is inextricably connected to the assessment process. In this way, the focus of assessment is not on the child's deficits or prior achievement, but is on the child's process of learn-ing, the barriers to the child's learning, and the child's individualized style of learning. This kind of strategy seems particularly appropriate for diverse populations because it avoids some of the culturally embedded assumptions involved in linking diagnosis to intervention that was endemic to the traditional medical model. Preliminary research supports the utility of dynamic assessment for ELM populations (e.g., Jitendra & Rohena-Diaz, 1996; Peña, 1998). This kind of assessment procedure seems particu-larly appropriate for behavioral assessment because behavioral observations could be used to monitor response to various interventions. These observations could be used to reconceptualize and individually tailor intervention strategies.

The second innovation involves reconceptualization of the role of examiner as an objective expert. In reaction to traditional views of the examiner's purported ob-jectivity and expertness, Fischer (1985) developed individualized assessment that emphasizes the examiner working collaboratively with clients in drawing conclusions and interpreting the assessment data. For example, she would provide copies of the assessment reports to clients for their reactions and include their reactions as an addendum to her reports. Additionally, resisting the general tendency of writing tech-nical assessment reports that were intended only for other professionals, Fischer writes reports so that clients could understand, respond to, and directly benefit from the findings. In this way, the examiner collaborated actively with clients at nearly every phase of the assessment process from prereferral, through collecting assessment re-sults, and finally disposition of the assessment report. These procedures described by Fischer (1985) seem particularly appropriate when working with ELM popula-tions. By instilling collaborative efforts, examiners could redress problems of disen-franchisement that can occur with ELM populations in the assessment process. Col-laborative efforts may also instill greater motivation for ELM populations in the interventions that are implicated by individualized assessment. Additionally, behav-ioral assessment is well suited to take advantage of individualizing assessment strat-egy discussed by Fischer. Indeed, the findings of behavioral assessment can usually be explained in nontechnical terms that can be readily understood by clients who have various educational backgrounds. Additionally, clients can be involved in the behavioral assessment in a collaborative manner. For example, clients (older chil-dren or parents) may be involved by making self-observations to supplement those made by others. In many other ways, clients could be involved in each phase of the behavioral assessment procedure.

Finally, the educational movement embracing authentic assessment also offers some innovations that could be easily incorporated within behavioral assessment and can have important implications for working with ELM populations. In authentic assessment, there is focus on (1) the skills and abilities that resemble those used outside of the classroom (i.e., "real-world" skills), (2) providing children with the opportu-nity to practice and learn those skills that will be assessed, (3) providing children with preliminary feedback on their performance as a way of attaining the desired skills, and (4) providing children with knowledge of the criteria used to evaluate their per-formance (Tombari & Borich, 1998). As in dynamic assessment, authentic assess-ment is used to facilitate performance and that feedback is provided to guide future performance. Additionally, the child is provided explicit information about what is going to be assessed and is involved directly in the process by which he/she is evaluated. These guidelines seem particularly applicable to behavioral assessment. Behavioral observations could be made in the child's environment with ongoing feedback being provided to the child and parents to assist the child in promoting his or her behavioral adjustment. Additionally, the behavioral criteria used to evaluate children could be communicated to them, thereby potentially instilling motivation and cooperation with the assessment process. Moreover, to integrate behavioral and authentic assessment approaches, it would be important that the behavioral criterion be formulated such that the behaviors reflect authentic or real-world adjustment. Criteria for authentic behavioral adjustment may need to be modeled after members of the child's cultural or ethnic group who are successful. Because of the novelty of these innovative procedures, more work is required in order to more fully integrate the implications of these innovations with behavioral assessment. These remain exciting avenues of research and treatment.

Culturally Centered Assessment Procedures

The innovations involved in individualized, dynamic, and authentic assessment procedures redress implicit cultural assumptions that made traditional assessment procedures problematic for ELM populations. In essence, these procedures address problematic cultural assumptions of the traditional procedures, thereby making assessment procedures less ethnocentric. Another assessment strategy recommended for ELM populations is to embed the assessment within the child's culture instead of stripping culture from the assessment procedures. Indeed, the cultural foundation of assessment procedures is not problematic per se—rather, problems occur when the cultural foundation for an assessment is inappropriately applied to another culture. One good example of embedding culture explicitly within the assessment procedures is the Tell Me A Story (TEMAS; Constantino, Malgady, & Rogler, 1986). Constantino and colleagues have developed and evaluated TEMAS, which is essentially a cultural revision and extension of the thematic apperception tests (e.g., Thematic Apperception Test, TAT; Murray, 1943; or Children's Apperception Test, CAT). The TEMAS, instead of stripping culture from the items, includes test material (pictures and scenes) that are particularly appropriate for the target population (in this case, inner-city children). Additionally, the TEMAS draws on the rich cultural foundation of folklore and story-telling traditions in ELM populations, especially among Puerto Rican populations. The TEMAS provides an example of the utility of centering the assessment procedures within the child's culture.

Multicultural Assessment Model

Ridley, Li, and Hill (1998) have proposed a model for multicultural assessment that describes a process for integrating cultural information into either traditional assessment or innovative assessment formats (see Table 15.4). This model includes four phases: (1) identify cultural data, (2) interpret cultural data, (3) incorporate cultural data, and (4) formulate a sound assessment decision. During the first phase cultural data are collected and identified. The cultural data can be obtained from children, parents, teachers, or others who are familiar with the child and his or her cultural environment. It is important that multiple data-collecting methods be used to avoid neglecting important kinds of information. To illustrate, consider an assessment conducted with a child using an alternation strategy to cope with cultural diversity. If data were only obtained from school, the child's other cultural frame of reference could not be incorporated into the assessment. Similarly, if a bilingual child was only observed while engaged in academic tasks, the child's linguistic preferences and abilities in social contexts may not be reflected in the assessment. Consequently, involving multiple sources in collecting cultural information can provide a more complete cultural context for the child.

The second phase involves interpreting the cultural data. Several features of the cultural data need to be considered and distinguished. The examiner must differentiate characteristics that are idiosyncratic to the child from characteristics that are specific to the child's cultural group (Ridley et al., 1998). This kind of differentiation may require the examiner to be intimately familiar with the child's cultural group. Examiners may also need to differentiate characteristics of the child's cultural group that have developed in response to acculturation experiences from those characteristics that occurred prior to contact with the nonminority cultural groups. For example, children of refugee parents might manifest many of the characteristics associated with the acculturation process whereas parents might manifest more strongly the primary cultural characteristics that occurred prior to their becoming refugees. While cultural data are being interpreted, the examiner may wish to consult with the child, the child's parents, and other members of the child's cultural group to add perspective to that of the examiner. Finally, during the interpretation phase, examiners formulate working hypotheses about the role of culture and language in the child's overall adjustment.

The third phase of the multicultural assessment model involves integrating the working hypotheses concerning the child's cultural context with the working hypothesis formulated from the findings of traditional sources of assessment. For example, when a child is referred for assessment by a teacher, the examiner may need to integrate the formulations about the role of culture in the child's life with the informa-

TABLE 15.4   Ridley et al.'s Multicultural Assessment System

Phase 1:	Identify cultural data
	Collect salient clinical information
Phase 2:	Interpret cultural data
	Formulate working hypotheses
Phase 3:	Incorporate cultural data
	Test working hypotheses
Phase 4:	Arrive at sound assessment decision

tion provided by the referral source. This is particularly important when the referral source has failed to adequately consider the cultural context of the child. In some cases, the cultural information may be more crucial than that provided by the traditional assessment sources. In other cases, the cultural information may have little relevance for the assessment (Ridley et al., 1998). Nonetheless, the process of identifying, formulating, and incorporating cultural information into the assessment process allows for the final phase in the multicultural assessment model—arriving at a sound assessment decision. This fourth phase represents the culmination of considering and integrating cultural information along with other personal and individual information about the child. Ridley and colleagues emphasize that at this phase, as well as each of the previous phases, it is critical that examiners invoke debiasing strategies. These debiasing strategies attempt to correct for some potential biases in the assessment process. Research into assessment decision making suggests pernicious problems (Spengler & Strohmer, 1994). Examiners may be particularly susceptible to a confirmatory bias in which their preliminary hypotheses are confirmed prior to searching for or reviewing disconfirming information. Consequently, it is important for examiners to withhold making conclusions or decisions about intervention until all of the information has been considered. Importantly, for our purposes, it is critical that examiners devote substantial effort to proceeding through the phases of the multicultural assessment model prior to reaching conclusion about the children they are assessing.

In summary, we recommend that behavioral assessments not be stripped of culture, but reflect the culture of the target population. Some of the ways in which culture may be reflected in the assessment process include the cultural background of the examiner, the language or linguistic style used by examiner, the contexts in which behavioral observations are made, the goal of the behavioral assessment, and the cultural framework used to interpret behavior. Ridley and colleagues' (1998) four phases could supplement more traditional assessment procedures by incorporating an explicit cultural framework for the assessment of ELM children. Several recent innovations in educational assessment provide useful heuristics for planning the assessment procedures. Dynamic, authentic, and individualized assessments provide promising guidelines. Finally, normative-based assessment using either explicit norms (standardized tests) or implicit norms need to be used very carefully with ELM children.

CULTURAL NATURE OF THE ASSESSMENT CONTEXT

Many have advocated the value of ecologically based or contextually based assessment procedures (e.g., Armour-Thomas & Gopaul-McNichol, 1997). Ecological assessment approaches emphasize the impact on children's behavior of the cultural nature of the various environments in which the child is engaged. An ecological, integrative model conceptualizing the developmental context of ethnic minority children has been articulated by García Coll et al. (1996). They have identified environmental factors that promote, but also inhibit children's adjustment and development. These ecological factors include environmental stress resulting from segregation (residential, economic, social, and psychological), discrimination (racism, oppression, and prejudice), local communities (neighborhoods and schools), and social services (medical care and psychological services). These ecological factors may impact the assessment process in important ways, either as a possible contributing factor to a behavioral problem, influencing the process for referral for behavioral assessment, and affecting recommendations, or interventions implicated by the assessment process. A review of each of these ecological factors is beyond the scope of this chapter, but we focus on two important ecological considerations for psychological assessment: (1) the school environment and (2) the ELM community.

Cultural Nature of School Environments

Culture influences school environments as much as it does children. Indeed, school environments can be classified according to the acculturation framework previously discussed. U.S. schools usually reflect assimilation orientations toward ELM populations (Rotheram-Borus, 1993; Fordham, 1988; Delpit, 1995). An assimilation orientation is reflected in the pressure within schools for ELM groups to assimilate to the behavior, language, values, and norms of the dominant group (Delpit, 1995; Fordham, 1988). This pressure to assimilate takes the forms of encouraging behaviors that conform to dominant cultural and linguistic norms (Delpit, 1995) or discouraging the maintenance of ELM culture or languages (Fordham, 1988). Assimilation orientations have been promoted by sociopolitical trends in the United States, including the passage of *English Only* legislation as well as the political undermining of effective bilingual education programs (Padilla et al., 1991). Cultural differences between school environments and ELM children potentially pose several kinds of problems in the assessment process.

First, educators use culturally derived behavioral norms that may reflect their own or the school's cultural orientation. These norms may conflict with those derived from the child's ELM community. Research has documented important differences across cultural groups in the determination of which behaviors are problematic as well as the bandwidth for behavioral norms (Crijnen, Achenbach, & Verhulst, 1997). For example, Lambert and colleagues (1992) found cultural differences in the threshold for behavioral problems as judged by Jamaican and U.S. parents, teachers, and clinicians. Jamaican raters were more tolerant of a wider range of behavior in children before considering the behavior problematic, compared to U.S. raters. Similarly, research has found that whereas white children prefer academic environments that are quiet and subdued over those that are vibrant and active, the reverse pattern was characteristic of African American children (Bell, 1994; Boykin & Allen, 1988). Moreover, Weisz and Weiss (1991) found significant cultural differences for "referability" of child problems. Referability refers to the ratio of the frequency of a behavior pattern being referred for professional attention divided by the incidence of the behavior pattern in the population. Undercontrolled behavioral problems (e.g., swearing, lying, cheating, arguing) were referred for treatment or assessment in the United States more often than in Thailand; there were no cultural differences for overcontrolled behavioral problems (e.g., depression). Hence, the U.S. culture in general, and school cultures within U.S. schools in particular, may be less tolerant of undercontrolled behavioral problems compared to other cultures. Psychological examiners could benefit from being cognizant of potential incompatibility between the cultural norms of the school and those of ELM communities — otherwise, a problem may be attributed exclusively to the child's behavior rather than being viewed as a conflict between the child's culture and the school's culture.

A second way in which cultural differences between the school and children's culture need to be considered in the assessment process is when there is pressure within the school environment for children to assimilate. Parents may resist this assimilation pressure by not cooperating with a school system that they may feel is undermining their culture. Children, especially youth in secondary schools, may resist assimilation pressure by accentuating cultural and linguistic differences between themselves and the larger school community as a way of expressing the sense of "differentness" that they feel (Davidson, 1996). This expression of differentness is the adolescent's way of maintaining a sense of identity that is threatened by the assimilation pressure of the school environment. This expression of differentness may take the form of noncompliance with the rules dictated by the school or instructor (Davidson, 1996).

Third, cultural differences between the school environment and children may increase the likelihood that children experience prejudice, discrimination, or other forms of oppression. Numerous surveys have documented the widespread prevalence of racism and discrimination toward ELM groups in U.S. society (e.g., Sears, 1988). Researchers have suggested that although the prevalence of blatant racial bias (i.e., old-fashioned racism) may be declining, it has not disappeared. Indeed, recent surveys have suggested the most common focus of hate crimes is racial bias. Nonetheless, researchers (e.g., Sears, 1988) have suggested that subtle, symbolic, or modern forms of racism may be more prevalent and pernicious. Modern forms of racism differ from old-fashioned racism in that the latter involves categorical rejection of persons based on racial status. Conversely, modern forms of racism do not involve this categorical rejection, but do involve selective denigration of persons based not on racial status per se, but on the extent to which persons manifest the perceived cultural characteristics of their racial group (Jhally & Lewis, 1992). To illustrate, modern racism involves denigrating an African American, for example, *not* because he or she is black per se, but because he or she may *act* "black." In this example, acting "black" is usually represented as those characteristics that are perceived as violating dominant values (e.g., work ethic), norms (e.g., law-abiding), and ideology (Sears, 1988; Jhally & Lewis, 1992).

Authorities within the school system are not likely to be immune to the biases and prejudices characteristic of the larger society. Research suggests that teachers may respond differently to ELM children than to white children (e.g., Simpson and Erickson, 1983; Aaron & Powell, 1982). Dusek and Joseph (1983) meta-analyzed 77 studies and found that teacher interactions with ELM children reflected lower expectations, less praise, and greater criticism when compared to teacher interactions with white children. Olsen (1988) reported that a third of her sample of Mexican American students reported being victims of prejudice from teachers. Children become aware of prejudice affecting their lives during elementary school (Quintana, 1994; 1998).

Research also suggests that psychologists' clinical judgments are susceptible to racial bias. For example, white psychologists ascribe greater pathology, more symptomology, and lower prognosis for African American clients, when compared to ratings of African American psychologists (e.g., Atkinson et al., 1996). Hence, racial bias may lead to the overdiagnosing of behavioral problems in ELM children, particularly those problems reflecting undercontrolled or externalizing behavioral expressions. It is important to note that although prejudice is most readily identifiable in its hostile, judgmental, or prejorative forms, prejudice can also be reflected in patronizing or paternalistic attitudes (Quintana, 1995). Patronizing attitudes may lead examiners to fail to identify legitimate problems in ELM children. This tendency is seen as being as much of a problem as is the problem of overdiagnosing ELM populations (Ortiz, 1997; Ridley et al., 1998).

Consequently, it is important that examiners consider the influence on the assessment process of cultural differences between the school environment and ELM children. Referrals for assessment may be made when behavioral norms differ between the person making the referral and the ELM children. In these situations, ELM children or their parents may believe the referral was inappropriate to label the child's behavior as problematic. In some situations, it may be appropriate for examiners to work with the school personnel to revise their cultural expectations for children's behavior or help them revise their pedagogy in order to be compatible with the ELM children in their school. It is also possible that some referrals reflect ethnic bias or stereotyping by the person making the referral. In these situations, it may be important for the examiner first to work with the person making the referral to address this bias. It may be helpful to have an examiner observe the child's behavior, using behavioral norms reflective of the child's ELM group, to detect the presence or absence of a behavioral problem independent of the referral source. It is also possible that prejudice or bias within the school environment is responsible for or contributes to the manifestation of behavioral problems. In these situations, it would seem incomplete for behavioral problems to be addressed in the assessment process without also addressing the prejudice or bias to which the children are exposed. Similarly, in situations in which children's resistance to assimilation pressures contribute to the manifestation of behaviors, it seems important that examiners supplement their assessment of the child with consideration of the assimilation pressures from the school culture.

ELM Communities' Reactions to School Environments

Given the sociopolitical climate in the United States, the prevalence of modern forms of discrimination, and the highly segregated nature of school neighborhoods, it is not unexpected that members of ELM communities would feel mistrust toward school personnel and educational systems. Ogbu (1994) has described historical and structural responses of ELM communities to dominant racial groups. These responses reflect mechanisms used by ELM communities to cope with assimilation pressures as well as perceived prejudice, discrimination, and bias. These coping mechanisms are considered secondary cultural characteristics because they evolve after contact with other ethnic groups and in response to the nature of the intergroup relations. These characteristics are distinguished from the primary cultural characteristics discussed previously, which occurred prior to cross-cultural contact. Conversely, secondary characteristics emerge in response to conflict between ethnic or racial groups. Several theorists have articulated the development of oppositional identities in ELM communities that are indicative of secondary cultural characteristics (e.g., Boykin, 1986; Cross, 1995; Davidson, 1996; Fordham, 1988; Ogbu, 1994). Oppositional identities are characterized by the development of a sense of identity that expresses opposition or resistance to the perceived characteristics of the dominant group. For example, academic achievement may be seen as reflective of the dominant culture and an oppositional identity would involve a disidentification with academic achievement (Steele, 1997). Academic disidentification reflects a disengagement of general self-esteem from academic performance. Osborne (1997) found that academic disidentification began to appear for African-American boys in the eighth grade. Similarly, Steele and Aronson (1995) found that African Americans were vulnerable to stereotype threat in which they underperformed on achievement tests when negative racial stereotypes were activated. Midgley, Arunkumar, and Urdan (1996) found support for the view that stigmatized groups may handicap themselves in anticipation of poor performance on, for example, academic assignments. Examples of handicapping strategies include procrastinating in doing homework and allowing peers to distract the student during class. These self-handicapping strategies function to offer an external source of attribution (e.g., "I didn't have the chance to do well"), rather than an internal attribution (e.g., "I am unable to do well"), which may threaten self-esteem or self-image. The development of oppositional identities and other coping strategies reflect the response to stigmatization and are not only found in groups which are stigmatized because of racial status. Indeed, Crocker and Major (1989) reviewed social-psychological research on the tendency for stigmatized groups to devalue those domains on which nonstigmatized groups are perceived to have superior performance (e.g., academic achievement). These responses have been found to emerge in a wide variety of stigmatization contexts: disability, physical unattractiveness, obesity, sexual orientation, and mental illness. Consequently, sociological, educational, and social-psychological research documents cultural mistrust within ELM communities as well as strategies used to cope with racial and cultural stigmatization.

Clearly, it is important that examiners consider the historical context of relations between ELM communities and the educational system. Indeed, Baker and O'Neil report on their experiences in attempting to enact educational reform (i.e., performance assessment) that they believed would increase the cultural fairness of the educational system for ELM children. They were surprised by the response from the ELM community when the reform was considered to be the "creation of the majority community intended to hold back the progress of disadvantaged children" (Baker & O'Neil, 1996, p. 185). Obviously, the response of the ELM community was not based solely on the nature of the proposed reform, but rather reflected a long history of relations between the ELM community and previous educational initiatives that were viewed as undermining the interests of the community. Psychological examiners are also likely to be perceived as being the latest representative of the educational system. This mistrust could undermine the educational goals being addressed by the behavioral assessment.

We recommend that during the behavioral assessment consideration be given to the roles of the reactions of ELM communities to the school environment in the development of behavioral problems, treatment acceptability, and other aspects of the assessment process. The examiner should consider children's coping with racism, stigmatization, and other ecological factors affecting their adjustment. Examiners should be prepared for ELM children, parents, and community to respond to them as members of the educational system with which there is a long history of interactions that were potentially marked by misunderstanding and mistrust. Examiners may need to make particular efforts to establish credibility before receiving the ELM member's trust and full cooperation. Ideally, examiners should have a history of visible involvement and participation in support of the community. Examiners may need to spend additional time and care in understanding the community's relationship with the educational system. Obviously, it may be improper to assume that the efforts of the examiner will be viewed as serving the interest and benefit of ELM children. Credibility with ELM community is not established simply by being careful not to be discriminatory. Rather, credibility is based on demonstrating that efforts are made to give priority to the welfare of the child. Finally, examiners may need to establish collaborative working relationships with children, parents, and other members of the ELM community in which the interests and welfare of the ELM child is central.

References

Aaron, R., & Powell, G. (1982). Feedback practices as a function of teacher and pupil race during reading groups instruction. *Journal of Negro Education, 51*, 50–59.

Armour-Thomas, E., & Gopaul-McNichol, S. (1997). In search of correlates of learning underlying "learning disability" using a bio-ecological assessment system. *Journal of Social Distress and the Homeless, 6*, 143–159.

Arredondo, P., Toporek, R., Brown, S. P., Jones, J., Locke, D. C., Sanchez, J., & Stadler, H. (1996). Operationalizing of the multicultural counseling competencies. *Journal of Multicultural Counseling and Development, 24*, 42–78.

Atkinson, D. R., Brown, M. T., Parham, T. A., Mattews, L. G., Landrum-Brown, J., & Kim, A. A. (1996). African American client skin tone and clinical judgments of African American and European American Psychologists. *Professional Psychology: Research and Practice, 27*, 500–505.

Baker, E. L., & O'Neil, Jr., H. F. (1996). Performance asssessment and equity. In M. B. Kane & R. Mitchell (Eds.), *Implementing performance assessment: Promises, problems, and challenges.* Mahwah, NJ: Erlbaum.

Bell, Y. R. (1994). A cultural sensitive analysis of Black learning style. *Journal of Black Psychology, 20*, 47–61.

Berry, J. (1993). Ethnic identity in plural societies. In M. E. Bernal & G. P. Knight (Eds.), *Ethnic identity: Formation and transmission among Hispanics and other minorities* (pp. 271–296). Albany, NY: SUNY Press.

Boykin, A. W. (1982). Population differences in the effect of format variability on task performance. *Journal of Black Studies, 12,* 469–485.

Boykin, A. W. (1986). The triple quandary and the schooling of Afro-American children. In V. Neisser (Ed.), *The school achievement of minority children.* Hilldale, NJ: Erlbaum.

Boykin, A. W., & Allen, B. A. (1988). Rhythmic-movement facilitation of learning in working class Afro-American children. *Journal of Genetic Psychology, 149,* 335–347.

Braken, B. A., & Barona, A. (1991). State of the art procedures for translating, validating and using psycho-educational tests in cross-cultural assessment. *School Psychology International, 12,* 119–132.

Coleman, H. L. K. (1995). Strategies for coping with cultural diversity. *Counseling Psychologist, 23,* 722–740.

Constantino, G., Malgady, R., & Rogler, L. (1986). *Standardization and validation of TEMAS, a pluralistic thematic apperception test.* New York: Fordham University, Hispanic Research Center.

Covington, M. V. (1992). *Making the grade: A self-worth perspective on motivation and school reform.* New York: Cambridge University Press.

Crijnen, A. A. M., Achenbach, T. M., & Verhulst, F. C. (1997). Comparisons of problems reported by parents of children in 12 cultures: Total problems, externalizing, and internalizing. *Journal of the American Academy of Child and Adolescent Psychiatry, 9,* 1269–1277.

Crocker, J. & Major, B. (1989). Social stigma and self-esteem: The self-protective properties of stigma. *Psychological Review, 96,* 608–630.

Cross, W. E., Jr. (1995). Oppositional identity and African American Youth: Issues and prospects. In W. D. Hawley & A. W. Jackson (Eds.), *Toward a common destiny: Improving peace and ethnic relations in America.* San Francisco: Jossey-Bass.

Cummins, J. (1984). *Bilingualism and special education: Issues in assessment and pedagogy.* Clevedon, Avon, England: Multilingual Matters.

Davidson, A. L. (1996). *Making and molding identity in schools.* Albany, NY: SUNY Press.

Delpit, L. (1995). *Other people's children: Sociocultural conflict in the classroom.* New York: New Press.

Dusek, J. B., & Joseph, G. (1983). The bases of teacher expectancies: A meta-anlaysis. *Journal of Educational Psychology, 75,* 327–346.

Fischer, C. T. (1985). *Individualizing psychological assessment.* Monterey, CA: Brooks/Cole.

Fordham. S. (1988). Racelessness as a factor in black students' success. *Harvard Educational Review, 58,* 54–84.

García Coll, C., Crnic, K., Lamberty, G., Wasik, B. H., Jenkins, R., García, H. V., & McAdoo, H. P. (1996). An integrative model for the study of developmental competencies in minority children. *Child Development, 67,* 1891–1914.

Gibbs, J. T., & Huang, L. N. (1998) *Children of color: Psychological interventions with culturally diverse youth.* San Francisco: Jossey-Bass.

Graham, S. (1994). Motivation in African Americans. *Review of Educational Research, 64,* 55–117.

Greenfield, P. (1994). Independence and interdependence as developmental scripts. In P. M. Greenfield & R. R. Cocking (Eds.), *Cross-cultural roots of minority child development* (pp. 1–40). Hillsdale, NJ: Erlbaum.

Greenfield, P. M., & Cocking, R. R. (1994). *Cross-cultural roots of minority child development.* Hillsdale, NJ: Erlbaum.

Hall, C. C. I. (1997). Cultural malpractice: The growing obsolescence of psychology with the changing U.S. population. *American Psychologist, 52,* 642–651.

Helms, J. E. (1992). Why is there no study of cultural equivalence in standardized cognitive ability testing? *American Psychologist, 47,* 1083–1101.

Herrnstein, R. J., & Murray, C. (1996). *The bell curve: Intelligence and class structure in American life.* New York: Simon & Schuster.

Jhally, S., & Lewis, J. (1992). *Enlightened racism.* Boulder, CO: Westview Press.

Jitendra, A. K., & Rohena-Diaz, E. (1996). Langauge assessment of students who are linguistically diverse: Why a discrete approach is not the answer. *School Psychology Review, 25,* 40–56.

LaFromboise, T., Coleman, H. L., & Gerton, J. (1993). Psychological impact of biculturalism: Evidence and theory. *Psychological Bulletin, 114,* 395–412.

Lambert, M. C., Weisz, J. R., Knight, F., Desrosiers, M., Overly, K., & Thesiger, C. (1992). Jamaican and American adult perspectives on child psychopathology: Further exploration of the threshold model. *Journal of Consulting and Clinical Psychology, 60*, 146–149.

Lidz, C. S. (1997). Dynamic assessment approaches. In D. P. Flanagan, J. L. Genshaft, & P. L. Harrison (Eds.), *Contemporary intellectual assessment: Theories, tests, and issues* (pp. 281–296). New York: Guilford Press.

Lopez, E. C. (1997). The cognitive assessment of limited English proficient and bilingual children. In D. P. Flanagan, J. L. Genshaft, & P. L. Harrison (Eds.), *Contemporary intellectual assessment: Theories, tests, and issues* (pp. 503– 516). New York: Guilford Press.

Lopez, E. C., & Rooney, M. (1997). A preliminary investigation of the roles of backgrounds of school interpreters: Implications for training and recruiting. *Journal of Social Distress and the Homeless, 6*, 161–175.

Malgady, R. G. (1998). Symptom severity in bilingual Hispanics as a function of clinician ethnicity and language of interview. *Psychological Assessment, 10*, 120–127.

McLoyd, V. C. (1998). Socioeconomic disadvantage and child development. *American Psychologist, 53*, 185–204.

McPhee, D., Kreutzer, J. C., & Fritz, J. J. (1994). Infusing a diversity perspective into human development courses. *Child Development, 65*, 699–715.

Midgley, C., Arunkumar, R., & Urdan, T. C. (1996). "If I don't do well tomorrow, there's a reason": Predictors of adolescents' use of academic self-handicapping strategies. *Journal of Educational Psychology, 88*, 423–434.

Murray, H. A. (1943). *Thematic apperception test manual.* Cambridge, MA: Harvard University Press.

Ogbu, J. U. (1994). From cultural difference to differences in cultural frame of reference. In P. M. Greenfield & R. R. Cocking (Eds.), *Cross-cultural roots of minority child development* (pp. 365–392). Hillsdale, NJ: Erlbaum.

Okagaki, L., & Sternberg, R. J. (1993). Parental beliefs and children's school performance. *Child Development, 64*, 36–56.

Olsen, L. (1988). *Crossing the schoolhouse border: Immigrant students and the California public schools.* Boston: California Tomorrow.

Ortiz, Al. a. (1997). Learning disabilities occurring concomitantly with linguistic differences. *Journal of Learning Disabilities, 30*, 321–332.

Osborne, J. W. (1997). Race and academic disidentification. *Journal of Educational Psychology, 89*, 728–735.

Padilla, A. M., Lindholm, K. J., Chen, A., Durán, R., Hakuta, K., Lambert, W., & Tucker, G. R. (1991). The English-only movement: Myths, reality, and implications for psychology. *American Psychologist, 46*, 120–130.

Padilla, A. M., & Medina, A. (1996). Cross-cultural sensitivity in assessment: Using tests in culturally appropriate ways. In L. A. Suzuki, P. J. Meller, & J. G. Ponterotto (Eds.), *Handbook of multicultural assessment* (pp. 3–28). San Francisco: Jossey-Bass.

Paniagua, F. A. (1994). *Assessing and treating culturally diverse clients: A practical guide.* Thousand Oaks, CA: Sage.

Peña, E. (1998). Dynamic assessment: The model and language applications. In K. Cole, P. Dale, and D. Thal (Eds.), *Advances in assessment of communication and language.* Baltimore: Paul H. Brookes.

Ponterotto, J. G., & Alexander, C. M. (1996). Assessing the multicultural competence of counselors and clinicians. In L. A. Suzuki, P. J. Meller, & J. G. Ponterotto (Eds.), *Handbook of multicultural assessment.* San Francisco: Jossey-Bass.

Quintana, S. M. (1994). A model of ethnic perspective-taking applied to Mexican-American children and youth. *International Journal of Intercultural Relations, 18*, 419–448.

Quintana, S. M. (1995). Acculturative stress: Latino immigrants and the counseling profession. *Counseling Psychologist, 23*, 68–73.

Quintana, S. M. (1998). Development of children's understanding of ethnicity and race. *Applied and Preventive Psychology: Current Scientific Perspectives, 7*, 27–45.

Quintana, S. M., & Bernal, M. E. (1995). Ethnic minority training in counseling psychology: Comparisons with clinical psychology and proposed standards. *Counseling Psychologist, 23*, 102–121.

Quintana, S. M., Vera, E., & Cooper, C. (1999). African-American children's racial identity and inter-racial coping strategies. Poster presentation at the American Psychological Association, Boston, August.

Ramirez, S. Z., Wassef, A., Paniagua, F. A., & Linskey, A. O. (1996). Mental health providers' perceptions of cultural variables in evaluating ethnically diverse clients. *Professional Psychology Research and Practice, 27,* 284–288.

Ridley, C. R., Li, L. C., & Hill, C. L. (1998). Multicultural assessment: Reexamination, reconceptualization and practical application. *Counseling Psychologist, 26,* 827–910.

Rollack, D., & Terrell, M. D. (1996). Multicultural issues in assessment: Toward an inclusive model. In J. L. DeLucia-Waack (Ed.), *Multicultural counseling competencies: Implications for training and practice* (pp. 113–153). Alexandria, VA: Association for Counselor Education and Supervision.

Rotheram-Borus, M. J. (1993). Biculturalism among adolescents. In M. E. Bernal & G. P. Knight (Eds.), *Ethnic identity: Formation and transmission among Hispanics and other minorities* (pp. 81– 102). Albany, NY: SUNY Press.

Rotheram-Borus, M. J., & Phinney, J. S. (1990). Patterns of social expectations among black and Mexican American children. *Child Development, 61,* 542–556.

Sears, D. O. (1988). Symbolic racism. In P. A. Katz, & T. Dalmas (Eds.), *Eliminating racism: Profiles in controversy* (pp. 53–84). New York: Plenum Press.

Simpson, A. W., & Erickson, M. T. (1983). Teacher's verbal and nonverbal communication patterns as a function of teacher race, student gender, and student race. *American Educational Research Journal, 20,* 183–198.

Spengler, P. M., & Strohmer, D. C. (1994). Clinical judgment biases: The moderation roles of clinical complexity and clinician client preferences. *Journal of Counseling Psychology, 41,* 1–10.

Steele, C. M. (1997). A threat in the air: How stereotypes shape intellectual identity and performance. *American Psychologist, 52,* 613–629.

Steele, C. M., & Aronson, J. (1995). Stereotype threat and the intellectual test performance of African Americans. *Journal of Personality and Social Psychology, 69,* 797–811.

Stockman, I. J. (1986). Language acquisition in culturally diverse populations: The black child as a case study. In O. L. Taylor (Ed.), *Nature of communication disorders in culturally and linguistically diverse populations* (pp. 117–155). San Diego: College-Hill.

Sue, S. (1998). In search of cultural competence in psychotherapy and counseling. *American Psychologist, 53,* 440–448.

Sue, D. W., Arredondo, P., & McDavis, R. J. (1992). Multicultural counseling competencies and standards: A call to the profession. *Journal of Counseling and Development, 70,* 477–486.

Suzuki, L. A., & Valencia, R. R. (1997). Race-ethnicity and measured intelligence: Educational implications. *American Psychologist, 52,* 1103–1114.

Tharp, R. G. (1994). Intergroup differences among Native Americans in socialization and child cognition: An ethnogenetic analysis. In P. M. Greenfield & R. R. Cocking (Eds.), *Cross-cultural roots of minority child development* (pp. 87–106). Hillsdale, NJ: Erlbaum.

Tombari, M. L. & Borich, G. D. (1998). *Authentic assessment in the classroom: Applications and practice.* Upper Saddle River, NJ: Prentice Hall.

Triandis, H. C., Bontempo, R., Villareal, M. J., Asai, M., & Lucca, N. (1988). Individualism and collectivism: Cross-cultural perspectives on self-ingroup relationships. *Journal of Personality and Social Psychology, 54,* 323–338.

Valencia, R. R., & Aburto, S. (1991). The uses and abuses of educational testing: Chicanos as a case in point. In R. R. Valencia (Ed.), *Chicano school failure and success: Research and policy agendas for the 1990s.* London: Falmer Press.

Valencia, R. R., & Guadarrama, I. (1996). High states testing and its impact on racial and ethnic minority students. In L. A. Suzuki, P. J. Meller, & J. G. Ponterotto (Eds.), *Handbook of multicultural assessment* (pp. 561–610). San Francisco: Jossey-Bass.

Velasquez, R., Ayala, G. X, & Mendoza, S. A. (1998). *Psychodiagnostic assessment of U.S. Latinos with MMPI, MMPI-2, and MMPI-A: A comprehensive resource manual.* East Lansing, MI: Julian Samora Research Institute.

Weisz, J. R., & Weiss, B. (1991). Studying the "referability" of child clinical problems. *Journal of Consulting and Clinical Psychology, 59,* 266–273.

CHAPTER 16

Educational and Psychiatric Classification Systems

THOMAS J. POWER
RICARDO B. EIRALDI
Children's Hospital of Philadelphia
University of Pennsylvania School of Medicine

Clinicians use behavioral assessment methods for many reasons; one of the most common objectives and intended outcomes of these procedures is the classification of children and adolescents. Several systems of classification have been developed for children and youth, but the ones that are most frequently used are the educational and psychiatric systems. The classification of young people has become increasingly controversial because of concerns about the stigmatizing effects of diagnostic labels, the disproportionate rates of diagnosis among minority children, inaccuracies in the use of diagnostic procedures, the questionable effectiveness of special education programming, and the movement toward full inclusion of children with educational impairments (Reschly, 1998). As an alternative, many experts have advocated for the development and use of functional approaches to assessment that lead to problem solving and obviate the need for diagnostic assessment and classification (Gresham & Gansle, 1992; Kratochwill & McGivern, 1996).

This chapter describes (1) the purposes of diagnostic classification, (2) methods of assessment used to make diagnostic decisions, (3) educational and psychiatric classification systems and behavioral methods that may be useful in classification, (4) the correspondence between these two systems of classification, (5) limitations of the educational and psychiatric systems, and (6) a proposed model for incorporating a classification model with functional approaches to problem solving. This chapter focuses primarily on the classification of emotional and behavioral disorders, which are the disorders most commonly classified using behavioral assessment methods. For a discussion of issues related to the classification of learning disorders using cognitive and academic methods of assessment, the reader is referred to Flanagan, Genshaft, and Harrison (1997), and Lyon (1996).

PURPOSES OF CLASSIFICATION

A major purpose of diagnostic classification systems is to organize a wide range of research and clinical findings into a manageable, coherent set of constructs. These formulations or diagnostic constructs can provide provisional meaning to clinical findings and thereby facilitate an understanding of an individual's problems and course of development. Research has demonstrated repeatedly that children and adolescents demonstrate several relatively discrete clusters of symptoms (e.g., autism, conduct disorders, anxiety disorders). The symptoms in each cluster generally occur simultaneously in an individual, persist for relatively long periods of time, and are often associated with specific developmental outcomes. For example, children with autism typically have severe deficits in language development, exhibit severe social impairments, and demonstrate repetitive, stereotyped patterns of behavior (American Psychiatric Association, 1994). These children have a high probability of experiencing significant social and language impairments throughout their lives (Gilberg & Steffenburg, 1987). When a referred child presents with many of the features of autism, a clinician who is familiar with this disorder will know to extensively evaluate communication and social problems. Information derived from the assessment can then be used to determine the extent to which the child fits the profile of autism and thereby can be expected to exhibit the characteristics of children with this symptom cluster.

Another important function of classification is to facilitate communication about an individual. Classification systems provide a uniform set of concepts and terms that can enable clinicians to communicate clearly and efficiently with one another as well as with family members. For example, when a clinician refers to a child as having attention-deficit/hyperactivity disorder (ADHD), combined type, there is an implicit communication that the child displays enduring problems paying attention and controlling behavior that have resulted in significant functional impairments in his or her life. Of course, a classification system can only facilitate communication if the parties involved are knowledgeable about the system and use the terms and concepts appropriately. For this reason, it is important for clinicians to carefully define diagnostic labels to laypersons, such as parents and children, when introducing these terms in the provision of clinical services.

Classification also serves the purpose of assisting with intervention planning. Classification may be useful in making decisions about eligibility for services or special programs. For example, educational classification is required to render a child eligible for special education services. Also, classification may have implications for the type of treatment approach to be used. For instance, physicians typically require a diagnosis of ADHD before they will prescribe stimulant medication for attention and impulse-control problems. Although classification systems are often used in intervention planning, many experts have questioned the practical significance of classification, that is, the usefulness of classification in planning interventions that really make a difference for children (Gresham & Gansle, 1992; Reschly & Ysseldyke, 1995). The extent to which the assignment of a classification or diagnosis to an individual has a positive impact on treatment outcome has been referred to as treatment utility or treatment validity (Hayes, Nelson, & Jarrett, 1987; Kratochwill & McGivern, 1996).

METHODS OF ASSESSMENT USED IN CLASSIFICATION

The essence of classification is to make a determination about the presence or absence of a diagnostic entity. Thus classification, by its very nature, necessitates the use of a categorical approach to assessment. The most commonly used methods for making categorical decisions about emotional and behavioral disorders are interview techniques and behavior rating scales.

Categorical Approach to Assessment

With the categorical approach to assessment, disorders are considered present or absent based on a set of diagnostic criteria that have been developed by a panel of experts after careful review of the research literature (Power & Eiraldi, 1998). For example, the *Diagnostic and Statistical Manual of Mental Disorders* (DSM) employs a categorical approach to the classification of emotional, behavioral, and developmental disorders (American Psychiatric Association, 1994). Diagnostic criteria for each of the disorders listed in the DSM was delineated by a panel of experts, mostly in the field of psychiatry, upon review of the literature and field testing of diagnostic symptoms and cut-off points (Lahey et al., 1994). Clinicians using the DSM are instructed to relate clinical findings to the descriptions in this manual to determine the presence of diagnostic entities, such as oppositional defiant disorder, generalized anxiety disorder, and obsessive–compulsive disorder.

The classification system espoused in the Individuals with Disabilities Education Act (IDEA) of 1997, the reauthorization of the original special education law known as the Education for All Handicapped Children Act of 1977, also utilizes a categorical method of assessment. Child Study Team members are required to relate assessment findings to classification criteria to determine whether a child meets criteria for one or more educational disabilities, including emotional disturbance, learning disabilities, autism, and mental retardation.

The categorical approach is often contrasted with the dimensional method, which provides an assessment of behavioral, emotional, and learning problems along a continuum from average to unusual without clear delimitation of the boundary between disordered and nondisordered (Achenbach & McConaughy, 1996). Unlike categorical approaches that only indicate whether an individual meets or does not meet criteria for a specific diagnostic entity, dimensional approaches indicate the severity of child problems on each of several important dimensions of functioning. Dimensional methods, which have been operationalized in the use of multiaxial behavior rating scales like the Child Behavior Checklist (CBCL; Achenbach, 1991a) and the Behavior Assessment System for Children (BASC; Reynolds & Kamphaus,

1992), yield profiles that are very useful in describing the externalizing and internalizing behavior of children and adolescents.

Diagnostic Interview Techniques

Interviewing parents, teachers, and children about problems at home and in school is a very useful tool for classifying emotional and behavioral disorders. Structured interviews are very commonly used in clinical practice and research in the classification of mental disorders described in the DSM. In fact, in the leading clinical psychology and psychiatry journals, structured interviews have become part of the gold standard for assessing and diagnosing emotional and behavioral disorders. The format and content of structured interviews generally map directly to the DSM, making it efficient to use these procedures in making DSM diagnoses. Clinicians are provided with very clear guidelines for administration and scoring that typically result in high rates of interrater agreement (Eiraldi, Power, & Nezu, 1997). Many excellent interview techniques are available; these include the Diagnostic Interview Schedule for Children (DISC; Shaffer et al., 1996), the Diagnostic Interview for Children and Adolescents (DICA; Reich, Leacock, & Shanfeld, 1995), and the Kiddic-Schedule for Affective Disorders—Present and Lifetime Version (K-SADS-PL; Kaufman, Birmaher, Brent, Rao, & Ryan, 1996). Each of these techniques provides a separate interview form for adults and children. Also, many of these techniques have been adapted for computerized administration and scoring, adding to the efficiency and utility of these procedures.

Despite their strengths, structured interviews have several limitations that are worth noting. These procedures can take between 50 and 90 minutes to administer, although newer versions are being developed that can be administered in less time. Structured interviews are not norm-referenced measures, and thereby do not yield information about the severity of symptoms and symptom clusters in relation to children of similar age and gender. Moreover, structured interviews use a uniform set of items and decision-making rules for diagnosing children across the full range of development, resulting in a system that may be insensitive to age, gender, and cultural differences (Power & Eiraldi, 1998).

The reliability and validity of structured interviews vary greatly depending on informant and disorder being evaluated. For example, research using the most recent DISC has revealed that the reliability and validity of this interview technique generally is poor with the child-reported version and much stronger with the parent-reported version, and that the parent-reported DISC is more valid and reliable is diagnosing externalizing as opposed to internalizing disorders (Schwab-Stone et al., 1996). Another limitation is that structured interviews typically yield a limited amount of information about family and school functioning. These procedures have been developed to facilitate decision making about the presence or absence of disorders and generally yield a limited amount of information about the family, school, and peer-oriented contexts within which symptoms are manifested.

Behavior Rating Scales

As indicated, behavior rating scales employ a dimensional approach to assessment that yields information about how a child is functioning on many dimensions of internalizing and externalizing functioning. Nonetheless, rating scales are being used increasingly for the purposes of diagnostic assessment. For example, researchers have investigated the ability of the Attention Problems subscale of the Child Behavior Checklist (CBCL; Achenbach, 1991a) to screen and diagnose children for ADHD and comorbid disorders (Chen, Faraone, Biederman, & Tsuang, 1994). More recently, studies have examined the discriminative validity and clinical utility of the CBCL and Teacher Report Form (TRF; Achenbach, 1991b) in relation to other multiaxial rating scales, in evaluating ADHD and comorbid disorders (Vaughn, Riccio, Hynd, & Hall, 1997; Eiraldi, Power, Karustis, & Goldstein, 2000).

A challenge that confronts clinicians who utilize multiple informants in conducting diagnostic assessments is the marked degree of disagreement among informant reports (Achenbach, McConaughy, & Howell, 1987). For example, psychologists are often confronted by the problem of discrepant reports between parents and teachers in the assessment of ADHD. Research with the ADHD Rating Scale–IV (DuPaul, Power, Anastopoulos, & Reid, 1998) has attempted to address this dilemma and to provide useful guidelines for practice. These researchers demonstrated that single-informant approaches generally are optimal for ruling out ADHD, but approaches that combine parent and teacher ratings are optimal for predicting or ruling in this disorder (Power, Andrews et al., 1998). These authors have suggested cutoff scores on parent and teacher versions of the ADHD Rating Scale–IV that are optimal for screening and diagnosing ADHD in clinical and school settings.

Behavior ratings scales also have important limitations. As useful as these measures can be in diagnostic assessment, their accuracy in predicting and ruling out diagnoses is not high enough to warrant their use in isolation without other techniques such as structured interviews (Power, Doherty et al., 1998). Relatedly, although behavior rating scales provide valuable information about the severity of symptom clusters in relation to children of similar age and gender, they typically do not provide sufficient information upon which to base a diagnosis. For example, most DSM diagnoses have age of onset and symptom duration criteria as well as a requirement that symptoms of the disorder be associated with significant levels of functional impairment. Ratings scales typically do not provide information about age of onset, duration of symptoms, and degree of functional impairment in a variety of domains of child functioning. Further, rating scales are subject to rater bias. Informants differ in their thresholds for determining that a behavior is a problem (Reid & Maag, 1994), and maternal depression has been linked with a bias to rate children high for internalizing and externalizing problems (Kolko & Kazdin, 1993). A further limitation is that most rating scales have been developed with and normed on primarily white children of middle-class background. These measures may not be appropriate in the diagnostic assessment of children from minority groups, particularly those from lower socioeconomic backgrounds (DuPaul et al., 1997; Reid, 1995).

EDUCATIONAL CLASSIFICATION SYSTEM

Behavioral assessment methods are commonly used in making classification decisions about emotional disturbance (ED), ADHD, and autism or pervasive developmental disorders (PDD). This section discusses these categories and how behavioral assessment techniques can be useful in diagnostic decision making related to each classification.

Emotional Disturbance

Educational criteria for classifying children with ED, specified in IDEA, have remained essentially unchanged since the late 1970s. A noteworthy change in the definition used in IDEA, 1997, is that the adjective "serious" has been omitted from the classification which may increase rates of classification of students with emotional and behavioral problems (Telzrow, 1999). This term refers to a relatively severe condition with a relatively long duration that adversely affects school performance and is characterized by one or more of the following: (1) an inability to learn, (2) an inability to establish or maintain social relationships, (3) inappropriate types of behavior or feelings, (4) depression, or (5) somatic problems or fears. This classification excludes children who are socially maladjusted unless it is determined that individuals with ED are also socially maladjusted.

Researchers have highlighted many problems with the classification of serious emotional disturbance (SED), which may contribute to the underidentification of children with this disorder (see Forness & Knitzer, 1992). The lack of specificity of the criteria pertaining to severity and duration is a frequently cited concern. Another problem is the lack of clarity with regard to the clause stating that the condition must adversely affect educational performance. Some school districts have narrowly defined this phrase to refer to a significant discrepancy between intellectual ability and academic achievement as measured by standardized tests. Wodrich, Stobo, and Trca (1998) suggested that the meaning of this clause be extended to include children who fail to master the curriculum as well as those who are chronically absent from school. Further, there has been considerable debate about the utility of the social maladjustment exclusion clause, given the high degree of comorbidity between conduct and mood disorders and that children with disruptive and aggressive behavior represent the largest subgroup of children in SED programs (McGinnis & Forness, 1988; Weinberg & Weinberg, 1990).

Problems with the SED classification criteria have created the need to develop alternative diagnostic criteria for children with emotional and behavioral disorders. A significant development in this regard was the proposed definition of Emotional or Behavioral Disorder advanced by the Workgroup on Definition of the National Mental Health and Special Education Coalition (see Forness, 1988; Forness & Knitzer, 1992). Highlights of this definition are that adverse educational performance refers to deficits in academic, social, vocational, and personal skills, and that a child's emotional or behavioral responses must be demonstrated to be markedly different from age and cultural norms. Also, this definition eliminated the social maladjustment exclusion clause and emphasized the need to demonstrate that interventions applied in the general education setting are not sufficient to address the child's problems. Although this definition addresses many of the problems with the educational classification of children with emotional and behavioral disorders, federal guidelines continue to reflect the traditional definition of SED.

The Workgroup on Definition recommended the use of norm-referenced methods to classify children with emotional and behavioral disorders, and behavior rating scales are being used with increasing frequency in the educational evaluation of children for ED (Cluett et al., 1998). The use of behavior rating scales in the evaluation of ED provides a method for determining the severity of the impact of a child's emotional and behavioral problems. Considerable research has demonstrated that behavior rating scales, in particular the CBCL, is quite successful in discriminating children with ED from those who are not classified, as well as in discriminating children with ED from those who are learning disabled (see McConaughy & Achenbach, 1990). Table 16.1 presents guidelines for employing commonly used multiaxial rating scales, including the Devereux Scales of Mental Disorders (Naglieri, LeBuffe, & Pfeiffer, 1994), to evaluate the severity of the six criteria, including schizophrenia, outlined in the IDEA definition of ED. As this table indicates, each of these rating scales has some utility in evaluating criteria pertaining to the classification of ED. For example, the Thought Problems subscale of the CBCL/TRF, the Atypicality subscale of the BASC, and the Acute Problems subscale of the DSMD can be used to provide evidence of "inappropriate types of behavior or feelings under normal circumstances." Similarly, the Anxious/Depressed subscale of the CBCL/TRF, the Depression subscale of the BASC, and the Depression subscale of the DSMD can be helpful in assessing "a general pervasive mood of unhappiness or depression."

The rating scale that relates most directly to the IDEA definition of ED is the Devereux Behavior Rating Scale—School Form (DBRS-SF; Naglieri, LeBuffe, & Pfeiffer, 1993). The DBRS-SF consists of four subscales, each with 10 items, that represent key criteria in the IDEA definition pertaining to ED. Recent research provides some support for the predictive validity of the DBRS-SF (Naglieri, Bardos, & LeBuffe, 1995). Naglieri and Gottling (1995) reported that the DBRS-SF was able to accurately classify over 75% of students with SED and they presented evidence of its superiority over the Teacher Report Form of the CBCL in classifying SED. Nonetheless, the relative paucity of predictive validity studies involving the use of rating scales to classify ED and the failure of these measures to attain high rates of prediction necessitate that school practitioners utilize multiple strategies in addition to rating scales in making classification decisions pertaining to SED.

Attention-Deficit/Hyperactivity Disorder

Educational law does not recognize ADHD as a separate disability. Nonetheless, children with ADHD are eligible for special-education services if they meet the cri-

TABLE 16.1 Multiaxial Rating Scales for the Assessment of Serious Emotional Disturbance as Defined in the IDEA

SED criteria	CBCL	TRF	BASC-PRS	BASC-TRS	DSMD	DBRS-SF
Inability to learn	School competence	Academic performance	—	Learning problems School problems	—	—
Inability to build or maintain relationships	Social problems Withdrawn	Social problems Withdrawn	Social skills Withdrawal	Social skills Withdrawal	—	Interpersonal problems
Inappropriate types of behavior or feelings	Thought problems	Thought problems	Atypicality	Atypicality	Acute problems	Inappropriate behaviors/ feelings
General pervasive mood of unhappiness/depression	Anxious/ depressed	Anxious/ depressed	Depression	Depression	Depression	Depression
Tendency to develop physical symptoms or fears	Somatic complaints	Somatic complaints	Somatization Anxiety	Somatization Anxiety	Anxiety	Physical symptoms/fears
Schizophrenic	Thought problems	Thought problems	Atypicality	Atypicality	Acute problems	—

Note. CBCL, Child Behavior Checklist; TRF, Teacher Report Form; EASC-PRS, Behavior Assessment System for Children—Parent Rating Scale; BASC-TRS, Behavior Assessment System for Children—Teacher Rating Scale; DSMD, Devereux Scales of Mental Disorders; DBRS-SF, Devereux Behavior Rating Scale—School Form.

teria for learning disabilities (LD) or ED. Based on a review of existing literature, Forness (1998) estimated that approximately 26% of children with learning disabilities and 43% of children with serious emotional disturbance meet criteria for ADHD. In addition, educational law recognizes that children with ADHD who do not meet criteria for LD or ED may still be eligible for special education under the classification of Other Health Impairment (OHI) if it can be demonstrated that their handicap significantly interferes with their educational performance. As with the ED classification, the meaning of the phrase "adversely affects educational performance" in the OHI definition is vague, which may result in disputes between parents and educational officials about the rights of these children. Since 1991 more and more children are being classified as OHI, presumably in response to the memo regarding ADHD. Current estimates are that about 40% of children classified as OHI meet criteria for ADHD (Forness, 1998).

Educational law contains additional protection for children with ADHD who do not meet criteria for OHI. Section 504 of the Rehabilitation Act of 1973 prohibits discrimination of persons on the basis of a handicapping condition. A handicapped person is defined as an individual who has a physical or mental impairment that significantly limits one or more major life activities. A memorandum from the Department of Education (Davila, Williams, & MacDonald, 1991) specified that a child with ADHD has a handicapping condition and thereby is eligible for protection under Section 504 if it can be demonstrated that this disorder results is a substantial impairment in the child's educational functioning.

The criteria used for diagnosing ADHD to determine eligibility for special education or to assess the applicability for protection under Section 504 is not specified under educational law. Diagnostic criteria outlined in DSM generally are used to make decisions about eligibility for educational services as a function of ADHD status. These criteria and behavioral methods used to assess ADHD are outlined in the next section. School officials vary widely in their perspectives about which professional groups should render the diagnosis of ADHD. Nonetheless, given the school-based psychologist's expertise in behavioral assessment and easy access to information about children's functioning in multiple, naturalistic settings, it is becoming increasingly clear that a psychologist working in schools can make very important contributions to the diagnostic assessment of ADHD (Power, Atkins, Osborne, & Blum, 1994).

Autism

Autism is recognized by educational law as a disabling condition. This classification requires a determination that a child demonstrates severe impairments in communication and social functioning. Also, a pattern of repetitive and restrictive behavior as well as abnormal responses to sensory stimuli are typically manifested. Although the educational classification recognizes a generic disorder of autism, many states provide sufficient latitude to warrant classification and educational placement of children with the wide range of PDDs outlined in the fourth edition of DSM (DSM-

IV). This classification often requires a diagnostic evaluation performed by a physician qualified in the area of autism in addition to an assessment by a school psychologist. Educational programming for children with autism or other PDDs can vary greatly, depending upon the level of cognitive and social impairment. For example, most children with autism function in the mentally retarded range and require highly intensive intervention for several years, preferably beginning in preschool (Stone, MacLean, & Hogan, 1995). In contrast, children with Asperger's Disorder typically have less severe cognitive and linguistic problems than those with autism, although their level of social impairment can be severe (Harris, Glasberg, & Ricca, 1996).

Several assessment tools are available to assist with the evaluation and classification of autism. Two highly useful parent-report structured diagnostic interviews are the Parent Interview for Autism (Stone & Hogan, 1993) and the Autism Diagnostic Interview—Revised (Lord, Rutter, & LeCouteur, 1994). Also, behavioral assessment data collected directly by clinicians also can contribute meaningfully to a comprehensive assessment of autism. For example, the Childhood Autism Rating Scale (Schopler, Reichler, & Renner, 1988) and the Autism Diagnostic Observation Schedule (Lord et al., 1989) are commonly used in the evaluation of this disorder.

PSYCHIATRIC CLASSIFICATION SYSTEM

Behavioral and Emotional Disorders

The DSM-IV provides the most commonly used system in this country for diagnosing behavioral and emotional disorders. The DSM-IV disorders that are most frequently used by clinicians to classify children, excluding ADHD, are oppositional defiant disorder (ODD), conduct disorder (CD), anxiety disorders, and mood disorders. DSM-IV criteria for ODD and CD were developed specifically for children, in contrast to criteria pertaining to the internalizing disorders. DSM-IV has been criticized for its failure to account for developmental variations in the presentation of anxiety and mood disorders, particularly among children and adolescents (Callahan, Panichelli-Mindel, & Kendall, 1996).

As indicated, structured diagnostic interviews can be very useful in the classification of behavioral and emotional disorders. Behavior rating scales are being used with increasing frequency in the diagnostic evaluation of emotional and behavioral disorders. Table 16.2 depicts how three commonly used multiaxial behavior rating scales can be employed in the assessment of DSM-IV disorders. Most of the research pertaining to the use of rating scales in diagnostic prediction has been conducted using the CBCL. The CBCL has been demonstrated to have an impressive level of discriminative validity and clinical utility in diagnosing conduct disorders (Lowe, 1998), depressive disorders (Biederman et al., 1996), and anxiety disorders (Biederman et al., 1993; Eiraldi et al., 2000). A potential problem with the use of the CBCL in the diagnostic assessment of internalizing problems is the clustering of items pertaining to both anxiety and depression into one subscale. In contrast, the BASC and

TABLE 16.2 Multiaxial Rating Scales for the Assessment of DSM-IV Psychiatric Disorders

DSM-IV disorder	CBCL/TRF	BASC-PRS/TRS	DSMD
Attention-deficit/ hyperactivity disorder	Attention problems	Attention problems Hyperactivity	Attention
Oppositional defiant disorder	Aggressive behavior	Aggression	Conduct
Conduct disorder	Delinquent behavior	Conduct problems	Conduct
Anxiety disorders	Anxious/depressed	Anxiety	Anxiety
Depressive disorders	Anxious/depressed	Depression	Depression
Schizoid personality disorder	Withdrawn	Withdrawal	—
Somatization disorder	Somatic complaints	Somatization	—
Psychotic disorders	Thought problems	Atypicality	Acute problems
Autism	Withdrawn	Withdrawal	Autism

Note. CBCL, Child Behavior Checklist; TRF, Teacher Report Form; BASC-PRS, Behavior Assessment System for Children—Parent Rating Scale; BASC-TRS, Behavior Assessment System for Children—Teacher Rating Scale; DSMD, Devereux Scales of Mental Disorders.

DSMD provide separate subscales for anxiety and depression. Research is beginning to evaluate the predictive validity of the BASC and the DSMD in diagnosing emotional and behavioral disorders (Doyle, Ostrander, Skare, Crosby, & August, 1997; Eiraldi et al., 2000). This research generally demonstrates that the BASC and DSMD are comparable to the CBCL in the prediction of emotional and behavioral disorders.

Attention-Deficit/Hyperactivity Disorder

Based on extensive empirical research, the DSM-IV recognizes two broad classes of behavior related to ADHD: Inattention and Hyperactivity–Impulsivity. The symptoms of these two dimensions listed in the DSM-IV are those behaviors that have been demonstrated empirically to be the best at discriminating children with ADHD from controls. The DSM-IV requires that a diagnosis of ADHD be rendered only when there is evidence of impairment related to inattention and/or hyperactivity in two or more major settings. The DSM-IV recognizes three subtypes of this disorder: (1) ADHD, inattentive type (ADHD/I); (2) ADHD, hyperactive–impulsive type (ADHD/HI); and (3) ADHD, combined type (ADHD/COM). Although there is considerable research support for the ADHD/I and ADHD/COM subtypes, the validity and utility of the ADHD/HI subtype has been questioned (Power & DuPaul, 1996).

Consensus is emerging that the "gold standard" for evaluating ADHD involves the use of structured interviews and behavior rating scales, and the collection of data from multiple informants, particularly teachers and parents (Biederman et al., 1995;

Loeber, Green, & Lahey, 1990). The importance of collecting self-report data from children and adolescents is more controversial, given the tendency of children with ADHD to underreport their symptoms (Loeber et al., 1990). Research has demonstrated that an approach to assessment that combines parent and teacher reports of child behavior is superior to a single-informant approach for evaluating ADHD (Power, Andrews et al., 1998; Power, Doherty et al., 1998). Further, when children are being taught by several teachers, diagnostic accuracy can be improved by including information from multiple educators (Molina, Pelham, Blumenthal, & Galiszewski, 1998).

A variety of multiaxial rating systems can be useful in the evaluation of ADHD (see Table 16.2). Several studies have affirmed the clinical utility of multiaxial scales in diagnosing ADHD (Chen et al., 1994; Eiraldi et al., 1999; Vaughn et al., 1997). A problem with the CBCL and DSMD is that these measures include only one factor related to ADHD, which is a heterogeneous grouping of items pertaining to inattention and hyperactivity–impulsivity. In contrast, the BASC includes separate subscales of Attention Problems and Hyperactivity that correspond closely with the two-factor delineation of ADHD in the DSM-IV. Research suggests that the BASC may be superior to the CBCL in differentiating children into subtypes of ADHD (Vaughn et al., 1997).

In addition, many narrowband rating scales have been developed for the behavioral assessment of ADHD. Perhaps the most commonly used of the narrowband measures is the Conners' Rating Scales—Revised (Conners, 1997), which have been updated to assist with diagnostic evaluations of ADHD using DSM-IV criteria. Another scale that was developed specifically for the purpose of evaluating ADHD according to DSM-IV is the ADHD Rating Scale–IV (DuPaul et al., 1998). The factor structure of both the parent and teacher versions of this scale closely correspond with the two-dimensional structure of the DSM-IV. The manual for the ADHD Rating Scale-IV provides extensive information about how to use ratings completed by parents and teachers, separately and in combination, in the diagnostic evaluation of ADHD.

Autism and the Pervasive Developmental Disorders

The DSM-IV reflects a major change in the classification of pervasive developmental disorders. The previous version of DSM recognized only autistic disorder (AD) and pervasive developmental disorder—not otherwise specified (PDD-NOS). In the DSM-IV three additional subtypes are identified: (1) Rett's disorder (RD), (2) childhood disintegrative disorder (CD), and (3) Asperger's disorder (AsD; American Psychiatric Association, 1994). With all of these subtypes, significant social impairment and restricted, stereotyped patterns of behavior are clearly present. The subtypes differ with regard to degree of cognitive and linguistic impairment, age of onset, and presence of a decline in functioning. With AD, RD, and CDD, severe impairments in social and language performance are manifested. Most children with AD, RD, and CDD perform in the mentally retarded range of cognitive functioning. However, unlike AD, there is a clear, marked decline in functioning with RD and CDD. Age of onset for AD and RD is typically before the age of 3, but older for CDD. Further, RD occurs only in girls and is characterized by distinctive pattern of purposeless, stereotypical hand movements (Harris et al., 1996).

Children with AsD are distinguished by generally normal cognitive functioning. Although these children often display language deficiencies and idiosyncracies, by definition they do not have severe impairments in the domain of communication (Eisenmajer et al., 1996). Some children with AD also manifest average to above-average intellectual ability, but they can be differentiated from children with AsD on the basis of the severity of their language impairments (Schopler & Mesibov, 1992).

The DSM-IV field trials for the PDDs revealed that experienced clinicians were able to distinguish among the various subtypes with a relatively high degree of reliability and validity (Volkmar et al., 1994). Diagnostic interview and observation procedures, such as the Autism Diagnostic Interview—Revised (Lord, Rutter, & LeCouteur (1994) and the Pre-Linguistic Autism Diagnostic Observation Schedule (DiLavore, Lord, & Rutter, 1995), are closely linked with DSM-IV and can be very useful in the diagnostic evaluation of the PDDs.

CORRESPONDENCE BETWEEN CLASSIFICATION SYSTEMS

Educational law does not specify criteria for ADHD and tacitly recognizes the DSM as the diagnostic system for this disorder. A DSM-IV diagnosis of ADHD does not automatically trigger educational classification or intervention. The school's Child Study Team must demonstrate that a child with ADHD has a handicapping condition that adversely affects educational performance to warrant classification as Other Health Impaired or protection under Section 504.

With regard to the PPDs, there is a high degree of correspondence between the educational and psychiatric classification systems. The criteria used in the educational system for classifying PDD is essentially modeled after DSM criteria. The DSM-IV specifies criteria for various subtypes of PDD that are not delineated in IDEA, but the guidelines in educational law generally are broad enough to include children with the full range of PDDs that demonstrate severe problems functioning in an educational setting.

The correspondence between the educational and psychiatric classification systems for diagnosing emotional and behavioral disorders is very limited. Research suggests that for children referred to Child Study Teams for evaluation of emotional and behavioral problems, there is a convergence between educational criteria for ED and DSM criteria for one or more diagnoses in about 50% of the cases (Tharinger, Laurent, & Best, 1986). The lack of specificity in the criteria for classifying children with ED and the DSM disorders contributes to this relatively low rate of agreement. Also, it is not clear how the DSM disorders are related to a diagnosis of ED. Although children with anxiety, mood, somatization, psychotic, and schizoid personality disorders display the types of problems that are described in the educational definition of ED, the criteria for determining whether problems related to these disorders are severe enough and of long enough duration to warrant this classification are very vague (McConaughy & Achenbach, 1990). Further, differences in how states interpret the social maladjustment clause in the ED definition can contribute to variations in whether children diagnosed with conduct disorder (CD) and oppositional defiant disorder (ODD) are eligible for a classification of ED (Forness & Knitzer, 1992).

CLASSIFICATION: A CRITICAL ANALYSIS

The classification of children and adolescents using educational and psychiatric systems is controversial. This section describes many of the advantages and limitations of the classification process.

Advantages to Classification

Facilitates an Understanding of Child Behavior

Classification systems delineate patterns of behavior that generally are consistent with theoretical formulations and empirical studies in the field of child and adolescent psychopathology. These systems can assist providers in organizing clinical information, determining the relationship between clinical findings and identified patterns of behavior, understanding the correlates of specified behavior patterns, and predicting the developmental outcomes of various disorders.

Facilitates Communication

Classification systems provide a set of terms and concepts that can facilitate communication among professionals. The accurate use of a diagnostic label can rapidly convey a wealth of information about a child's pattern of behavior and likely developmental outcomes.

Identifies Risk Factors

The presence of a diagnosis often provides a signal that a child is at risk for comorbid conditions that further impair functioning. For example, ADHD is known to be associated with a variety of comorbidities, including ODD, CD, anxiety disorders, and mood disorders (Jensen, Martin, & Cantwell, 1997). The presentation of ADHD symptoms in a clinical or school setting should alert the professional to the possible presence of coexisting conditions that might be exacerbating the child's problems. Further, the presence of a diagnosis often signals that the child is at-risk for negative outcomes later in life. For example, the emergence of ODD in childhood often is a precursor of severe conduct problems in adolescence, particularly among children from families of lower socioeconomic background where the parents are abusing drugs and alcohol (Loeber, Green, Keenan, & Lahey, 1995).

Provides a Framework for Assessment

Classification systems provide diagnostic criteria that can serve as guidelines for the assessment of various patterns of child and adolescent psychopathology. These systems inform clinicians about (1) domains of functioning that are important to evaluate, (2) specific behaviors that need to be assessed, (3) cut-offs for determining when problems are likely to be severe and clinically important, and (4) alternative hypotheses to consider when evaluating patterns of behavior. For example, DSM-IV criteria pertaining to separation anxiety disorder (SAD) indicate that several domains of functioning, including clinical symptoms, duration of problems, age of onset, and extent of functional impairment, need to be considered during an evaluation. Further, the criteria for SAD specify critical behaviors that need to be evaluated (e.g., recurrent excessive stress when separation from a major attachment person occurs), and the number of symptoms (at least three of eight) that need to be manifested to suggest that the child's problems require clinical attention. Further, DSM-IV suggests competing explanations for problems related to SAD (e.g., PDD, schizophrenia, panic disorder) that should be considered during the diagnostic evaluation.

As indicated, numerous clinical tools have been developed to assist with the evaluation of child and adolescent psychopathology as defined by the major classification systems, particularly the DSM-IV. Structured diagnostic interviews are particularly useful for the evaluation of DSM-IV entities, because the content of these measures maps directly to this diagnostic system (Power & Eiraldi, 1998).

Facilitates Access to Treatment

Classifying children can be useful in identifying children who may benefit from specific types of intervention. The presence of a DSM diagnosis or special education classification generally indicates not only that a child is manifesting a particular cluster of symptoms, but that he or she is experiencing substantial functional difficulties coping as a result of these problems. Although failure to meet diagnostic criteria does not mean that a child does not require intervention, the presence of a diagnosis usually highlights the need for specialized treatment. For example, a diagnosis of PDD typically indicates that the child is in need of intensive educational intervention. Assigning a diagnosis of PDD can justify the need for specialized school-based interventions through IDEA (Harris et al., 1996).

The diagnostic evaluation of a child often has implications for the use of psychopharmacological interventions. Given that the single most effective intervention for ADHD is stimulant medication (Klein & Abikoff, 1997; Pelham et al., 1993), the presence of this disorder generally signifies the need for a trial of stimulants. The presence of comorbid conditions also may be useful in predicting response to medication. For example, children with an anxiety disorder in addition to ADHD have been shown to have a less robust response to stimulants than children with ADHD without this comorbidity (Pliszka, 1989; Tannock, Ickowicz, & Schachar, 1995).

The assignment of a diagnosis may also be useful to parents. This information may direct parents to a literature that helps them to better understand their child and the interventions needed to address their child's problems. Further, the classification may direct parents to support groups that can prevent social isolation among families coping with disabilities and help to maintain the effects of parent training and family therapy.

Limitations of Classification

Identifies the Child as Source of Problem

Classification systems generally are based on a medical model that posits that pathology is based within the individual (Gresham & Gansle, 1992). Such a view fails to reflect a transactional model of psychopathology that has gained increasing acceptance in psychology; this model posits that the behavior of an individual is reciprocally determined by the individual and psychosocial contexts in which the person functions. Assigning a diagnosis fails to recognize important relationship and contextual variables that contribute to a child's pattern of behavior and that are critical to understand in developing intervention plans. Classification may also have stigmatizing effects, particularly in educational settings.

Oversimplifies the Child's Problems

Although diagnostic terms may be used to convey important information about a child, these labels describe common patterns of behavior and may not represent adequately the unique combination of symptoms a particular child displays, the idiosyncratic manner in which each child manifests these symptoms, and the severity of symptom presentation. Further, diagnostic systems generally fail to acknowledge strengths about the child that are not consistent with diagnostic criteria. As a result, clinicians must guard against using these systems in a way that leads to stereotyping children and highlighting child weaknesses as opposed to strengths and resources.

Fails to Account for Age and Gender Differences

Classification systems typically employ a uniform set of diagnostic criteria across the life span and between genders. The use of a uniform set of classification criteria has not been supported by empirical research in the case of certain disorders. For example, age and gender differences in the presentation of ADHD symptoms has been documented by many researchers (DuPaul, Power et al., 1997; Trites, Blouin, & LaPrade, 1982). The marked decline in symptoms of hyperactivity–impulsivity during the adolescent years appears to warrant a reduction in the number of symptoms required by DSM-IV to diagnose ADHD, Combined or Hyperactive–Impulsive Types among youths in this age range. Similarly, the relatively high prevalence of inattention and hyperactivity–impulsivity symptoms among preschoolers appears to warrant a higher threshold for this age group (Barkley, 1998). Variations in symptom presentation between genders also should be accounted for in diagnostic systems (Arnold, 1996).

Fails to Provide Specific Guidelines for Assessment

Although diagnostic systems like the DSM-IV provide a broad framework for assessment, they generally fail to specify informants needed for assessment and useful tools for evaluating disorders. For example, the criteria for oppositional defiant disorder indicate symptoms of the disorder and the threshold of symptoms needed for diagnosis, but the system offers no recommendations about informants and how to acquire assessment information. Further, the DSM-IV in many instances indicates diagnoses that should be considered and ruled out in making a diagnosis, but it provides no recommendations for how to conduct a differential diagnosis (Power & DuPaul, 1996).

Has Limited Treatment Utility

Classification systems have been strongly criticized on the grounds that they are not linked directly to intervention and do not result in treatment plans that are useful for children (Gresham & Gansle, 1992). Although classification systems are often used to make eligibility decisions, the evidence is not clear that children who meet criteria for certain classifications (e.g., ED) are any more likely to benefit from treatment than those who do not meet the criteria. Also, the presence of emotional and behavioral disorders typically indicates that a behavioral or cognitive–behavioral approach to treatment is indicated, but it does not specify the strategies to be used. For example, knowing that a child has ADHD may not be helpful in determining the approach to behavioral intervention. The effectiveness of a positive reinforcement/response cost approach versus a time-out strategy generally depends on the function or purpose of a child's behavior (DuPaul, Eckert, & McGoey, 1997). Diagnostic systems provide no information about the function of behavior; a functional analysis of behavior is more helpful in this regard.

An Alternative to Classification: The Functional Approach

As described above, the classification approach to problem solving requires that diagnostic criteria be applied to determine the types of disorders present; this information then is used to determine what approaches ought to be used to treat the child. In contrast, a functional approach to problem solving bypasses the classification process; decisions about placement and intervention strategies are based on an assessment of the needs of the child, and a determination about whether a placement or intervention approach could help the child to attain important goals (Ikeda, Tilly, Stumme, Volmer, & Allison, 1996). The functional approach to problem solving has emerged largely in response to limitations in the traditional, classification approach to solving problems, specifically its failure to link assessment with intervention.

Numerous functional models of problem solving have been developed. Perhaps the model that has had the most influence on the practice of psychology in schools is the behavioral consultation approach (Bergan & Kratochwill, 1990), involving problem identification and behavioral assessment, intervention planning, ongoing outcome evaluation, and modification of interventions. Recent variations of the behavior consultation model have included a systematic functional analysis of behavior to identify antecedents that prompt target behaviors and consequences that maintain the behaviors (Dunlap et al., 1993; DuPaul & Ervin, 1996). Also, progress monitoring procedures used in curriculum-based measurement are very useful in problem solving, particularly in the design and evaluation of instructional interventions (Shinn, 1998).

Although a functional model of problem solving has many advantages, a potential limitation is the time and training required to conduct an in-depth analysis of behavior (DuPaul, Eckert, & McGoey, 1997). Relatedly, research has not yet evaluated the relative merits of a functional versus a classification model for solving children's problems (Kratochwill & McGivern, 1996).

INTEGRATING THE CLASSIFICATION AND FUNCTIONAL MODELS

Given that the classification and functional approaches to problem solving each have strengths and limitations and that these approaches to some extent are complementary, attempts have been made to integrate these models. For example, Zentall and Javorsky (1995) recommended that a functional approach to assessment be utilized initially to address the problems of children with ADHD. If symptoms of ADHD persist despite the use of behavior-analytic techniques, these authors recommended that a diagnostic evaluation of ADHD be conducted. Power and Ikeda (1996), utilizing a similar approach, developed a school-based model for assessing and treating ADHD that more fully links the processes of functional and diagnostic assessment (see Figure 16.1).

Upon referral to the Instructional Support Team (IST), team members identify critical target problems and gather important background information. The team then considers whether the child is presenting with problems related to ADHD requiring a screening for this disorder. If so, the team conducts a screening for ADHD, which might entail behavior ratings completed by the teacher and a brief classroom observation. Regardless of whether the child has problems related to ADHD, the team

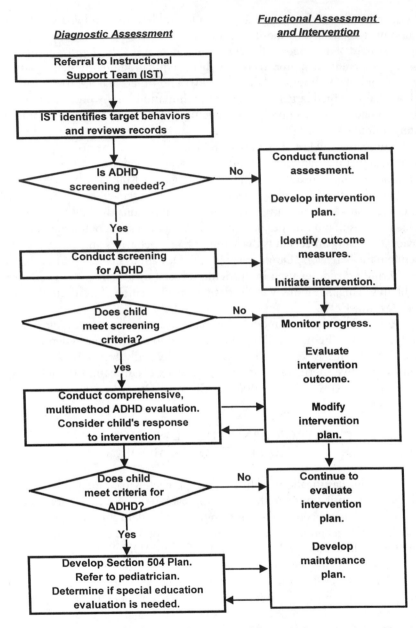

FIGURE 16.1   The relationship between diagnostic and functional assessment in addressing the needs of inattentive, overactive students.

initiates a functional analysis of behavior for the purposes of developing an intervention plan. The team also selects useful, multiple methods for monitoring progress and evaluating intervention outcome, and then initiates the process of intervention. Pending the results of progress monitoring and outcome evaluation, the interventions are modified or maintained.

If the child meets screening criteria for ADHD and the behavioral interventions derived through functional analysis do not adequately address the child's problems, then a comprehensive, multimethod evaluation of ADHD is indicated. Once the evaluation has been completed, if the child's behavior meets DSM criteria and functional impairments related to ADHD persist despite the use of behavioral interventions, then the evaluation team can consider a diagnosis of ADHD. If the child has ADHD, services outlined under Section 504 should be implemented. Also, the team should consider whether the child's problems could be better addressed through IDEA, which involves a consideration of several factors, including (1) the severity of the child's problems, (2) the effectiveness of medication, if used, and (3) the team's assessment of the effectiveness of behavioral interventions implemented in a general education context.

CONCLUSIONS

Educational and psychiatric classification systems have been developed for multiple purposes including the organization of clinical findings to assist in understanding and prognosticating an individual's behavior, the facilitation of communication among professionals and between providers and family members, and the development of useful and effective interventions. Several tools have been developed to assist with classification, most notably structured interviews and behavior rating scales. Although these methods have noteworthy limitations, they serve to complement each other in conducting a diagnostic evaluation. There is considerable overlap between the educational and psychiatric classification systems with regard to the pervasive developmental disorders and ADHD. However, the relationship between the educational classification of ED and the psychiatric classification of emotional and behavioral disorders is generally poor and very unclear. Classification systems, despite their advantages, have been widely criticized for their limitations in the area of treatment utility. Alternative approaches to problem solving, notably the functional method, have emerged recently and have demonstrated strong potential with regard to treatment utility. Functional approaches also have limitations, notably the time and expertise required to use these methods. Further, the superiority of the functional model as compared to the classification model of problem solving, particularly in the domain of treatment utility, has yet to be empirically demonstrated. At this time, a model of problem solving that fully integrates classification and functional approaches appears to be the optimal way of addressing problems that arise in the course of school practice.

References

Achenbach, T. M. (1991a). *Manual for the Child Behavior Checklist/4–18 and 1991 Profile*. Burlington: University of Vermont, Department of Psychiatry.

Achenbach, T. M. (1991b). *Manual for the Teacher's Report Form and 1991 Profile*. Burlington: University of Vermont, Department of Psychiatry.

Achenbach, T. M., & McConaughy, S. H. (1996). Relations between DSM-IV and empirically-based assessment. *School Psychology Review, 25*, 329–341.

Achenbach, T. M., McConaughy, S. H., & Howell, C. T. (1987). Child/adolescent behavioral and emotional problems: Implications of cross-informant correlations for situational specificity. *Psychological Bulletin, 101*, 213–232.

American Psychiatric Association. (1994). *Diagnostic and statistical manual of mental disorders* (4th ed.). Washington, DC: Author.

Arnold, L. E. (1996). Sex differences in AD/HD: Conference summary. *Journal of Abnormal Child Psychology, 24*, 555–570.

Barkley, R. A. (1998). *Attention deficit hyperactivity disorder: A handbook for diagnosis and treatment* (2nd ed.). New York: Guilford Press.

Bergan, J. R., & Kratochwill, T. R. (1990). *Behavioral consultation and therapy*. New York: Plenum Press.

Biederman, J., Faraone, S. V., Doyle, A., Lehman, B. K., Kraus, I., Perrin, J., & Tsuang, M. T. (1993). Convergence of the Child Behavior Checklist with structured interview-based psychiatric diagnoses of ADHD with and without comorbidity. *Journal of Child Psychology and Psychiatry, 34*, 1241–1251.

Biederman, J., Faraone, S., Mick, E., Moore, P., & LeLon, E. (1996). Child Behavior Checklist findings further support comorbidity between ADHD and major depression in a referred sample. *Journal of the American Academy of Child and Adolescent Psychiatry, 35*, 734–742.

Biederman, J., Wosniak, J., Kiely K., Ablon, S., Faraone, S., Mick, E., Mundy, E., & Kraus, I. (1995). CBCL clinical scales discriminate prepubertal children with structured interview-derived diagnosis of mania from those with ADHD. *Journal of the American Academy of Child and Adolescent Psychiatry, 34*, 464–471.

Callahan, S. A., Panichelli-Mindel, S. M., & Kendall, P. C. (1996). DSM-IV and internalizing disorders: Modifications, limitations, and utility. *School Psychology Review, 25*, 297–307.

Chen, W. J., Faraone, S. V., Biederman, J., & Tsuang, M. T. (1994). Diagnostic accuracy of the Child Behavior Checklist Scales for attention-deficit hyperactivity disorder: A receiver-operating characteristics analysis. *Journal of Consulting and Clinical Psychology, 62*(5), 1017–1025.

Cluett, S. E., Forness, S. R., Ramey, S. L., Ramey, C. T., Hsu, C., Kavale, K. A., & Gresham, F. M. (1998). Consequences of differential diagnostic criteria on identification rates of children with emotional or behavior disorders. *Journal of Emotional and Behavioral Disorders, 6*, 130–140.

Conners, C. K. (1997). *Manual for the Conners' Rating Scales—Revised*. North Tonawanda, NY: Multi-Health Systems.

Davila, R., Williams, M. L., & MacDonald, J. T. (1991). Clarification of policy to address the needs of children with attention deficit disorder within general and/or special education. Memorandum from the U.S. Department of Education. Washington, DC: Department of Education.

DiLavore, P. C., Lord, C., & Rutter, M. (1995). The Pre-Linguistic Diagnostic Observation Schedule. *Journal of Autism and Developmental Disorders, 25*, 355–379.

Doyle, A., Ostrander, R., Skare, S., Crosby, R. D., & August, G. J. (1997). Convergent and criterion-related validity of the Behavior Assessment System for Children—Parent Rating Scale. *Journal of Clinical Child Psychology, 26*(3), 276–284.

DuPaul, G. J., & Ervin, R. A. (1996). Functional assessment of behaviors related to attention-deficit/hyperactivity disorder: Linking assessment to intervention. *Behavior Therapy, 27*, 601–622.

DuPaul, G. J., Eckert, T. L., & McGoey, K. E. (1997). Interventions for students with attention-deficit/hyperactivity disorder: One size does not fit all. *School Psychology Review, 26*, 369–381.

DuPaul, G. J., Power, T. J., Anastopoulos, A. D. & Reid, R. (1998). *ADHD Rating Scale–IV: Checklists, norms, and clinical interpretation*. New York: Guilford Press.

DuPaul, G. J., Power, T. J., Anastopoulos, A. D., Reid, R., McGoey, K., & Ikeda, M. J. (1997). Teacher ratings of attention-deficit/hyperactivity disorder symptoms: Factor structure, normative data, and psychometric properties. *Psychological Assessment, 9,* 436–444.

Dunlap, G., Kern, L., dePerczel, M., Clarke, S., Wilson, D., Childs, K. E., White, R., & Falk, G. D. (1993). Functional analysis of classroom variables for students with emotional and behavioral disorders. *Behavioral Disorders, 18,* 275–291.

Eiraldi, R. B., Power, T. J., Karustis, J. L., & Goldstein, S. G. (2000). Assessing ADHD and comorbid disorders in children: The Child Behavior Checklist and the Devereux Scales of Mental Disorders. *Journal of Child Clinical Psychology, 29,* 3–16.

Eiraldi, R. B., Power, T. J., & Nezu, C. M. (1997). Patterns of comorbidity associated with subtypes of attention-deficit/hyperactivity disorder among 6–12 year old children. *Journal of the American Academy of Child and Adolescent Psychiatry, 36,* 503–514.

Eisenmajer, R., Prior, M., Leekam, S., Wing, L., Gould, J., Welham, M., & Ong, B. (1996). Comparison of clinical symptoms in autism and Asperger's disorder. *Journal of the American Academy of Child and Adolescent Psychiatry, 35,* 1523–1531.

Flanagan, D. P., Genshaft, J. L., & Harrison, P. L. (Eds.). (1997). *Contemporary intellectual assessment: Theories, tests, and issues.* New York: Guilford Press.

Forness, S. R. (1988). Planning for the needs of children with serious emotional disturbance: The national special education and mental health coalition. *Behavioral Disorders, 13,* 127–133.

Forness, S. R. (1998). The impact of attention deficit hyperactivity disorder on school systems. In National Institutes of Health (Eds.), *NIH consensus development conference on diagnosis and treatment of attention deficit hyperactivity disorder.* Bethesda, MD: National Institutes of Health.

Forness, S. R., & Knitzer, J. (1992). A new proposed definition and terminology to replace "serious emotional disturbance" in Individuals with Disabilities Education Act. *School Psychology Review, 21,* 12–20.

Frick, P. J., Lahey, B. B., Applegate, B., Kerdyck, L., Ollendick, T., Hynd, G. W., Garfinkel, B., Greenhill, L., Biederman, J., Barkley, R. A., McBurnett, K., Newcorn, J., & Waldman, I. (1994). DSM-IV field trials for the disruptive behavior disorders: Symptom utility estimates. *Journal of the American Academy of Child and Adolescent Psychiatry, 33,* 529–539.

Gillberg, C., & Steffenburg, S. (1987). Outcome and prognostic factors in infantile autism and similar conditions: A population-based study of 46 cases followed through puberty. *Journal of Autism and Developmental Disorders, 17,* 273–287.

Gresham, F. M., & Gansle, K. A. (1992). Misguided assumptions of DSM-III-R: Implications for school psychological practice. *School Psychology Quarterly, 7,* 79–95.

Harris, S. L., Glasberg, B., & Ricca, D. (1996). Pervasive developmental disorders: Distinguishing among subtypes. *School Psychology Review, 25,* 308–315.

Hayes, S. C., Nelson, R. O., & Jarrett, R. D. (1987). The treatment utility of assessment: A functional approach to evaluating assessment quality. *American Psychologist, 42,* 963–974.

Ikeda, M. J., Tilly, W. D., Stumme, J., Volmer, L., & Allison, R. (1996). Agency-wide implementation of problem solving consultation: Foundations, current implementation, and future directions. *School Psychology Quarterly, 11,* 228–243.

Jensen, P. S., Martin, D., & Cantwell, D. P. (1997). Comorbidity in ADHD: Implications for research, practice, and DSM-V. *Journal of the American Academy of Child and Adolescent Psychiatry, 36,* 1065–1079.

Kaufman, J., Birmaher, B., Brent, D., Rao, U., & Ryan, N. (1996). *Kiddie-Schedule of Affective Disorders—Present and Lifetime Version.* Pittsburgh: Western Psychiatric Institute and Clinic.

Klein, R. G., & Abikoff, H. (1997). Behavior therapy and methylphenidate in the treatment of children with ADHD. *Journal of Attention Disorders, 2,* 89–114.

Kolko, D. J., & Kazdin, A. E. (1993). Emotional/behavioral problems in clinic and nonclinic children: Correspondence among child, parent, and teacher reports. *Journal of Child Psychology and Psychiatry and Allied Disciplines, 34,* 991–1006.

Kratochwill, T. R., & McGivern, J. F. (1996). Clinical diagnosis, behavioral assessment, and functional analysis: Examining the connection between assessment and intervention. *School Psychology Review, 25,* 342–355.

Lahey, B. B., Applegate, B., Barkley, R. A., Garfinkel, B., McBurnett, K., Kerdyk, L., Greenhill, L., Hynd, G. W., Frick, P. J., Newcorn, J., Biederman, J., Ollendick, T., Hart, E. L., Perez, D., Waldman, I., & Shaffer, D. (1994). DSM-IV field trials for oppositional defiant disorder and conduct disorder in children and adolescents. *American Journal of Psychiatry, 151,* 1163–1171.

Loeber, R., Green, S. M., Keenan, K., & Lahey, B. B. (1995). Which boys will fare worse? Early predictors of the onset of conduct disorder in a six-year longitudinal study. *Journal of the American Academy of Child and Adolescent Psychiatry, 34,* 499–509.

Loeber, R., Green, S. M., & Lahey, B. B. (1990). Optimal informants on childhood disruptive behaviors. *Development and Psychopathology, 1,* 317–337.

Lord, C., Rutter, M., Goode, S., Heemsbergen, J., Jordan, H., Mawhood, L., & Schopler, E. (1989). Autism Diagnostic Observation Schedule: A standardized observation of communicative and social behavior. *Journal of Autism and Developmental Disorders, 19,* 185–212.

Lord, C., Rutter, M., & LeCouteur, A. (1994). Autism Diagnostic Interview—Revised: A revision of the diagnostic interview for caregivers of individuals with possible pervasive developmental disorders. *Journal of Autism and Developmental Disorders, 24,* 659–685.

Lowe, L. A. (1998). Using the Child Behavior Checklist in assessing conduct disorder: Issues of reliability and validity. *Research on Social Work, 8*(3), 286–301.

Lyon, G. R. (1996). Learning disabilities. *The future of children: Special education for students with disabilities, 6,* 56–76.

McConaughy, S. H., & Achenbach, T. M. (1990). Contributions of developmental psychopathology to school services. In T. Gutkin & C. R. Reynolds (Eds.), *The handbook of school psychology (2nd ed.).* New York: Wiley.

McGinnis, E., & Forness, S. R. (1988). Psychiatric diagnosis: A further test of the special education hypothesis. *Monographs in Behavioral Disorders, 11,* 3–10.

Molina, B. S. G., Pelham, W. E., Blumenthal, J., & Galiszewski, E. (1998). Agreement among teachers' behavior ratings of adolescents with a childhood history of attention deficit hyperactivity disorder. *Journal of Clinical Child Psychology, 27,* 330–339.

Naglieri, J. A., Bardos, A. N., & LeBuffe, P. A. (1995). Discriminant validity of the Devereux Behavior Rating Scale School Form for student with serious emotional disturbance. *School Psychology Review, 24*(1), 104–111.

Naglieri, J. A., & Gottling, S. A. (1995). Use of the Teacher Report Form and the Devereux Behavior Rating Scale—School Form with learning disordered/emotionally disordered students. *Journal of Clinical Child Psychology, 24*(1), 71–76.

Naglieri, J. A., LeBuffe, P. A., & Pfeiffer, S. I. (1993). *Devereux Behavior Rating Scale–School Form.* San Antonio, TX: The Psychological Corporation.

Naglieri, J. A., LeBuffe, P. A., & Pfeiffer, S. I. (1994). *Manual for the Devereux Scales of Mental Disorders.* San Antonio, TX: The Psychological Corporation.

Pelham, W. E., Carlson, C., Sams, S. E., Vallano, G., Dixon, M. J., & Hoza, B. (1993). Separate and combined effects of methylphenidate and behavior modification on boys with attention-deficit-hyperactivity disorder in the classroom. *Journal of Consulting and Clinical Psychology, 61,* 506–515.

Pliszka, S. (1989). Effect of anxiety on cognition, behavior, and stimulant response in ADHD. *Journal of the American Academy of Child and Adolescent Psychiatry, 28,* 882–887.

Power, T. J., Andrews, T. A., Eiraldi, R. B., Doherty, B. J., & Ikeda, M. J. (1998). Evaluating attention deficit hyperactivity disorder using multiple informants: The incremental utility of combining teacher with parent reports. *Psychological Assessment, 10,* 250–260.

Power, T. J., Atkins, M. S., Osborne, M. L., & Blum, N. J. (1994). The school psychologist as manager of programming for ADHD. *School Psychology Review, 23,* 279–291.

Power, T. J., Doherty, B. J., Panichelli-Mindel, S. M., Karustis, J. L., Eiraldi, R. B., Anastopoulos, A. D., & DuPaul, G. J. (1998). The predictive validity of parent and teacher reports of ADHD symptoms. *Journal of Psychopathology and Behavioral Assessment, 20,* 57–81.

Power, T. J., & DuPaul, G. J. (1996). Attention-deficit/hyperactivity disorder; The re-emergence of subtypes. *School Psychology Review, 25,* 284–296.

Power, T. J., & Eiraldi, R. B. (1998). Using interviews and rating scales to collect behavioral data. In M. Mercugliano, T. J. Power, & N. J. Blum, *The clinician's practical guide to attention-deficit/ hyperactivity disorder*. Baltimore: Paul H. Brookes.

Power, T. J., & Ikeda, M. J. (1996). A clinic–school partnership in managing elementary school students with ADHD. In G. Stoner (Chair), *Prevention and intervention for students with ADHD: Models for effective practice across levels of schooling*. Paper presented at the annual meeting of the National Association of School Psychologists, Atlanta, March.

Reich, W., Leacock, N., & Shenfeld, K. (1995). *Diagnostic Interview for Children and Adolescents — Parent Version*. St. Louis, MO: Washington University, Division of Child Psychiatry.

Reid, R. (1995). Assessment of ADHD with culturally different groups: The use of behavior rating scales. *School Psychology Review, 24*, 537–560.

Reid, R., & Maag, J. W. (1994). How many fidgets in a pretty much: A critique of behavior rating scales for identifying students with ADHD. *Journal of School Psychology, 32*, 339–354.

Reschly, D. J. (1998). Utility of individual ability measures and public policy choices for the 21st century. *School Psychology Review, 26*, 234–241.

Reschly, D. J., & Ysseldyke, J. E. (1995). School psychology paradigm shift. In A. Thomas & J. Grimes (Eds.), *Best practices in school psychology — III* (3rd ed.; pp. 17–31). Washington, DC: National Association of School Psychologists.

Reynolds, C. R., & Kamphaus, R. W. (1992). *Manual for the Behavior Assessment System for Children*. Circle Pines, MN: American Guidance Service.

Schopler, E., & Mesibov, G. B. (Eds.) (1992). *High functioning individuals with autism*. New York: Plenum Press.

Schopler, E., Reichler, R. J., & Renner, B. R. (1988). *The Childhood Autism Rating Scale*. Los Angeles: Western Psychological Services.

Schwab-Stone, M. E., Shaffer, D., Dulcan, M. K., Jensen, P. S., Fisher, P., Bird, H. R., Goodman, S. H., Lahey, B. B., Lichtman, J. H., Canino, G., Rubio-Stipec, M., & Rae, D. S. (1996). Criterion validity of the NIMH Diagnostic Interview Schedule for Children Version 2.3 (DISC-2.3). *Journal of the American Academy of Child and Adolescent Psychiatry, 35*, 878–888.

Shaffer, D., Fisher, P., Dulcan, M. K., Davies, M., Piacentini, J., Schwab-Stone, M. E., Lahey, B. B., Bourdon, K., Jensen, P. S., Bird, H. R., Canino, G., & Regier, D. A. (1996). The NIMH Diagnostic Interview Schedule for Children Version 2.3 (DISC-2.3): Description, acceptability, prevalence rates, and performance in the MECA study. *Journal of the American Academy of Child and Adolescent Psychiatry, 35*, 865–877.

Shinn, M. R. (Ed.). (1998). *Advanced applications of curriculum-based measurement*. New York: Guilford Press.

Stone, W. L., & Hogan, K. L. (1993). A structured parent interview for identifying young children with autism. *Journal of Autism and Developmental Disorders, 23*, 639–652.

Stone, W. L., MacLean, W. E., & Hogan, K. L. (1995). Autism and mental retardation. In M. C. Roberts (Ed.), *Handbook of pediatric psychology* (2nd ed.). New York: Guilford Press.

Tannock, R., Ickowicz, A., & Schachar, R. (1995). Differential effects of methylphenidate on working memory in ADHD children with and without comorbid anxiety. *Journal of the American Academy of Child and Adolescent Psychiatry, 34*, 886–896.

Telzrow, C. F. (1999). IDEA amendments of 1997: Promise or pitfall for special education reform. *Journal of School Psychology, 37*, 7–28.

Tharinger, D. J., Laurent, J., & Best, L. R. (1986). Classification of children referred for emotional and behavioral problems: A comparison of PL 94-142 SED criteria, DSM III, and the CBCL system. *Journal of School Psychology, 24*, 111–121.

Trites, R. L., Blouin, A. G., & LaPrade, K. (1982). Factor analysis of the Conners Teacher Rating Scale based on a large normative sample. *Journal of Consulting and Clinical Psychology, 50*, 615–623.

Vaughn, M. L., Riccio, C. A., Hynd, G. W., & Hall, J. (1997). Diagnosing ADHD (Predominantly Inattentive and Combined Type subtypes): Discriminant validity of the Behavior Assessment System for Children and the Achenbach parent and teacher rating scales. *Journal of Clinical Child Psychology, 26*, 349–357.

Volkmar, F. R., Klin, A., Siegel, B., Szatmari, P., Lord, C., Campbell, M., Freeman, B. J., Cicchetti, D. V., Rutter, M., Kline, W., Buitelaar, J., Hattab, Y., Fombonne, E., Fuentes, J., Werry, J., Stone, W., Kerbeshian, J., Hoshino, Y., Bregman, J., Loveland, K., Szymanski, K., & Towbin, K. (1994). Field trial for autistic disorder in DSM-IV. *American Journal of Psychiatry, 151,* 1361– 1367.

Weinberg, L. A., & Weinberg, C. (1990). Seriously emotionally disturbed or socially maladjusted? A critique of interpretations. *Behavioral Disorders, 15,* 149–158.

Wodrich, D. L., Stobo, N., & Trca, M. (1998). Three ways to consider educational performance when determining serious emotional disturbance. *School Psychology Quarterly, 13,* 228–240.

Zentall, S. S., & Javorsky, J. (1995). Functional and clinical assessment of ADHD: Implications of DSM-IV in the schools. *Journal of Psychoeducational Assessment: Special ADHD Issue,* 22–41.

Author Index

Aaron, R., 457
Abbott, R. D., 161
Abbott, S. P., 161
Abikoff, H., 478
Ablon, S., 474
Aburto, S., 437, 438
Achenbach, T. M., 84, 111, 226, 234, 235, 236, 239, 240, 243, 251, 253, 257, 289, 292, 293, 294, 295, 296, 297, 298, 305, 310, 311, 323, 324, 334, 336, 337, 338, 339, 340, 341, 342, 347, 358, 360, 370, 456, 468, 470, 476
Adams, C. D., 310
Adams, H. E., 4
Afflerbach, P., 154
Ageton, S. S., 311, 312
Agran, M., 206, 214, 219, 226
Ahern, W., 97
Air, A., 360, 371, 382
Aitken, T. L., 83
Akiskal, H. S., 300
Akkerhuis, G. W., 235
Albano, A. M., 107
Albers, A. E., 53
Alberto, P. A., 233
Albin, R. W., 85, 360, 371, 382
Alcala, J., 126
Alcorn, M. B., 302
Alegria, M., 261
Alessi, G., 19, 26, 39
Alessi, N. E., 293, 300, 303
Alexander, C. M., 440
Allaire, A., 91, 120
Allen, B. A., 456
Allen, D., 169
Allen, S. J., 357, 371. 375, 380
Allinder, R. M., 170, 171, 179
Allison, R., 481
Almond, P., 424, 425

Alper, S., 206, 213, 214, 218
Aman, M. G., 84, 309
Ambrosini, P. J., 328
Anastasi, A., 363, 364, 365, 419, 420
Anastopoulos, A. D., 468, 469, 475, 480
Andelman, H. S., 409, 412
Anderson, G., 302
Anderson, J. C., 300
Anderson, K. E., 298
Anderson, T. K., 276, 283, 345
Andrews, D. A., 51
Andrews, T. A., 468, 475
Angle, H. V., 27
Angold, A., 293, 326, 327, 328, 329, 330, 336
Applegate, B., 154, 466
Apter, S. J., 257
Archbald, D. A., 182, 183
Ardoin, S. P., 59, 61
Armour-Thomas, E., 455
Armstrong, M., 79
Armstrong, S. W., 208
Arnold, K. D., 126
Arnold, L. E., 480
Aronson, J., 459
Arredondo, P., 401, 440
Artiles, A. J., 406
Arunkumar, R., 459
Asai, M., 445, 446
Aschbacher, P. R., 155
Asher, S. R., 124
Ashworth, R., 215
Asmus, J. A., 59, 82, 84, 87, 88, 89, 96
Asmus, J. M., 60, 87, 96
Assaire, A., 381, 382
Atkins, M. S., 472
Atkinson, D. R., 458
August, G. J., 474
Ault, M. F., 79, 85, 86
Ault, M. H., 57, 58

Subject Index